DRIPPS / ECKENHOFF / VANDAM

INTRODUCTION TO ANESTHESIA

NINTH EDITION

David E. Longnecker, MD
Robert D. Dripps Professor and Chair
Department of Anesthesia
University of Pennsylvania Health System
Philadelphia, Pennsylvania

Frank L. Murphy, MD
Associate Professor of Anesthesia
Hospital of the University of Pennsylvania
Philadelphia, Pennsylvania

W. B. SAUNDERS COMPANY
A Division of Harcourt Brace & Company

Philadelphia   London   Toronto   Montreal   Sydney   Tokyo

W. B. SAUNDERS COMPANY
A Division of Harcourt Brace & Company
The Curtis Center
Independence Square West
Philadelphia, Pennsylvania 19106

Library of Congress Catalog Card Number: 96-70362

Dripps, Eckenhoff, Vandam
INTRODUCTION TO ANESTHESIA

ISBN 0-7216-6279-X

Printed in the United States of America

Last digit is the print number: 9   8   7   6   5   4   3   2   1

Contributing Authors

Christian M. Alexander, MD
Assistant Professor of Anesthesia
Veterans Affairs Medical Center
Philadelphia, Pennsylvania
Positioning the Surgical Patient

Stanley J. Aukburg, MD
Associate Professor of Anesthesia
Hospital of the University of Pennsylvania
Philadelphia, Pennsylvania
The Anesthesia Machine

James E. Baumgardner, MD, PhD
Assistant Professor of Anesthesia
University of Pennsylvania Health System
Philadelphia, Pennsylvania
Interpretation of Arterial Blood Gas and Acid-Base Data

Elizabeth C. Behringer, MD
Assistant Professor of Anesthesia
Hospital of the University of Pennsylvania
Philadelphia, Pennsylvania
Postanesthesia Care

Eugene K. Betts, MD
Associate Professor of Anesthesia
Department of Anesthesia and Critical Care
The Children's Hospital of Philadelphia
Philadelphia, Pennsylvania
Pediatric Anesthesia

Frederick W. Campbell, MD
Professor of Anesthesiology
Allegheny University Hospital, East Falls
Campus
Philadelphia, Pennsylvania
Cardiopulmonary Resuscitation

Angelina D. Castro, MD
Associate Professor of Anesthesia
Hospital of the University of Pennsylvania
Philadelphia, Pennsylvania
Management of Anesthesia for Specialty Procedures

Theodore G. Cheek, MD
Associate Professor of Anesthesia
Hospital of the University of Pennsylvania
Philadelphia, Pennsylvania
Obstetric Anesthesia and Perinatology

Albert T. Cheung, MD
Assistant Professor of Anesthesia
Hospital of the University of Pennsylvania
Philadelphia, Pennsylvania
Inhaled Anesthetics

Thomas J. Conahan, III, MD
Associate Professor of Anesthesia
Hospital of the University of Pennsylvania
Philadelphia, Pennsylvania
Outpatient Anesthesia

Ray H. d'Amours, MD
Assistant Professor of Anesthesia
Hospital of the University of Pennsylvania
Philadelphia, Pennsylvania
Nerve Blocks

Clifford S. Deutschman, MD
Associate Professor of Anesthesia
Hospital of the University of Pennsylvania
Philadelphia, Pennsylvania
Metabolic and Endocrine Disorders

John J. Downes, MD
Professor of Anesthesia
Department of Anesthesia and Critical Care
Children's Hospital of Philadelphia
Philadelphia, Pennsylvania
Pediatric Anesthesia

Roderic G. Eckenhoff, MD
Associate Professor of Anesthesia
University of Pennsylvania Health System
Philadelphia, Pennsylvania
The Medical Gases

F. Michael Ferrante, MD
Associate Professor of Anesthesia
Hospital of the University of Pennsylvania
Philadelphia, Pennsylvania
Chronic Pain

Dennis M. Fisher, MD
Professor of Anesthesia and Pediatrics
University of California Medical Center
San Francisco, California
Muscle Relaxants

Robert R. Gaiser, MD
Assistant Professor of Anesthesia
Hospital of the University of Pennsylvania
Philadelphia, Pennsylvania
Pharmacology of Local Anesthetics; Spinal, Epidural, and Caudal Anesthesia

Ralph T. Geer, MD
Associate Professor of Anesthesia
Hospital of the University of Pennsylvania
Philadelphia, Pennsylvania
Critical Care of the Surgical Patient

Brett B. Gutsche, MD
Professor of Anesthesia
Hospital of the University of Pennsylvania
Philadelphia, Pennsylvania
Obstetric Anesthesia and Perinatology

C. William Hanson, III, MD
Associate Professor of Anesthesia
Hospital of the University of Pennsylvania
Philadelphia, Pennsylvania
Anesthesia and Respiratory Disease; Managing the Desperately Ill Patient

David R. Jobes, MD
Professor of Anesthesia
Hospital of the University of Pennsylvania
Philadelphia, Pennsylvania
Managing Fluids, Electrolytes, and Blood Loss

Sean K. Kennedy, MD
Associate Professor of Anesthesia
Hospital of the University of Pennsylvania
Philadelphia, Pennsylvania
Pharmacologic Principles of Anesthesia; Nonopioid Intravenous Anesthetics

Thomas H. Kramer, Pharm.D.
Assistant Professor of Anesthesia
Hospital of the University of Pennsylvania
Philadelphia, Pennsylvania
Opioids in Anesthesia Practice

David E. Longnecker, MD
Robert D. Dripps Professor and Chair
Department of Anesthesia
University of Pennsylvania Health System
Philadelphia, Pennsylvania
Anesthesia as a Medical Specialty

Bryan E. Marshall, MD
Professor of Anesthesia
University of Pennsylvania Health System
Philadelphia, Pennsylvania
Inhaled Anesthetics

Ronald M. Meyer, MD
Assistant Professor of Anesthesiology
Northwestern University Medical School
Attending Anesthesiologist
Columbus Hospital
Chicago, Illinois
Airway Management

Stanley Muravchick, MD, PhD
Professor of Anesthesia
Hospital of the University of Pennsylvania
Philadelphia, Pennsylvania
Geriatric Patients

Frank L. Murphy, MD
Associate Professor of Anesthesia
Hospital of the University of Pennsylvania
Philadelphia, Pennsylvania
Conduct of General Anesthesia; Hazards of Anesthesia; The Further Study of Anesthesiology

Constance F. Neely, MD
Assistant Professor of Anesthesia
University of Pennsylvania Health System
Philadelphia, Pennsylvania
Cardiovascular Disease

Gordon R. Neufeld, MD
Associate Professor of Anesthesia
Department of Anesthesia
Veteran's Administration Hospital
Philadelphia, Pennsylvania
Anesthesia and Respiratory Disease

Alan J. Ominsky, MD
Bernstein, Silver and Gardner
Philadelphia, Pennsylvania
The Law and Anesthesia Practice

Andranik Ovassapian, MD
Professor of Anesthesia
Northwestern University Medical School
Veteran's Administration Lakeside Medical Center,
Chicago, Illinois
Airway Management

Ivan S. Salgo, MD
Assistant Professor of Anesthesia
Hospital of the University of Pennsylvania
Philadelphia, Pennsylvania
Monitoring the Anesthetized Patient

Joseph S. Savino, MD
Associate Professor of Anesthesia
Hospital of the University of Pennsylvania
Philadelphia, Pennsylvania
Monitoring the Anesthetized Patient

Harry A. Seifert, MD
Assistant Professor of Anesthesia
University of Pennsylvania Health System
Philadelphia, Pennsylvania
Neuroanesthesia and Neurologic Diseases

David S. Smith, MD, PhD
Associate Professor of Anesthesia
University of Pennsylvania Health System
Philadelphia, Pennsylvania
Neuroanesthesia and Neurologic Diseases

Mitchell D. Tobias, MD
Assistant Professor of Anesthesia
Hospital of the University of Pennsylvania
Philadelphia, Pennsylvania
*Premedication: Drugs to Start, Continue, or Withhold;
Patients with Hepatic and Renal Disease*

Karen B. Traber, MD
Assistant Professor of Anesthesia
Hospital of the University of Pennsylvania
Philadelphia, Pennsylvania
Preoperative Evaluation

Timothy R. VadeBoncouer, MD
Assistant Professor of Anesthesiology
University of Illinois
Chicago, Illinois
Management of Postoperative Pain

Kathleen M. Veloso, MD
Assistant Professor of Anesthesia
Hospital of the University of Pennsylvania
Philadelphia, Pennsylvania
Chronic Pain

Stuart J. Weiss, MD, PhD
Assistant Professor of Anesthesia
Hospital of the University of Pennsylvania
Philadelphia, Pennsylvania
Cardiovascular Disease

Marie L. Young, MD
Associate Professor of Anesthesia
Hospital of the University of Pennsylvania
Philadelphia, Pennsylvania
Outpatient Anesthesia

Lester A. Zuckerman, MD
Lecturer in Anesthesia
Hospital of the University of Pennsylvania
Philadelphia, Pennsylvania
Premedication: Drugs to Start, Continue, or Withhold

Preface

Introduction to Anesthesia had its origins in a 1949 manual for anesthesia residents at the Hospital of the University of Pennsylvania. The intent was to provide a concise source of current practice for those entering the specialty. The editors of the first seven editions, Robert D. Dripps, James E. Eckenhoff and Leroy D. Vandam, established fundamental goals for this text that still apply. This book is intended for those entering the specialty, or for those who seek a concise summary of current practice as they prepare for qualifying examinations or the management of a specific patient. The approach emphasizes medical management and the essential scientific basis of anesthesia practice, as technical matters are best learned in the clinical environment. The editors have organized the book so that scientific principles are presented together with discussions of clinical management.

As before, this book represents contemporary anesthesia practice. Thus, it offers increased emphasis on pain management, preoperative evaluation, trauma, and the care of very ill patients for major procedures. The conflicting goals of brevity versus broad coverage have been resolved in favor of the beginning student of anesthesia. Advanced topics, such as anesthesia for cardiac surgery, operations on neonates, or lung and liver transplantation, have been omitted. Other topics, such as the use of the laryngeal mask airway, received emphasis.

Experts in the subspecialties of anesthesia practice provided many of these chapters, but we edited their work to assure broad but concise coverage and some uniformity of style. Several anesthesia residents from the University of Pennsylvania reviewed chapters for this volume. We are grateful to Ms. Irene Soroka for her unstinting efforts in preparing the manuscripts. Errors that remain are the responsibility of the editors, not Ms. Soroka, the authors, or the resident consultants.

David E. Longnecker
Frank L. Murphy

Acknowledgments

The editors acknowledge these resident physicians from the Department of Anesthesia at the Hospital of the University of Pennsylvania who served as consultants in the writing of this edition.

Christine M. Cillis, MD
Robert F. G. deQuevedo, MD
James E. Hughes, MD
Nathaniel Carl Law, MD
Margaret A. Pitts, MD
Diane G. Portman, MD
Jonathan W. Tanner, MD, PhD
Mark A. Taylor, MD
Douglas A. Arbittier, MD
Paul Sanders, MD
Andrew J. Mannes, MD
Ivan S. Salgo, MD
Michael C. Thorogood, MD

Contents

1

Anesthesia as a Medical Specialty

David E. Longnecker

Anesthesiology as a Medical Specialty

Anesthesiology has continued to advance as a medical specialty over the past decade. Anesthesiologists now participate actively in both inpatient and outpatient care, working in operating rooms, recovery rooms, outpatient clinics, outpatient surgery centers, and intensive care units (ICUs). Anesthesiologists are also active in medical research, in the administration of their hospitals, and in national organized medicine. However, this was not always the case. Earlier, the specialty experienced significant difficulties in establishing its position in medical practice, in medical schools, and in organized medicine. The limited number of medical personnel in the specialty contributed greatly to these problems. A restricted view of anesthesia practice held by some anesthesiologists (and others in the medical community) also presented barriers to growth of the specialty. The key to the continued development of the specialty lies not so much in the development of new drugs or techniques but in the continued development of a philosophy that anesthesiology is the practice of perioperative medicine.

Anesthesiology will thrive as long as its practitioners fulfill a commitment to care for all patients who may benefit from the medical expertise of anesthesiologists. The application of this expertise is most evident in the classic practice of anesthesia, the care of surgical patients in operating rooms. However, this expertise extends into other areas, including the pre-operative and postoperative care of surgical patients, management of the critically ill or injured, the care of those with chronic pain, and the treatment of acute drug overdose. Anesthesiologists are partners in the care of medical and surgical patients, not simply technical consultants who participate in specific procedures only. Wherever the partnership philosophy prevails, anesthesiologists are valued and respected by their patients and colleagues. Indeed, the recent development of anesthesiology as a specialty, the promise for its continued development, and the satisfaction that its practitioners experience all reflect the application of this comprehensive form of practice.

A Concise View of the Development of Anesthesiology in the United States

Although surgical anesthesia was discovered in the 1840s, the real emergence of the specialty began in the early 1900s. The importance of the specialty was enhanced greatly during World War II, when the influence of anesthesia care on the survival of surgical patients was especially apparent.

The first organization of anesthesia practitioners in the United States was the nine-member Long Island Society of Anesthetists, formed in 1905. The name was changed to the New York Society of Anesthetists in 1911 because interest in the society extended well

3

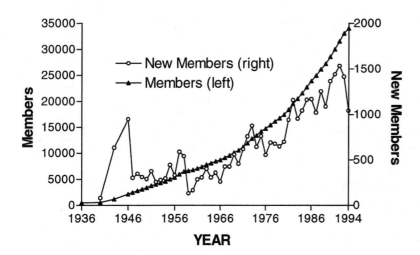

Figure 1-1

Annual and cumulative growth in membership of the American Society of Anesthesiologists. Values for initial years are discontinuous because data by year are not available.

beyond Long Island. Efforts to form a section of anesthesiology within the American Medical Association were begun by the New York Society in 1912, but despite repeated efforts, the section was not approved until 1940. Although numerous factors contributed, this long delay reflected attitudes about the value of the specialty in the first part of the twentieth century. The fact that large numbers of both medical and nonmedical personnel were allowed to administer anesthesia without formal clinical training marred the reputation of the specialty.

The years immediately before, during, and after World War II were associated with great changes in the discipline and with the introduction of organizations that today represent the specialty. The New York Society of Anesthetists became the American Society of Anesthetists in 1936 and the American Society of Anesthesiologists in 1945. The growth of this orga-

nization has been dramatic, from 568 members in 1940 to 34,033 in 1994 (Fig. 1-1). The American Board of Anesthesiology (ABA) was formed in 1938 as an affiliate board of the American Board of Surgery (nine diplomats were certified after the first examination); the ABA became an independent board in 1941. The number of ABA diplomats increased from 105 to 25,084 between 1940 and 1994 (Fig. 1-2).

While graduate medical education in the specialty paralleled the growth in numbers of practitioners, the overall academic development of the specialty lagged behind that of many other disciplines in universities and medical schools. The first certificate for formal graduate medical training in anesthesiology was awarded at the University of Iowa in 1923. Dr. Ralph Waters, of the University of Wisconsin, became the first university professor of anesthesiology in 1927. However, most institutions did not establish depart-

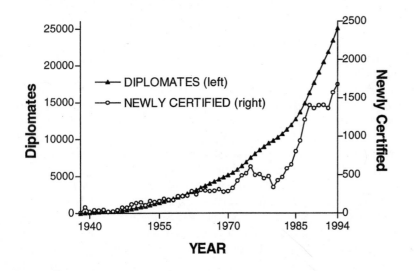

Figure 1-2

Annual and cumulative growth in numbers of diplomats certified by the American Board of Anesthesiology.

ments of anesthesiology until the 1940s to the 1960s, and many university departments have had no more than two or three chairpersons. (The Veterans Administration has only accepted the concept of independent departments of anesthesiology very recently, and anesthesiology remains a section of surgery in many Veterans Administration hospitals).

The value and prowess of physician anesthesiologists were recognized most dramatically during World War II, when the importance of anesthesia became evident in the care of wounded soldiers. Many physicians returned from World War II to enter training programs in anesthesiology, and these individuals became leaders during the emergence of the specialty in the 1950s and 1960s. A small number of individuals developed elite university departments that supplied large numbers of leaders and practitioners to the specialty during this interval; prominent among these were Robert D. Dripps of the University of Pennsylvania (one of the editors of the earlier editions of this textbook), Emanuel M. Papper of Columbia University, and Stuart F. Cullen of the University of Iowa and later the University of California at San Francisco. These men, and a small group of others, formed the nucleus for the development of the scientific foundations of the specialty in the three decades immediately after World War II. Several of these pioneers in anesthesiology achieved leadership positions in university medical centers, and this recognition among their peers further enhanced the stature of the discipline.

Breadth of the Specialty

Initially, nearly all anesthesiologists practiced in all areas of the discipline, an understandable necessity in a new specialty with few practitioners. This remains the basis of practice for the vast majority of anesthesiologists, but there is a growing trend for subspecialization in major universities and medical centers. The principal subdisciplines include obstetric anesthesia, pediatric anesthesia, cardiothoracic anesthesia, neuroanesthesia, anesthesia for outpatient surgery, and acute and chronic pain management.

■ Obstetric Anesthesia

Obstetric anesthesia has emerged as a subdiscipline that is highly regarded by patients and obstetricians alike. Anesthesia-related factors such as anesthetic

mishaps or associated factors such as pulmonary aspiration of gastric contents have been prominent causes of maternal morbidity and mortality for many years, emphasizing the need for subspecialty practice in obstetric anesthesia. The role of anesthesiologists in preventing neonatal morbidity and in resuscitating newborns has become established in recent years. Further, the dramatic pain relief and safety provided by epidural analgesia for labor and delivery are well recognized by large numbers of patients. Indeed, hospital administrators even use the presence of obstetric anesthesia subspecialty practice as evidence of the quality of their hospitals and as enticements for patients in their marketing programs. Anesthesiologists also have played a prominent role in neonatal care; one of the most prominent among these was Virginia Apgar, the creator of the Apgar score, which is used internationally to evaluate the condition of newborns. Obstetric anesthesiologists have formed a society for their subdiscipline, and fellowship training in obstetric anesthesia is offered by many training programs.

■ Pediatric Anesthesia

Pediatric anesthesia is a highly developed subspecialty that focuses on the perioperative care of neonates, infants, and children. Pediatric anesthesiologists have achieved positions of prominence in the training of both anesthesiologists and pediatricians who practice pediatric critical care medicine. Many prominent pediatric anesthesiologists have training and board certification in both pediatrics and anesthesiology, and fellowships in pediatric anesthesia are available to those who have completed anesthesiology training programs. Pediatric anesthesia is a recognized section within the American Academy of Pediatrics, and pediatric anesthesiologists have formed their own subspecialty society as well.

■ Cardiothoracic Anesthesia

Cardiothoracic anesthesia is one of the largest subdisciplines within the specialty of anesthesiology. Anesthesiologists have contributed prominently to the quality and safety of cardiac and thoracic surgery. The development of narcotic anesthesia, a technique that permitted cardiac operations even in those with poor myocardial function, is an example of the role of anesthesia care in cardiac surgery; others include recent studies that defined the influences of anesthetic techniques or underlying myocardial ischemia on the morbidity and mortality associated with cardiac operations. Cardiothoracic anesthesiologists have continued to lead in the transfer of technology into the operating room; a current example is the intraoperative use of transesophageal echocardiography (TEE). There are two major organizations for cardiothoracic anesthesiologists, and fellowships in cardiothoracic anesthesia are offered in numerous major universities and medical centers.

■ Neuroanesthesia

Neuroanesthesia is a smaller subdiscipline of anesthesia practice. Although neuroanesthesiologists participate in all the operations performed by neurosurgeons, their special expertise usually involves intracranial procedures. Anesthetics have significant influences on cerebral blood flow, cerebral metabolism, intracranial pressure, and the extent of tissue hypoxia that is tolerated by the central nervous system. Anesthesiologists have been leaders in studying the influences of these factors on outcome following cerebral ischemia or hypoxemia. Neuroanesthesiologists also care for patients in ICUs, since many of the principles of neuroanesthesia practice apply in the postoperative period. Neuroanesthesiologists and their colleagues in neurosurgery have formed a combined society, evidencing their common interests in the care of neurosurgical patients. Fellowships in neuroanesthesia are offered at major universities and centers and may well become even more common with the further development of vascular neurosurgery, an area that tests the skills of both neurosurgeons and neuroanesthesiologists.

■ Anesthesia for Outpatient Surgery

Anesthesia for outpatient surgical procedures has developed rapidly in recent years as outpatient surgical practice has become increasingly common. These initiatives were developed in response to efforts to lower costs by reducing the length of hospital stays for surgical patients. Procedures that were once restricted to hospital inpatients are now performed routinely on outpatients. The development of new anesthetic drugs and techniques that are associated with rapid induction and emergence from general anesthesia has done much to expand the range of possible candidates for outpatient procedures. Anesthesiologists interested in outpatient surgery have formed a society devoted to their subdiscipline, and some training programs offer extended subspecialty training in outpatient anesthesia.

■ Pain Management

Pain management has become increasingly prominent in recent years. Chronic pain management developed in the 1970s, whereas acute pain management gained popularity in the late 1980s. The importance of the subdiscipline of pain management was recognized by the American Board of Anesthesiology, which has offered subspecialty board certification in pain management since 1991.

Chronic Pain Management

Chronic pain management is directed to the care of those with chronic pain due to malignancy, musculoskeletal disorders, or other causes or those with acute pain that is known to lead to chronic pain and disability (such as the pain associated with reflex sympathetic dystrophy). The subdiscipline requires an understanding of medical oncology, neurologic disease, and musculoskeletal disease, as well as expertise in regional anesthesia, behavioral medicine, exercise physiology (many treatment plans include an important exercise component), and the pharmacology of sedatives, antidepressants, narcotics, and analgesics. Multidisciplinary training is an important component of the fellowship training in pain management, and multidisciplinary clinics that incorporate the expertise of several disciplines are often staffed by anesthesiologists.

Acute Pain Management

Acute pain management is now a major component of many anesthesiology departments. The most prominent activity involves the management of acute postoperative pain, although other types of acute pain are managed as well. The many techniques of acute pain management include patient-controlled intravenous narcotic analgesia, epidural analgesia with combinations of narcotics and local anesthetics, and less common regional anesthesia approaches such as intrapleural analgesia. These techniques provide remarkable relief from postoperative pain and decrease the duration of postoperative ICU care and overall hospital stay as well.

■ Critical Care Medicine

Critical care medicine is a natural extension of the intensive care that anesthesiologists provide in operating rooms. The American Board of Anesthesiology certified more than 600 subspecialists in critical care medicine during the first decade (1985–1994) of such recognition. Anesthesiologists care for patients, teach, and provide administrative direction in surgical, pediatric, and medical ICUs.

■ Preanesthetic Evaluation

Modern anesthesiology departments provide preanesthetic evaluation for patients scheduled to come to the hospital on the day of operation, who otherwise would not be seen by an anesthesiologist in advance of the procedure. This ensures that the patients are evaluated medically for the demands of anesthesia and operation and that they understand the plans for anesthesia care. It may be a cost-saving mechanism as well, for it eliminates delays and cancellations in the operative schedule, and the anesthesiologist may limit preoperative tests and consultations to those which are essential for quality care.

Anesthesiologists are also active in clinical hyperbaric medicine, blood banking, and trauma care.

Anesthesia Practice and Managed Care

Health care reform and managed care provide an opportunity for anesthesiologists to contribute in several important areas of health care delivery. *Cost-effectiveness* is a common theme among all the various approaches to health care delivery. This goal is shared by health maintenance organizations (HMOs), governmental initiatives, commercial health insurance companies, and local hospitals and clinics. Anesthesiologists are well positioned to contribute to this theme because they practice in areas that have an enormous impact on hospital budgets, including operating rooms, postoperative care units, delivery suites, ICUs, and radiology suites. In addition, perioperative anesthesia care affects length of hospital stay through programs such as preoperative preparation of

the surgical patient and postoperative pain management. Others look to our discipline to take a leadership role in these areas as well. In a recent article in the *British Medical Journal*, Wickham speculated that "the traditional specialty alignments will be revised. . . . The anesthetist will be responsible for preoperative and postoperative care."

The Anesthesia Care Team

Nurse anesthetists are an important part of anesthesia practice in the United States. In Great Britain, anesthesia was administered from the first by physicians, who made frequent use of chloroform, a dangerous anesthetic that was difficult to administer. In the United States, few physicians took up the practice of anesthesiology, and the administration of anesthetics often was left to medical students, nonspecialist physicians, or other hospital workers who happened to be available when an anesthetic was required. This unsatisfactory state of affairs was improved when registered nurses became involved in the practice of anesthesia. Today, certified registered nurse anesthetists (CRNAs) work in both academic and private practice settings, where teams of anesthesiologists and nurse anesthetists provide a model for other specialties of productive cooperation between physicians and nurses in delivering safe and effective medical care.

Research

Anesthesiologists have become increasingly involved in clinical and laboratory research. The breadth of clinical research ranges from health care policy and health services research to drug and device testing for perioperative or intensive care. Laboratory research spans similarly broad areas, ranging from cardiopulmonary physiology to molecular genetics. Future advances in anesthesiology depend to a great extent on the discoveries made by those in clinical or laboratory research.

BIBLIOGRAPHY

American Board of Anesthesiology. Quality anesthesia care: A model of future practice of anesthesiology. *Anesthesiology* 1977; 47:488-489.

Eckenhoff JE. A wide-angle view of anesthesiology. Emory A. Rovenstine Memorial Lecture. *Anesthesiology* 1978;48:272-279.

Little DM Jr. The founding of the specialty boards. *Anesthesiology* 1981;55:317-321.

Little DM Jr, Betcher AM. *The Diamond Jubilee 1905-1980.* Park Ridge, Ill: American Society of Anesthesiologists, 1980.

Vandam LD. Anesthesiologists as clinicians. American Society of Anesthesiologists Rovenstine Lecture, 1979. *Anesthesiology* 1980;53:40-48.

Volpitto PP, Vandam LD. *The Genesis of Contemporary American Anesthesiology.* Springfield, Ill: Charles C Thomas, 1982.

Wickham JEA. Minimally invasive surgery. *Br Med J* 1994;309:193-196.

Preparing to Administer Anesthesia

CHAPTER **2**

Preoperative Evaluation

Karen B. Traber

Preoperative evaluation is the initial step in the preparation of a patient for the operating room. It consists of a review of previous medical records, a survey of past and present medical and surgical problems, and a well-directed physical examination. Laboratory tests augment the findings of the history and physical examination. At the conclusion of the evaluation, the anesthesiologist develops a plan for anesthesia and perioperative management and discusses it with the patient. Beyond gathering information, the anesthesiologist establishes a doctor-patient relationship that reduces patient anxiety by building a foundation of trust and respect. Educating the patient about anesthesia, outlining a schedule of upcoming events, and discussing risks and options in an objective manner lead naturally to informed consent for the anesthetic management plan. The task is to have the patient in the best possible condition, both mental and physical, prior to operation, with the ultimate goal of reduced perioperative morbidity and mortality (Table 2-1).

Table 2-1

Objectives of Preanesthetic Evaluation
Review database
Medical history
Consultations
Laboratory and diagnostic studies
Perform physical examination directed at anesthetic concerns
Develop anesthesia management plan
Obtain consent
Establish doctor-patient relationship

Review of Medical Records

Preoperative evaluation begins with review of the patient's medical records, including relevant medical history, previous consultations and diagnostic testing, and records of prior anesthetics. This shortens the preoperative interview and reduces costly duplication of consultation and testing. Prior anesthetic records can describe such problems as difficult mask ventilation or endotracheal intubation, difficulty with vascular access, unusual responses to anesthetics, or other perioperative complications, some of which may not appear elsewhere in the medical records or may not be remembered by the patient.

History and Physical Examination

The anesthesiologist's history and physical examination do not replicate those of the admitting physician. Instead, they have a specific goal: to discover and assess any abnormalities that may affect the perioperative course and the plan for anesthesia. Components of the preoperative anesthetic history and physical examination are outlined in Table 2-2.

■ History

The medical history may be elicited by questioning the patient directly and by asking the patient to complete a questionnaire. Questionnaires include a brief review of systems and provide information regarding the patient's medications, allergies, and prior hospitalizations and operations. This permits

Table 2-2

Preanesthetic History and Physical Examination

Present illness (including age, sex, problem, planned procedure, including whether it is elective, urgent, or emergent)
Past medical history
  List of medical problems with brief history
  Medications
  Allergies with specific reactions and exposure to related compounds
  List of past surgical history with type of operation, date or age of patient, type of anesthetic, and anesthetic-related problems
  Family history, including history of anesthetic-related problems
  Social history, including history of smoking, drug use, hepatitis, or HIV
  Review of systems, including a general review with exercise tolerance and a functional approach to major organ systems
Physical examination
  Vital signs, including height, weight, blood pressure, heart rate, and temperature
  Dental examination documenting loose, chipped, absent, or bonded or prosthetic teeth
  Airway, including overall appearance, mouth (opening and tongue size), movement, trachea palpation, and nares patency
  Pulmonary, including presence of wheezing, rales, or rhonchi
  Cardiac rhythm and presence of murmurs
  Neurologic examination when appropriate documenting baseline prior to intervention
  Other physical markers pertinent to the history and planned procedure

the anesthesiologist to focus on abnormal findings. Computer-based history and physical examination systems may improve on conventional questionnaires and generate large databases for managed care and outcome research.

The interview focuses on the severity and treatment of health problems and the impact these have on the patient's activities, especially exercise tolerance. Can the patient walk up stairs, play sports, or perform household chores? If exercise tolerance is adequate, advanced cardiopulmonary testing often is unnecessary.

Medications

A patient's medications can alter anesthetic requirements, potentiate muscle relaxants, induce an exaggerated response to sympathomimetics, or alter the metabolism of other medications. As a rule, most medications are continued unchanged, but it may be

appropriate to alter the dose, change to a shorter-acting preparation, or even discontinue the drug temporarily (see Chap. 4). Table 2-3 lists some common medications with their anesthetic implications and management recommendations.

Allergies

Allergic reactions to drugs are sometimes misunderstood by patients, and appropriate documentation may be lacking. Severity ranges from asymptomatic rashes to life-threatening anaphylaxis, but often the reported allergy represents only drug intolerance, usually to an opioid. The preoperative evaluation records all drug reactions with a comment as to potential for serious allergic response, including all reactions to adhesive tape, iodine soap, and latex. If an allergic response seems likely, the offending drug is not repeated without formal immunologic testing or pretreatment with antihistamines, H_2 blockers, or corticosteriods.

Previous Surgical and Anesthesia History

Review of the patient's previous surgical and anesthetic experience may be invaluable in planning a subsequent anesthetic. Patients easily recall awakening with an endotracheal tube in place or experiencing severe nausea and vomiting, although they usually cannot recall more critical life-threatening events, which may consist only of the patient's recollection of an unplanned stay in the intensive care unit (ICU) or of prolonged hospitalization. After recovery from a difficult intubation or other unexpected complications, the patient should be informed of the problem. Enrolling the patient in the Medic Alert Difficult Airway/Intubation Registry provides detailed information for anesthesiologists later involved in the patient's care. If the patient wears a Medic Alert bracelet or carries a card, the anesthesiologist may contact the registry at 1-800-432-5378.

Family and Social History

A family history of anesthetic complications may reveal inheritable diseases such as malignant hyperthermia, pseudocholinesterase abnormalities, or glucose-6-phosphate dehydrogenase (G6PD) deficiency. A history of smoking or drug use may prompt further questioning or diagnostic testing to assess respiratory, cardiovascular, and liver disease. Women of child-bearing age should be questioned regarding the likelihood of pregnancy. In case of doubt, preoperative pregnancy testing is indicated.

Table 2-3

Medications, Anesthetic Implications, and Recommendations for Preoperative Management

Medication	Anesthetic Implication	Recommended Management
Aspirin	Platelet dysfunction, bleeding potential	Consider preoperative discontinuation for at least 10–14 days; discuss with surgeon and prescribing physician regarding risk for stroke, MI, or thrombosis with discontinuation
Aminoglycosides	Can potentiate nondepolarizing relaxants	Monitor neuromuscular relaxants carefully
Clonidine	Acute withdrawal can cause hypertensive crisis; decreases anesthetic requirements	Continue therapy the day of surgery; can use dermal delivery perioperatively; decrease anesthetic requirements intraoperatively
Insulin	Hypoglycemia if not monitored	Depends on time of surgery and serum glucose range; recommend to continue partial dose (one-half or one-third) of long-acting insulin and delete short-acting insulin the day of surgery; monitor serum glucose closely perioperatively; watch for combined long- and short-acting preparations.
Lithium	Potentiate neuromuscular blockers, induce hypothyroidism in some patients; lithium concentrations increase with decreased serum sodium	Monitor neuromuscular blockade carefully; obtain thyroid function tests preoperatively if indicated; monitor serum sodium and avoid sodium wasting diuretics
Monoamine oxidase inhibitors (isocarboxazid, pargyline, phenelzine, tranylcypromine)	Increased catecholamine stores; hepatoxicity; rare but potentially fatal reactions with opioids, especially meperidine	Avoid indirect-acting sympathomimetics and use reduced doses of direct-acting agents; serum liver function tests if not done; avoid opioids, especially meperidine; for elective surgery, request psychiatrist to discontinue for 14 to 21 days unless suicide risk; less time needed for pargyline and tranylcypromine since reversibly bound
Warfarin	Excessive intraoperative bleeding	Manage with prescribing physician; withdrawal in advance; substitute heparin; heparin may be stopped immediately preoperatively and restarted postoperatively

Review of Systems

A review of organ systems, modified to suit the individual patient's general state of health, is an important component of a comprehensive preoperative evaluation. A well-done review of systems is a dynamic process that may be brief or lengthy, depending on the patient. A guide for a complete review of organ systems is listed in Table 2-4.

Discovery of an abnormality in the review of systems requires further investigation. For example, patients who have suffered myocardial infarctions or congestive heart failure may benefit from delay of operation, treatment of pulmonary edema, more invasive cardiovascular monitoring, or postoperative intensive care. Similarly, patients with chronic obstructive pulmonary disease (COPD) and a productive cough may benefit from diagnostic testing, preoperative antibiotics, bronchodilator drugs, and chest physiotherapy.

■Physical Examination

The extent of the physical examination is based on the patient's history and the planned anesthetic technique. Healthy patients may require only the basic elements of airway and cardiopulmonary evaluation.

Vital Signs

Documentation of preoperative vital signs is important, especially in patients with cerebrovascular or cardiovascular disease. Determining blood pressure on several occasions may reveal a range of values that are safe. The cause of abnormal vital signs must be determined. For example, tachycardia may be due to

Table 2-4

General Review of Organ System Function

General: exercise tolerance, weakness, fatigue, fever, weight change
Skin: rashes, sores, lesions, change in hair or nails
Head: frequent headaches, head injury
Eyes: double, blurred, loss of vision, glaucoma, cataracts
Ears: limited hearing, tinnitus, vertigo, discharge, pain
Nose and throat: sinusitis, sore throat, epistaxis, dysphagia
Mouth: lesions, bleeding gums, dentures, bridges, caps, loose or damaged teeth
Cardiac: history of hypertension, myocardial infarction, congestive heart failure, rheumatic heart fever, heart murmurs, angina, palpitations, dyspnea, orthopnea, paroxysmal nocturnal dyspnea, peripheral edema
Respiratory: cough, sputum, hemoptysis, asthma or wheezing, bronchitis, emphysema, pneumonia, tuberculosis
Gastrointestinal: hiatal hernia, heartburn, reflux, nausea, vomiting, diarrhea, constipation, hematemesis, melena, jaundice, hepatitis
Urinary: frequency, urgency, nocturia, dysuria, hematuria, incontinence, change in stream
Female: last menstrual period, likelihood of current pregnancy
Extremities: claudication, thrombophlebitis, joint pain or swelling, back pain
Neurologic: seizure, TIA, stroke, paralysis, syncope, numbness, loss of consciousness
Hematologic: anemia, easy bruising, bleeding, past transfusion
Endocrine: thyroid abnormalities, diabetes
Psychiatric: emotional illness, hospitalizations for psychiatric care
Prosthetics: glasses, contacts, hearing aid

fever, pain, hypovolemia, anemia, or hyperthyroidism; a different anesthetic plan is required for each.

The anesthesiologist also must account for compensatory physiologic mechanisms when evaluating the patient's vital signs. A young patient with a ruptured spleen after a motor vehicle accident may have vital signs within normal limits despite massive blood loss. An arterial pressure of 110/70 may represent hypotension in a patient whose blood pressure is usually 170/90.

Airway Examination

The airway examination distinguishes the anesthesiologist's evaluation from those of most other consultants. The primary goal of the airway examination is to describe the anatomy and anticipate difficulties maintaining the airway or intubating the trachea. The medical history may provide clues, such as a history of

snoring, obstructive sleep apnea, head or neck surgery, radiation therapy, stridor or hoarseness, neck pain, or loose or prominent teeth. When available, previous anesthesia records can provide valuable information about the airway. Physical examination of the airway includes the teeth, mouth, and neck, including determination of range of motion of the mandible and neck and palpation of the trachea. Documentation of the airway examination is described in Table 2-5 (see Chap. 13 for more).

Pulmonary Examination

A complete pulmonary examination assesses the severity of illness and guides the anesthesia plan. For example, if a patient with COPD complains of dyspnea on exertion, inspection may reveal a barrel chest, pursed-lip breathing, use of accessory muscles, and prolonged exhalation. Pertinent negative findings, such as wheezing in a patient with asthma, may be as important as positive findings. Pulmonary function testing is indicated when it is important to quantitate the degree of impairment.

Cardiac Examination

Physical examination of the heart includes an assessment of the rate, rhythm, and murmurs. Palpation of the radial pulse can determine the rate and rhythm of the heart, which can be confirmed later by direct auscultation. Understanding the cause of a dysrhythmia is necessary prior to induction of anesthesia. For example, atrial fibrillation in a patient may be due to thyrotoxicosis, ischemic or valvular heart disease, or pulmonary embolism; the anesthesia plan accounts for each differently. Examination of the heart may reveal a murmur known from the history or not previously suspected. The type of murmur and the extent of dysfunction affect the choice of anesthetic agents and technique. For example, spinal anesthesia may be dangerous in a patient with severe aortic stenosis. Antibiotic prophylaxis must be considered in all patients with valvular or congenital heart disease.

Neurologic and Musculoskeletal Examination

A neurologic examination to document preexisting abnormalities is important when planning a regional anesthetic and before procedures with possible neurologic complications, such as carotid endarterectomy or thoracic aneurysm repair. Examination of the site of a proposed nerve block may reveal unsuspected problems such as a skin infection. Musculoskeletal

Table 2-5

Documenting the Examination of the Airway

Overall appearance
  Neck: stout or thin, long or short?
  Sunken cheeks suggesting poor mask fit
Dentition
  Dental damage (loose, chipped, absent)
  Dental prostheses (bonding, caps, bridges)
  Use numeric charting to describe teeth

	Right Molars								Incisors							Left Molars		
maxilla	1	2	3	4	5	6	7	8	m i d	9	10	11	12	13	14	14	16
mandible	32	31	30	29	28	27	26	25	l i n e	24	23	22	21	20	19	18	17

Mouth
  Opening, anterior displacement of the mandible, tongue size, visibility of uvula, protruding incisors
Movement
  Flexion, extension, and lateral movement of the neck
Palpation
  Trachea midline or fixed, distance from mentum to hyoid
Nose
  Nares patent, septum deviated

---

evaluation may detect ankylosing spondylitis, scoliosis, or severe rheumatoid arthritis, which may make intubation of the trachea or placement of a regional anesthetic more difficult.

Additional Physical Examination

The remainder of the physical examination depends on the patient's history and the procedure planned. For example, if a patient is scheduled for an abdominal hernia repair, examination of the location and size of hernia may aid in the decision for local infiltration with intravenous sedation or regional or general anesthesia. Similarly, knowing the site for placement of an arteriovenous fistula in a patient is important in planning an interscalene or axillary block.

Laboratory Testing

Few quibble over laboratory testing for an appropriate clinical indication. However, the routine preoperative use of laboratory testing to screen asymp-

tomatic patients has contributed little to medical management or to outcome. The costs and the poor yield argue against such testing. In one study of 5003 preoperative screening tests performed on 1010 asymptomatic patients undergoing cholecystectomy, 225 were found to be abnormal. Of these, 104 were of potential importance; 17 abnormalities resulted in changes in medical management, but only 4 patients received significant benefit from the random screen. Routine preoperative laboratory testing provides little information beyond the results of history and physical examination to alter the management of otherwise healthy patients.

The value of laboratory tests is also limited by the statistics of the result. That is, the prevalence of the disease and the sensitivity, specificity, and positive predictive value of the proposed test must be known so that the test results can be interpreted. No currently available diagnostic test is 100 percent sensitive (always positive in the presence of the disease) or 100 percent specific (always negative in the absence of the disease). Therefore, test results must be evaluated by their ability to predict the disease accurately; that is,

Table 2-6

University Hospital Consortium (UHC) Preoperative Diagnostic Testing Recommendations	
Test	**UHC Recommendation**
Chest x-ray	All patients over age 60
	All other patients with a specific clinical indication (e.g., HTN, malignancy, acute pulmonary symptoms)
ECG	All men age 40 and older, women age 50 and older
	All other patients with a specific clinical indication (e.g., HTN, palpitations, previous MI)
CBC	Specific clinical indications (e.g., renal disease, anticoagulant use, malignancy)
Serum chemistries	Specific clinical indications (e.g., hepatitis, renal disease, diabetes)
Urinalysis	Specific clinical indications (e.g., urinary tract symptoms)
PT and PTT	Clinical history or specific clinical indications (e.g., bleeding history, anticoagulant use)
Platelet count	Clinical history or specific clinical indications (e.g., malignancy, bleeding history)
Use of Prior Test Results	
Chest film	A chest film showing normal results that was performed within 1 year can be used if there has been no intervening clinical event
ECG	An ECG showing normal results that was performed within 6 months can be used if there has been no intervening clinical event
Blood tests	Tests performed within 6 weeks that show normal results can be used if there has been no intervening clinical event

Source: Adapted from *Technology Assessment: Routine Preoperative Diagnostic Evaluation in University Hospital Consortium Advancement Center,* Oak Brook, Ill, June 1994, p 39.

they must have a great positive predictive value {positive predictive value = [true positive/(true positive + false positive)] × 100}.

The positive predictive value of the test decreases dramatically as the prevalence of the disease decreases because the number of false-positive test results overwhelms the number of true-positive results, even though the test is highly sensitive and specific. These calculations often yield startling results when a test such as the partial thromboplastin time (PTT) is examined closely. The PTT has a sensitivity of 99 percent and a specificity of 72 percent for detecting clotting disorders. Since the prevalence of significant asymptomatic clotting disorders is 1 in 100,000 patients, only one individual with real disease will be found out of 100,000 patients, but 28,000 patients will be falsely labeled by an abnormal PTT test as having a coagulation defect. The burden imposed by unnecessarily delaying or canceling operations after so many false-positive results and retesting to determine if any bleeding disorder does exist argues against the use of this test in asymptomatic patients.

To contain the rising costs in light of the lack of benefit of routine preoperative laboratory screening, the University Hospital Consortium (UHC), a nonprofit alliance of leading academic medical centers, developed recommendations for preoperative diagnostic testing (Table 2-6). These recommendations

were based on a review of the literature and a survey of current practices. In addition, based on the work of Roizen, Kaplan and Blery, the UHC proposed a strategy for preoperative testing (Table 2-7). Although the portion of the strategy proposed by Blery has been tested prospectively, this modified version awaits clinical trials of the impact of reduced laboratory testing on outcome.

Advanced Cardiopulmonary Testing

The need for advanced cardiopulmonary testing is based on the patient's historical risk factors, functional status, and the complexity of the surgical procedure. If a patient suffers no complaints, is active and healthy, and is undergoing a low-risk surgical procedure, further testing is rarely needed. In patients undergoing high-risk procedures, which include intrathoracic, vascular, and major abdominal operations, historical markers and exercise tolerance are not good predictors of perioperative cardiac risk, and these patients frequently require additional cardiac evaluation. If noninvasive tests are abnormal, a decision must be made regarding the risk of coronary angiography (and possibly angioplasty or coronary revascularization prior to the operation) versus accepting the risk of possible myocardial infarct and

Table 2-7

Strategy for Preoperative Testing

Preoperative Condition	HGB M	HGB F	WBC	PT/ PTT	PLT BT	Electro- lytes	CREAT/ BUN	Blood GLU	AST/ ALK	Chest film	ECG	Preg	T/S
Procedure with blood loss	X	X											X
Procedure without blood loss													
Neonates	X	X											
Age < 40		X											
Age 40–49		X									M		
Age 50–64		X									X		
Age ≥ 65	X	X								±	X		
Cardiovascular disease							X			X	X		
Pulmonary disease										X	X		
Malignancy	X	X	*	*						X			
Radiation therapy			X							X	X		
Hepatic disease				X					X				
Exposure to hepatitis									X				
Renal disease	X	X				X	X						
Bleeding disorder				X	X								
Diabetes						X	X	X			X		
Smoking ≥ 20 pack-yr	X	X								X			
Possible pregnancy												X	
Diuretic use						X	X						
Digoxin use						X	X				X		
Steroid use						X		X					
Anticoagulant use	X	X		X									
CNS disease			X			X	X	X			X		

Note: Not all diseases are included in this table. The physician's own judgment is needed regarding patients with diseases not listed. To use chart to guide in ordering tests, select all rows that apply to the given patient and order all tests that appear in any row selected. *Symbols:* ± = perhaps obtain; * = obtain for leukemias only; X = obtain; M = men only. *Abbreviations:* HGB = hemoglobin; WBC = white blood count; PT = prothrombin time; PTT = partial thromboplastin time; PLT = platelet count; BT = bleeding time; elect = electrolytes; CREAT/BUN = creatinine or blood urea nitrogen; AST = serum glutamic-oxaloacetic transaminase; ALK = alkaline phosphatase; T/S = blood typing and screen for unexpected antibodies.

Source: Adapted from *Technology Assessment: Routine Preoperative Diagnostic Evaluations in University Hospital Consortium Advancement Center,* Oak Brook, Ill, June 1994, p 59.

Table 2-8

Risk Factors Associated with Increased Pulmonary Morbidity

Patient factors
  Old age
  Obesity
  Past and present smoking
  Respiratory infection
Surgical factors
  Proximity of operation to diaphragm
  Vertical abdominal incision
  Duration of operation

proceeding directly to the operation. This decision is based on the mortality of angioplasty or coronary revascularization and the mortality of the surgical procedure without those preoperative interventions within one's institution.

Preoperative risk factors that have been associated with postoperative pulmonary complications are listed in Table 2-8. The proximity of the operative site to the diaphragm is the most consistent risk factor in the development of postoperative pulmonary complications. Reduced preoperative pulmonary function does not necessarily predict postoperative pulmonary complications, except for patients with severe COPD and those undergoing thoracic operations. Likewise, normal pulmonary function does not preclude pulmonary morbidity. Pulmonary function testing is ordered only to quantify the degree of impairment, assess appropriate therapy, or aid in planning perioperative care in patients who have functional limitations.

Informed Consent

Before undertaking an anesthetic, the anesthesiologist is obliged to obtain the patient's informed consent. A prudent approach is to inform the patient of the anesthetic options, to cite the risks and benefits as plainly as possible, and to agree on a course of action that covers most common contingencies. The patient's response to this discourse may range from a request for more specifics to an expression of trust with no further doubts concerning the procedure. The anesthesiologist must be prepared to answer all questions posed by the patient in a manner that provides the appropriate information for a reasonable and educated decision. Written documentation of the informed consent is included in the patient's chart.

Physical Status Classification

At the conclusion of the preanesthetic evaluation, every patient is assigned an American Society of Anesthesiologists (ASA) physical status classification (Table 2-9). This serves as a general measure of the well-being of the patient. Although studies of anesthetic mortality show a correlation with ASA physical status classification, this categorization does not describe risk directly. The risks of any operation are determined not only by patient-related factors but also by the risk of the specific operative procedure, the experience of the surgical team and of the medical institution with the procedure, whether the procedure is elective or emergent, and to a degree, the choice of anesthetic agents and techniques. The efficacy of various means proposed for reducing patient risk, such as invasive monitoring or postoperative ICU stay, remains unknown.

Table 2-9

Physical Status Modified Slightly from ASA Definition

1. The patient has no systemic disease, including the pathologic process for which operation is needed, which is localized. Example: A healthy young man requires inguinal herniorrhaphy.
2. The patient suffers mild or moderate systemic disease due either to the surgical condition or to a concomitant disease. Example: The patient describes taking oral medication for diabetes but has no end-organ damage and has never suffered severe ketoacidosis.
3. Severe systemic disease limits the patient's activity. Example: The patient above had a myocardial infarction last year and now has angina usually controlled by medical treatment.
4. Severe life-threatening disease markedly limits the patient. Example: The patient has congestive heart failure and can walk less than half a block.
5. The moribund patient has a 50 percent 24-hour mortality, regardless of the planned operation. Example: Our patient has infarcted bowel and is anuric, comatose, and has a blood pressure of 70/40 with a dopamine infusion.
6. The patient is declared dead and will undergo operation for organ donation. Example: 72 hours after a motorcycle accident, a PS 1 patient comes to the OR for liver and kidney donation.
E. When the patient requires emergency operation, an E is appended to the PS number. Example: The diabetic patient described suffered a strangulated hernia during the years before he developed coronary occlusion, and sought attention promptly; he was rated PS 2E.

Table 2-10

Components of the Anesthetic Impression and Plan

1. Brief summary of the patient's history and physical findings as they pertain to anesthesia management, organized in a problem list, paralleling any existing problem list used by the primary physician
2. Planned anesthetic technique including special techniques discussed (e.g., fiberoptic intubation, invasive monitoring)
3. Planned postoperative pain management, if appropriate
4. Special postoperative issues when indicated (e.g., ICU stay)
5. Request for further medical evaluation if indicated
6. Statement of risks, informed consent, and statement that all questions were answered
7. Physical status classification and brief justification

Anesthetic Impression and Plan

Preoperative evaluation includes writing a concise note summarizing the history and physical examination, laboratory data, the ASA physical status classification, and a description of the anesthetic plan. This includes the need for special techniques such as rapid-sequence or fiberoptic intubation, proposed intraoperative monitoring, postoperative pain management, and other perioperative care. If necessary, the need for further medical evaluation or testing is clearly stated. Preoperative management of the patient's medications, oral intake, and other therapy is included in the physician's orders. See Table 2-10 for an outline of the written anesthetic impression and plan.

Conclusion

The classic preoperative visit, conducted at the patient's bedside on the evening before the operation, is passing. Now patients with major medical problems come to the hospital on the day of even complex operations and may go home that same day. Nevertheless, three essential elements of the preoperative visit remain: a thorough consultant's history and physical examination, good rapport between patient and physician, and selection of tests and anesthetic techniques indicated by the medical history and clinical judgment.

BIBLIOGRAPHY

Blery C, Szatan M, Fourgeaux B, et al. Evaluation of a protocol for selective ordering of preoperative tests. *Lancet* 1986;1:139-141.

Fleisher LA, Barash PG. Preoperative cardiac evaluation for noncardiac surgery: A functional approach. *Anesth Analg* 1992;74:586-596.

Fleisher LA, Skolnick ED, Holroyd KJ, Lehmann HP. Coronary artery revascularization before abdominal aortic aneurysm surgery: A decision analytic approach. *Anesth Analg* 1994;79:661-669.

Kaplan EB, Sheiner LB, Boeckman AL, et al. The usefulness of preoperative screening. *JAMA* 1985;253:3576-3581.

Malhotra N, Roizen MF. Laboratory testing. *Probl Anesth* 1991;5:575-590.

Mangano DT. Perioperative cardiac morbidity. *Anesthesiology* 1990;72:153-184.

Narr BJ, Hansen TR, Warner MA. Preoperative laboratory screening in healthy Mayo patients: Cost-effective elimination of tests and unchanged outcomes. *Mayo Clin Proc* 1991;66:155-159.

Stein M, Cassara EL. Preoperative pulmonary evaluation and therapy for surgery patients. *JAMA* 1970;211:787-790.

Turnbull JM, Buck C. The value of preoperative screening investigations in otherwise healthy individuals. *Arch Intern Med* 1987;147:1101.

Zibrak JD, O'Donnell CR. Indications for preoperative pulmonary function testing. *Clin Chest Med* 1993;2:227-236.

3

Interpretation of Arterial Blood Gas and Acid-Base Data

James E. Baumgardner

Arterial blood gas measurements make it possible to manage scientifically respiratory and acid-base disorders in anesthetized and critically ill patients. This chapter provides a pragmatic introduction to interpreting data obtained from the blood gas laboratory. Related material is covered in later chapters on medical gases (Chap. 12), respiratory disease (Chap. 22), and critical care (Chap. 33).

Arterial Oxygen Tension

Arterial oxygen tension (PaO_2) is defined as the partial pressure of oxygen present in a hypothetical gas phase in equilibrium with a sample of arterial blood. Normal values of 90 to 100 mmHg decrease with age (see Chap. 27). Although intraarterial measurement is possible, most often a sample of arterial blood is drawn into a syringe and taken to the blood gas laboratory, where it is placed in a chamber separated by an oxygen-permeable membrane from an electrolyte solution bathing a platinum cathode and a silver anode. The electric current flowing through this polarographic oxygen electrode at a fixed potential is a function of the oxygen tension. Errors in obtaining and handling the blood sample may invalidate the data. First, blood may be drawn from a vein by mistake. Second, large air bubbles left in the syringe containing

the blood sample may exchange oxygen and carbon dioxide with the sample. Third, if the syringe is not placed in ice, cell metabolism may consume enough oxygen to decrease the PaO_2; because white cells are especially metabolically active, this problem is accentuated in patients with leukocytosis.

Although there are hazards to increased arterial oxygen tension, especially in neonates, usually the patient's PaO_2 is less than expected. Thus the interpretation of arterial oxygen tension commonly requires explaining a decreased PaO_2. The difference between inspired oxygen tension and the PaO_2 mainly reflects factors involving regional pulmonary blood flow, regional ventilation, and gas diffusion (see Chaps. 12, 22, and 33).

Hypoventilation usually is described in pulmonary physiology texts as an unlikely cause of arterial hypoxemia, which is quite true in a normal subject whose minute ventilation changes slowly. In the practice of anesthesia, the patient's minute ventilation often changes rapidly and profoundly, such as after the intravenous administration of muscle relaxants, narcotics, sedatives, or anesthetics. Because the body stores of oxygen are very small and primarily limited to the oxygen stores in the functional residual capacity of the lung, sudden depression of ventilation commonly leads to hypoxia; hypoventilation must be considered in the differential diagnosis of decreased PaO_2.

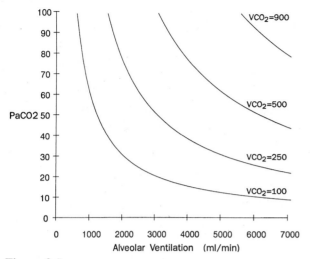

Figure 3-1

The relationship between arterial CO_2 tension and alveolar ventilation is a hyperbola for each value of minute CO_2 production ($\dot{V}_{CO_2}$).

Arterial Carbon Dioxide Tension

The partial pressure of carbon dioxide in an arterial blood sample ($PaCO_2$), like the PaO_2, represents the partial pressure in a hypothetical gas phase in equilibrium with the blood. In the Severinghaus CO_2 electrode, carbon dioxide in the blood sample diffuses through a membrane to a bicarbonate solution; the change in the pH of this solution, measured by a pH electrode, corresponds to the $PaCO_2$.

$PaCO_2$ is closely regulated around a normal value between 37 and 43 mmHg. Deviations may reflect changes in minute ventilation, rate of CO_2 production, and the efficiency of gas exchange in the lungs (see Chap. 22).

Causes of hypercarbia include increased CO_2 production, decreased minute ventilation, and decreased efficiency of ventilation (i.e., how well the lung uses the minute ventilation to exchange gases). Conversely, a low $PaCO_2$ can be the result of decreased CO_2 production or increased minute ventilation, but supranormal lung efficiency does not occur. Decreased CO_2 production most commonly results from hypothermia, whether induced or unintentional. Patients receiving mechanical ventilation who are in shock, with reduced cardiac outputs and peripheral vasoconstriction, may become hypocarbic and give the appearance of decreased CO_2 production

because of failure to deliver carbon dioxide from the unperfused tissue to the lungs. Physiologic compensation for metabolic acidosis or alkalosis includes increased or decreased minute ventilation and hypocarbia or hypercarbia, respectively.

Isolated abnormalities of $PaCO_2$ are relatively well tolerated as long as associated hypoxemia or extreme alterations in pH are avoided. When time permits, successful treatment of the underlying abnormality corrects the $PaCO_2$ as well. In more urgent circumstances, the patient is likely to be receiving controlled ventilation; altering minute ventilation promptly changes $PaCO_2$ (Fig. 3-1). Therapy for abnormalities of $PaCO_2$ is directed toward changes in minute ventilation. Thus, even when an increased CO_2 is the result of increased production, increases in $PaCO_2$ by definition represent hypoventilation and are treated by increasing the minute ventilation, usually mechanically.

Arterial pH

A complex array of mechanisms involving the lungs, blood, and kidneys, which are integrated with other physiologic systems, regulates acid-base status. To describe the patient's acid-base status, first define the pathophysiology (respiratory or metabolic; acidosis or alkalosis), then assess the severity of the disorder, and finally deduce from the overall clinical picture the pathologic process that led to the acid-base derangement.

The variables we measure to define acid-base status are arterial CO_2 tension and hydrogen ion concentration or, more commonly, pH, the negative logarithm to the base 10 of the hydrogen ion concentration. Serum bicarbonate concentration ($[HCO_3^-]$) is not measured but is calculated from the arterial pH and CO_2 measurements; the values are accurate as long as the plasma bicarbonate buffer system is near equilibrium, which is usually the case.

■ Respiratory Acidosis and Alkalosis

Interpretation of respiratory acid-base status is straightforward and depends solely on the measured $PaCO_2$. An increased $PaCO_2$ is by definition respiratory acidemia, and reduced CO_2 tension is by definition respiratory alkalemia. As long as minute ventilation, CO_2 production, and pulmonary function do not change for several minutes before the arterial blood sample is obtained, it is reasonable to assume that arterial CO_2 tension reflects PCO_2 throughout the body.

Assessing the degree of derangement is also straightforward. The fraction of alveolar gas present as CO_2 ($FACO_2$), CO_2 production ($\dot{Q}_{CO2}$), and alveolar ventilation ($\dot{V}A$) are related by

$$\dot{Q}_{CO2} = FACO_2 \times \dot{V}A \qquad (3.1)$$

Over the short term, alveolar CO_2 and arterial CO_2 are directly related, as are the alveolar and expired minute volumes. Because CO_2 production also changes little over the short term in anesthetized patients or those in the intensive care unit (ICU), this equation also may be written as

Expired minute ventilation $\times$ arterial CO_2

$$= \text{constant}$$

or

$$\dot{V}E \times PaCO_2 = k \qquad (3.2)$$

Thus, for a constant CO_2 production, $PaCO_2$ and alveolar ventilation are inversely related (Fig. 3-1). This relationship quantitates derangements of the respiratory acid-base status and dictates adjustment of mechanical ventilators. For example, if arterial CO_2 is found to be twice normal, then ventilation is half the needed value.

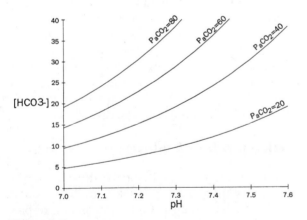

Figure 3-2

Plots of the Henderson-Hasselbach relationship. $[HCO_3^-]$ can be uniquely determined for any $PaCO_2$ and pH.

■ Metabolic Acidosis and Alkalosis

It would be convenient if the patient's metabolic acid-base status could be quantified by comparing the serum bicarbonate concentration ($[HCO_3^-]$) with its normal value, 26 mM. The $[HCO_3^-]$ does respond to changes in the metabolic acid-base status, but buffering of metabolic acids and bases by noncarbonate buffers, especially hemoglobin, complicates the relationship. These noncarbonate buffers necessitate a correction (usually fairly small) to the deviation of bicarbonate concentration from normal, as outlined below. The most common such corrected value is the *base excess*, a term used frequently yet often misunderstood.

The Bicarbonate Buffer System

The bicarbonate buffer system figures in any discussion of metabolic acid-base status not only because of its physiologic role but also because two important variables, arterial pH and $PaCO_2$, are readily measured. Recall that carbonic acid (H_2CO_3) is in equilibrium with its conjugate base, bicarbonate (HCO_3^-):

$$CO_2 + H_2O \rightleftarrows H_2CO_3 \rightleftarrows HCO_3^- + H^+ \quad (3.3)$$

Therefore, the concentrations of ions in this reaction are related by the equation

$$[H^+] \times [HCO_3^-]/[CO_2] = K \qquad (3.4)$$

In logarithmic notation, this is the familiar Henderson-Hasselbach relationship:

$$pH = pK + \log [HCO_3^-]/\alpha PCO_2 \qquad (3.5)$$

where α is a solubility coefficient for CO_2 in plasma.

For plasma, in which CO_2, hydrogen ion, and HCO_3^- are in equilibrium, any of the three variables is uniquely determined by the other two. For example, if this equation is plotted as in Figure 3-2, with separate curves for each value of $PaCO_2$, for any given pH and $PaCO_2$, the $[HCO_3^-]$ is uniquely determined. Therefore, by knowing PCO_2 and pH, one can calculate $[HCO_3^-]$ regardless of any other buffers of the system. The curves of Figure 3-2 always hold as long as the system includes H^+, HCO_3^-, and CO_2 in equilibrium.

However, the Henderson-Hasselbach relationship does not reveal how $[HCO_3^-]$ and pH change when

PaCO$_2$ increases or decreases from normal, corresponding to hypo- or hyperventilation. For example, without any additional information, we cannot tell in Figure 3-3 if a patient whose CO$_2$ increases from 40 to 50 mmHg will be represented by point A, B, or C. We see from Equation (3.3) that adding CO$_2$ to the buffer system will increase both HCO$_3^-$ and H$^+$ (i.e., decrease pH).

Adding CO$_2$ in the physiologic range of pH, however, has practically no effect on [HCO$_3^-$] if there are no other buffers in the system. At a pH of 7.4, the absolute concentration of H$^+$ is about 4 x 10^{-8} mol/liter, whereas the concentration of HCO$_3^-$ is around 2.6 x 10^{-2} mol/liter, a ratio of 6.5 x 10^5, or nearly 1 million. If there were no other buffers, the equal amounts of H$^+$ and HCO$_3^-$ formed from the added H$_2$CO$_3$ would change the pH much more than the [HCO$_3^-$]; in fact, the change in [HCO$_3^-$] could be neglected completely. Therefore, if the system included only the HCO$_3^-$ buffer, the buffer line for CO$_2$ would be flat, as in Figure 3-4.

If changes in PaCO$_2$ do not change the [HCO$_3^-$] for a pure bicarbonate buffer system, the corollary is that at any PaCO$_2$ the [HCO$_3^-$] reflects only the amount of metabolic acid added to or subtracted from the system. For a pure bicarbonate system at a pH around 7.4, the [HCO$_3^-$] alone would be a simple indicator of metabolic acid-base status. The buffer lines for CO$_2$ titration would be a family of flat curves with the vertical distance between the curves reflecting metabolic acid-base status.

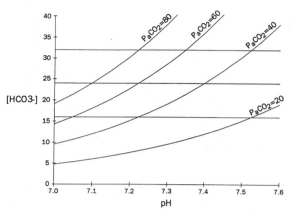

Figure 3-4

The *buffer curve* for a CO$_2$ titration determines the results of PaCO$_2$ changes. The buffer curves are the nearly horizontal lines, each corresponding to a given [HCO$_3^-$]. For a pure bicarbonate buffer system at physiologic pH, the slopes of the buffer curves are nearly zero; for example, a bicarbonate buffer system with [HCO$_3^-$] of 24 (middle line) had a pH of 7.4 at a PaCO$_2$ of 40 mmHg, as shown at the intersection of the lines. If CO$_2$ is added to bring the PaCO$_2$ to 60 mmHg, the pH decreases to 7.2. Bicarbonate concentration is changed only by adding or removing metabolic acid.

Other Buffers

In reality, however, there are other buffers for H$^+$ in the body, each obeying a relationship similar to Equation (3.6):

$$H^+ + B^- \rightleftharpoons HB \qquad (3.6)$$

where B$^-$ represents buffer species. As metabolic acid is added to the system, some of the hydrogen ions (H$^+$) are bound to these other bases (B$^-$) and not to bicarbonate. Since concentrations of these other buffers are not measured in assessing metabolic acid-base status, how can one determine how much hydrogen ion has been added or taken away from the system? Even though the amount of HB or B$^-$ is unknown, if the system were somehow adjusted to a normal hydrogen ion concentration, then the ratio B$^-$:HB also would be normal. In addition, if this titration of H$^+$ were performed with an acid that produces a change of one HCO$_3^-$ for every H$^+$ ion, then the change in [HCO$_3^-$] during this titration would directly reflect how much H$^+$ had been in the system as HB. The acid to use for this imaginary titration is CO$_2$.

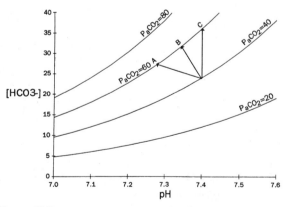

Figure 3-3

As PaCO$_2$ is increased from 40 to 60 mmHg, Equation (3.4) predicts an increase in both [HCO$_3^-$] and [H$^+$]. However, the Henderson-Hasselbach relationship does not predict whether the result is point A, B, or C.

Base Excess

This is one way of viewing the concept of base excess. Base excess is the difference between a normal $[HCO_3^-]$ and the $[HCO_3^-]$ that would result from titrating the blood sample to a normal pH by adjusting the $PaCO_2$. The deviation of this corrected $[HCO_3^-]$ from normal can be viewed as having two components: the amount $[HCO_3^-]$ has changed from normal due to buffering of metabolic acid by the bicarbonate system (recall that this component will not change during the CO_2 titration because the $[HCO_3^-]$ for a pure bicarbonate system is independent of $PaCO_2$) and the amount $[HCO_3^-]$ has changed from normal due to buffering by other buffers. This latter component can be considered a correction factor to the measured bicarbonate concentration, and although much has been written on the best way to correct the $[HCO_3^-]$, in reality, this correction is usually small.

Of course, one cannot carry out this titration in the patient, so the correction factor is calculated. Given the actual slope of the CO_2 buffer line, one can then imagine correcting any measured arterial blood gas to a normal pH by adding or removing CO_2. For a pure HCO_3^- system (see Fig. 3-4), the slope of this line is essentially zero; the buffer line is steeper when there are more noncarbonate buffers in the system, as found in patients (Fig. 3-5).

Unfortunately, in any given patient, the slope of the buffer line is unknown. Typical slopes for typical patients, the slope for normal whole blood, and how the slope for whole blood changes with variations in hemoglobin concentration are all known, but there is

no assurance that in a particular patient the buffers will be typical or present in normal concentrations. In fact, the slope varies depending on the duration of the acid-base disturbance, and the buffer curve is not really linear even in normal subjects. The end result is that despite the importance frequently attached to the base excess, the number is always calculated, not measured, and the calculation is always approximate. It is inappropriate to prescribe bicarbonate therapy based only on a quantitative interpretation of the base excess.

In summary, if the $PaCO_2$ has increased, the patient has a respiratory acidosis; if it has decreased, the patient has a respiratory alkalosis. The degree of ventilatory abnormality is proportional to the deviation of $PaCO_2$ from normal. If the base excess is positive, the patient has a metabolic alkalosis; if negative, a metabolic acidosis. The magnitude of the base excess reflects the severity of the abnormality, but only approximately.

Defining the direction and severity of the acid-base abnormality, however, is only the first part of interpreting the data. Each of these disturbances may be primary or compensatory, and in mixed disturbances, several processes occur simultaneously, with combinations of primary and secondary changes. The underlying pathology is not defined by the blood gas and pH data alone but by an understanding of the patient's overall condition. Some examples may help to clarify the importance of assessing other clinical data in determining the causes of acid-base disturbances.

Case Histories

■ Case 1

A 72-year-old man with a history of chronic obstructive pulmonary disease (COPD) and peripheral vascular disease presents to the emergency room with the sudden onset of abdominal pain, breathing at a respiratory rate of 28. As an anesthesiologist, you go to the emergency room to evaluate the patient before a planned exploratory laparotomy. Among the data is the analysis of an arterial blood sample taken while the patient was breathing room air: PaO_2, 57; $PaCO_2$, 40; pH, 7.12; $[HCO_3^-]$, 12.

One can estimate the alveolar PO_2 from an approximate form of the alveolar gas equation (see Chap. 22):

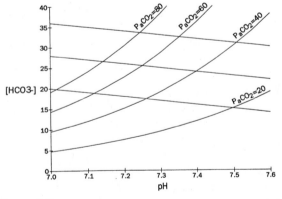

Figure 3-5

In a patient, the slope of the CO_2 buffer curve is small but not negligible because of the effects of nonbicarbonate buffers.

$$PaO_2 = FiO_2 \times 713 - (PaCO_2/R)$$

where R is the respiratory quotient.

$$PaO_2 = 0.21 \times 713 - (40/0.8) = 100$$

The alveolar-arterial O_2 difference is $100 - 57 = 43$ mmHg, clearly increased (normal is less than 10 mmHg). The PaO_2 is much decreased; given the history of COPD, this is likely due to ventilation-perfusion mismatch and an unknown degree of shunt. The $PaCO_2$ is normal, but much more respiratory compensation (hyperventilation, diminished $PaCO_2$) might be expected for this degree of metabolic acidosis (see below).

To assess the metabolic acid-base status, estimate the base excess. One convenient estimate predicts that for every increase in pH of 0.1 as the CO_2 is decreased, the $[HCO_3^-]$ will decrease by 1. In this patient, one would like to increase the pH from 7.12 to 7.42 by removing CO_2, a change of 0.3 pH units, predicting that $[HCO_3^-]$ would decrease by 3 mEq during this hypothetical titration. The corrected $[HCO_3^-]$ would be $12 - 3 = 9$. The base excess is given by (base excess) = (corrected $[HCO_3^-]$) − (normal $[HCO_3^-]$), or base excess = $9 - 26 = -17$. This patient has a severe metabolic acidosis.

This defines the patient's acid-base and oxygen disorders and the severity of each, but determining the causes of these disorders requires considering other data. The severe metabolic acidosis suggests organ ischemia, especially if the anion gap is large or the measured lactate is increased. The pain and the patient's history suggest a dissecting aortic aneurysm, mesenteric artery occlusion, bowel obstruction, or pancreatitis. The patient very likely will come to the operating room soon.

The patient's tachypnea and inability to compensate for severe metabolic acidosis suggest significant COPD, abdominal splinting, fatigue, and impending respiratory failure. He may benefit from immediate mechanical ventilatory support despite his normal $PaCO_2$. Also, bicarbonate therapy would be futile and possibly hazardous before ventilation is controlled, since the patient may not be able to excrete the additional CO_2 load owing to his lung disease.

Although there is no way to be certain without baseline data, the suggestion of severe COPD raises the possibility that this patient chronically retains CO_2. Also, the PaO_2 would be decreased even more if the CO_2 were increased, raising the possibility that this patient chronically depends on hypoxic stimulus to ventilation. Both these points will be important in planning weaning from mechanical ventilation after the operation.

■ Case 2

A 45-year-old woman with controlled hypertension and morbid obesity undergoes an uneventful open cholycystectomy. Anesthetic management includes inhalation anesthesia with administration of parenteral narcotics prior to skin closure for postoperative analgesia. Postoperatively, an arterial blood gas obtained while the patient breathes 50% oxygen by face mask reveals: PaO_2, 62; $PaCO_2$, 52; pH, 7.31; and $[HCO_3^-]$, 26. On your way to examine the patient, you begin to define the nature of the disorder. By the alveolar gas equation, the alveolar-arterial O_2 difference is $291 - 62 = 229$ mmHg, substantially increased. The increased $PaCO_2$ represents respiratory acidemia. By our simple estimate of the slope of the buffer line, increasing the pH from 7.31 to 7.42 by removing CO_2 would require a change of 0.11 pH units, predicting a decrease in HCO_3 of 1.1 mEq, so the base excess is estimated at $24.9 - 26 = -1.1$, within the normal range. The disturbance of the arterial blood gas values can therefore be defined as respiratory acidosis with no metabolic acid-base abnormalities and impaired oxygenation.

Compromise of both CO_2 and O_2 exchange could represent respiratory failure, but examination of the patient suggests otherwise. Your patient is breathing at a rate of 16 breaths per minute, with no evidence of distress. She is sleepy but easily aroused. When specifically questioned, she does say that she has moderate pain, but with coaching she is able to take deep breaths, and after the deep breaths her pulse oximeter reading increases from 92 to 97 percent. Your diagnosis is postoperative pain with splinting and atelectasis (with resulting hypoxemia due to pulmonary shunt), combined with depression of central respiratory drive from narcotic analgesia. The clinical history and physical examination provided the explanation of the underlying cause of the arterial blood gas abnormalities.

■ Case 3

A previously healthy 22-year-old student, struck by a motor vehicle, is brought to the operating room for laparotomy and repair of multiple fractures.

After securing the airway, establishing large-bore intravenous access, and rapidly restoring central blood volume with salt solutions and type-specific blood, you place an arterial catheter and send a sample for arterial blood gas determination (during controlled ventilation with 100% oxygen), which reveals: PaO_2, 472; $PaCO_2$, 49; pH, 7.21; and $[HCO_3^-]$, 17. You then begin to define the nature of the disorder: oxygenation is only mildly impaired (note that the alveolar gas equation is not readily applied here because the respiratory quotient cannot be assumed to be 0.8 in this setting); there is a mild respiratory acidosis; and the base excess can be estimated to be −11.1, indicating a severe metabolic acidosis. By the clinical history, the most likely cause of the metabolic acidosis is lactic acidosis, with a small contribution due to citrate in the blood preservative. Upon restoration of tissue perfusion and a return to aerobic glycolytic pathways, the normal fate of lactate is to be metabolized, and bicarbonate administered during the acute event carries some risk of rebound alkalosis. Current recommendations in this setting are to avoid bicarbonate therapy unless the acidosis is so severe that cardiac output and catecholamine sensitivity are compromised. A very simple and effective way to increase arterial pH is to increase minute ventilation, compensating for the metabolic acidosis with respiratory alkalosis.

BIBLIOGRAPHY

Astrup P, Severinghaus JW. *The History of Blood Gases, Acids, and Bases.* Copenhagen: Munksgaard International Publishers, 1987.

Cohen RD. Roles of the liver and kidney in acid-base regulation and its disorders. *Br J Anaesth* 1991;67:154-164.

Davenport HW. *The ABCs of Acid-Base Chemistry,* 6th ed. Chicago: University of Chicago Press, 1974.

Fencl V, Leith DE. Stewart's quantitative acid-base chemistry: Applications in biology and medicine. *Respir Physiol* 1993; 91:1-16.

Hindman BJ. Sodium bicarbonate in the treatment of subtypes of acute lactic acidosis: Physiologic considerations. *Anesthesiology* 1990;72:1064-1076.

Oeseburg B, Rolfe P, Siggaard Andersen O, et al. Definition and measurement of quantities pertaining to oxygen in blood. *Adv Exp Med Biol* 1994;345:925-930.

Shapiro BA, Cane RD. Blood gas monitoring: Yesterday, today, and tomorrow. *Crit Care Med* 1989;17:573-581.

Shapiro BA, Harrison RA, Walton JR. *Clinical Application of Blood Gases,* 3rd ed. Chicago: Year Book Medical Publishers, 1982.

Tobin MJ. Respiratory monitoring. *JAMA* 1990;264:244-251.

CHAPTER

4

Premedication: Drugs to Start, Continue, or Withhold

Mitchell D. Tobias and Lester A. Zuckerman

Premedication, the practice of giving patients special medications before anesthesia and operation, originally was required to make it safe and practical to induce anesthesia with agents such as ether and chloroform. Although modern intravenous anesthetics permit the rapid and pleasant induction of anesthesia without premedication, perioperative care of the surgical patient still begins with treatment before the induction of anesthesia (Table 4-1). Such therapy can increase the patient's comfort, blunt harmful reflexes, reduce the risk of aspiration of gastric contents, and ensure that patients receive the medications needed to treat chronic illnesses, allergies, or perioperative infections (Table 4-2). This chapter considers these issues for adults; for children, see Chap. 25.

Patient Safety and Preoperative Medication

Premedication is not without risks, for all preoperative medications may produce side effects. Opioids and hypnotics present special hazards, especially in combination, because they can cause loss of consciousness, respiratory depression, and airway obstruction, leading to hypoxemia or hypercarbia. Patients at special risk include the elderly and the very young and those who suffer from obesity, sleep apnea,

shock, or cardiopulmonary disease. When medications are given orally or intramuscularly so that absorption is delayed and unpredictable and the patient is left unobserved without supplemental oxygen, the risks increase.

To minimize the hazards of preoperative sedatives and opioids, these medications are avoided completely or used in reduced doses in patients at special risk. Sedatives and hypnotics can be given incrementally in small intravenous doses with appropriate monitoring by a trained observer so that an unanticipated relative overdose can be avoided or treated. Supportive preoperative visits and reassurance, along with the routine use of lesser doses of these drugs, reduce the risk of overdose and avoid the potential for serious side effects. Undertreated patients can receive additional sedatives intravenously in a holding area or before entering the operating room.

Alleviating Anxiety

Relief from preoperative anxiety is of unquestioned humanitarian importance; by reducing sympathetic nervous activity, important physiologic benefits also may accrue. There is conflicting evidence that reducing the patient's anxiety improves patient outcome, as measured by postoperative pain, analgesic require-

27

Table 4-1

Common Problems Amenable to Treatment before Anesthesia and Operation

Anxiety
Amnesia
Pain
Salivation and airway secretions
Vagal reflexes
Hypertensive responses
Seizures
Aspiration of gastric contents
Nausea and vomiting
Infection
Reactions to intravenous contrast media
Latex allergy
Continuation of preoperative therapy

ments, blood pressure and heart rate, and length of hospital stay. In some studies, patients who worried preoperatively were more realistic, dealt actively with their situation, and left the hospital sooner.

Most patients suffer anxiety before operations, especially those undergoing genitourinary, cosmetic, or cancer-related procedures. Depending on the patient, anxiety may not be apparent to the observer, or it may produce frantic regressive or combative behavior. Prevention and treatment depend on speaking to the patient and on the use of drugs.

■ Relieving Anxiety without Drugs

Not all patients are calmed by sedatives. Some may be rendered sleepy so that they appear calm to a casual observer, but questioning reveals that they are anxious nonetheless. Others who are most comfortable when in control of themselves and their surroundings may respond paradoxically and experience increased anxiety. Patients' anxieties are greatly relieved by a skilled preoperative visit that includes sympathy, reassurance, direct and frank discussion of the patient's concerns, and careful description of what is to come. Sedation can then be prescribed if the patient requests it or if some specific benefit is anticipated. Alternatively, medication can be withheld if that seems appropriate.

■ Drugs to Relieve Anxiety

Moderate doses of barbiturates are likely to cause drowsiness but not to relieve anxiety, whereas benzodiazepines have specific antianxiety effects. Benzodiazepines are well absorbed from the stomach, so the discomfort of intramuscular injection can be avoided.

Effective relief of anxiety depends greatly on the timing of drug administration. Sedative premedications given orally or intramuscularly just before the patient comes to the operating room are likely to exert no beneficial effects before the induction of anesthesia, but they delay emergence from anesthesia and

Table 4-2

Commonly Used Premedications

Drug Group	Drug Name	Adult Dose (mg)	Route
Benzodiazepines	Diazepam	5–20	Oral
	Flurazepam	15–30	Oral
	Lorazepam	2–4	Oral, IM
	Midazolam	2–5	IM/IV
	Triazolam	0.125–0.250	Oral
Tranquilizers	Droperidol	0.625–2.5	IM/IV
Antihistamines	Diphenhydramine	25–75	Oral, IM/IV
	Hydroxyzine	50–100	IM
Opioids	Fentanyl	0.05–0.2	IM/IV
	Hydromorphone	1.0–2.0	IM/IV
	Morphine	5–15	IM/IV
	Meperidine	50–100	IM/IV
Anticholinergics	Atropine	0.2–0.6	IM/IV
	Glycopyrrolate	0.2–0.6	IM/IV
	Scopolamine	0.2–0.4	IM/IV
Gastrokinetics	Metoclopramide	10–20	Oral, IM/IV
H_2 antagonists	Cimetidine	300	Oral, IM/IV
Alpha-2-agonists	Clonidine	0.20–0.40	Oral
5-HT antagonist	Ondansetron	4.0–8.0	IM/IV

exacerbate postoperative respiratory depression. Medication can be given both the night before the operation and several hours before the patient goes to the operating room; appropriate times are on awakening for morning operations and a few hours later in the morning for afternoon operations.

Midazolam

Because it is water soluble and does not produce pain on intravenous or intramuscular injection, midazolam is used widely in anesthesia practice. Like other benzodiazepines, it possesses antianxiety, sedative, amnestic, and anticonvulsant properties. Midazolam is stored in acidic solution (pH < 4.0), which opens its ring structure, rendering it water soluble. At physiologic pH, the molecule closes, becoming the lipid-soluble active form. Small amounts given intravenously (1 to 5 mg in adults) produce the rapid onset of sedation of brief duration, although care is required to guard against respiratory depression and airway obstruction in susceptible patients. Larger doses, 0.05 to 0.1 mg/kg, are given orally or intramuscularly.

Diazepam

Diazepam, about one-third to one-half as potent as midazolam, is commonly administered orally. The usual dose is 0.15 mg/kg of body weight, given several hours before operation. In patients habituated to benzodiazepines or those who are unusually anxious, up to 0.25 mg/kg can be used. Smaller doses are appropriate for older or frail patients. Diazepam is unsuited for parenteral use because of inconsistent absorption from intramuscular sites and pain and phlebitis after intravenous injection.

Lorazepam

Lorazepam, twice as potent as midazolam, is well absorbed orally and is so long acting in its effects that it may produce unwanted sedation and amnesia after surgical procedures. It is most useful for patients undergoing lengthy procedures following which prompt emergence is not desirable. Lorazepam produces remarkable amnesia in many patients.

Amnesia

Amnesia for perioperative events may or may not add to patient comfort. Some patients fear that they may say or do something embarrassing during their amnesia, although this is a rare occurrence. For uncomfortable procedures such as awake intubation, insertion of central venous catheters, long operations under regional anesthesia, or when a patient asks not to recall events, anterograde amnesia is most reliably produced by midazolam, lorazepam, or scopolamine (0.4 to 0.6 mg intravenously); there is no reliable way to produce retrograde amnesia for events preceding drug administration.

Amnesia after midazolam is dose-related: after receiving 0.05 mg/kg intravenously, 60 percent of patients do not remember endoscope insertion; after 0.15 mg/kg, 96 percent lack recall. The amnesia from midazolam is greatest 2 to 5 minutes after intravenous injection and reliably lasts only 20 to 30 minutes; after intravenous lorazepam, the onset of amnesia is delayed 15 to 20 minutes but can last up to 6 or 8 hours.

Analgesia

Patients in pain may receive opioids for analgesia as part of their premedication. For those not in pain, adding opioids increases respiratory depression without a concomitant gain in sedation; opioids are not the best choice if only sedation is required. Morphine is used commonly. Thoughtful timing of the administration of the drug can increase safety. For example, if opioid premedication is needed to make comfortable such procedures as placement of an epidural or internal jugular catheter, morphine may be given intravenously in the operating room. This allows close monitoring so that an effective dose can be administered without the risk of untreated respiratory depression.

Reducing Salivation and Bronchial Secretions

Inducing anesthesia by the inhalation of ether or cyclopropane leads to the release of copious saliva and airway secretions. Modern inhaled agents are less liable to produce this effect, but the accumulation of saliva and bronchial secretions, particularly in smokers, still can provoke coughing or laryngospasm. These secretions also interfere with the actions of topical local anesthetic solutions used to anesthetize the airway mucosa before procedures such as sedated laryngoscopy or intubation of the trachea. Thirty minutes after the intravenous or intramuscular administration of 0.2 to 0.4 mg of glycopyrrolate to an adult, the mouth will be dry. Glycopyrrolate is less liable to cross the blood-brain barrier and cause somnolence and confusion than are scopolamine or atropine. Atropine also produces more tachycardia than does glycopyrrolate, an important consideration in some patients with cardiac disease.

Blocking Vagal Reflexes

Intubation of the trachea or other airway manipulations may produce profound and abrupt bradycardia, although this reflex is more common in children than in adults. Premedication with an anticholinergic drug such as atropine prevents this reflex, although tachycardia may follow.

Prevention of Hypertension

Patients with hypertension respond to laryngoscopy, intubation, and pain with exaggerated increases in blood pressure. Important measures to control these responses include continuing the patient's usual antihypertensive therapy until the induction of anesthesia and providing an adequate depth of anesthesia to blunt noxious stimuli. Adding additional drugs to the premedication regimen also may help. Alpha and beta sympathetic blockers, opioids, and alpha-2 sympathetic agonists such as clonidine all diminish these responses and have been used for this purpose. These drugs can produce unwanted hypotension, bradycardia, or respiratory depression, so they are often given intravenously after the patient reaches the operating room.

■ Clonidine

Clonidine blunts perioperative catecholamine responses through its central alpha-2-adrenergic action; it also reduces the requirement for inhaled anesthetic agents and opioids during and after the operation. The drug is given orally 60 to 90 minutes before anesthesia in a dose of 5 μg/kg. Side effects include sedation, dry mouth, hypotension, and bradycardia.

Anticonvulsants

Patients with seizure disorders should continue taking their anticonvulsant medications throughout the perioperative period. There is no need to increase the dose or change the drugs used.

Premedication with benzodiazepines may reduce the chance of central nervous system toxicity (seizures) from local anesthetics. In mice, moderate doses of benzodiazepines that did not cause sedation or loss of the righting reflex reduced the incidence of deaths and convulsions from local anesthetics given intraperitoneally. Benzodiazepines may be used to treat seizures due to local anesthetics, but the benefits of prophylaxis for this purpose have not been proven in humans. Optimal effects can be expected from intravenous administration just before the local anesthetic is administered, not from intramuscular or oral administration.

Aspiration of Gastric Contents

Skilled anesthesia management includes identifying patients at increased risk for pulmonary aspiration of gastric contents and the use of special precautions, such as the immediate intubation of the trachea, to decrease these risks. Few cases of severe aspiration pneumonitis occur in modern anesthesia practice. Nevertheless, the risk is always present. As many as 80 percent of patients undergoing elective operations have gastric contents of pH less than 2.5, and many have gastric volumes greater than 25 ml. These threshold values for the development of acid aspiration pneumonitis are based on incomplete animal and human data, but there is no doubt that aspiration of larger volumes of gastric fluid of greater acid content is more dangerous than aspiration of smaller volumes of less acidity. Despite the lack of large-scale outcome studies to justify the practice, it is logical to employ at least the simpler treatments that reduce gastric acidity or the volume of gastric contents.

■ Fasting

The least costly and simplest of the treatments designed to reduce the risk of aspiration is fasting. Common practice dictates that adult patients take nothing by mouth for 8 hours prior to the induction of anesthesia. Nevertheless, the stomach of a fasting patient often contains clear acidic fluid. Ingestion of 150 ml of water actually improves gastric emptying so that gastric volume and acid content decrease over the subsequent hour. In contrast, gastric emptying is prolonged after eating fats and solids, and the pulmonary aspiration of solid food particles is particularly dangerous. Since the discomfort of an overnight fast is slight and the damage done by pulmonary aspiration is great, it is wise to prescribe that healthy adult patients scheduled for elective operations abstain from solid food for 8 hours. Clear liquids may be taken until 3 hours before the operation unless there is some reason to expect delayed gastric emptying, as with pain, anxiety, or associated conditions (e.g., diabetes) or medication (e.g., opioids). Oral medications with up to 30 ml of water are permitted until anesthesia begins. Children, who are more susceptible to dehydration, may take fluids more freely (see Chap. 25).

▪ Gastric Antisecretory Agents

H_2 Receptor Antagonists

Gastric pH can be maintained greater than 2.5 by giving H_2 histamine receptor-blocking agents. The least expensive of these, cimetidine, decreases the hepatic metabolism of diazepam, phenytoin, lidocaine, theophylline, and propranolol, causes sedation, and can be associated with arrhythmias. Ranitidine and famotidine are newer, more expensive agents that exert more prolonged effects and are relatively free of these side effects.

Prostaglandin E_1 Analogues

Misoprostol is a synthetic prostaglandin E_1 analogue that reduces gastric acid secretion via a direct action at the parietal cells, increasing gastric pH without altering the volume. The effect of a 200-μg oral dose on gastric acid secretion is similar to that of 300 mg cimetidine. Inhibition of gastric acid secretion persists for 2 to 3 hours.

Omeprazole

Omeprazole is a potent gastric antisecretory agent chemically unrelated to H_2 receptor antagonists or the prostaglandin analogues. It blocks the final step in the secretion of hydrochloric acid by parietal cells. Because the drug binds irreversibly, inhibition of gastric acid secretion persists for up to 72 hours. For short-term use, omeprazole appears to be as well tolerated as ranitidine. Taken orally, 20 mg once daily is effective.

▪ Antacids

Orally administered antacids buffer the contents of the stomach and may be used as premedicants,

especially immediately before emergency operations, although complete mixing with stomach contents may take up to 20 minutes. Between 10 and 20 ml of magnesium citrate, sodium citrate, or a commercially available combination of the two reliably neutralizes gastric contents, as do a few milliliters of sodium bicarbonate 8.4%. Particulate antacids, which contain magnesium and aluminum hydroxides, cause serious pneumonitis if aspirated and are not used before anesthesia.

Because aspiration pneumonitis is rare in healthy patients without risk factors, it is difficult to determine what prophylactic measures beyond fasting are justified. Cost may preclude the routine use of prophylactic medication. Patients predicted to be at increased risk, such as those who are obese or pregnant, who suffer from diabetes with gastroparesis, who require emergency operations, or who experience gastroesophageal reflux, may benefit from rational combinations of therapies. For elective operations, a combination of an antisecretory therapy beginning the night before and metoclopramide (see next section) on the morning of the operation is effective in reducing volume and acidity of gastric contents. For emergency procedures, a soluble antacid taken 15 to 30 minutes before induction reduces acidity. Metoclopramide is also appropriate if enhanced gastric emptying and stimulated bowel motility will not harm the patient, as might occur with bowel obstruction. When anesthesia and operation are urgent, H_2 blockers can do little when administered just before induction, but they may serve to increase the intragastric pH by the end of the operation.

Nausea and Vomiting

Nausea, retching, and vomiting are common before and after operations; the incidence reported in various studies ranges from 10 to 55 percent. In addition to the distress it causes patients, retching and vomiting can endanger the results of eye, ear, facial, or neurologic operations by increasing the chance of venous bleeding or by increasing intraocular and intracranial pressures. Vomiting can predispose to aspiration of gastric contents, particularly at the time of anesthesia induction and emergence. Antiemetic premedicants may help to reduce the incidence of this distressing complication.

■ Ondansetron

Ondansetron is a selective 5-hydroxytryptamine (5-HT, serotonin) receptor-blocking drug. The details of the mechanism by which it inhibits vomiting are unclear, although 5-hydroxytryptamine receptors are located on the vagus nerve and within the chemoreceptor trigger zone (CTZ) of the area postrema. The drug is used to reduce nausea and vomiting associated with cancer chemotherapy. To prevent perioperative emesis, the intravenous dose is typically 4 mg in adults, one-eighth that recommended for chemotherapy. One 8-mg tablet 30 minutes prior to the operation may be effective.

■ Metoclopramide

Metoclopramide increases the resting tone and phasic contractile activity of gastrointestinal smooth muscle, increasing lower esophageal sphincter pressure and accelerating gastric emptying. Unlike nonspecific cholinergic stimulation of upper gastrointestinal smooth muscle, metoclopramide produces coordinated gastric, pyloric, and duodenal motor activity that enhances gastric emptying and reduces the stasis that precedes vomiting. Dopamine antagonism in the CTZ also contributes to the antiemetic effects of metoclopramide. This drug can be administered orally or parenterally. In awake patients, each intravenous dose (typically 10 to 20 mg) is administered over 1 to 2 minutes to avoid transient but intense cramping and restlessness.

■ Droperidol

Droperidol, a butyrophenone, has been shown to have significant antiemetic effects. It reduces the incidence of nausea or vomiting from 50 to 10 percent among children undergoing strabismus operations. Droperidol is not used commonly as a premedicant because it often causes dysphoria and agitation, even leading to refusal of the operation on occasion. Small doses (0.125 to 0.25 mg) given intravenously during the anesthetic to avoid the possibility of preoperative dysphoria reduce the incidence of postoperative nausea and vomiting. This approach is especially useful for patients with a history of severe postoperative nausea and vomiting and those who are at special risk for complications, such as patients in whom the upper and lower teeth are wired together after dental or oral operations. Ondansetron may be more effective, but it is expensive and often is unnecessary when the preceding regimen is used.

Premedication to Prevent Infection

Antibiotics reduce the rate of wound infections if given just prior to surgical incision. It is necessary to consult the surgeon about the dose and timing of prophylactic antibiotics used for this purpose. Patients with cardiac valvular disease or prosthetic devices are susceptible to endocarditis or infection of the prosthesis during procedures that produce bacteremia of 15 minutes' or more duration. The current recommendations of the American Heart Association (AHA) outline the patients considered to be at risk (Table 4-3). The AHA antibiotic regimen or one recommended by an appropriate consultant may be used.

The administration of some antibiotics requires special precautions. About 10 percent of patients with penicillin allergies also react to cephalosporins. Rapid intravenous administration of vancomycin (over less than 60 minutes) may cause histamine release with flushing, edema, rash, and hypotension. Excessive blood concentrations of aminoglycoside antibiotics may cause ototoxicity or nephrotoxicity. These drugs

Table 4-3

Prophylaxis of Endocarditis
1. *For dental, oral or upper respiratory procedures:* amoxicillin 3.0 g PO 1 hour preoperatively and 1.5 g 6 hours after initial dose
For amoxicillin-PCN allergic patients: erythromycin 800 mg PO, 2 hours preoperatively and 400 mg 6 hours after initial dose or clindamycin 300 mg PO 1 hour preoperatively and 150 mg 6 hours after initial dose
2. *Alternatives for dental, oral, or upper respiratory procedures:* ampicillin 2.0 g IV/IM 30 min preoperatively; then 6 hours later, ampicillin 1.0 g IV/IM or amoxicillin 1.5 g PO. A second option: clindamycin 300 mg IV 30 min preoperatively, then in 6 hours, 150 mg IV.
3. *For GI/GU procedures:* IV/IM ampicillin 2.0 g plus gentamicin 1.5 mg/kg (not to exceed 80 mg) 30 minutes preoperatively; then repeat parenteral ampicillin and gentamicin 8 hours later, or substitute amoxicillin 1.5g PO 6 hours later.
For ampicillin/amoxicillin/PCN allergic patients: vancomycin and gentamicin: IV vancomycin 1.0 g plus IV/IM gentamicin 1.5 mg/kg (not to exceed 80 mg) 1 hour preoperatively; may repeat 8 hours after initial dose

also may potentiate the actions of nondepolarizing neuromuscular blockers.

Premedication to Prevent Reactions to Intravenous Contrast Media

Radiocontrast media contain iodinated organic molecules and may be administered orally or injected parenterally. About 5 percent of intravascular contrast administrations result in adverse systemic reactions, of which one-third require immediate treatment. Most reactions respond well to therapy, but there are an estimated 500 fatalities per year in the United States related to intravenous contrast media.

Contrast media are hypertonic, so predictable hemodynamic effects occur. Serum osmolarity may increase 10 percent or more, and circulating blood volume may increase transiently. This results in hypertension, increased central venous, systemic, and pulmonary artery pressures, and increased cardiac output. The diuresis that follows may lead to hypovolemia and renal failure, especially in patients with previously compromised renal function. Newer nonionic media of lesser osmolalities (400 to 800 mOmol/kg) may be less likely to provoke this adverse reaction.

■ Idiosyncratic Reactions to Intravenous Contrast Media

Idiosyncratic reactions range from mild inconveniences such as nausea, vomiting, and facial flushing to moderate or severe problems such as an anaphylactoid-like response (immunoglobulin E or immune complexes are not generally recoverable from an affected patient's serum). Moderate symptoms of increased capillary permeability, hypotension, and bronchospasm may progress to arrhythmias and cardiovascular collapse. More than 50 percent of idiosyncratic reactions can be classified as mild. A history of atopy, asthma, or allergy (particularly to iodine or seafood) is associated with an incidence of allergic reactions of 10 to 15 percent; after a previous reaction to intravenous contrast media, the subsequent risk is 35 percent.

■ Treatment of Reactions to Iodinated Contrast Media

In addition to oxygen and intravenous fluids, five classes of drugs are used to treat moderate to severe anaphylactoid reactions (Table 4-4). Mild reactions (nausea, flushing, itching, rash) require only observation and reassurance. Oxygen, intravenous fluids, and epinephrine in large doses may be required to treat such reactions as bronchospasm, airway obstruction, pulmonary edema, and shock.

■ Prophylaxis against Iodinated Contrast Media Reactions

Testing for intravenous contrast media allergy has been of little value, but prophylactic treatment of high-risk patients with prednisone prior to the administration of contrast media has been successful (Table 4-5). An effective regimen is to administer three 50-mg doses of prednisone 6 hours apart, followed by 50 mg diphenhydramine and 300 mg cimetidine intravenously just prior to exposure.

Table 4-4

Treatment for Anaphylactic Reactions

1. Discontinue intravenous contrast media, latex, or other allergen exposure.
2. Monitor ECG and blood pressure.
3. Administer supplemental oxygen.
4. Administer fluids as required to maintain blood pressure.
5. IV drug regimen: as needed

Anticholinergics	Atropine	0.5 mg IV
Antihistamines	Diphenhydramine	25–50 mg IV
Methylxanthines	Aminophylline	5 mg/kg IV loading dose
Steroids	Methylprednisolone	Up to 1 g IV
Catecholamines	Epinephrine	3–5 µg/kg IV bolus
		1–4 µg/kg/min IV infusion

6. Be prepared for full resuscitative measures including endotracheal intubation and cardiac defibrillation.

Table 4-5

Anaphylaxis Prophylaxis Regimen Suggested for High-Risk Patients

1. Prednisone 50 mg PO every 6 hours, begin 24 hours before procedure, continue for 24 hours after procedure.
2. Diphenhydramine 50 mg IV immediately prior to procedure.
3. Cimetidine 300 mg IV every 6 hours, or ranitidine if patient is receiving anticonvulsants, theophylline, oral contraceptives, or other medications that require hepatic p450 metabolism.

Latex Allergy

Severe anaphylactic reactions to latex were recognized initially in patients with histories of spina bifida or bladder exstrophy who had been exposed to latex from an early age. The problem is now recognized in hospital workers and others exposed frequently to latex. Treatment is that usually employed for allergic reactions (see Table 4-4). Management of patients known to be allergic to latex depends on scrupulous avoidance of contact with latex, including not only gloves and airway equipment but also intravenous equipment. Hospitals, operating suites, and anesthesia departments must develop policies and protocols in advance, because ad hoc arrangements are difficult and often incomplete. The efficacy of corticosteroid premedication as prophylaxis is not defined at present.

Continuation of Preoperative Therapy

Almost any medication that the patient requires routinely should be continued before anesthesia and operation. It is especially important to continue those drugs which are associated with serious acute withdrawal syndromes; clonidine, beta-adrenergic blockers, barbiturates, and opioids are examples. The patient on methadone maintenance can be given methadone as a premedicant. Drugs given for angina, hypertension, or arrhythmias should be continued through anesthesia and operation. Patients dependent on alcohol receive benzodiazepines to prevent withdrawal symptoms.

■ Diuretics

Loop diuretics, such as furosemide, are sometimes discontinued before operations to avoid intravascular volume depletion and electrolyte imbalance. However, withdrawing diuretics from a diuretic-dependent patient may precipitate hypervolemia, pulmonary edema, and congestive heart failure. Intravascular volume may be managed effectively by careful intravenous fluid administration while the diuretic therapy is continued throughout the perioperative interval.

■ Antidepressants

Patients taking monoamine oxidase inhibitors (MAOIs) may suffer unpredictable or exaggerated responses to adrenergic drugs or experience wide variations in blood pressure intraoperatively. For most MAOIs, elimination of their effect requires weeks of abstinence. If the patient is taking the MAOI for depression, the patient's psychological condition may worsen during this interval, and severe depression or even suicide is a real risk. Fortunately, experience has shown that patients taking MAOIs can be managed successfully for major and minor procedures. Only direct-acting sympathomimetics, such as phenylephrine, are used to treat hypotension; close monitoring and reduced doses allow these drugs to be used safely. Meperidine must not be used in patients taking MAOIs because it has been associated with acute vascular collapse, hyperthermia, coma, and death with even a single administration. Morphine is safe. Tricyclic antidepressants also block uptake of norepinephrine, but their effects largely dissipate within 3 days of being discontinued. Precautions for their use are similar to those for MAOIs.

■ Glucocorticoids

Full consideration of perioperative glucocorticoid use is found in Chapter 24. Continuation or augmentation of chronic steroid regimens is still recommended for patients at risk for adrenal suppression.

■ Insulin Regimens

Operations present significant metabolic challenges to diabetic patients. Fasting leads to hypoglycemia if the usual regimen of insulin or oral hypoglycemics is continued, yet the hormonal response to the stress of operation tends to increase blood glucose. Successful regimens for the perioperative management of diabetic patients adhere to several principles. First, glucose is provided as an energy-yielding substrate; second, insulin is administered to prevent catabolism; and third, the customary morning insulin dose is reduced to decrease the risk of hypoglycemia.

Insulin-dependent diabetic patients have been managed successfully for elective operations with a number of regimens: withholding all morning insulin, providing a portion of the patient's regular insulin, or providing the usual insulin dose with supplemental glucose infusions. Minor procedures especially are best done early in the day to allow minimum disruption of the patient's insulin and dietary schedule. In general, hyperglycemia is better tolerated than is hypoglycemia, so a safe rule is to err on the side of mild hyperglycemia and adjust therapy according to perioperative blood glucose determinations. Management of the poorly controlled or brittle diabetic patient requires attention to treatment of potential acidosis, electrolyte imbalance, and dehydration, as well as frequent blood glucose determinations.

A conservative yet well-tested approach involves the administration of one-half the usual morning insulin dose. Glucose is administered as intravenous D_5W at the rate of 100 ml/h beginning when the insulin is given. Blood glucose is determined upon arrival to the operating room and every 4 to 6 hours for the next day. Regular insulin is provided on a sliding scale for blood glucose concentrations above 300 mg/dl.

BIBLIOGRAPHY

Egbert LD, Battit GE, Turndorf H, Beecher HK. The value of the preoperative visit by an anesthetist. *JAMA* 1963;185:553-555.

Gold M, Swartz JS, Braude BM, et al. Intraoperative anaphylaxis and association with latex sensitivity. *J Allergy Clin Immunol* 1991;87(3):662-666.

Goldberg M. Systematic reactions to intravascular contrast media. *Anesthesiology* 1984;60:46-56.

Goresky GV, Maltby JR. Fasting guidelines for elective surgical patients (Editorial). *Can J Anaesth* 1990;37:493-495.

Maltby JR, Reid CR, Hutchinson A. Gastric fluid volume and pH in elective inpatients: II. Coffee or orange juice with ranitidine. *Can J Anaesth* 1988;35(1):16-19.

Maltby JR, Lewis P, Martin A, Sutheriand LR. Gastric fluid volume and pH in elective patients following unrestricted oral fluid until three hours before surgery. *Can J Anaesth* 1991;38(4 Pt 1): 425-429.

McCammon RL. Prophylaxis for aspiration pneumonitis. *Can Anaesthesiol Soc J* 1986;33:S47-S53.

Palazzo MGA, Strunin L. Anaesthesia and emesis: I. Etiology. *Can Anaesthesiol Soc J* 1984;31:178-187.

Palazzo MGA, Strunin L. Anaesthesia and emesis: II. Prevention and management. *Can Anaesthesiol Soc J* 1984;31:407-415.

Phillips S, Daborn AK, Hatch DJ. Preoperative fasting for paediatric patients. *Br J Anaesth* 1994;73(4):529-536.

Scuderi P, Wetchler B, Sung Y, et al. Treatment of postoperative nausea and vomiting after outpatient surgery with 5-HT$_3$ antagonist ondansetron. *Anesthesiology* 1993;78:15-20.

Slater J. Rubber anaphylaxis. *N Engl J Med* 1989;320(17):1126-1129.

Vaughan RW, Bauer S, Wise L. Volume and pH of gastric juice in obese patients. *Anesthesiology* 1975;43:686-689.

Weber L, Hirshman CA. Cimetidine for prophylaxis of aspiration pneumonitis: Comparison of intramuscular and oral dosage schedules. *Anesth Analg* 1979;58:426-427.

CHAPTER **5**

The Anesthesia Machine

Stanley J. Aukburg

The anesthesia machine delivers anesthetic gases and vapors to the patient and permits spontaneous or controlled ventilation. The machine serves the anesthesiologist as a desk and storage cabinet and often contains devices such as capnographs, pulse oximeters, and other physiologic monitors as described in Chap. 6. The anesthesia machine includes the gas delivery system, which provides mixtures of oxygen, other gases, and anesthetics via the fresh gas outlet, the patient breathing circuit, and the ventilator. This chapter describes the components of the anesthesia machine and the devices that monitor their function.

Anesthesia Gas Cylinders and Central Gas Supply Connections

The cylinders mounted on anesthesia machines are usually "E" size. Oxygen and air cylinders contain compressed gas at a pressure of 2200 lb/in^2 (psi) and can deliver 650 to 700 liters of gas at atmospheric pressure. Cylinders filled with nitrous oxide contain liquid and gas in equilibrium at 750 lb/in^2; they deliver about 1550 liters of gas.

Cylinders are attached to the anesthesia machine by yokes equipped with pin indexing systems that permit attaching only cylinders containing the intended gas. The positions of the pins on the yoke and matching holes in the cylinder outlet are specific for each gas. The indexing system must not be compromised by altering the fittings or using adapters to attach inappropriate gas cylinders. Yokes include check valves to prevent the reverse flow of gases from

the machine, as might occur when replacing an empty cylinder.

The anesthesia machine is fitted with connectors to receive gases from a central supply also. These connectors incorporate gas-specific fittings analogous to the pin indexing system for cylinders. Check valves similar to those in the yoke prevent escape of gas when a hose is disconnected from the machine.

Cylinders, supply hoses, pressure gauges, flow control valves, and flow indicators share a common color coding system. In the United States and Canada, oxygen is assigned the color green; nitrous oxide, blue; and air, yellow. These colors differ from the international standard.

Pressure-Reducing Valves

The pressure within gas cylinders varies with temperature and decreases as the gas is used. Pressure regulators convert the cylinder pressure to a working pressure of about 45 lb/in^2, which remains constant as the tank empties. The pressure regulator contains an outlet chamber and a smaller inlet chamber separated by a valve. The valve is held open by pressure from a spring, which is adjusted to set the desired pressure in the outlet chamber. Gas pressure in the outlet chamber acts through a diaphragm to close the valve. When downstream pressure decreases, the valve opens to supply more gas and maintain the pressure constant. Gauges display the pressures found in gas cylinders and supply lines.

Control of Gas Flow

Gases at the regulated pressure pass through flow controllers, each of which contains a needle valve and a flowmeter. The needle valve employs a screw with a fine thread to drive a gently tapered stem that fits into a seat with a matching taper, providing precise control of the resistance to gas flow. In addition to being color coded, the oxygen flow control knob is fluted as well, to make it easier to identify.

Anesthesia machines meeting current design guidelines deliver 150 to 500 ml/min of oxygen when the oxygen flow control knob is in the full "off" position to provide a minimum supply of oxygen to the breathing circuit. The minimal oxygen flow is achieved by placing a fixed-flow bypass in parallel with the needle valve (Fig. 5-1).

Flowmeters are calibrated glass tubes with a barely perceptible internal taper mounted vertically with the narrowest end at the bottom; a float rides freely in the bore of the tube. Gas, flowing from the bottom upward in the tube, buoys the float. The resistance to the flow of gas through the gap between the float and the wall of the tube creates a pressure drop across the float. At an equilibrium position, the force created by the pressure difference across the float equals the weight of the float, and the gas flow can be read from the adjacent calibrated scale. A spherical float is read at its center; all other shapes are read at the top of the float. The more rapid the flow through the tube, the greater is the cross-sectional area of the gap between the float and the inner wall of the glass tube at equilibrium and hence the higher is the float.

The minimum flow that can be determined accurately from a flow tube with a linear taper is approximately one-tenth its full scale, which may not provide adequate resolution or accuracy for both high and low flow rates. This limitation can be overcome by using a single tube with a dual taper or a pair of flow tubes for a single gas. In modern machines, each gas flows through a pair of tubes in series. One tube is calibrated for lesser flows, and the other is for greater. Gas flow is read from the tube giving the best estimate (see Fig. 5-1).

Flow tubes are calibrated for 20°C and sea-level atmospheric pressure and are accurate to ±10 percent of the reading under these conditions. Flowmeters read falsely high at a high altitudes and falsely low when ambient pressures exceed 760 mmHg. The

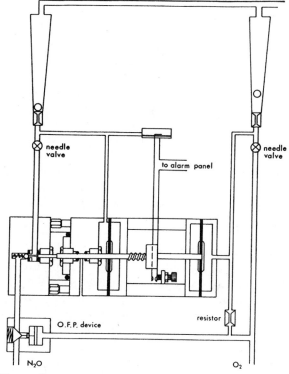

Figure 5-1

Gas flow control and safety systems. The high-pressure gas system includes the needle valves, flow tubes, bypass resistor for oxygen, the oxygen-nitrous oxide ratio controller and the oxygen pressure fail-safe device (O.F.P. device). Oxygen enters at the lower right corner from a pressure regulator. The oxygen pressure fail-safe system stops the flow of N_2O if the O_2 supply pressure fails. The bypass resistor allows a small flow of oxygen, even when the oxygen needle valve is closed.

(Reproduced with permission from Technical Service Manual, *North American Drager, Telford, Pa, 1985.)*

changes in outlet pressure during positive-pressure breathing cause the float to bob up and down; accurate flows are indicated at end-expiration. Each flowmeter must be used only with the specific gas for which it is calibrated and with the calibrated scale supplied with the tube.

The outflows of the various flowmeters are mixed in a manifold and then delivered to the vaporizer assembly. By convention, gases flow from left to right within the manifold, with O_2 always at the right. This reduces the chance that a gas leak will decrease the delivered concentration of oxygen and provides a standard position for the O_2 flowmeter.

Additional Safety Features

The risk of hypoxia is reduced further by other design features of the gas delivery system.

■ Oxygen Flush

The oxygen flush valve delivers about 50 liters/min of oxygen directly to the common gas outlet, bypassing flowmeters and vaporizers. Intermittent flushes of oxygen may be used to compensate for large leaks in the breathing system while the cause of the leak is corrected, to increase rapidly the inhaled oxygen concentration and decrease the inhaled anesthetic concentration, and to speed the emergence from anesthesia by allowing rapid refilling of the breathing system reservoir bag after venting the exhaled gas into a scavenger system. Because of the very high flow rates, pressing the O_2 flush button during the inspiratory phase of mechanical ventilation can result in dangerous peak airway pressures.

■ O_2-N_2O Flow Ratio Controller

An oxygen "fail-safe" system stops the flow of all gases but oxygen if oxygen supply pressure fails. This does not guard against setting the flowmeters to deliver a hypoxic mixture, as might happen when the oxygen flow control valve is turned off by mistake. Design standards now require that anesthesia machines deliver gas mixtures of O_2 and N_2O containing at least 25% oxygen. This is accomplished manually by a nitrous oxide-oxygen flow ratio monitor or automatically by a flow ratio controller.

The flow ratio monitor incorporates flow detectors for N_2O and O_2. When the N_2O-O_2 flow ratio exceeds a predetermined value (usually 7:3), the device sounds an alarm signal, alerting the operator to correct the flows. Nitrous oxide-oxygen flow ratio controllers automatically adjust the flow of the other gas to maintain the oxygen concentration at no less than 25% (see Fig. 5-1).

■ Oxygen Analyzers

Although fail-safe devices are effective, a malfunction still might allow the delivery of a hypoxic gas mixture. To guard against this, an oxygen analyzer monitors the oxygen content of the gases in the patient breathing circuit. A self-polarizing polarographic electrode is used most commonly. It consists of a lead anode, an alkaline electrolyte solution, and a gold cathode, separated from the gas phase by a Teflon membrane. The reduction of oxygen produces hydroxyl ions, which react with the lead anode to induce a voltage proportional to the oxygen concentration. For reliability, oxygen analyzers include reserve power supplies, they are calibrated against room air daily, and the low-oxygen alarm cannot be switched off. Because condensation of liquid on the barrier membrane slows the response time of these cells, they are mounted above the path of the dry gas in the inspired limb of the breathing circuit.

Vaporizers

Modern precision vaporizers convert liquid anesthetics such as halothane, enflurane, and isoflurane into metered amounts of vapor that are added to the fresh gas mixture to produce known concentrations of anesthetic. The first such vaporizers were the "copper kettles." Using a needle valve and flowmeter, a known flow of oxygen was passed through a kettle that produced a saturated vapor mixture of oxygen and anesthetic. Knowing the oxygen flow and the saturated vapor pressure of the anesthetic at the temperature of the kettle allowed calculation of the amount of vapor produced. Diluent gases were supplied by other needle valves and flowmeters. Determination of the anesthetic concentration required calculation, and misadjustment could cause delivery of excessive concentrations of anesthetic. Because of these problems, kettle-type vaporizers are no longer offered for sale, although some are still in use.

Kettles have been replaced by agent-specific vaporizers, which supplement the fresh gas mixture with the concentration of volatile anesthetic indicated on the dial of the vaporizer. The combined gas output from all flowmeters is delivered to the vaporizer, which proportions it into two streams, a vaporizer stream and a bypass stream, according to the setting on the dial. Gas flowing in the vaporizer stream becomes saturated with the anesthetic and is automatically diluted to the set concentration by the bypass stream (Fig. 5-2).

Inaccuracies can be introduced by a number of factors. Changes in room temperature and cooling of the anesthetic liquid due to vaporization alter the vapor pressure of the anesthetic and thereby the amount of anesthetic vapor added to the vaporizer stream. Modern vaporizers provide nearly constant

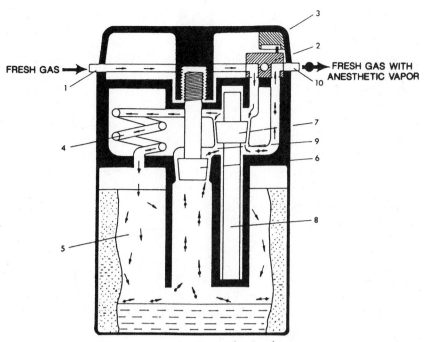

1 fresh gas inlet
2 turn on and turn off control (actuated by concentration knob)
3 concentration knob
4 pressure compensation (patented)
5 vaporizing chamber
6 control cone
7 vaporizing chamber by-pass cone
8 expansion member for temperature-compensation
9 mixing chamber
10 fresh gas outlet

Figure 5-2

Precision vaporizer. The precision vaporizer allows output concentration to be set with a single concentration knob. Gas delivered to the fresh gas inlet is proportioned into two streams that flow through two parallel passages. Each passage contains a control cone that creates resistance to flow. The bypass cone resistance is fixed. The vaporization chamber cone resistance is controlled by rotating the concentration knob. Gas flowing through the vaporizing chamber becomes saturated with the anesthetic agent and is diluted by the bypass stream. The anesthetic concentration increases with counterclockwise rotation of the concentration knob.

(Reproduced with permission from Technical Service Manual, *North American Drager, Telford, Pa, 1984.)*

output over a wide range of temperatures by employing materials with appropriate temperature expansion coefficients in the bypass valve assembly. The new agent desflurane, because of its low boiling point at atmospheric pressure, presents a special problem. Small changes in vaporizer temperature produce large changes in desflurane vapor pressure. To overcome this, desflurane vaporizers employ a thermostatically controlled heater requiring electric power, are internally pressurized, and contain their own alarm systems.

The composition of the gas mixture influences the output of agent-specific vaporizers by at least two mechanisms. First, the solubility of nitrous oxide in halogenated agents (approximately 4 ml of N_2O gas per milliliter of volatile liquid per atmosphere) causes the volatile liquid to act as a reservoir when the N_2O

concentration is changed. After an increase in delivered N_2O concentration, N_2O is taken up by the volatile liquid, transiently decreasing the volume of gas flowing through the vaporization chamber and thus decreasing the output concentration of volatile anesthetic. Conversely, decreases in the concentration of N_2O cause a temporary increase in output. Second, changes in the viscosity of the carrier gas alter the performance of the flow-dividing valve, also causing anesthetic output concentration to decrease when N_2O concentration is increased. Changes in carrier gas flows and backpressure have negligible effects on the output of modern, well-designed vaporizers.

Even the best-designed vaporizers can be unsafe if used improperly. Filling an agent-specific vaporizer with the wrong agent causes it to deliver not only the wrong agent but the wrong concentration as well.

This is most dangerous when a vaporizer designed for an anesthetic of lesser vapor pressure is filled with one having a greater vapor pressure. A system of vaporizer filling ports that are keyed to matching rings on bottles of liquid anesthetic can prevent using the wrong agent, but it has proven impractical and unpopular. Agent-specific gas analyzers (see Chap. 6) can identify both the type and concentration of anesthetic emanating from a vaporizer, protecting against filling the vaporizer with the wrong anesthetic or against a vaporizer malfunction. Vaporizers have low-mounted filling ports to prevent overfilling, and they are mounted rigidly to the machine to prevent overturning. Both these accidents can introduce liquid anesthetic into the output of the machine. When a machine has several vaporizers, they are linked by a system that prevents switching on more than one at a time to avoid contamination of the downstream vaporizer by vapor from the one upstream. Vaporizers require calibration and service at regular intervals.

The most prevalent misuse of vaporizers consists simply of administering a greater concentration of anesthetic than the patient requires. An agent-specific vaporizer is limited to delivering a concentration no more than a few times the minimum alveolar concentration (MAC), a safety feature not offered by the older kettles, but this does not prevent delivery of anesthetic concentrations that are too great for some patients.

After passing through the vaporizer assembly, the gas mixture is piped to the common gas outlet of the anesthesia machine and then to the breathing circuit.

Breathing Circuits

Breathing circuits supply the lungs with gas of appropriate composition, volume, and pressure, allowing either spontaneous, assisted, or controlled ventilation. They also may conserve heat, water vapor, and anesthetics by allowing rebreathing of exhaled gas from which CO_2 has been removed. Two breathing circuit designs dominate modern anesthesia practice: circle systems and various modifications of the Mapleson D system. Both systems employ reservoir bags, breathing tubes, a fresh gas inlet, and an adjustable positive-pressure relief (APR) valve for release of excess gas; the circle system also incorporates respiratory valves and a CO_2 absorption canister.

■ Reservoir Bags

Although a normal adult patient rarely requires a total minute ventilation greater than 12 liters/min, the instantaneous inspiratory flow often exceeds 30 liters/min. Because the anesthesia machine delivers fresh gas at lesser flow rates, these transitory peak demands are met by supplementing fresh gas flow with gas from a compliant reservoir bag. The bag also serves as a safety device because its distensibility limits circuit pressures to less than 60 cmH_2O, even when the APR valve is closed.

■ Breathing Tubing

The reservoir bag is connected to the patient's mask or endotracheal tube by wide-bore rubber or plastic breathing tubing about 1 m in length, with a volume of 400 to 500 ml/m. Corrugations in the wall of the tubing provide flexibility, resist kinking, and promote turbulent flow instead of laminar flow. During positive-pressure ventilation, some of the delivered gas distends the tubing and some is compressed within the breathing circuit, resulting in a tidal volume entering the lungs that is less than the delivered gas volume. Because of its wide bore, a breathing tube offers little resistance to breathing (less than 1 cmH_2O/liter per minute). Breathing tubing is connected to the patient by a fitting having an outside diameter of 22 mm to fit standard face masks and an inside diameter of 15 mm to fit endotracheal tube connectors.

The possibility that breathing circuits might transmit bacterial infections from one patient to the next has led to the use of disposable tubing and rebreathing bags and bacterial filters. Postoperative respiratory infections seem to occur no less frequently with disposable equipment than with reusable circuits that have been cared for properly. Proper care includes washing with soap and water or germicides, followed by thorough drying.

■ Respiratory Valves

Respiratory valves in the breathing tubing of the circle breathing circuit limit gas flow to one direction, preventing unintended rebreathing of exhaled gas. The large orifices of the valves are closed by light disks of mica, ceramic, or plastic so that resistance to breathing is negligible. The valves are enclosed in a clear dome housing so that the operator can monitor their function.

■ CO$_2$ Absorption Canisters

In a circle system, gas that is to be rebreathed is cleared of carbon dioxide by passing it through a canister containing a chemical CO$_2$ absorbent. Hydroxides of potassium, sodium, lithium, barium, and calcium all have clinical use. The reaction between CO$_2$ and the alkaline metal hydroxides NaOH and KOH involves the intermediate formation of a hydrate and thus requires water:

$$2NaOH + 2H_2O \rightarrow 2NaOH \cdot H_2O \quad (5.1)$$

$$2NaOH \cdot H_2O + CO_2 \rightarrow Na_2CO_3 + 3H_2O \quad (5.2)$$

The reaction produces both heat and water. Solid granules of calcium hydroxide combine with CO$_2$ through a different reaction, too slow to be of practical use. However, a combination of 70 to 80 percent Ca(OH)$_2$, 3 to 5 percent NaOH (or KOH), and 10 to 20 percent water with small amounts of sodium silicate produces a granule with acceptable reaction speed, capacity, and durability. A pH-sensitive dye is added to indicate when the chemical absorbent has been consumed. Although other agents have been used, this mixture, sold as soda lime, is the most popular.

The 2-liter two-part (top and bottom) canister in modern absorbers has a gas volume of nearly 1 liter when filled with granules of CO$_2$ absorbent. It contains about 1000 g of absorbent and is capable of eliminating more than 100 liters of CO$_2$, giving a fresh canister more than 8 hours of useful life in a low-flow system employed for a normal adult. Resistance is typically less than 1 cmH$_2$O for gas flows up to 60 liters/min. Flow direction through the canister is from top to bottom, with a dust and moisture trap at the bottom to avoid introduction of dust or wet alkali into the inspiratory limb of the breathing circuit. The dye changes color in the top canister first; when the color change reaches the bottom canister, it is moved to the top, and the top canister is refilled with fresh absorbent and moved to the bottom.

■ The Circle System

A circle breathing system contains an inspiratory and an expiratory breathing tube, each with an oppositely directed one-way valve, connecting the patient to a reservoir bag (Fig. 5-3). Three more components make up a functional system: a carbon dioxide absorber, a fresh gas inflow site, and an APR valve. These may be placed anywhere within the circle, but only a few locations are practical. In practice, the valves usually reside on the absorber.

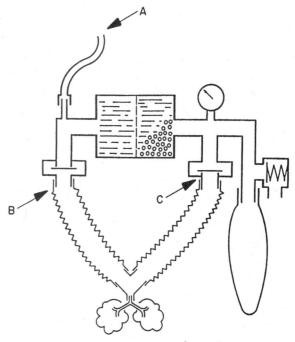

Figure 5-3

Circle breathing system. The circle breathing system derives its name from the two limbs of breathing tubing linking the patient's airway to a compliant reservoir (rebreathing bag or ventilator bellows) in which exhaled gas is collected. One-way valves in the breathing tubing divide the circle into patient and reservoir sides and limit each limb of tubing to either inhalation or exhalation. A CO$_2$ absorption canister allows for safe rebreathing of the exhaled gas. The composition of inhaled gas is altered by the introduction of fresh gas (A) to the circle. An APR valve exhausts excess gas to the atmosphere via a scavenging system. To provide efficient replenishment of oxygen and anesthetic gas, fresh gas is introduced close to the inspiratory valve (B) on its bag side. The inspiratory and expiratory valves are mechanically attached to the absorber for durability and convenience. For efficient CO$_2$ elimination, the APR valve is positioned on the bag side of the expiratory valve (C).

(Reproduced with permission from Schreiber P, Anesthesia Systems, Telford, Pa: North American Drager, 1985, p 27.)

The CO_2 absorption canister removes CO_2 from the expired gas, allowing minimal fresh gas flows with almost complete rebreathing of the exhaled volume (closed system). As fresh gas flows are increased, rebreathing is reduced; when fresh gas flow exceeds the minute ventilation, rebreathing of expired gas approaches nil, and the canister is unnecessary.

The absorber offers some resistance to breathing; so that the operator can assist inspiration, the absorber is placed in the inspiratory limb on the bag side of the inspiratory valve. Fresh gas is introduced to the inspiratory limb, upstream of the inspiratory valve. This provides fresh gas for most or all of the inspired gas in high-flow techniques and efficiently restores oxygen and anesthetic gas to the inspired gas mixture in low-flow techniques.

The APR valve usually resides on the bag side of the expiratory valve opposite the bag mount. During spontaneous ventilation, it is usually left wide open to minimize end-exhaled pressure as gas leaves the circuit via the APR valve during the latter phases of exhalation. When manually controlled or assisted ventilation is desired, the valve is partially closed so that some gas enters the patient's lungs and some leaves the system via the APR valve during positive-pressure inspiration.

■ Mapleson D Circuits

The Mapleson D breathing system consists of a reservoir bag connected to the patient's airway by a single breathing tube with a fresh gas inlet at the patient end of the tube and an APR valve at the bag end (Fig. 5-4). This configuration places the APR valve in the position for most efficient CO_2 elimination. With the Mapleson D system, alveolar CO_2 tension depends on both minute ventilation and fresh gas flow rates, enabling reduction in alveolar CO_2 tension during hyperventilation to be limited by careful selection of the fresh gas flow rate. Owing to this property, their light weight, and their mechanical simplicity, Mapleson D-based systems are popular for pediatric use.

■ Humidity and Heat Exchange in Breathing Circuits

Tracheal intubation bypasses the natural heat and water exchange that occurs in the nose and pharynx, placing the burden of humidification on the tracheobronchial tree. Breathing only the cool, dry gas

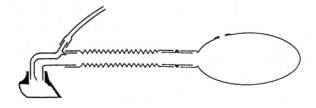

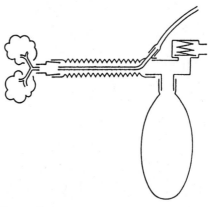

Figure 5-4

Mapleson D breathing systems. Two variations of Mapleson D systems are depicted, the Jackson-Rees *(above)* and the Baine modification *(below)*. The Jackson-Rees version vents excess gas through an aperture in the rebreathing bag; in the Baine version, a spring-loaded APR valve serves this function.

(Reproduced with permission from Shreiber P, Anesthesia Systems, Telford, Pa: North American Drager, 1985, p 27.)

from the anesthesia machine results in water losses of about 10 ml/hr, with a concomitant heat loss due to evaporation of about 5 kcal/hr. This is enough to reduce the temperature of an average adult about 0.1°C per hour. With circle systems and minimal fresh gas flows, water loss can be reduced to as little as 3 ml/hr and heat loss to 1 kcal/hr. Conservation of heat and humidity arises from both the reuse of relatively warm, humid exhaled gas and the exothermic water-producing reaction between CO_2 and alkali. Because systems based on the Mapleson D circuit require high flows to eliminate CO_2, devices for actively heating and humidifying inspired gas are commonly employed, especially in pediatric anesthesia.

■ Pressure and Flow Monitors in the Breathing Circuit

In addition to monitoring the oxygen content of the gas in the breathing circuit, modern anesthesia machines also display airway pressure and expiratory flow, employing both an obligatory mechanical pressure gauge and electronic transducers as well. A microprocessor provides automatic monitoring of peak, plateau, and end-expiratory pressures, as well as alarms for apnea, breathing circuit disconnections, or sustained high or negative pressures. Sustained high pressure occurs most frequently when a spontaneously breathing patient is mistakenly connected to a circuit with a fully closed APR valve.

Scavenging of Excess Gas

Gases escaping from the APR valve or around a loose-fitting face mask can contaminate the operating room atmosphere with measurable concentrations of anesthetics. To reduce exposure of operating room workers, modern APR valves and ventilator relief valves discharge exhaust gas to a waste gas scavenger. Excess gas is usually aspirated from the scavenger by the operating room suction system at flows of 15 to 20 liters/min. Because APR flow rates may reach brief peaks of 50 liters/min, the scavenger includes a reservoir of capacity greater than a single tidal volume. To protect the breathing circuit from the negative pressure of the suction system or from excessive positive pressure from obstruction of the vacuum system, scavengers provide for both positive and negative pressure relief. Scavenger systems with compliant reservoirs require valves for pressure relief. Rigid reservoir systems employ only orifices to achieve the same protection.

The Anesthesia Ventilator

Patient breathing circuits permit assisted or controlled ventilation by manual compression of the reservoir bag; this not only allows control of the ventilatory pattern but also provides tactile clues to changes in chest wall compliance and airway resistance. Using a mechanical ventilator removes this valuable source of information but in return frees the operator for other tasks.

Anesthesia ventilators are simpler than their intensive care unit counterparts. They consist of three elements: a bellows assembly enclosed in a sealed box, an APR valve, and a pneumatic drive (Fig. 5-5). The bellows is the functional equivalent of the rebreathing

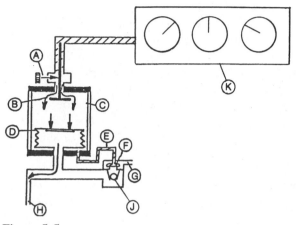

Figure 5-5

A typical anesthesia ventilator. The bellows (D) in its sealed chamber (C) empties into a T-connector. One arm of the connector (H) is attached to the anesthesia breathing circuit. The other arm is connected to the mushroom valve (F), which is closed during inspiration by pressure delivered via tubing arriving from the sealed chamber (E). The valve discharge port (G) permits venting of excess gas to the atmosphere at end-expiration. A ball valve (J), in series with the mushroom valve, prevents entrainment of room air during spontaneous breathing and ensures sufficient airway pressure to raise the bellows during exhalation. The bellows is driven by oxygen metered into the chamber via a conduit (B) by the control circuitry (K). A stop (A) regulates tidal volume by limiting bellows excursion.
(Adapted from Technical Service Manual, *North American Drager, Telford, Pa, 1985.)*

bag. The pneumatic drive applies pressure to the inside of the box, compressing the bellows and substituting for manual compression of the bag. The box is usually a clear plastic cylinder so that the bellows is visible. An adjustable stop limits the excursion of the bellows, thereby determining the volume to be delivered. The mouth of the bellows is attached to one limb of a T-connector. The second limb incorporates an automatic APR valve, and the remaining limb connects to the bag mount of the breathing circuit. By means of a selector valve, the breathing circuit is attached either to the ventilator bellows with its integral APR valve or to the usual rebreathing bag and manual APR valve.

If the bellows is mounted with its opening pointing upward, refilling during exhalation is aided by gravity. When small partial disconnections or leaks occur, this design helps maintain bellows volume, a minor theoretical benefit. However, major leaks or disconnections may go unnoticed because the bellows fills passively with each breathing cycle. If the bellows opening faces downward, any leak in excess of fresh gas flow leads to emptying of the bellows, providing a visible signal. It is preferable to mount the bellows with its opening facing downward. The positive pressure required to fill the bellows during exhalation creates an obligatory positive end-expiratory pressure (PEEP) of 1 to 3 cmH_2O.

The automatic APR valve found in an anesthesia ventilator resembles a one-way dome valve, but with a flexible membrane walled chamber ("mushroom valve") replacing the rigid disk. The chamber is connected by tubing to the cylinder enclosing the bellows. During inhalation, the valve chamber is pressurized by the same pressure source that compresses the bellows, occluding the annulus of the valve and directing the gas discharged from the bellows into the breathing circuit.

Anesthesia ventilators use oxygen from the regulated supply forced through an air-entraining Venturi to compress the bellows. If leaks in the bellows develop, the breathing circuit will be contaminated with oxygen-enriched air, thus offering a margin of safety. The driving gas is metered into the bellows housing through valves and solenoids controlled by logic and timing circuitry that vents the chamber to the atmosphere to allow passive exhalation.

The switch from inhalation to exhalation may be triggered either by the appearance of a large pressure difference between the inside and outside of the bellows or by a timer. While the bellows is in motion, the pressure difference is limited to a few centimeters of H_2O, but the transmural pressure increases sharply when the bellows is fully compressed, providing a signal to begin exhalation. If the change from inhalation to exhalation is controlled by a timer, the flow rate from the pneumatic drive must be adequate to fully compress the bellows during t he inspiratory phase. Adequate exhalation time must be allowed for passive exhalation of the entire tidal volume without trapping air in the lungs.

Although tidal volume is adjusted by setting the volume displaced from the bellows, the bellows displacement is not the same as the tidal volume. Volume is lost to compression of gas in the breathing system and to expansion of the breathing tubing. Also, fresh gas inflow from the common gas outlet during the inspiratory phase augments tidal volume. A flowmeter placed as close to the tracheal tube connector as possible is required for accurate measurement of tidal volume.

■ Disconnection Alarms

As mentioned, use of a mechanical ventilator removes the tactile feedback provided during manual ventilation, eliminating one source of warning of inadvertent breathing circuit disconnection. Listening continuously to breath sounds and observing chest wall movement are part of good practice, but lapses occur. Monitoring of exhaled volume in the breathing circuit and of airway CO_2 concentration helps overcome this problem, but a pressure-based disconnection alarm also is provided with anesthesia ventilators. When the ventilator is functioning, this alarm senses the periodic positive-pressure excursions that exceed a threshold somewhat below the peak inspiratory pressure. If no pressure excursion is detected during a given interval, then an alarm is sounded.

The Anesthesia Machine Check

Before administering anesthesia, one completes a checklist procedure to ensure that the anesthesia machine is in working order and that all necessary equipment and supplies are available. Failure to inspect the anesthesia machine is a critical factor in many anesthesia accidents, and a written checklist reduces the chance of overlooking an important item (see Appendix 5A). An abbreviated check may be sufficient between patients when the same anesthesia machine is to be reused immediately, but it is never proper to induce anesthesia without first examining the breathing circuit, oxygen supply, suction, and airway equipment. A thorough testing of an unfamiliar machine will reveal its important idiosyncrasies and make safe operation possible.

Regular preventive maintenance of anesthesia machines is required by state and national hospital-certifying agencies. Hospital biomedical engineering departments, manufacturers, and independent service agencies all may offer service contracts that include regular inspection. Detailed checks of the anesthesia machine provide opportunities to identify deficiencies between preventive maintenance visits. Each malfunction must be recorded in writing, and defective machines must be removed from service immediately until repaired. Malfunctions must be reported as required by the Safe Medical Device Act of 1990 (Public Law 101-629).

Conclusion

The complexity of a modern anesthesia machine incorporating safety devices, ventilators, and physiologic monitors can overwhelm an inexperienced operator. Although these machines can assist with some vigilance tasks, operators must understand the system thoroughly and interpret the data correctly. When first encountering an unfamiliar machine, study the manual supplied by the manufacturer, and complete an approved machine checkout procedure supplied by the manufacturer or use the one given in this chapter (see Appendix 5A). Perform the complete checkout procedure daily and an abbreviated version between patients. These approaches will provide familiarity with the equipment and detect malfunctions, thereby enhancing safety.

If a machine malfunction occurs or an alarm sounds during an operation, the anesthesiologist must focus attention on the patient's condition and ensure that the patient is well ventilated with oxygen and has normal vital signs. The availability of an alternate sources of oxygen and positive-pressure ventilation can be lifesaving if the breathing system or the anesthesia machine should fail. A regular program of maintenance and repair will forestall machine failures.

When used by a knowledgeable and vigilant clinician, a modern, well-maintained anesthesia machine is a safe and reliable device; without these precautions, it is a dangerous instrument.

BIBLIOGRAPHY

American Society of Anesthesiologists. *Check-Out: A Guide for Preoperative Inspection of an Anesthesia Machine*. Park Ridge, Ill: ASA Patient Safety Videotape Program, 1993.

Dorsch JA, Dorsch SA, eds. *Understanding Anesthesia Equipment*. Baltimore: Williams & Wilkins, 1994.

Eger EI, Ethans CT. The effects of inflow, overflow and valve placement on economy of the circle system. *Anesthesiology* 1968;29:93.

Petty C, ed. *The Anesthesia Machine*. New York: Churchill-Livingstone, 1987.

Schreiber P. *Anesthesia Equipment: Performance, Classification, and Safety*. New York: Springer-Verlag, 1972.

Appendix 5A

■ Anesthesia Apparatus Checkout Recommendations, 1993

This checkout, or a reasonable equivalent, should be conducted before administration of anesthesia. These recommendations are only valid for an anesthesia system that conforms to current and relevant standards and includes an ascending bellows ventilator and at least the following monitors: capnograph, pulse oximeter, oxygen analyzer, respiratory volume monitor (spirometer), and breathing system pressure monitor with high- and low-pressure alarms. This is a guideline that users are encouraged to modify to accommodate differences in equipment design and variations in local clinical practice. Such local modifications should have appropriate peer review. Users should refer to the operator's manual for the manufacturer's specific procedures and precautions, especially the manufacturer's low-pressure leak test (step 5).

Emergency Ventilation Equipment

* **1.** Verify that backup ventilation equipment is available and functioning.

High Pressure System

* **2.** Check oxygen cylinder supply.
  a. Open O_2 cylinder and verify that it is at least half full (about 1000 lb/in^2).
  b. Close cylinder.
* **3.** Check central pipeline supplies.
  a. Check that hoses are connected and pipeline gauges read about 50 lb/in^2.

Low-Pressure System

* **4.** Check initial status of low-pressure system.
  a. Close flow control valves and turn vaporizers off.
  b. Check fill level and tighten vaporizers' filler caps.

---

*If an anesthesia provider uses the same machine in successive operations, these steps need not be repeated or may be abbreviated after the initial checkout.
Source: FR FDA 07/11/94 N 59 FR 35373. *Anesthesia apparatus checkout recommendations, 1993;* availability 94-1661859 FR 35373, Vol 59, No 131 Monday, July 11, 1994, p 35373 (Notice), Food and Drug Administration (Docket No 86B-0058).

* **5.** Perform leak check of machine low-pressure system.
  - **a.** Verify that the machine master switch and flow control valves are off.
  - **b.** Attach "suction bulb" to common (fresh) gas outlet.
  - **c.** Squeeze bulb repeatedly until fully collapsed.
  - **d.** Verify that bulb stays fully collapsed for at least 10 seconds.
  - **e.** Open one vaporizer at a time and repeat steps c and d as above.
  - **f.** Remove suction bulb and reconnect fresh gas hose.

* **6.** Turn on machine master switch and all other necessary electrical equipment.

* **7.** Test flowmeters.
  - **a.** Adjust flow of all gases through their full range, checking for smoother operation of floats and undamaged flow tubes.
  - **b.** Attempt to create a hypoxic O_2-N_2O mixture and verify correct changes in flow and/or alarm.

Scavenging System

* **8.** Adjust and check scavenging system.
  - **a.** Ensure proper connections between the scavenging system and both APL (pop-off) valve and ventilator relief valve.
  - **b.** Adjust waste gas vacuum (if possible).
  - **c.** Fully open APL valve and occlude Y-piece.
  - **d.** With minimum O_2 flow, allow scavenger reservoir bag to collapse completely and verify that absorber pressure gauge reads about zero.
  - **e.** With the O_2 flush activated, allow the scavenger reservoir bag to distend fully and then verify that absorber pressure gauge reads <10 cmH_2O.

Breathing System

* **9.** Calibrate O_2 monitor.
  - **a.** Ensure that monitor reads 21% in room air.
  - **b.** Verify that low O_2 alarm is enabled and functioning.
  - **c.** Reinstall sensor in circuit and flush breathing system with O_2.
  - **d.** Verify that monitor now reads greater than 90%.

10. Check initial status of breathing system.
  - **a.** Set selector switch to "bag" mode.
  - **b.** Check that breathing circuit is complete, undamaged, and unobstructed.
  - **c.** Verify that CO_2 absorbent is adequate.
  - **d.** Install breathing circuit accessory equipment (e.g., humidifier, PEEP valve) to be used during the operation.

11. Perform leak check of the breathing system.
  - **a.** Set all gas flows to zero (or minimum).
  - **b.** Close APL (pop-off) valve and occlude Y-piece.
  - **c.** Pressurize breathing system to about 30 cmH_2O with O_2 flush.
  - **d.** Ensure that pressure remains fixed for at least 10 seconds.
  - **e.** Open APL (pop-off) valve and ensure that pressure decreased.

Manual and Automatic Ventilation Systems

12. Test ventilation systems and unidirectional valves.
  - **a.** Place a second breathing bag on Y-piece.
  - **b.** Set appropriate ventilator parameters for next patient.
  - **c.** Switch to automatic ventilation (ventilator) mode.
  - **d.** Fill bellows and breathing bag with O_2 flush and then turn ventilator on.
  - **e.** Set O_2 flow to minimum and other gas flows to zero.
  - **f.** Verify that during inspiration bellows delivers appropriate tidal volume and that during expiration bellows fills completely.
  - **g.** Set fresh gas flow to about 5 liters/min.
  - **h.** Verify that the ventilator bellows and simulated lungs fill and empty appropriately without sustained pressure at end-expiration.
  - **i.** Check for proper action of unidirectional valves.
  - **j.** Exercise breathing circuit accessories to ensure proper function.
  - **k.** Turn ventilator off and switch to manual ventilation (bag/APL) mode.
  - **l.** Ventilate manually and ensure inflation and deflation of artificial lungs and appropriate feel of system resistance and compliance.
  - **m.** Remove second breathing bag from Y-piece.

Monitors

13. Check, calibrate, and/or set alarm limits of all monitors:
  a. Capnometer
  b. Pulse oximeter
  c. Oxygen analyzer
  d. Respiratory volume monitor (spirometer)
  e. Pressure monitor with high and low airway alarms

Final Position

14. Check final status of machine.
  a. Vaporizers off.
  b. APL valve open.
  c. Selector switch to "bag."
  d. All flowmeters to zero.
  e. Patient suction level adequate.
  f. Breathing system ready to use.

CHAPTER 6

Monitoring the Anesthetized Patient

Joseph S. Savino and Ivan Salgo

Monitoring during anesthesia includes monitoring of the anesthesia machine and ventilator, discussed in the preceding chapter, and monitoring of the patient, the subject of this chapter. Careful observation of the anesthetized patient serves several purposes. First, patients respond to anesthesia and operation with changes in breathing, heart rate, blood pressure, or other variables. Monitoring these responses and the inspired and end-tidal concentrations of anesthetic gases allows one to regulate the depth of anesthesia appropriately. Second, treatment of such physiologic derangements as blood loss, hypothermia, hypertension, arrhythmias, organ ischemia, metabolic changes, or pulmonary dysfunction requires systematic assessment. Third, vigilant observation supplemented by automatic alarms detects unexpected catastrophes such as myocardial infarction and airway obstruction.

The most basic monitors are the senses of touch, hearing, sight, and smell. Monitoring devices supplement the anesthetist's perceptions with sensors that provide more sensitive and continuous assessment. These sensors are transducers that respond to such variables as electrical signals, gas flows, temperatures, and/or pressures and produce signals that can alert the anesthetist or be processed further by a computer. These systems must be accurate during both stable and changing conditions, precise, reliable, safe, inexpensive, and practical.

The selection of monitors takes into account the usefulness of the data, expense, and risk. Routine essential monitors include pulse oximeters, noninvasive blood pressure devices, capnographs, temperature probes, electrocardiograms, precordial or esophageal stethoscopes, and oxygen analyzers. These monitors and inspection of the patient are essential because they impose minimal risk and offer potential for lifesaving information. Present standards are summarized in Table 6-1. Other noninvasive and invasive monitors are used for clear indications.

Modern monitoring devices are expensive. The complex balance among cost, added risks of monitoring, and possible improved patient safety governs not only the use of a technique in a given patient but also the decision to invest in equipment and training. Whereas a monitor that does not influence medical or surgical management cannot be justified, even some quite expensive techniques can save money for patients, physicians, hospitals, and insurance companies. Improved safety implies lessened morbidity and mortality for patients, reduced costs of complications, diminished legal costs, and less costly insurance premiums and malpractice settlements.

Invasive monitors penetrate the body through the skin or via an orifice, but the distinction between these and noninvasive monitors is not rigid. A peripheral nerve stimulator is considered noninvasive, but it is rarely used while the patient is awake. Likewise,

Table 6-1

Essential Monitors for All Patients Undergoing Anesthesia

Observation
  A trained individual present at all times
  Observe movement, skin color, pattern of breathing, tearing, position, events in the surgical field, blood loss
  Patient's report of comfort or discomfort
  Monitor, interpret, and act on all data listed below
Stethoscope
  Breath sounds
  Heart sounds: amplitude, rhythm
Pulse oximeter
  Heart rate
  Peripheral oxygen saturation
Oximeter
  Inspired oxygen concentration (not used if patient not breathing from breathing circuit)
Capnograph
  End-tidal CO_2
  Shape of capnogram
  Respiratory rate
  Delivery of CO_2 to lungs by cardiac output
ECG
  Cardiac rate
  Rhythm
  Ischemic changes
Blood pressure
  Continuous or intermittent, according to need
Airway pressure (if applicable)
  Cyclic changes indicate breathing
  Disconnection of endotracheal tube
  Breathing circuit malfunction
Temperature for all but the briefest of general anesthetics and most regional anesthetics
Neuromuscular
  Peripheral nerve stimulator, if muscle relaxants are in use
Fluid balance
  Blood, urine, and estimated blood loss
  Blood and other fluids given
Other
  The automatic alarms provided with the anesthesia machine and ventilator
Anesthesia record
  A contemporaneous record, complete and accurate, for all the above data, the drugs given, and the events of the
    operation

Note: These recommendations are more stringent than those of the American Society of Anesthesiologists' House of Delegates (1989) but reflect a careful standard of practice. When patients are breathing room air or receiving oxygen by nasal cannula, it may not be practical to measure inspired oxygen tension or airway pressure. For short procedures, temperature monitoring may not be needed.

although the standard echocardiogram is noninvasive, transesophageal echocardiography (TEE) is invasive but is associated with little morbidity and mortality.

Monitors do not interpret data and do not substitute for sound clinical judgment. In this sense, the most important monitor of the patient's condition is a vigilant and thoughtful observer. To make the most of the data available, one must constantly integrate and interpret the information in light of the clinical situation.

Precordial or Esophageal Stethoscope

Those administering anesthesia often wear a custom-molded earpiece that is connected either to a stethoscope placed on the chest (precordial) or to a sealed tube inserted into the midesophagus (esophageal). This provides continuous monitoring without sophisticated electronics; it is noninvasive, inexpensive, and easy to use. Listening continuously to heart tones warns of changes in stroke volume or cardiac contractility (loudness and pitch), venous air embolism (mill-wheel murmur), and the onset of dysrhythmias. As a monitor of ventilation, the stethoscope detects wheezing, rhonchi, and stridor. During anesthetic induction, the precordial stethoscope provides information about heart sounds, airway patency, secretions, respiratory rate, and depth of anesthesia.

A conventional binaural stethoscope provides better-quality sound transmission, which is useful when listening closely to breath or heart sounds or when verifying positioning of an endotracheal tube but is impractical for continuous use.

Blood Pressure

The repeated measurement of arterial blood pressure is standard practice during anesthesia because operations and anesthetics are associated with changes in blood pressure great enough to do harm unless anticipated and treated. Blood pressure and the pressure waveform are not uniform throughout the arterial tree. The influence of gravity produces a net hydrostatic pressure in a column of fluid such as blood. A 1-cm column of blood exerts hydrostatic pressure equal to 0.74 mmHg (mercury is 13.6 times more dense than water). In the upright or sitting position, arterial blood pressure in the head may be 20 or 30 mmHg less than central aortic pressure. Likewise, blood pressure in dependent extremities is increased by the weight of the fluid column from the heart to the site of measurement. These differences in blood pressure are negligible in the recumbent position.

Blood is a fluid in motion. Under the simplifying assumptions of constant laminar flow, the flow Q along a vessel depends on the radius r, the length L, the viscosity μ, and the pressure difference ΔP along the vessel (for laminar flow):

$$Q = \frac{\Delta P \pi r^4}{8 \mu L} \qquad (6.1)$$

Differences in vessel diameter account for the differences in blood pressure in the aorta and radial artery. With each cardiac cycle, a stroke volume of blood is ejected into the aorta, creating a pressure wave that propagates downstream and is reflected back at the artery-arteriole junction. The contour of the arterial pressure wave at a specific site represents the sum of these incident and reflected pressure waves compared with the wave of the ascending aorta, but peripheral

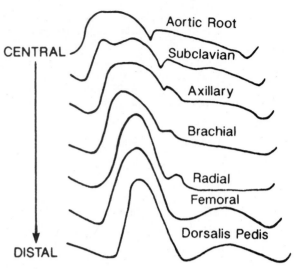

Figure 6-1

As compared with the aortic trace, the pressure waveform from the radial artery is changed by a delay in transmission, steeper upstroke, loss of high-frequency components, increases in systolic and pulse pressures, and a decrease in mean arterial pressure.

(Reproduced with permission from Bedford R, Invasive blood pressure monitoring. In Blitt CD, ed. Monitoring in Anesthesia and Critical Care Medicine, *New York: Churchill-Livingstone, 1990.)*

sites for blood pressure measurement are closer to the artery-arteriole interface and are more affected by reflected waves (Fig. 6-1).

Noninvasive blood pressure monitoring suffices for most patients during routine operations. A cuff wrapped around the patient's arm or leg is connected to a manometer and is inflated to a pressure greater than systolic blood pressure; during gradual deflation, the observer detects signs of blood flow distal to the cuff. The simplest method of detection is palpation of a distal artery with the return of a pulse corresponding to the systolic blood pressure. Listening for Korotkoff sounds provides systolic and diastolic blood pressures. Unfortunately, the auscultatory method requires a quiet workplace and is insensitive at lesser pressures because the Korotkoff sounds are faint.

Oscillometry bypasses the need for auscultation. The oscillometric method senses cyclic variations in cuff pressure as the cuff is deflated. When the pressure in the cuff is just below systolic blood pressure, the cuff pressure begins to oscillate at the same frequency as the pulse rate. Further deflation yields an increasing amplitude of oscillation; the maximum oscillation occurs at the mean arterial pressure. The oscillations dissipate with further deflation because the volume changes are not transmitted to the more loosely fitting cuff. The oscillation of the cuff pressure disappears when the cuff pressure is less than diastolic pressure. Although reliable for determining systolic and mean blood pressure, oscillometric instruments are less reliable for determining diastolic pressure.

Automatically measuring blood pressure at frequent intervals decreases the incidence of undetected hypotension. The devices that measure blood pressure noninvasively automatically inflate and deflate the cuff and detect distal flow, usually by oscillometry. The major disadvantage is sensitivity to motion artifact. Other automated techniques include Doppler ultrasonography to detect motion in the walls of the artery, a microphone and amplifier to detect Korotkoff sounds, and finger plethysmography to detect changes in the volume of digital arteries with each pulse.

The size of the blood pressure cuff influences the pressure reading. The minimum cuff width is approximately 40 percent of the circumference of the extremity. A cuff that is too narrow does not transmit the pressure uniformly to the underlying artery and results in a falsely increased blood pressure reading. A cuff that is too wide does not distort the pressure measurement but may compress neural structures at the axilla or elbow.

Cuff measurements of systolic and mean arterial pressure are accurate when compared with invasive methods. However, fluctuations in blood pressure related to respiration are common. Because the slowly deflating cuff measures the systolic and diastolic pressures during different portions of the respiratory cycle, the pulse pressure may be inaccurate. This is true whether a manual or automated device is used.

Continuous intraarterial monitoring of blood pressure is useful when small changes in blood pressure may produce organ ischemia (as in unstable angina pectoris) and when major operations produce large, rapid changes in blood pressure. The measuring system includes an intraarterial catheter, low-compliance pressure tubing, a pressurized low-flow continuous flush system, a transducer with a pressure-sensing diaphragm, and a display unit that converts the electrical signal into a numerical value. The risk of infection with reusable transducers has led to the use of disposable systems. After it is assembled and filled with heparin-saline solution, all air bubbles must be cleared from the system to prevent damping of the signal or arterial air embolism.

Small arterial cannulas are likely to kink and damp the waveform or limit the rate of blood sampling. Twenty-gauge Teflon catheters are preferred for the radial artery because, compared with large catheters, they are less likely to cause thrombosis and vascular injury (Fig. 6-2).

If cannulation results in thrombosis of the radial artery, it is feared that inadequate ulnar blood flow or an incomplete palmar arch may lead to ischemia of the hand. Often, Allen's test is performed before placing a radial artery catheter to assess ulnar and palmar arch blood flow. However, the predictive value of Allen's test has been challenged by reports in which the ulnar artery was cannulated after multiple punctures of the ipsilateral radial artery, with no evidence of subsequent hand ischemia, and by reports that indicate few complications occur when it is not employed. Available evidence does not indicate that estimating adequacy of ulnar flow by Allen's test improves the safety of the technique.

Allen's Test

The operator compresses the patient's radial and ulnar arteries at the wrist while the patient makes a tight fist for 10 to 20 seconds. After the patient relaxes the hand, it remains blanched until the ulnar artery is released. If the entire hand, including the thumb and thenar eminence, does not appear well perfused within 5 seconds, the ulnar supply is inadequate. A pulse oximeter on the thumb can be used instead of skin color to judge adequate perfusion.

The pressure-sensing transducer consists of a stiff diaphragm that is displaced by intravascular pressure. The displacement is sensed by a strain gauge that is connected to electronic circuitry that displays the pressure waveform and the systolic, mean, and diastolic pressures. The mean pressure is determined by calculating the area under several pulse waveforms, averaged over time. This represents the closest value to the true average pressure. Computing a mean pressure as a weighted average of the systolic and diastolic blood pressures yields a less accurate approximation.

Transducers require a zero reference point. The height of the column of fluid from the catheter tip to the strain gauge of the pressure transducer affects the net pressure sensed by the system. The typical zero reference point is the level of the right atrium. If the

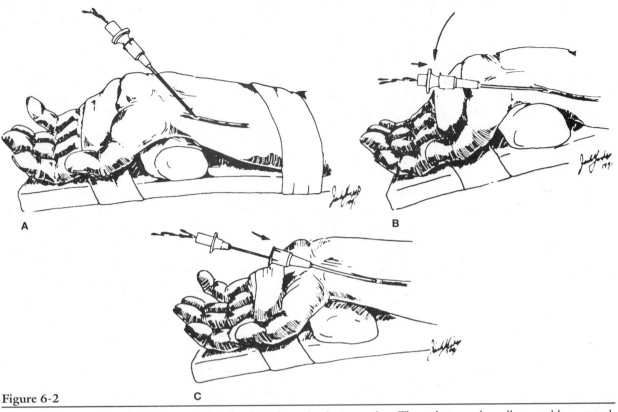

Figure 6-2

Radial artery cannulation. (*A*) A small pad under the wrist maintains extension. The catheter and needle assembly approach the artery at about a 30-degree angle from the horizontal. (*B*) After the needle enters the artery, the hub of the needle is depressed; then it and the catheter are advanced together a few millimeters into the lumen. (*C*) With the needle fixed, the catheter is advanced fully into the artery.

Placing a Catheter in the Radial Artery

Cannulas may be placed in the other arteries, but the radial artery is a popular site because of safety and ease of access.

A large number of acceptable techniques have been described for placing a catheter in the radial artery; none is foolproof, and all depend on skill and experience. The following paragraphs describe one workable method.

Gently fix the patient's hand and forearm to a board, with the wrist held in moderate dorsiflexion by a bolster under it (see Fig. 6-2). To reduce the risk of local infection and to eliminate contact with the patient's blood, prepare the skin aseptically and use appropriate sterile precautions, including gloves. Infiltrate the skin over the radial artery at the middle or proximal skin crease, where it is prominent. If the artery is small or puncture is difficult, make a small aperture in the skin with an 18- or 19-gauge needle to reduce drag on the arterial catheter. Using a 20-gauge catheter-over-needle assembly, advance the needle directly at the artery, with the hub raised at an angle of 30 degrees from the horizontal, until the pulsatile flow of blood into the hub

of the needle signals that the tip of the needle has entered the artery.

At this point, two techniques are possible. If it seems easy to do so, depress the hub of the needle, advance the needle in the artery for a few millimeters, and slide the catheter into the artery, just as when placing an intravenous catheter. If this is not feasible, pass the needle through the artery, transfixing it, and then remove the needle from the catheter. Withdraw the catheter slowly until arterial blood appears; the catheter sometimes can be threaded into the artery or a flexible wire (0.025-in for the usual 20-gauge catheter) advanced into the lumen to serve as a guide. If the first attempt fails, apply pressure to the artery for a few minutes before trying again, to prevent the formation of a large hematoma. The connection between the hub of the catheter and the tubing leading to the transducer must be secure; accidental disconnection can cause disastrous bleeding. Apply a transparent sterile dressing and remove the bolster under the wrist or replace it with a smaller one to prevent compression of the median nerve.

measurement of perfusion pressure to a specific organ (such as the brain) is indicated, then the zero reference is adjusted accordingly (such as to the base of the skull). Mounting the transducer at the zero reference level can be cumbersome; an alternate method uses a pressure offset. During "zeroing," fluid- filled tubing is connected between the transducer and the desired zero point. This creates an offset zero pressure level that is valid until the patient or the transducer is moved.

"Ringing" occurs in pressure-measuring systems when their natural resonant frequencies (20 to 25 Hz) are near those found in the arterial tree at the site of cannulation, thereby producing an exaggerated systolic peak. Ringing does not significantly change the diastolic value or the area under the pressure waveform and so has little effect on the mean arterial blood pressure. Higher natural resonant frequencies give less trouble with ringing and are produced by using tubing that is larger in diameter, less compliant, or shorter.

If peaks are blunted instead of accentuated, the signal is said to be "damped," usually due to constriction in the tubing produced by stopcocks or kinks or to air bubbles in the tubing or transducer. Overdamped systems underestimate systolic blood pressure and overestimate diastolic blood pressure. An underdamped system does not distort pressure waveforms if the natural frequency of the system is high enough to prevent ringing. When long lengths of tubing lead to ringing, deliberate damping may improve the accuracy of the arterial waveform. Miniature transducers placed at the tips of intraarterial catheters produce high-fidelity signals that are independent of the catheter, extension tubing, and stopcocks. They are not used routinely for arterial pressure monitoring because of expense.

Central Venous Pressure

Cannulating the central venous circulation can provide access for the rapid administration of fluids, a port for blood sampling, a route for the passage of catheters into the heart, and a means to measure the central venous pressure (CVP). Numerous anatomic approaches have been used. In anesthesia practice, cannulation of the right internal jugular vein is popular because of the ease of access to the neck and the straight path from the internal jugular

vein to the right side of the heart (Fig. 6-3). The subclavian route or an antecubital vein is sometimes used. As with arterial cannulas, the intravascular pressure is displayed on a physiologic monitor in both analog and digital forms. Complications occur infrequently but include pneumothorax, hemothorax, and inadvertent puncture of the subclavian or carotid artery.

Central venous pressure is an index of the circulating blood volume and preload to the right ventricle. The pulsatile characteristics of the CVP are a function of the uninterrupted return of venous blood to the right atrium, right atrial size and compliance, intrathoracic pressure, and the mechanical properties of the tricuspid valve and right ventricle (Fig. 6-4).

A decreased CVP suggests hypovolemia or an increase in venous capacitance, as with vasodilatation following sympathetic blockade. An increased CVP with normal cardiac function suggests hypervolemia, vasoconstriction, or increased intrathoracic pressure. Central venous pressure is increased by positive-pressure ventilation and positive end-expiratory pressure and is measured only at end-expiration. An increased CVP in the presence of arterial hypotension suggests cardiac dysfunction, but left ventricular dysfunction may not be reflected promptly by increased CVP. Disorders that increase right ventricular afterload (pulmonary emboli, pulmonary hypertension) or impair diastolic filling (cardiac tamponade) also increase CVP, as does incompetence of the tricuspid valve, which also results in large *v* waves.

Pulmonary Artery Pressure

Pulmonary artery (PA) catheters provide measures of pulmonary artery pressure (PAP), pulmonary artery occlusion pressure (PAOP), cardiac output, mixed venous oxygen saturation, and the derived values of systemic and pulmonary vascular resistance (Fig. 6-5). In addition to the risks of jugular puncture, the pulmonary artery catheter itself may cause right ventricular perforation, pulmonary embolus, pulmonary artery rupture, dysrhythmia, infection, and pulmonary infarction.

The pulmonary artery occlusion pressure is an indirect measure of left atrial pressure and an index of left ventricular preload. Usually, changes in PAOP

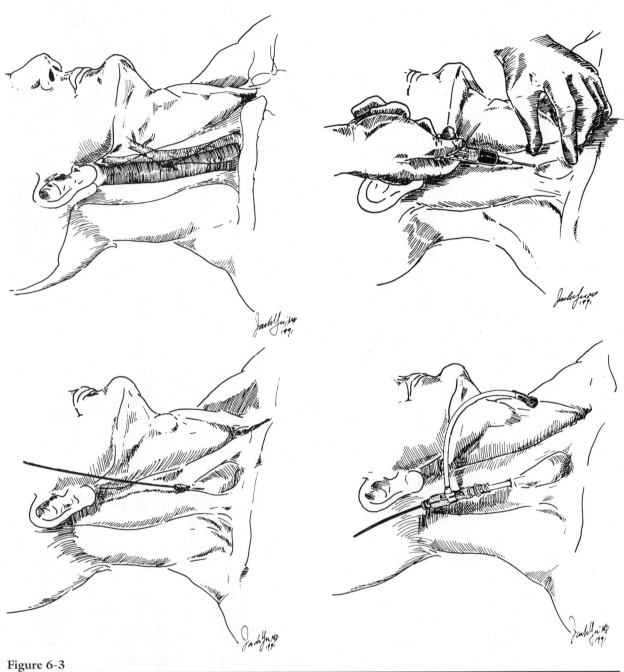

Figure 6-3

Anatomic relationship between internal jugular vein, carotid artery, and sternocleidomastoid muscle. Cannulation of the internal jugular vein and passage of a guidewire in the Seldinger technique.

Technique of Placing Pulmonary Artery Catheter: Right Internal Jugular Route

Most PA catheters used for intraoperative monitoring are inserted via the right internal or external jugular vein. The internal jugular vein is located immediately lateral to the carotid artery and beneath the medial border of the clavicular head of the sternocleidomastoid muscle (see Fig. 6-4). Ultrasound imaging allows a direct view of the internal jugular vein and carotid artery. The needle may be placed while the operator watches the image.

Place the patient head down to distend the jugular vein, with the head turned to the left. Using sterile technique and local anesthesia, insert a 20-gauge catheter-over-needle assembly, with a syringe attached, near the apex of the triangle formed by the lateral border of the medial head and the medial border of the lateral head of the sternocleidomastoid muscle. Direct the needle posteriorly, in the direction of the ipsilateral nipple, advancing while aspirating until venous blood flows freely into the syringe; then advance the cannula into the vein. When this or any other catheter is open from the air to the central circulation, precautions to prevent air embolism include the head-down position, Valsalva maneuver, or occluding the hub of the catheter with the gloved finger. Connect the catheter via a fluid-filled tube to the transducer, and verify that the pressure trace is not that of the carotid artery. Then pass

a wire to serve as a guide for a dilator and a no. 8.5 French introducer that will accommodate a no. 7 French PA catheter.

Flush the PA catheter with heparinized saline, cover it with a catheter contamination shield, test the distal balloon for asymmetry or leaks, and connect the lumen from the distal opening to a transducer. Insert the catheter to a depth of 20 cm (the junction of the right atrium and superior vena cava), inflate the balloon, and watch the pressure trace while advancing the catheter into the right ventricle and pulmonary artery until a PAOP tracing is obtained (see Fig. 6-5). Advance the catheter only while the balloon is inflated; do not pass the catheter deeper than 60 cm; after attaining the PAOP tracing, withdraw the deflated balloon a few centimeters to remove redundancy or loops in the right atrium or right ventricle.

To avoid dangerous pulmonary hemorrhages, do not leave the balloon inflated for longer than is needed to obtain a PAOP reading or exceed the manufacturer's recommended volume of inflation (1.0 to 1.5 ml). Because PA catheters tend to migrate distally, monitor pressure at the tip of the catheter; if a PAOP trace appears with the balloon deflated, withdraw the catheter and do not inflate the balloon until a PA waveform again is obtained.

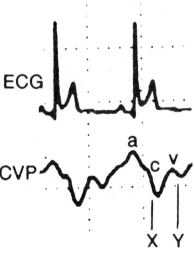

Figure 6-4

The ECG and a simultaneous central venous waveform. The *a* wave represents right atrial contraction; the *x* descent, right atrial relaxation; the *c* wave, bulging of the tricuspid valve into the right atrium during right ventricular contraction; the *v* wave, passive filling of the right atrium; the *y* descent, rapid emptying of the right atrium into the right ventricle.

precede changes in CVP, but the two change in the same direction (hypovolemia, heart failure). Isolated right-sided heart failure is an exception and produces an increase in the CVP and a decrease in the left atrial pressure.

Pulmonary artery catheters detect myocardial ischemia but lack sensitivity and specificity. Myocardial ischemia results in a decrease in ventricular compliance and an increase in left ventricular end-diastolic pressure (LVEDP). In the absence of mitral stenosis, the increased LVEDP results in an increase in PAOP and PAP. In addition, mitral regurgitation due to ischemia of the papillary muscles may be detected by the appearance of a *v* wave on the PAOP tracing. Although commonly used for ischemia monitoring, the PA catheter is a less sensitive monitor for myocardial ischemia than the electrocardiograph (ECG) or transesophageal echocardiography (TEE). Increases in PAP and PAOP are not specific for myocardial ischemia and are affected by changes in intravascular volume, sympathetic nervous system activity, and the mode of ventilation.

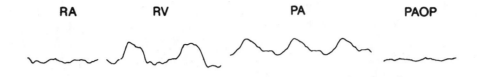

RA   RV   PA   PAOP

Figure 6-5

The typical waveform recorded from the distal port of a PA catheter as it is advanced from the right atrium (RA), to the right ventricle (RV), to the pulmonary artery (PA), and to the pulmonary occlusion position (PAOP). Notice the increase in diastolic pressure after passing from RV to PA.

Cardiac Output

The usual estimate of cardiac output is obtained by measuring pulmonary blood flow by thermodilution. Other methods, not dependent on an indwelling PA catheter, include dye dilution, aortic pressure pulse methods, transthoracic bioimpedance, and echocardiography, but all have proven cumbersome, impractical, or unreliable for routine intraoperative use. The thermodilution pulmonary artery catheter is equipped with multiple ports and a tip thermistor to measure the change in blood temperature at the pulmonary artery after injection of a cold solution into the central venous circulation. Cardiac output is related to the volume of blood in which the indicator (cold solution) is diluted and is measured by integrating the change in pulmonary blood temperature over time. The measurements are not continuous and are influenced by the speed of injection, the relationship of injection to the phase of the respiratory cycle, the volume of injectate, the concomitant administration of cold intravenous fluids, and technical errors. Further, the pulmonary artery catheter measures right ventricular cardiac output, which is not an accurate estimate of left ventricular cardiac output in patients with intracardiac shunts.

Calculating Peripheral Resistance

$$SVR = 80(MAP - CVP)/CO$$

where SVR = systemic vascular resistance (1200 to 1500 dyn · cm/s^5)*

CO = cardiac output (2.5 to 4.0 liters/min/m^2)*

MAP = mean arterial pressure (80 to 120 mmHg)*

CVP = mean central venous pressure (0 to 8 mmHg)*

*Normal values.

The most important application of intraoperative cardiac output monitoring is in the management of hypotension. Hypotension is caused either by reduced cardiac output (heart failure, hypovolemia) or by decreased systemic vascular resistance (sepsis, spinal or epidural anesthesia, drug effects). Cardiac output monitoring differentiates these categories of hypotension. Diminished cardiac output is treated with volume expansion, inotropes, or chronotropes. Decreased systemic vascular resistance may be treated with a vasoconstrictor (phenylephrine) or left untreated if tissue perfusion is adequate.

The continuous cardiac output catheter intermittently heats blood adjacent to a proximal portion of the catheter and senses changes in blood temperature at the catheter tip using a fast-response thermistor. Little heat is applied, requiring a special algorithm to detect the subtle changes in temperature. Cardiac output is calculated using the same principle as the thermodilution technique (i.e., indicator dilution). This technique requires no manual injections; averaged measurements are updated automatically every several minutes.

Pulmonary artery catheters also permit the measurement of mixed venous oxygen saturation, either by sampling or by continuous measurements using oximetric pulmonary artery catheters. These measurements are useful in evaluating shock states and determining optimal positive end-expiratory pressure (PEEP) settings.

Anesthetic Gas Monitoring

A commonly employed instrument to measure the concentration of anesthetic gases is the mass spectrometer. A gas sample is retrieved from the breathing circuit and analyzed in a central off-line spectrometer. The ionized molecules from the sample are deflected as they pass through a magnetic field and dispersed onto a collecting plate. Because deflection by the magnet is a function of the mass and charge of the ions, the site of impact is specific for a given gas species, and the number of impacts at each site represents the relative concentration in the sample. Mass spectrometers are used to measure concentrations of oxygen, nitrogen, carbon dioxide, and anesthetic gases. The anesthetic concentration in the airway during the plateau (end-tidal) phase of the carbon dioxide expirogram reflects the alveolar concentration of anesthetic.

A mass spectrometer can be placed in each anesthetizing location, providing continuous measurements. Shared systems sample gas from the separate operating rooms sequentially, resulting in intervals of several minutes between successive measurements for each patient in a large system.

Other methods used to measure anesthetic and respiratory gases include infrared spectroscopy, Raman spectroscopy, electrochemical and polarographic sensors, and piezoelectric adsorbtion. Most anesthetic gases and carbon dioxide absorb light in the infrared spectrum. The concentration of a known gas can be derived from the light energy absorbed, the path length of the emitted signal, and the extinction coefficient of the gas. Conventional infrared spectroscopy cannot identify specific anesthetic vapors in a breathing circuit because their absorption spectra overlap considerably. More sophisticated (and expensive) light sources are available that emit light in the far-infrared range and permit identification of the specific halogenated agents by their characteristic absorption patterns. Symmetrical molecules (i.e., those with no net electrical dipole) such as O_2 and N_2 cannot be detected by infrared spectrophotometry.

Molecules of gas can absorb light and reemit it in the same direction and at the same wavelength as incident light. However, certain vibrational and rotational energy states can produce a reemission with a different direction and wavelength and at a reduced energy. This phenomenon is known as *Raman scattering*. By measuring this scattered light, Raman spectroscopy can detect gases that do not have a net dipole. The Raman spectrometer can distinguish and measure the concentration of potent anesthetic vapors, nitrous oxide, and carbon dioxide, as well as oxygen and nitrogen.

Monitoring the inspired, expired, and end-tidal concentrations of anesthetic gases adds precision to their administration. At moderate fresh gas flows of 3 liters/min or more, estimating the inspired concentration of anesthetic vapor to be equal to the vaporizer

setting suffices for clinical purposes, especially in view of the need to adjust concentrations pragmatically to account for intermittent variability. With lesser flows and closed breathing systems, analyzers are necessary if one wants to determine the inspired concentration of anesthetic agent. Analyzers also guard against inadvertent overdose of anesthetics regardless of the fresh gas flow. Detection of nitrogen (Raman scattering and mass spectrometry) can warn of air embolism or a leak in the breathing system.

Oxygen

Monitoring of inspired oxygen tension is described in Chapter 5. Although anesthesia machines are reliable, separate and specific monitoring of the concentration of oxygen in the inspired gas is necessary and dictated by present standards of care. This provides a final protection against using hypoxic gas mixtures or against gas supply errors (e.g., a piping connection error of the central supply or a cylinder misfilled with the wrong gas).

Carbon Dioxide

Carbon dioxide in respiratory gases can be measured by infrared light absorption or mass spectrometry. Nitrous oxide strongly absorbs infrared light near the same wavelength as carbon dioxide, and its presence in the gas mixture must be taken into account. The sample chamber may lie within the breathing circuit (mainstream) or be connected to the breathing circuit by a sampling tube through which a pump aspirates a small flow of gas (sidestream).

End-tidal PCO_2 approximates arterial PCO_2 in normal people. However, end-tidal PCO_2 underestimates arterial PCO_2 when physiologic deadspace is increased. The difference changes significantly with induction of anesthesia, changes in position, or pathologic factors that affect matching of pulmonary ventilation and perfusion, such as pulmonary embolism.

The capnogram is the graphic display of airway PCO_2 as a function of time. Changes in its contour reflect disorders of ventilation. Many factors influence the shape of the capnogram, including the expiratory flow rate, the distribution of pulmonary blood flow, the distribution of ventilation, and the gas sampling rate when using a sidestream analyzer. The interplay

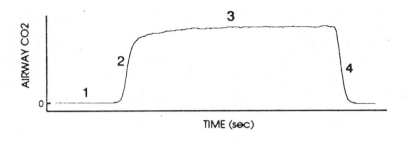

Figure 6-6

A typical capnogram: (1) inspired CO_2 is zero; (2) washout of anatomic deadspace and appearance of alveolar CO_2 create upslope; (3) plateau represents alveolar gas CO_2 content; and (4) downslope begins with inspiration.

of all these factors renders capnography a relatively nonspecific monitor of disease. Nonetheless, abrupt changes in the shape of the capnogram always signify an acute change in the patient's physiologic state (Fig. 6-6).

Capnography effectively detects many breathing circuit problems. Breathing circuit disconnections during mechanical ventilation, accidental extubation, and airway obstruction produce acute changes in the CO_2 expirogram. Tracheal intubation can be distinguished from esophageal intubation by the consistent concentration of CO_2 in the exhaled gas from the trachea. A slow increase in the exhaled CO_2 concentration suggests partial airway obstruction, either mechanical (tube kinking) or physiologic (bronchospasm). A progressive decrease in the end-tidal CO_2 occurs with hyperventilation, failing cardiac output, increased physiologic deadspace ventilation (pulmonary emboli consisting of air or thromboemboli), or decreased CO_2 production (hypothermia). A progressive increase in end-tidal PCO_2 occurs with hypoventilation or an increase in CO_2 production (malignant hyperthermia). If the inspired CO_2 is increased above zero, malfunction in the breathing circuit (valves) or exhaustion of the CO_2 absorbent is the usual cause.

Pulse Oximetry

Hypoxemia results in irreversible organ injury if not detected and treated within minutes. Pulse oximeters continuously measure arterial hemoglobin saturation, warning of deteriorating peripheral hemoglobin oxygen saturation before changes in the color of the patient's skin or blood are evident. Pulse oximeters are noninvasive, cost-effective, and reusable.

These devices were adopted almost immediately and universally in the United States, without the benefit of studies showing that they improve outcome, because they are inexpensive when compared with the human and financial costs of hypoxic episodes. Further, a number of studies using them have demonstrated unexpected hypoxemia during sedation for local anesthesia and following general anesthesia.

Pulse oximetry is likely to decrease the incidence and duration of perioperative hypoxemia and is useful in the titration of oxygen therapy, weaning of patients from ventilators, reducing the risk of retrolental fibroplasia in neonates, and monitoring pulse rate. Other controversial uses include measuring systolic blood pressure in combination with a sphygmomanometer, detecting perfusion in Allen's test, and detecting brachial or subclavian artery compression during shoulder or chest procedures. These are questionable applications because these devices were designed to detect oxygen saturation despite poor blood flow, not to detect inadequate perfusion.

The pulse oximeter is not an early warning monitor for esophageal intubation, breathing circuit malfunctions, or the administration of hypoxic gas mixtures. Capnography, pressure-volume alarms, and inspired oxygen concentration monitors permit earlier recognition of these common critical incidents.

Pulse oximetry measures the oxygen saturation of hemoglobin in arterial blood by measuring the absorption of light at 660 and 940 nm, which indicate the relative proportions of oxyhemoglobin and deoxyhemoglobin. The contribution of arterial hemoglobin to this absorption is isolated by examining only the pulsatile component of the transmitted signal, which is due to incoming arterial blood and is independent of the light absorbance from venous blood and tissue. Arterial hemoglobin saturation is calculated from data obtained in healthy volunteers. Accuracy fails at lesser saturations because these experiments were not conducted at hemoglobin oxygen saturations of less than 70 percent.

Dyshemoglobins adversely affect oximetry accuracy. Since the pulse oximeter uses only two wavelengths, it can only distinguish two species: oxy- and deoxyhemoglobin. The instrument cannot account for other hemoglobin species altering the absorbed light. Methemoglobin (ferric hemoglobin instead of ferrous hemoglobin) yields similar absorbances at both emitted wavelengths (660 and 940 nm) and results in an erroneous saturation of 85 percent regardless of the true value. Carbon monoxide poisoning yields a falsely increased value for oxyhemoglobin saturation because the pulse oximeter cannot distinguish between carboxyhemoglobin and oxyhemoglobin absorption at 660 nm. Co-oximeters, which require arterial blood samples, use enough different wavelengths to account for the extra hemoglobin species and can be used when dyshemoglobinemia is suspected.

Pulse oximeter signal processing is affected by electrical interference and motion. Oximeter probes need not be shielded from ambient light because the oximeter detects and corrects for background light by interspersing short intervals when no signal is emitted. Motion artifact is common and difficult to filter if it occurs at a frequency similar to that of the arterial pulse.

Electrocardiography

The intraoperative monitoring of the electrocardiogram (ECG) was described in 1918 and remains the most sensitive and practical monitor for the detection of disorders of cardiac rhythm and conduction. Multilead monitoring and the ability to select a frequency response range have improved its diagnostic value, as have computerized signal processing and automated ST-segment analysis. Permanent (paper) recording permits more leisurely analysis, comparison with the preoperative ECG, and documentation of findings. The inability to monitor 12 leads continuously, the lack of specificity of ST- and T-wave changes, interference associated with shivering and electrocautery, and the filtering used to reduce this interference are the major limitations of intraoperative ECG monitoring.

Using the ECG

Standardization of the ECG tracing is required before evaluating ST-segment changes; a 1-mV signal must produce a 10-mm deflection. The configuration of the ECG waveform frequently is distorted by extraneous electrical activity. A baseline trace width of greater than 2 mm suggests electrical interference, most commonly caused by 60-Hz power lines. The true ECG waveform consists of several frequency components. Filters used to "clean" the ECG signal usually eliminate a portion of the true ECG signal. Filtering modes on the electrocardiograph are selected by the user. The mode selected with the least amount of filtering is generally referred to as the *diagnostic mode*. The diagnostic mode eliminates signals with a frequency of less than 0.05 Hz; in the *monitor mode*, filters pass only frequencies greater than 0.5 and less than 40 Hz. The monitor mode minimizes baseline drift and the effects of respiration and muscle movement on the ECG but may result in distortion of the ST segment and T wave. *Filter mode* (0.5 to 25 Hz with a 60-Hz notch filter) eliminates stray power supply noise. The restricted bandwidth of the monitor mode alters the spectral power of certain component frequencies comprising the ST segment and can produce artifactual ST-segment elevation or depression. The diagnostic mode is used in patients at risk for myocardial ischemia. Other filters with even narrower bandwidths are useful when electrical interference produces an unrecognizable ECG but leave little information of value in the ST segments.

Operating room ECG equipment estimates heart rate by averaging several RR intervals. This is unreliable in patients with irregular rhythms such as atrial fibrillation. The device may not sense R waves if the electrical vector of the heart is isoelectric in the monitored lead. Because the R and T waves have the same electrical axis in normal patients, it is not unusual for the beat detector to be triggered by both waves, resulting in a calculated heart rate of twice the actual rate. Adjusting sensitivity or monitoring a different lead resolves both these problems.

Analysis of intervals and QRS configuration permits the detection and diagnosis of conduction disorders. Conduction blocks, such as ectopic electrical activity, can be acute or chronic in onset, variant of normal (right bundle branch block), or associated with severe disease (see Chap. 21).

ST segments are examined for their shape and position relative to the preceding TP interval. Normal

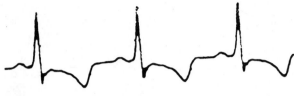

Figure 6-7

ST-segment depression and inverted T wave in a patient with myocardial ischemia.

ST segments are slightly curved with a smooth transition to the T wave. ST-segment depression of greater than 1 to 2 mm is associated with myocardial injury and is never normal (Fig. 6-7). ST-segment elevation results from transmural ischemia but also may occur after direct-current (DC) cardioversion and in normal adults; marked ST-segment elevation in the precordial leads has been described in otherwise healthy young black men. The automated ST-segment trending monitor measures the vertical distance between the ECG's baseline and the J point. Appropriate operation therefore depends on accurate identification of these ECG loci. If the cursor that defines the J point is misplaced onto the S wave, the displayed reading will suggest ST-segment depression. Factors other than myocardial ischemia that produce abnormal ST segments include drug therapy, electrolyte disturbance, cardiomyopathy, pericarditis, myocarditis, mitral valve prolapse, and cerebrovascular accidents. The most sensitive lead for the detection of perioperative myocardial ischemia is V_5. The simultaneous display of leads II and V_5 permits monitoring of a large portion of the left ventricle. The presence of left or right bundle branch block (BBB) places significant limitations on the diagnostic value of ST-segment analysis. Finally, a normal ECG does not exclude the presence of coronary artery disease or myocardial ischemia.

The T wave represents ventricular repolarization and has the same general direction (50 degrees) as the QRS axis. Inverted T waves with an upright QRS complex are almost always associated with a myocardial abnormality. The normal T wave has a smooth contour. The height of a T wave is compared with the amplitude of the R wave. Tall T waves may occur with myocardial ischemia, infarction, hyperkalemia, or stroke. Small or flat T waves and U waves occur with hypokalemia.

QT-interval measurement is practical only if a printed tracing of the ECG is available. A normal QT interval is less than half the RR interval, although the QT interval must be corrected for heart rates greater than 90 or less than 65 beats per minute. Prolongation of the QT interval may be idiopathic or associated with hypokalemia, stroke, hypothermia, mitral valve prolapse, and drug effect (quinidine, procainamide, and phenothiazines). Prolonged QT intervals are associated with increased risk of reentrant ventricular tachydysrhythmias because of the delay in ventricular repolarization.

Rhythm Disturbances under Anesthesia

Disturbances of rhythm in patients under anesthesia may be supraventricular or ventricular. The differentiation is important because rhythm disturbances differ in their etiology, effect on the cardiovascular system, treatment, and prognosis. Tachycardia caused by atrial or A-V node reentry is common during anesthesia and usually not associated with significant hemodynamic instability. Ventricular tachycardia is a medical emergency, associated with hypotension and poor cardiac output and requiring immediate intervention. Supraventricular arrhythmias originate in the atria or A-V junction and, unless associated with aberrant conduction, are characterized by QRS complexes of normal axis and duration. Ventricular arrhythmias originate in the lower conduction system or ventricular myocardium and appear as wide QRS complexes. Ventricular arrhythmias most commonly have a left bundle branch block (LBBB) pattern. The association of P waves and QRS complexes does not exclude the possibility of ventricular arrhythmias if the ectopic focus is high in the conduction system or there is retrograde conduction to the atria. QRS complexes with constantly related upright P waves suggest a supraventricular origin. All available leads are inspected when diagnosing a rhythm disorder. Lead II and V_1 are the most useful because P waves have the largest amplitude in these leads and lead II is parallel to the electrical vector of the heart.

The ECG is most valuable if monitoring begins before induction of anesthesia. Any abnormal or marginal ECG finding is less worrisome if it is present in the preoperative ECG and remains unchanged throughout the perioperative period; it is more troubling if it first appears or worsens intraoperatively.

Temperature

Temperature regulation by the hypothalamus is impaired during general anesthesia. Hypothermia is common during major operations in modern, cold operating rooms and may produce cardiac dysrhythmias, potentiation of anesthetic drugs and neuromuscular blockade, coagulopathy, increased vascular resistance, decreased availability of oxygen, and postoperative shivering. Small children and infants are especially prone to hypothermia because of their increased ratio of body surface area to weight; the elderly are susceptible because of their limited compensatory mechanisms. Intraoperative hyperthermia is less common and may result from malignant hyperthermia, fever, and inappropriate efforts to warm the patient.

Temperature monitoring is appropriate in all patients unless the procedure is very brief (less than 15 minutes). However, increases in body temperature do not provide the earliest warnings of malignant hyperthermia, whose first sign is increased CO_2 production.

Temperature is measured with electronic thermometers. The site of temperature measurement is important because body temperature is not uniform. Core temperature reflects the temperature of vital organs and is measured in the nasopharynx, external auditory canal, midesophagus, or central blood. Rectal temperature is not a reliable measure of core temperature. Temperature measurements at peripheral sites reflect perfusion and heat loss at the site being monitored. Disposable surface devices that detect temperature change chemically reflect only the heat given off by the skin and are not an accurate reflection of intrinsic core temperature.

Even temperature monitoring is not without risk. Temperature probes meant to lie in the external auditory canal may perforate the tympanic membrane if placed too deep. Nasopharyngeal probes may cause epistaxis. Esophageal temperature measurement may be in error if the probe is left high in the esophagus, exposed to the cooling effect of gases in the adjacent trachea.

Echocardiography

Transesophageal echocardiography (TEE) is expensive but can be a useful continuous perioperative

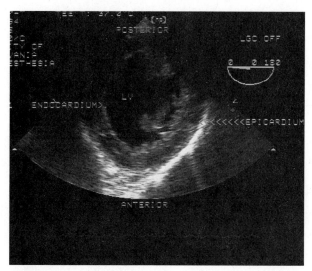

Figure 6-8

TEE transgastric short-axis view of the left ventricle (LV) in diastole. The endo- and epicardium are demarcated. The two structures within the LV are the papillary muscles.

monitor of heart anatomy and function. The retrocardiac position of the TEE probe permits high-resolution two-dimensional imaging of the myocardium, atria, valves, and great vessels of the mediastinum (Fig. 6-8). These images and the Doppler measurement of flows provide assessment of valvular function, invaluable during cardiac operations, and of global and regional wall motion (Table 6-2).

A decrease in coronary blood flow or an increase in myocardial oxygen demand that results in myocardial ischemia produces an abrupt change in ventricular

Table 6-2

Clinical Applications for Intraoperative TEE
Global ventricular size and function
Systolic
Diastolic
Regional ventricular wall motion
Valvular anatomy and function
Congenital and acquired anatomic heart defects
Intracardiac air
Pericardial disease and cardiac tamponade
Aortic atheroma, aneurysm, and dissection
Endocarditis
Cardiomyopathy
Cardiac tumors
Thrombus and foreign bodies
Trauma

wall motion. Although wall motion abnormalities may be produced by disorders other than myocardial ischemia, such as rheumatic heart disease, reperfusion injury, valve disease, and ventricular pacing, these changes occur early in the course of myocardial ischemia and provide more sensitive warnings than do changes in the ECG and pulmonary artery occlusion pressure. Also, innovative edge-detection algorithms permit continuous display of left ventricular (area) ejection fraction and chamber size, making TEE useful in differentiating hypovolemia from poor myocardial contractility as a cause for depressed cardiac output syndromes and allowing analysis of regional motion.

TEE is most often used during heart operations when abrupt changes in cardiac function and anatomy are common and frequently unexpected. In addition to the assessment of myocardial function and ischemia described above, anatomic and functional disorders of heart valves are frequently best assessed in the operating room with TEE. Aortic, mitral, and tricuspid valves are assessed for their suitability for repair versus replacement. Repairing a valve is associated with better long-term ventricular function (for mitral valves) and spares the patients the need for lifelong anticoagulation (both mitral and aortic valves). The ability to assess the competency of the reconstructed valve with intraoperative TEE enables the surgeon to ensure the adequacy of the repair before closing the chest.

BIBLIOGRAPHY

Barker SJ, Tremper KK. Pulse oximetry: Application and limitations. *Int Anesthesiol Clin* 1987;25:155-175.

Blitt CD, Hines RL. *Monitoring in Anesthesia and Critical Care Medicine*, 3rd ed. New York: Churchill-Livingstone, 1995.

Gravenstein JS, Paulus DA. *Clinical Monitoring Practice*, 2nd ed. Philadelphia: JB Lippincott, 1987.

Hutton P, Prys-Roberts C. *Monitoring in Anaesthesia and Critical Care*. Philadelphia: WB Saunders, 1994.

Kelleher JF. Pulse oximetry. *J Clin Monit* 1989;5:37-62.

Norton HN. *Biomedical Sensors, Fundamentals and Application*. Park Ridge, Ill: Noyes Publications, 1982.

Wagner GS. *Marriott's Practical Electrocardiography*, 9th ed. Baltimore: William & Wilkins, 1994.

Weinfurt PT. Electrocardiographic monitoring: An overview. *J Clin Monit* 1990;6:132-128.

Wiedermann HP, McCarthy K. Noninvasive monitoring of oxygen and carbon dioxide. *Clin Chest Med* 1989;10:239-254.

SECTION 3

Drugs Used in Anesthesia

CHAPTER **7**

Pharmacologic Principles of Anesthesia

Sean K. Kennedy

Anesthetic drugs may be administered in a single dose or titrated in a series of smaller increments to achieve a desired effect. In either case, the anesthesiologist must be aware of the factors that determine how the administered dose will achieve a resulting blood concentration of drug (pharmacokinetics) and how that concentration of drug will affect the patient (pharmacodynamics). The relationship between a dose of drug and the resulting physiologic effect, the *dose-response curve*, represents the summation of both pharmacokinetics and pharmacodynamics.

The factors governing responses to even a single drug are complex. The practice of anesthesia requires administering multiple drugs, demanding considerable understanding of pharmacologic principles.

Pharmacokinetics

The pharmacokinetics of a drug may be separated into three categories: absorption, distribution, and elimination. All these processes involve the movement of a drug across cell membranes, controlled by such physical-chemical properties as the drug's molecular size, the solubility of the drug at the site of administration, its lipid solubility and the ease with which it crosses the cell membrane, and the fraction of drug in the ionized and un-ionized forms.

The cell membrane is a dynamic fluid mosaic of globular proteins penetrating either partially or completely through a phospholipid bilayer. The mobile lipid molecules make the bilayer a flexible structure. Although the phospholipid bilayer is impermeable to polar molecules, specific hydrophobic or hydrophilic channels are formed by lipid or protein complexes in the membrane. Water diffuses easily through most physiologic membranes and may take with it small (molecular weight < 100 to 200) water-soluble compounds such as urea.

Larger, nonpolar molecules may diffuse passively across the cell membrane driven by the concentration gradient across the membrane and depending on the lipid solubility of the drug, expressed as the lipid:water partition coefficient of the drug. The greater the lipid:water partition coefficient, the greater is the concentration of drug in the membrane and the faster equilibrium is achieved. At equilibrium, the concentrations of polar compounds is equal on the two sides of the membrane. Differences in pH across the membrane influence the ionization of the molecule on each side, producing an electrochemical gradient that affects the final equilibrium concentrations (Fig. 7-1).

Drugs also may be carried across the cell membrane by carrier-mediated active transport. In contrast to passive diffusion, this process is specific for certain molecules, requires energy, may move compounds against an electrochemical gradient, and may be inhibited competitively. Facilitated diffusion is a similar process that requires no energy input but cannot move compounds against an electrochemical gradient.

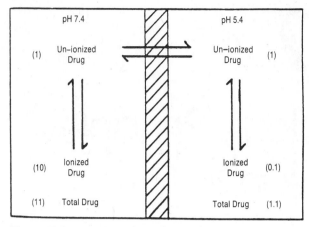

Figure 7-1

A concentration difference of total drug can develop on two sides of a membrane that separates fluids with different pH values. At steady state, the nonionized (un-ionized) drug concentration on both sides of the membrane is similar, but the concentration of ionized drug differs.

(From Hug CC, Pharmacokinetics of drugs administered intravenously. Anesth Analg *1978;57:704-723. Reproduced by permission of the author and the International Anesthesia Research Society.)*

■ Absorption

In its broadest sense, *bioavailability* refers to the fraction of administered drug that reaches either the site of action or a biologic fluid with access to the site of action. For example, after oral administration, a large fraction of drug absorbed from the gastrointestinal tract and then through the portal circulation may be inactivated by the liver. This phenomenon, called the *first-pass effect*, results in decreased bioavailability of the drug.

Molecular properties of a drug may influence absorption. Most drugs are weak acids or bases in a solution containing both ionized and un-ionized forms. The pK of the drug and the pH of the environment determine how much of the drug is in the un-ionized lipid-soluble form available to cross cell membranes. In the stomach, for instance, weak acids exist predominantly in their un-ionized, readily absorbable forms. In the intestine, at pH 7 to 8, the same drugs are ionized and do not readily cross the membrane.

The route of administration determines bioavailability. The oral route is often the simplest for the patient but offers several impediments to absorption, including the first-pass effect discussed earlier. Variations in gastric pH, gastrointestinal motility, and the presence of food and enzymes all modify the extent of absorption. Some drugs may be dissolved and absorbed in the mouth, minimizing the first-pass effect and destruction by gastric enzymes. Similarly, rectal administration reduces the impact of the first-pass effect.

Subcutaneous injection usually results in a gradual absorption of the drug. Drugs in aqueous solutions are more rapidly absorbed from intramuscular sites than after subcutaneous injection. The intravenous route eliminates impediments to absorption, providing drug to the circulation immediately upon injection. This is the fastest way to provide drug effect and is usually the route chosen for drugs given during anesthesia (except inhalation anesthetic agents). The inhalation route is nearly as fast as the intravenous because of the large alveolar surface area and its ready access to the pulmonary blood flow. In an emergency, epinephrine instilled through an endotracheal tube reaches the circulation nearly as quickly via mucosal absorption as via the intravenous route.

Other factors influence the rate of absorption. Drugs in aqueous solution are more rapidly absorbed than solids, suspensions, or oily solutions. Drugs given in greater concentration are absorbed more rapidly, as are those exposed to a large surface area for absorption. Blood flow at the site of drug administration influences the rate of absorption as well. For example, local anesthetics are taken up especially rapidly from well-perfused areas such as the face or scalp, but the addition of vasoconstrictors such as epinephrine slows absorption.

■ Distribution

Once a drug has reached the systemic circulation, either through absorption or intravenous injection, it distributes throughout the body, ultimately coming to equilibrium within all accessible tissues. Immediately following administration, distribution is determined principally by lipid solubility and regional blood flow. Thus lipid-soluble drugs are rapidly distributed to the brain, heart, and kidney, all organs with substantial blood flow. With more time, muscle tissue receives its share, and much later, the poorly perfused fat and bone tissue. (See Fig. 9-3, which depicts the phases in the distribution of thiopental.) While it is possible at equilibrium for peripheral tissue to have a greater drug concentration than blood (from ion trapping, tissue binding, or tissue solubility, for instance), the blood concentration usually exceeds tissue concentration during this early phase of distribution.

For a drug that equilibrates freely between blood and its site of action (the effect compartment), the effects of small intravenous doses dissipate because the circulation redistributes the drug to other more slowly equilibrating compartments, not because of metabolism or elimination. This is often the case for drugs given in anesthesia practice; a good example is thiopental, which has a pK_a of 7.6 and is quite lipid soluble (see Fig. 9-3). Following initial intravenous administration, effective brain concentrations are achieved almost immediately, because cerebral blood flow is great and the drug remains mostly un-ionized and lipid-soluble. As the drug distributes into other, less well-perfused organs, the blood concentration declines, and thiopental diffuses out of brain tissue and back into the central circulation. As the brain concentration decreases, the patient regains consciousness. The brevity of the effect of thiopental is the result of redistribution, not metabolism or elimination.

Protein binding, usually reversible, also influences the distribution of drugs. Plasma albumin is the most important binding agent, especially for acidic drugs; alpha-1-acid glycoprotein tends to bind basic drugs. Because the bound fraction of the drug is unavailable for pharmacologic activity or metabolism, only the free fraction determines drug effect. The bound portion, in effect, functions as a drug reservoir, releasing drug as the plasma concentration decreases through redistribution or metabolism and prolonging the effect as well as the half-life of the drug. Plasma proteins have only a limited number of binding sites, and protein-bound drugs tend to compete for those sites. Administration of a new drug with affinity for the same binding sites displaces a previously administered protein-bound drug, effectively increasing the blood concentration of free drug. Such effects are seen after thiopental (70 to 85 percent bound to plasma albumin) is administered to a patient taking other protein-bound drugs, such as phenylbutazone or aspirin. Similarly, patients with severe liver disease may have markedly decreased plasma protein concentrations. With less protein available to bind with thiopental, a greater amount of free drug is present in the circulation (see Chap. 9).

Fat tissue also may act as a reservoir of fat-soluble compounds. After prolonged administration, fat stores may accumulate a large amount of drug, which will be released to the central circulation as the concentration in the blood decreases from drug metabolism. The blood supply to fat is relatively poor, so accumulation of the drug takes a long time and the subsequent release of the drug is slow. This effect accounts for the small but measurable concentrations of anesthetics found in blood for days after anesthesia, which in turn may produce prolonged impairment of cognitive function or significant degrees of hepatic metabolism of the drug.

■ Elimination

The elimination of drugs from the body is usually a two-step process of metabolism and excretion. In some cases, such as modern inhalation anesthetics, metabolism is a minor element, and elimination depends almost exclusively on excretion via the lungs.

Most metabolism of drugs takes place in the liver. Phase I reactions convert the drug to a more polar metabolite by oxidation, reduction, or hydrolysis, an important mechanism for inactivating such drugs as succinylcholine and procaine. Usually, the metabolite is inactive, but it may be even more active than the parent compound. Phase II synthetic reactions join the drug or its metabolite to an endogenous molecule (e.g., glucuronate, sulfate), creating a water-soluble substance that is more readily excreted.

Most drugs are eliminated via renal or hepatobiliary excretion. Renal excretion is the net result of filtration, reabsorption, and excretion of substances in the kidney. Driven by arterial pressure, the ultrafiltrate of plasma in Bowman's capsule contains water and low-molecular-weight substances filtered from the blood. Hydrophilic substances remain in the tubule and are excreted. Lipophilic substances are reabsorbed across the tubule and reenter the systemic circulation along with any substances that are actively reabsorbed. Passive reabsorption of lipophilic substances occurs in the presence of a concentration gradient, enhanced by tubular reabsorption of water in the tubules. Small molecules that are not ionized tend to be easily reabsorbed; the usually acidic environment of the renal tubule provides for ready reabsorption of weak acids.

Clinical Pharmacokinetics

Simple physiologic and mathematical models that may fail to represent all the complexities of pharmacokinetics nevertheless make it possible to understand

and predict the behavior of drugs in the body. These models group together organ systems according to their role in the pharmacokinetics of the specific drug being modeled. For instance, to simplify predicting the behavior of inhaled anesthetics, organs are grouped together depending on their relative blood supply rather than by category of organ function. Thus organs of the vessel-rich group, including the heart and brain, tend to show similar patterns of drug accumulation and distribution. Similarities of drug solubility and blood perfusion are the common denominators that define organ groups in physiologic models, but these complex models require extensive analysis and may be difficult to apply to individual patients.

Mathematical models, on the other hand, do not follow anatomic definitions when assigning compartments. Rather, the models describe observed drug concentrations over time in hypothetical pharmacokinetic compartments that do not have any direct anatomic correlates. The apparent volume of distribution, for instance, may be larger than or smaller than the blood volume or the extracellular fluid compartment.

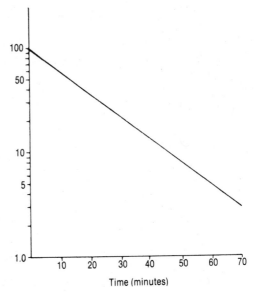

Figure 7-3

Plotting the logarithm of the drug concentration on the ordinate yields a straight line for monoexponential decay of drug concentrations in a single-compartment model with first-order kinetics.

(Reprinted with permission from Stanski DR, Watkins WD, Drug disposition in anesthesia. New York: Grune & Stratton, 1982, p 7.)

■ One-Compartment Model

In the simplest one-compartment model, the concentration of drug in the blood decreases by a fixed fraction from the equilibrium concentration during each equal time period. In Figure 7-2, a hypothetical curve demonstrates this relationship of drug concentration to time. Figure 7-3 shows the same data with drug concentration displayed on a logarithmic scale; decay of drug concentration at constant rates (single exponential decline) is portrayed as a straight line on such a plot. The *elimination half-life* is the time required for the concentration to decrease by one-half. After five half-lives, the drug concentration decreases to about 3 percent of its original value.

■ Two-Compartment Model

The pharmacokinetics of most anesthetic drugs given intravenously can be described with a two-compartment model. Figure 7-4 illustrates the simulated behavior of a drug in two compartments. Two distinct phases are apparent: The first is a sharp decline from the peak concentration following administra-

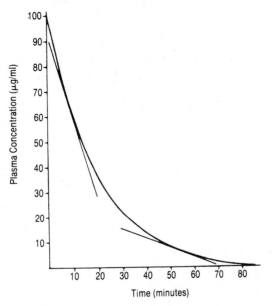

Figure 7-2

The exponential decay of drug concentrations at a fixed rate from a single compartment generates the curve shown. The tangents represent the slopes, or rates of decay, of drug concentration at 10 and 50 minutes after injection.

(Reprinted with permission from Stanski DR, Watkins WD, Drug disposition in anesthesia. New York: Grune & Stratton: 1982, p 7.)

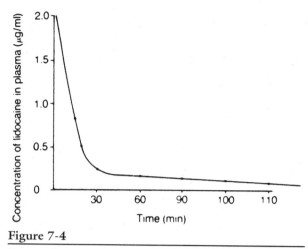

Figure 7-4

Expected concentrations over time for an intravenously administered drug with kinetics that fit a two-compartment model.

tion, representing rapid distribution of the drug into tissue spaces; the second is a much slower decay representing elimination.

The distribution phase resembles the introduction of a drug into a central compartment of relatively small volume (analogous to, but not anatomically equivalent to, the blood and richly perfused organs such as the heart, lung, and brain). The slower phase of elimination corresponds to the behavior of a drug in a peripheral compartment of much larger volume. In Figure 7-5, the same data are presented with drug concentrations plotted on a logarithmic scale. The two distinct phases are defined by the equation

$$C_p = Ae^{-\alpha t} + Be^{-\beta t}$$

where C_p = plasma concentration at time t
α = rate constant of the distribution phase
β = rate constant of the elimination phase
A = intercept at time 0 of the distribution phase line
B = intercept at time 0 of the elimination phase line
t = time

■ Elimination

Although distribution of anesthetic drugs often requires a two-compartment model to describe behavior, elimination usually follows first-order kinetics; that is, a constant fraction of the drug is eliminated in a given time period. As long as the mechanisms for

metabolism and excretion are not saturated, this is generally the case. Should those mechanisms become saturated, then elimination would follow zero-order kinetics; that is, a constant amount of drug would be eliminated during each time period. This situation might occur during constant infusion of a drug such as vecuronium, a nondepolarizing neuromuscular blocking agent.

Because elimination follows first-order kinetics, the *elimination rate constant k* is equal to the fraction of drug eliminated in that time period. If 15 percent of a barbiturate is eliminated each hour, then $k = 0.15$ hour. For many anesthetic drugs, such as the inhalation agents, elimination is often described in terms of the *elimination time constant* $T_{1/e}$. In one time constant, the drug concentration changes by a factor of $1/e$, or 63 percent. The elimination time constant (measured in units of time) is equal to the reciprocal of the elimination rate constant:

$$T_{1/e} = 1/k$$

The half-life of the drug is related to the time constant by

$$t = 0.693\,T_{1/e}$$

■ Clearance

In pharmacokinetic terms, clearance of a drug is analogous to the concept of creatinine clearance in renal physiology. *Creatinine clearance* does not refer to the amount of creatinine cleared in a given time period; rather, it defines the volume of blood that

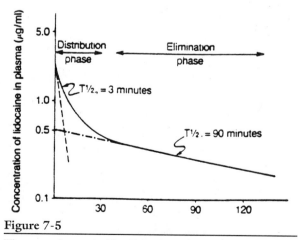

Figure 7-5

The same data as in Fig. 7-4, plotted on logarithmic scale.

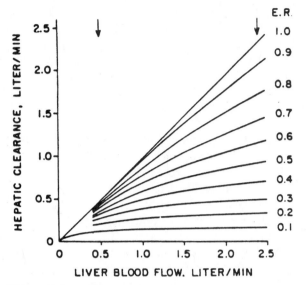

Figure 7-6

Hepatic blood flow varies between 0.5 and 2.5 liters/min, denoted by the arrows. Within this range, hepatic clearance of drugs poorly extracted by the liver [low extraction ratio (E.R.)] are not much affected by changes in blood flow; the clearances of those with larger values for E.R. do change with hepatic blood flow.

(Reproduced with permission from Wilkinson GR, Shjand DG, A physiologic approach to hepatic drug clearance. Clin Pharmacol Ther 1975;18:377.)

would have to be cleared of its creatinine in a given time period in order to account for all the creatinine excreted in that period. *Drug clearance*, expressed as volume per unit time (flow), similarly describes that volume of a biologic fluid (plasma) that would have to be totally cleared of the drug in order to account for all the drug eliminated in that time period. Total drug clearance is the sum of all the component clearance rates, such as renal, hepatic, etc., and represents that part of the volume of distribution cleared of drug per unit time:

$$Cl = V_d \times k$$

where Cl = clearance
$\quad V_d$ = the volume of distribution
$\quad k$ = the elimination rate constant

Drugs with larger hepatic extraction ratios ($ER > 0.7$) are cleared at a rate that depends on hepatic blood flow and not changes in enzyme activity, a phenomenon referred to as *perfusion-dependent elimination*. Hepatic disease tends not to influence the extraction ratio. Drugs with a small extraction ratio ($ER < 0.3$) are not greatly influenced by changes

in hepatic blood flow. With small hepatic extraction, a large amount of drug remains available for metabolism by hepatic enzyme systems. A decrease in hepatic blood flow does not have much influence on clearance because the altered flow results in only a slight change in the amount extracted (low extraction ratio), and the amount available for metabolism is already excessive. Thus total clearance changes very little. An increase in enzyme activity, however, produces a corresponding increase in hepatic clearance. Hepatic elimination of drugs with lesser extraction ratios is referred to as *capacity-dependent elimination*. Figure 7-6 demonstrates the effect of liver blood flow on hepatic clearance at various values of the hepatic extraction ratio.

Pharmacokinetics and Disease

Renal disease with resulting loss of glomerular filtration reduces renal clearance of drugs, the decreased drug clearance usually paralleling the decrease in creatinine clearance. Many nondepolarizing neuromuscular blockers are excreted unchanged in the urine, and decrease in creatinine clearance predicts the decreased excretion seen with these drugs in patients with renal disease (Fig. 7-7). If the only effect of renal disease is on elimination, then the initial dose of the

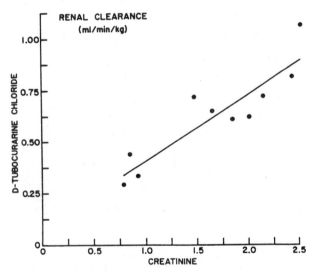

Figure 7-7

Renal curare clearance parallels creatinine clearance.
(Reproduced with permission from Shanks CA, Avram MJ, Ronai AK, Bowsher DJ. The pharmacokinetics of d-Tubocurarine with surgery involving salvaged autologous blood. Anesthesiology 1985;62:161.)

drug need not be reduced, but subsequent maintenance doses are reduced to take into account the decreased elimination of drug. In fact, renal disease may affect pharmacokinetics by mechanisms other than diminished renal clearance of drugs. Urea competes with other drugs for protein-binding sites, especially on albumin. In some forms of renal disease there is protein wasting. Both these features of renal disease reduce the number of protein-binding sites available for drugs, making more free drug available in the plasma. Uremic patients have a reduced dose requirement for thiopental because of decreased protein binding of the drug.

Hepatic disease also may influence drug action. Decreased production of albumin may decrease plasma protein concentrations and make more free drug available, as described earlier. Such patients would be unusually sensitive to usual doses of a protein-bound drug. On the other hand, patients with cirrhosis or ascites are more resistant to initial doses of pancuronium because of an increased apparent volume of distribution. This increased volume of distribution leads to a prolonged elimination half-life as well.

Hepatic enzyme and synthetic function tests are unreliable predictors of decreased capacity to metabolize and excrete drugs. The functions of the liver are numerous and complex, making any one synthetic test an unreliable predictor of other hepatic functions. Hepatic clearance may be unaffected by hepatic disease, probably owing to the large margin of reserve in hepatic function. Decreased clearance of diazepam and midazolam (metabolized by phase I oxidation) is seen in viral hepatitis and cirrhosis, while clearance of oxazepam and lorazepam (metabolized by phase II glucuronide conjugation) is unchanged.

In cases of decreased cardiac output, hepatic blood flow is likely to decrease, so clearance of drugs with greater hepatic extraction ratios decreases. For instance, infusion rates of lidocaine (ER = 0.7 to 0.9) must be reduced in patients with congestive heart failure. Similar reductions in subsequent doses are made with fentanyl (ER = 0.6), etomidate (ER = 0.9), propofol (ER = 1.0), ketamine (ER = 1.0), and methohexital (ER = 0.5).

Pharmacodynamics

Once a drug has been delivered to the target organ, it can exert its pharmacologic effect. The *pharmacodynamics* of a drug describe the interaction of that drug with the target cell, usually in the form of a specific interaction with a protein macromolecule, a *receptor*. Receptors are classified on the basis of observed responses to specific agonists and antagonists. Multiple subtypes of receptors are often identified, such as alpha-1- and alpha-2-adrenergic receptors. Some receptors, such as the steroid hormone receptors, are located in the cytoplasm, but most are within the cell membrane. Their receptor sites face outward from the cell membrane; substances with poor lipid solubility do not need to cross the cell membrane in order to exert their effect. (Many endogenous catecholamines and polypeptide hormones have poor lipid solubilities.)

Because the density of receptors in the cell membrane may change, the response to a given concentration of drug may vary widely, depending on the status of receptors on the target cells. An excess of drug or endogenous substance (e.g., catecholamines in pheochromocytoma) leads to a decreased concentration of receptors in the cell membrane (downregulation) and a decreased pharmacologic effect at the same drug concentration. Tachyphylaxis to exogenous catecholamines may occur for the same reason. Chronic antagonist therapy leads to the opposite condition, an increase in receptor concentration (upregulation). This probably explains the rebound seen after abrupt cessation of beta-antagonist therapy. Endogenous catecholamines, now unopposed by an antagonist, produce exaggerated responses because of the increased number of available receptors.

The *intrinsic pharmacologic activity* of a substance refers to the nature of its interaction with a receptor (agonist, partial agonist, antagonist), the nature of the interacting receptor (histamine receptor, catecholamine receptor), and more precisely, the receptor subtype (H_1 or H_2, α_1, α_2, β_1, β_2, etc.). The intrinsic activity determines the potential pharmacologic effect exerted by the substance (i.e., the efficacy of the drug).

The affinity of a substance for its corresponding receptor determines the concentration of substance necessary to occupy and activate receptor sites. This determines the potency of the drug. Changes in receptor density also may influence the potency of a drug, as described earlier.

■ Dose-Response Relationships

Because all drugs have multiple effects, a single dose-response curve describes only one effect of a drug. A family of dose-response curves, each describing one of the many distinct pharmacologic effects of the drug, must be considered when assessing a drug. A narcotic drug has one curve describing its analgesic properties, another describing its respiratory depressant effect, another describing its effect on vasodilatation, and so on.

Assuming that a drug exerts its pharmacologic effect by binding reversibly with receptors and that the effect of a given dose is linearly related to the fraction of receptors occupied, then the effect of a drug concentration [D] can be described by the following equation:

$$\text{Fraction of maximum effect} = [D]/(K_D + [D])$$

where [D] = concentration of free drug
K_D = dissociation constant (k_2/k_1) of the drug-receptor complex

This is the same analysis applied to enzyme substrate interactions described in the Michaelis-Menten equation. The effect plotted against dose results in the curve shown in Figure 7-8. As in the Michaelis-Menten model, when [D] = 0, there is no effect; when [D] = K_D, half the receptors are occupied, and the effect is half maximal; as the dose increases, the effect approaches the maximum as the asymptote. Because a wide range of doses is often studied, it is more convenient to display the log dose on the abscissa. This produces the familiar sigmoid-shaped dose-response curve seen in Figure 7-9.

Four important parameters are considered when analyzing the dose-response curve: potency, slope, efficacy or power, and individual variation (see Fig. 7-9).

Potency

Potency is not a description of the magnitude of the pharmacologic effect produced but merely a

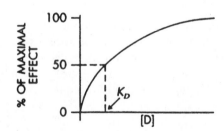

Figure 7-8

The relationship of the concentration of a drug and the magnitude of the response to it, with arithmetic abscissa and ordinate.

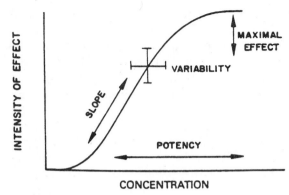

Figure 7-9

Plot of the magnitude of a drug effect against the logarithm of the concentration, showing the four characteristics of the dose-response curve: efficacy, or maximum effect; potency, or the amount of drug required to produce the effect; slope, or the rate at which effect changes with respect to dose; and variability.

statement of how much of the drug is required. Lack of potency becomes a limiting factor only when so much drug is required to produce an effect that it is difficult to administer.

If the potency of a drug is judged from dose-response curves, then pharmacokinetic factors such as absorption, distribution, and elimination affect the results. If concentration response curves are examined, these confounding effects are eliminated, but there is still considerable interpatient variability. The potencies of two drugs can be compared only if their dose-response curves are parallel. Otherwise, the curves would be closer together on the dose axis (similar potency) at one point and farther apart (different potency) at another. The curves might even cross. In such a case, at a lesser dose one drug is more potent, while at greater dose the other drug is more potent.

The potencies of drugs used in anesthesia are often characterized in terms of the ED_{50}, or *median effective dose*, which is the dose necessary to produce a specific response in 50 percent of subjects. When dealing with binary drug effects, such as awake or asleep, the dose is plotted against the percentage of subjects who displayed the specific drug effect being studied. The *lethal dose* of a drug is often expressed in similar terms; the LD_{50} is the dose of drug that is fatal to 50 percent of subjects.

An inherently safe drug has an LD_{50} that is much greater than the ED_{50}. The *therapeutic index* is the ratio of the median lethal to the median effective doses (LD_{50}/ED_{50}); a large therapeutic index implies a greater margin of safety, but only for a particular pharmacologic effect of the drug. Thus, if the drug effect desired is antiplatelet effect, aspirin has a large therapeutic index; if the effect desired is relief of severe rheumatoid arthritis, the ED_{50} is greater and the therapeutic index correspondingly less. Likewise, the conditions under which the drug is used must be specified to define lethality. In unattended patients, a muscle relaxant would have small LD_{50}; when mechanical ventilation is supplied, the LD_{50} and the therapeutic index are much greater. As compared with safe drugs such as aspirin, the drugs used to produce anesthesia possess small therapeutic indices. Lethal alveolar concentrations of potent inhaled anesthetics such as halothane are only a few times those required to produce anesthesia. Because 1.05 atm of nitrous oxide is required to produce surgical anesthesia in half the population, the LD_{50} for this drug (as the result of hypoxia) is actually less than its ED_{50} for surgical anesthesia.

Slope

The slope of the dose-response curve is related to the number of receptors that must be occupied to produce the pharmacologic effect. If a drug must occupy a large fraction of receptors before any effect is seen, the slope will be steep once the effect begins to appear. This is characteristic of nondepolarizing neuromuscular blockers as well as inhaled inhalation anesthetics. A steep slope implies that small increments in dose produce large increases in pharmacologic effect. It is also likely that the difference between therapeutic dose and toxic dose will be small. Drugs with steeply sloped dose-response curves demand careful titration to achieve the desired effect in all patients.

Efficacy

The efficacy of a drug is the maximum pharmacologic effect that the drug can produce and is unrelated to potency. Efficacy is determined by the intrinsic activity of the drug in its interaction with cell membrane receptors. In practice, the efficacy of a drug may be limited by the appearance of side effects within the dose range needed to produce the desired effect, as the dose-response curves for the desired effect and the undesired side effect overlap.

Individual Variation

Whereas the usual dose-response curves describe the behavior of a population, interpatient variation may make an individual patient's response unpredictable. All the factors described above that influence pharmacokinetics (bioavailability, renal and hepatic function, age) or pharmacodynamics (genetic differences, receptor density) come into play to enhance the variability of patients' responses, along with coexisting diseases and drug interactions. The combination of interpatient variability, steep dose-response curves, and small therapeutic indices make the drugs used in anesthesia particularly dangerous.

These hazards are overcome in several ways. Precise monitoring of the effect of the drug (e.g., nerve stimulators with neuromuscular blockers) or of the amounts of drugs used (e.g., precision vaporizers, mass spectrometers, or oximeters) add to safety. Knowledge of the patient factors that alter responses allows the anesthesiologist to adjust doses accordingly and to choose drugs with side effects that are least harmful for a specific patient. Combinations of drugs, each chosen to achieve a specific effect, may produce fewer side effects than a large dose of a single drug given to achieve the same spectrum of effects. This is the argument in favor of combinations of nitrous oxide, opioids, sedatives, muscle relaxants, and sometimes small amounts of inhaled anesthetics ("balanced anesthesia"). Unfortunately, the side effects as well as the therapeutic effects of drugs used in combination summate too; the technique is not a guarantee of freedom from unwanted anesthetic side effects.

The practice of administering drugs in divided doses and allowing time to assess the effects of one dose before giving the next adds greatly to safety, as does the analogous habit of decreasing at intervals the rate of a drug infusion or the concentration of an inhaled agent to ascertain whether less anesthetic might be needed. Most new anesthetic drugs are introduced not because they produced a novel therapeutic effect but because they offer the promise of a better therapeutic index. Newer muscle relaxants do not produce more profound muscle relaxation than does curare, but they can be applied more easily to a wider range of patients without producing side effects such as prolonged paralysis, hypotension, or tachycardia. Similar principles apply to the introduction of newer narcotics and even inhalation anesthetics.

■ Choosing the Dose

An understanding of the dose-response curve and its potential variability allows the anesthesiologist to estimate the magnitude of dose required to elicit the desired effect. When using drugs with relatively rapid onset and a small therapeutic index, the safest method is usually titration, the successive administration of small aliquots, separated by time intervals that permit assessment of the clinical effect on the patient. When a predetermined endpoint is reached, such as respiratory depression signaled by a respiratory rate of 6 to 8 breaths per minute, no further drug is given.

A novel approach to selecting doses, especially with synthetic narcotics, is computer-guided constant infusion based on the known pharmacokinetics and pharmacodynamics of the particular drug. A target plasma concentration is selected based on knowledge of the dose-response curve. The loading dose needed to achieve the target plasma concentration (during the distribution phase of the two-compartment model) equals the product of the volume of distribution and the target plasma concentration. Once the target concentration is achieved, a maintenance dose of additional drug is supplied to replace the drug eliminated (during the elimination phase; see Fig. 7-5). The maintenance dose is a function of the target concentration and systemic clearance rate. Computer programs based on two-compartment mathematical models, as described above, regulate a pump that delivers the drug at the rate necessary to maintain the desired concentration. Such systems do not replace clinical judgment. Patient variability, coexisting disease, and surgical situations all influence how a particular patient responds to the doses administered.

BIBLIOGRAPHY

Eger EI II, ed. *Anesthetic Uptake and Action*. Baltimore: Williams & Wilkins, 1974.

Gilman AG, Goodman LS, Rall RW, Murad F, eds. *The Pharmacological Basis of Therapeutics*, 9th ed. New York: Macmillan, 1995.

Stanski DR, Watkins WD. *Drug Disposition in Anesthesia*. Orlando, Fla: Grune & Stratton, 1982.

CHAPTER **8**

The Inhaled Anesthetics

Albert T. Cheung and Bryan E. Marshall

The discovery of general anesthesia ranks among the great achievements in medicine, for it enabled surgical operations to be performed without pain. Despite an incomplete understanding of their mechanisms of action, the inhaled anesthetics are universally effective in all living organisms and are sufficient alone to provide complete anesthesia. The uptake and elimination of these drugs are unique, depending on equilibrium between the gas and blood across the alveolar membrane. Modern techniques control precisely the delivered concentrations of the anesthetic to achieve desired effects.

The anesthetic action of nitrous oxide was first described in 1799 and its medical importance was recognized by Horace Wells in 1844, but its lack of potency limited its initial use and range of applications. The first successful public demonstration of general anesthesia was performed by William Morton in 1846 using diethyl ether. Over the succeeding years, other compounds were adopted and subsequently replaced by newer agents chosen to avoid adverse side effects (Fig. 8-1). Thus diethyl ether was supplanted because it was flammable, induced copious airway secretions, and caused severe postoperative nausea and vomiting. Chloroform (1847) was hepatotoxic and produced severe cardiovascular depression. Cyclopropane (1929) was highly flammable. Trichloroethylene (1934) reacted with soda lime to form the toxic gas phosgene. Fluroxene (1954), the first fluorinated volatile anesthetic, was flammable and produced nausea and vomiting. Methoxyflurane (1959) was metabolized in the liver to release free fluoride ions that were nephrotoxic. Although ether is still in use in some parts of the world, the only inhaled anesthetics employed in the United States are nitrous oxide, halothane, isoflurane, enflurane, desflurane, and sevoflurane.

Despite the effectiveness of the inhaled anesthetics, they are among the most difficult drugs to use. Because of their narrow margins of safety and variations among patients, constant attention to the dose and continuous physiologic monitoring of the anesthetized patient are required. Concentrations of anesthetic only slightly less than the effective concentration may fail to produce general anesthesia and adequate operating conditions. Concentrations effective for producing surgical anesthesia frequently cause significant depression of central nervous, respiratory, circulatory, and neuromuscular function that require continuous life support.

Chemical Structure and Physical Properties

The chemical structure and physical properties of the anesthetic gases determine how they are stored, the equipment required for administration, their pharmacokinetic behavior, and in part their pharmacologic actions (Fig. 8-2 and Table 8-1).

Nitrous oxide is a gas at room temperature and atmospheric pressure. It is supplied in pressurized steel tanks. At a pressure of 50 atm (745 lb/in^2), it remains a liquid at temperatures up to 36°C. As nitrous oxide is used, the pressure within a tank remains at 745 lb/in^2 until all the liquid has been vaporized, so the amount of nitrous oxide remaining in the tank is measured by weight, not pressure. Though it is not flammable, nitrous oxide supports combustion.

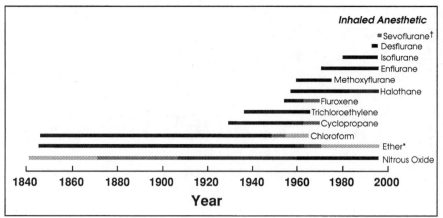

Figure 8-1

Year of clinical introduction and approximate year of discontinuation of selected inhaled anesthetics. *Ether is still used in parts of the world but not in the United States. †Sevoflurane was approved in 1995 for clinical use in the United States.

Halothane, enflurane, and isoflurane are colorless liquids at room temperature with vapor pressures at 20°C of 243, 172, and 238 mmHg, respectively. Anesthetic vaporizers (see Chap. 5) control precisely the concentrations of vaporized gases that are delivered in the breathing mixture.

Halothane is stored as a liquid in tinted glass bottles with 0.01% thymol and 0.00025% ammonia as stabilizing agents to prevent photochemical decomposition. Some metal, plastic, and rubber components of the anesthesia machine are damaged by prolonged exposure to the anesthetic, and halothane vaporizers require periodic cleaning to prevent the accumulation of thymol deposits. Halothane undergoes biotransformation by mixed-function oxidases in the liver, so as much as 20 percent of the administered dose can be recovered as nonvolatile byproducts in the urine (mainly bromide ions and trifluoroacetic acid).

Enflurane (1972) and isoflurane (1981) differ from halothane by the replacement of bromine with fluorine and by the introduction of an ether link into the structure of the anesthetic molecule. The strong carbon-fluoride bond increases the stability of these agents, eliminating the requirement for stabilizing agents and decreasing biotransformation and the release of potentially toxic metabolites. The ether link is associated with a reduced incidence of cardiac arrhythmias.

Desflurane (1993) was synthesized by substituting fluorine for the chlorine in enflurane. This enhances stability, lessens biotransformation, and decreases solubility in blood. Because the boiling point of desflurane is very close to ambient temperature, it is stored in bottles sealed by a valve that only opens when it is attached to the filler port of the vaporizer.

The desflurane vaporizer heats the liquid in a sealed chamber to form gaseous desflurane that is added to the carrier gas in metered proportions.

Sevoflurane (1995), like nitrous oxide and desflurane, is not very soluble in blood, permitting rapid induction and recovery from general anesthesia. Sevoflurane is less pungent than desflurane and does not require a special apparatus for administration. In some circumstances, significant concentrations (>50 μM/liter) of free fluoride have been detected in adults anesthetized with sevoflurane, suggesting the

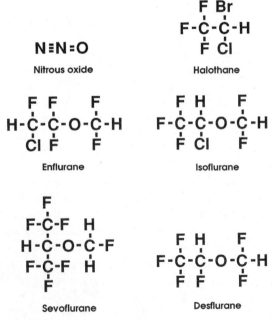

Figure 8-2

Chemical structures of the inhaled anesthetics. Note that isoflurane and enflurane are structural isomers.

Table 8-1

General Properties of Inhaled Anesthetics

	Nitrous Oxide	Isoflurane	Enflurane	Halothane	Desflurane	Sevoflurane
Molecular wieght	44	184.5	184.5	197.4	168	200.1
Boiling point (°C) at 1 atm	−89	48.5	56.5	50.2	23.5	58.6
Vapor pressure at 20°C (mmHg)	Gas	238	172	243	664	157
Partition coefficients at 37°C						
Blood:gas	0.47	1.4	1.8	2.3	0.42	0.66
Brain:blood	1.1	2.6	1.4	2.9	1.3	1.7
Muscle:blood	1.2	4	1.7	3.5	2	3.1
Fat:blood	2.3	45	36	60	27	51
Rubber:gas	1.2	62	74	120	19	11
MAC in 100% oxygen (%)*	105	1.2	1.8	0.75	6	1.6–2.5
MAC in 70% nitrous oxide (%)*	—	0.5	0.57	0.29	2.8	0.9–1.4
MAC, awake (%)*	68	0.43	0.51	0.41	2.4	0.63
Stability						
Alkali	Stable	Stable	Stable	Some instability	Stable	Some instability‡
Ultraviolet light	Stable	Stable	Stable	Unstable	Stable	Stable
Metal	Stable	Stable	Stable	Corrosive	Stable	Stable
Preservative	None	None	None	Thymol	None	None
Percent recovered as metabolites	0†	0.2	2.4	20	0	5§

*Values apply to adults ranging in age from 25 to 60 years.
†Trace metabolism by gut flora.
‡Breakdown products formed in presence of soda lime (compound A: 32 ppm; compound B: <1.5 ppm) and Baralyme (compound A: 61 ppm; compound B: <1.5 ppm).
§Inorganic fluoride concentrations >50 μmol/liter detected in 7 percent of adults.

potential for nephrotoxicity. Sevoflurane reacts with soda lime to form degradation products that in large doses cause organ toxicity in animals.

Pharmacokinetics of the Inhaled Anesthetics

◾Anesthetic Uptake, Distribution, and Elimination

The inhaled anesthetic gases move rapidly across the pulmonary blood-alveolar gas interface. The partial pressure of the anesthetic in the alveolar gas determines the partial pressure of the anesthetic in the blood and consequently in the central nervous system and other potential sites of anesthetic action. The pharmacokinetics of anesthetic gases depend on the partial pressure of the anesthetic in the inspired gases, alveolar ventilation, the distribution and volume of pulmonary blood flow, the transfer of anesthetic from the alveoli into pulmonary capillary blood, uptake from the blood into body tissues, and elimination by ventilation, metabolism, and percutaneous diffusion.

The dose of an inhaled anesthetic is controlled by adjusting the vaporizer to change the concentration of the gas mixture entering the breathing circuit. Changes in the alveolar concentration of anesthetic follow changes in the vaporizer setting after a delay that depends on several factors. First, the gas already in the anesthesia breathing circuit must be replaced with fresh gas containing the new anesthetic concentration. This occurs quickly in nonrebreathing circuits but may take several minutes (depending on the rate of fresh gas flow) in a circle system (Fig. 8-3). Second, the anesthetic in the inspired limb of the circle system is diluted by the rebreathing of exhaled gas. Third, anesthetic uptake by soda lime and other components of the breathing circuit may reduce transiently the inspired concentration of the gas.

The delivery of gases from the breathing circuit to the alveoli depends on the minute ventilation. Increasing the minute ventilation decreases the time needed for the alveolar gas concentration to reach equilibrium with the inspired gas concentration. Airway obstruction, increased anatomic deadspace, an increased ratio of body weight to minute ventilation and perfusion, or depressed respiration also increase the time required to reach equilibrium. Finally, a

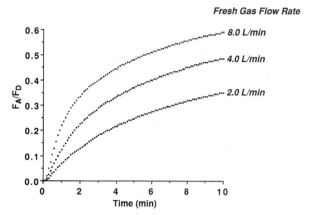

Figure 8-3

The increase in the alveolar concentration of isoflurane (FA) as a proportion of the concentration delivered from the anesthetic vaporizer (FD) at three different fresh gas flows. Increasing the fresh gas flow increases the rate of equilibration between the delivered and end-tidal anesthetic concentrations. The data were derived from a pharmacokinetic simulation of an adult patient breathing from an anesthetic machine circle system with a circuit volume of 6 liters.

phenomenon referred to as the *second-gas effect* alters anesthetic uptake and elimination when nitrous oxide is administered together with a volatile anesthetic. The rapid uptake of nitrous oxide increases the effective minute ventilation during the induction of anesthesia by increasing the flow of gases into the alveoli from the tracheobronchial tree. Further, the uptake of nitrous oxide from the alveoli decreases the volume of gas remaining within the alveoli and thus increases the concentrations of the remaining gases within the alveoli, speeding the induction of general anesthesia. The reverse also occurs and is responsible for diffusion hypoxia when nitrous oxide administration is discontinued. The rapid diffusion of nitrous oxide from the blood into the alveoli decreases the alveolar oxygen tension and can cause a brief period of hypoxia. Diffusion hypoxia can be prevented by administering supplemental oxygen.

The partitioning of anesthetics between the alveoli and the pulmonary capillary blood depends on the solubility of the anesthetic in blood, described by the *blood:gas solubility coefficient*. This is the ratio of the anesthetic concentrations in the blood and gas phases at equilibrium when the partial pressures of the anesthetic are same in the blood and in the gas phase. For example, at 37°C, blood in equilibrium with 1% enflurane contains 1.8 vol% enflurane (i.e., a blood: gas solubility coefficient of 1.8). During induction, the rate of increase in the alveolar concentration of the

anesthetic is more rapid for agents with lesser blood: gas solubility coefficients (Fig. 8-4). Insoluble anesthetics such as nitrous oxide, desflurane, and sevoflurane are notably faster acting than are soluble anesthetics such as halothane or ether. Similarly, during emergence, less soluble anesthetics are cleared more quickly than are more soluble ones.

The transfer of anesthetics from the alveoli to the blood is also determined by the pulmonary blood flow, the matching of ventilation to perfusion within the lung, the presence of shunt flow, and the concentration of the anesthetic in the mixed venous blood. Diminished pulmonary blood flow or reduced cardiac output decreases the rate at which anesthetic is removed from the lungs, thus promoting a more rapid increase in the alveolar anesthetic concentration. Mismatching of ventilation to perfusion and right-to-left shunts decrease the arterial concentration of anesthesia.

Uptake and accumulation of inhaled anesthetics also occur as the anesthetic is transported to body tissues from the arterial blood. The tissue concentrations of the anesthetic depend on tissue blood flow,

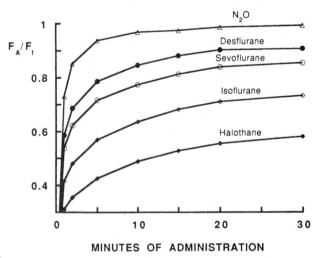

Figure 8-4

Increase in the alveolar concentration (FA) toward the inspired concentration (FI) of inhaled anesthetics over time. The least soluble anesthetics (N_2O, desflurane, and sevoflurane) show the most rapid increase in their alveolar concentrations during the induction of general anesthesia. The rapid increase in the alveolar concentration of nitrous oxide is explained in part by the second-gas effect (see text). The rate of increase in FA/FI for enflurane (not shown) lies between that of halothane and isoflurane.

(From Eger EI, New inhaled anesthetics. Anesthesiology 1994;80:907.)

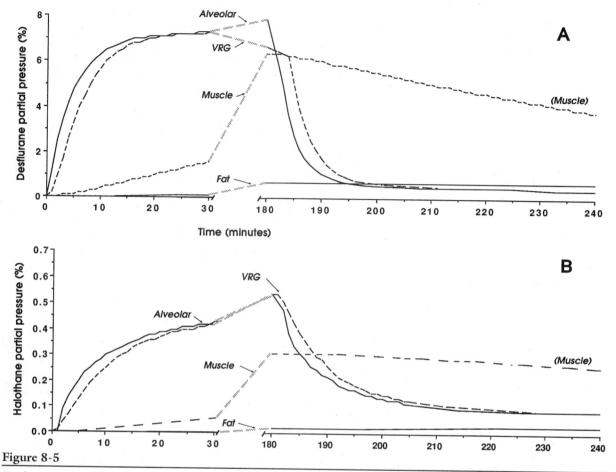

Figure 8-5

Desflurane (*A*) and halothane (*B*) concentrations in the alveoli, vessel-rich organ group (VRG), muscle, and fat as a function of time during the course of an anesthetic in a typical adult patient. The inhaled anesthetic was administered at a concentration of 1.5 MAC into a circle system with a fresh gas flow of 3 liters/min for 180 minutes and then discontinued. The fresh gas flow was increased to 6 liters/min during the elimination phase. Inhaled anesthetics such as halothane that have greater blood:gas and tissue:blood partition coefficients exhibit a more gradual increase in tissue anesthetic concentrations during administration and a more gradual decrease in tissue anesthetic concentrations during elimination.

the tissue:blood solubility coefficient, and the duration of exposure to the anesthetic (Fig. 8-5). Anesthetics are soluble in fat and accumulate because of the constant but slow blood flow to this tissue compartment.

Volatile anesthetics diffuse into gas-filled cavities within the body; this is most troublesome with nitrous oxide, which is administered in concentrations as great as 80%. The principal gas within body cavities is usually nitrogen. Because nitrous oxide is more soluble in blood than is nitrogen, the influx of nitrous oxide into a gas-filled cavity exceeds the rate of elimination of nitrogen from the cavity. The resulting increase in volume and pressure may worsen the consequences of air embolism, pneumothorax, or pneumocephalus. This process is inconsequential for the halogenated anesthetics, which are administered only in dilute concentrations.

The elimination of the inhaled anesthetics occurs primarily through the lungs and is governed by the same principles that apply to their uptake (see Fig. 8-5). Other elimination pathways such as biotransformation and diffusion through the skin contribute minimally.

■ Clinical Application of Pharmacokinetic Principles

Applying these pharmacokinetic principles allows some control over the speed of induction and emer-

Table 8-2

Factors that Affect the Rate of Uptake and Elimination of Inhaled Anesthetics

Factors that increase the rate of anesthetic induction
  Increased anesthetic concentration entering the breathing circuit
  Increased fresh gas flow
  Increased alveolar ventilation
  Diminished cardiac output
  Second gas effect
  Nonrebreathing circuits
  Low blood:gas solubility coefficient

Factors that increase the rate of recovery from anesthesia
  Increased fresh gas flow
  Increased alveolar ventilation
  Nonrebreathing circuits
  Low blood:gas solubility coefficient
  Low tissue:gas solubility coefficient
  Decreased duration of anesthetic

gence from anesthesia. Induction can be hastened by selecting an insoluble agent, increasing the inspired concentration of the anesthetic, increasing fresh gas flow, eliminating rebreathing, assisting ventilation, and employing the second-gas effect (Table 8-2), but careful monitoring is required to avoid overdose.

The physiologic actions of anesthetics also affect their pharmacokinetics. Depression of respiration in a spontaneously breathing patient slows induction and emergence; increased minute ventilation due to pain or arousal hastens these processes. Increases in cardiac output due to pain, excitement, or light anesthesia enhance the removal of the anesthetic from the lungs and thus retard induction.

During maintenance, an appropriate depth of general anesthesia is maintained by administering an inspired concentration slightly greater than the end-expired anesthetic concentration so that anesthetic transfer into body tissues is balanced by anesthetic uptake in the lungs. Because tissue uptake is greater for more soluble agents, the disparity between inspired and expired anesthetic concentrations is greatest for soluble agents and least for insoluble anesthetics. As the inspired and blood concentrations of the anesthetic equalize, anesthetic delivery is less affected by the rate of fresh gas flow.

Anesthetics accumulate in body tissues over time. The total body content of anesthetic depends on the duration of anesthesia, body mass, and the tissue:blood solubility coefficients of the anesthetic. Increased body fat content, increased fat solubility of the anesthetic, and increased duration of anesthesia all-

prolong the elimination of the anesthetic. Administering nitrous oxide, which is relatively insoluble in fat, decreases the amount required of the more lipid soluble volatile anesthetics, thereby lessening tissue accumulation of the fat-soluble volatile anesthetic during lengthy operations.

Emergence from anesthesia begins with discontinuing the anesthetic and can be facilitated by increasing the fresh gas flow, decreasing rebreathing, and increasing minute ventilation (see Table 8-2). The relatively gradual decrease in the alveolar concentration of a typical volatile agent may leave the patient in an intermediate depth of anesthesia (stage II), too deep to permit safe extubation of the trachea yet too light to block reflex responses to pain. This problem can be obviated by relying during this phase of the anesthetic on an insoluble anesthetic such as nitrous oxide that will permit rapid emergence when it is discontinued.

Efficient delivery of inhaled anesthetics can reduce costs. When fresh gas flows exceed uptake, excess gas leaves the breathing circuit via the pressure relief valve and is lost to the scavenging system. Closed or low-flow breathing systems reduce these losses to a minimum and are convenient to use during anesthetic maintenance when anesthetic concentrations are close to steady-state levels. Oxygen and agent monitors eliminate uncertainty about the concentrations of gases in the breathing circuit when using low-flow techniques.

Pharmacologic Actions of the Inhaled Anesthetics

■ Depth of Anesthesia

Establishing dose-response relationships requires measuring both the dose of a drug and the magnitude of its effects. For inhaled anesthetics, it is easy to measure the dose precisely but difficult to define the effect. It has proven impossible to make a single numerical measurement that is related to the amount of anesthesia produced; the anesthetic state is a composite of many effects. Further, the site of action of inhaled anesthetics has not been established. In 1965, Eger introduced the *minimum alveolar concentration* (MAC) as a standard measure of the potency of inhaled anesthetics. MAC is defined as the equilibrium end-tidal anesthetic concentration, expressed as a fraction of 1 atm, that prevents movement in response to surgical skin incision in 50 percent of human subjects. This defines the therapeutic effect of anesthetics as the prevention of movement in response to surgical stimulation.

The MAC for each of the inhaled anesthetics has been determined under standard conditions (see Table 8-1), providing a reasonable estimate of anesthetic requirements. At an alveolar concentration of approximately 1.3 MAC, 99 percent of subjects do not move in response to surgical stimulation. Further, if the MAC values of several anesthetics in a mixture sum to 1 MAC, the mixture prevents movement in 50 percent of subjects, just as 1 MAC of a single agent would. In practice, an anesthetic mixture consisting of 55% nitrous oxide (0.5 MAC) and 3% desflurane (0.5 MAC) is as effective as 6% desflurane.

The potency of an anesthetic (assessed as MAC) varies with the patient's age and health, clinical conditions, and the administration of other drugs (Table 8-3). MAC is approximately 10 percent greater in infants and young children than in young adults and is decreased by approximately 6 percent in the elderly. Chronic alcohol use, hyperosmolar states, and the acute ingestion of central nervous system stimulants, such as dextroamphetamine and cocaine, increase MAC. Pregnancy, decreased body temperature, and hypo-osmolar states decrease MAC. Intravenous anesthetics, sedatives, hypnotics, tranquilizers, and analgesics acutely decrease anesthetic

Table 8-3

Factors that Modify MAC	
Increase MAC	**Decrease MAC**
Young age	Old age
Hyperthermia	Hypothermia
CNS hypo-osmolality	CNS hyperosmolality
Habituation to alcohol	Acute effects of alcohol
CNS stimulants	CNS depressants
Dextroamphetamine	Benzodiazepines
Cocaine	Barbiturates
	Propofol
Physostigmine	Tranquilizers
	Chlorpromazine
	CNS effects of local anesthetics
	Narcotics
	Pregnancy
	Alpha-2-adrenergic agonists
	Clonidine
	Dexmedetomidine

requirements and decrease the MAC of the inhalational anesthetics.

The use of anesthetic adjuvants and patient-to-patient variability make it impossible to predict the concentration of inhaled anesthetic required for a given patient. The physical signs (decreases in heart rate and blood pressure, regular shallow breathing, and conjugate miotic pupils) used traditionally to gauge the depth of anesthesia with drugs such as diethyl ether are of limited use with the halogenated hydrocarbon anesthetics. These signs of anesthetic depth are often obscured by other drug effects. Antihypertensive medications and beta-adrenergic antagonists modify circulatory responses; narcotics and anticholinergic drugs change pupillary size; muscle relaxants and controlled ventilation eliminate respiratory signs.

A more rational way of determining the dose of anesthetic drugs is to abandon the idea of a univariate function called the *depth of anesthesia* (whether MAC or some other description) and assess simultaneously the several effects that make up the anesthetic state. These include attenuated physiologic responses to surgical stress, adequate operating conditions, analgesia, amnesia, and unconsciousness. Controlling the physiologic responses may entail regulating heart rate or contractility, blood pressure, and muscle tone. Adequate operating conditions may range from simple immobility to control of intracranial pressure or providing hypothermic cardiac arrest as needed. Assessing consciousness may be simple, if the patient receives no muscle relaxants and does not respond to verbal stimuli or to surgical incision; at other times, it may be almost impossible to determine whether the paralyzed, narcotized patient is amnestic or unconscious.

The concentration of inhaled anesthetic required to block the autonomic responses to nociceptive stimuli is about 1.7 to 2.0 times the MAC and is sometimes referred to as the *MAC-beta-adrenergic response* (MAC-BAR). However, at these concentrations, inhaled anesthetics often produce other unwanted effects, such as arrhythmias, tachycardia, hypotension, and delayed emergence.

No single anesthetic, whether inhaled or given intravenously, provides all the components of satisfactory anesthesia, as defined in the modern context, without some unwanted side effect. To overcome their individual limitations, inhaled anesthetics are often combined or used with other drugs and techniques. Nitrous oxide provides additional analgesia and partial anesthesia. Narcotics provide analgesia, muscle relaxants prevent movement, and regional anesthetic techniques block nociception. Applied in this context, the primary role of the inhaled anesthetics may be to ensure unconsciousness and blunt cardiovascular reflexes. The dose of inhaled anesthetic necessary to produce unconsciousness is about half the MAC for preventing movement and is sometimes referred to as *MAC-awake*.

■ Nervous System

General anesthesia with inhaled anesthetics entails the loss of consciousness and the suppression of normal reflexes, but other effects on the central nervous system occur as well. Cerebral metabolic activity is depressed, most effectively by isoflurane, desflurane, and sevoflurane and to a lesser extent by halothane and enflurane. Accounting for much of this metabolic depression is progressive depression of both spontaneous and stimulated neural electrical activity. Isoflurane, at an end-tidal concentration of 2.5%, produces an isoelectric electroencephalographic (EEG) pattern, and the potent inhaled anesthetics generally decrease the amplitude and increase the latency of somatosensory, motor, auditory, and visual evoked potentials. Synaptic conduction is slowed during anesthesia as well; the speed and amplitude of action potentials decrease progressively as they travel toward the cerebral cortex. The role of neuronal depression in the mechanism of general anesthesia is unclear, but these effects must be taken into account in using intraoperative neurophysiologic monitoring.

Neural electrical activity is not always depressed during anesthesia. Concentrations of nitrous oxide that produce unconsciousness cause rapid EEG activity. Especially with hyperventilation, enflurane occasionally may cause generalized tonic-clonic seizures accompanied by high-voltage EEG activity and increased cerebral oxygen demand. Although it usually produces a dose-dependent decrease in EEG fast activity, most practitioners avoid enflurane in patients with seizure disorders.

All the inhaled anesthetics cause dose-dependent dilation of the cerebral vasculature. Cerebral vasodilation may increase intracranial pressure as a consequence of increased intracranial blood volume, perhaps increasing the risk of cerebral herniation in susceptible patients with intracranial mass lesions. Concentrations of isoflurane or desflurane in the range of 0.2 to 0.6 MAC do not change the cerebrovascular responsiveness to CO_2 and can be used in combination with hyperventilation to anesthetize patients with increased intracranial pressure.

Abnormalities such as the Babinski sign and decerebrate or decorticate posturing, shivering, depressed cognitive function, and impaired ability to perform fine motor tasks often appear as patients recover from general anesthesia. The duration of these deficits varies depending on the duration and concentration of the anesthetic administered, the lingering effects of adjuvant anesthetic drugs, and the physical condition of the patient. Sensitive psychomotor testing reveals that minimal impairment of thinking may persist for several days, but patients may resume tasks such as driving 24 hours after recovery from general anesthesia.

■ Respiration and Gas Exchange

Inhaled anesthetics depress a broad range of respiratory functions. These include blunted or absent ventilatory responses to hypercarbia and hypoxia (Fig. 8-6), decreased minute ventilation, and increased arterial CO_2 tension; hypoxic ventilatory drive is inhibited markedly at 0.1 MAC and abolished at 1.0

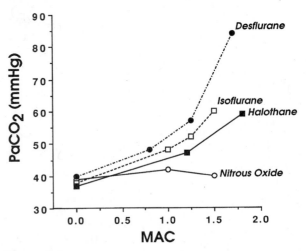

Figure 8-6

The relationship between arterial carbon dioxide tension ($PaCO_2$) and inhaled anesthetic dose (MAC) in anesthetized, spontaneously breathing volunteers. Except for nitrous oxide, all the potent inhaled anesthetics cause a dose-dependent decrease in respiratory drive.

(Modified from Eger EI, Desflurane: A Compendium and Reference. Rutherford, NJ: Healthpress Publishing Group, 1993, p 31.)

MAC. Spontaneous ventilation with inhaled agents is rapid, regular, and shallow; although the accompanying use of opioids may slow and deepen breathing, they further depress ventilation. Shallow breathing, lack of sighing, and absence of coughing may contribute to atelectasis in patients breathing spontaneously under anesthesia. Relaxation of skeletal muscles leads to upper airway obstruction and decreased diaphragmatic strength. These depressant effects of the inhaled anesthetics can be treated by controlled or assisted ventilation and by maneuvers to maintain airway patency during anesthesia. Effects persist during recovery until all residual anesthetics have been eliminated. Narcotic analgesics, sedative and hypnotic agents, residual neuromuscular blocking drugs, and pulmonary diseases all worsen these effects.

Most inhaled anesthetics are pungent and irritating to awake or partially anesthetized patients, accounting for such problems during induction as coughing, breath holding, excessive airway secretions, and laryngospasm. Desflurane is particularly pungent and not recommended for use to induce general anesthesia by mask. Isoflurane is less irritating, and halothane and sevoflurane are well tolerated. Nitrous oxide causes virtually no airway irritation.

Inhaled anesthetics cause bronchodilation by direct action on the tracheobronchial tree and by inhibiting airway reflexes that mediate bronchoconstriction. At surgical levels of anesthesia, patients with reactive airway disease almost always benefit from this effect. A few patients with asthma have experienced exacerbations during and after enflurane anesthesia. Fear of the irritating effects of pungent agents may lead to choosing halothane or sevoflurane, but desflurane and isoflurane can provide satisfactory anesthesia for these patients also.

Pulmonary arterial vasodilation by inhaled anesthetics may impair hypoxic pulmonary vasoconstriction, a process by which blood flow is diverted from poorly ventilated regions to maintain even distribution of ventilation and perfusion in the lungs. Impaired hypoxic pulmonary vasoconstriction is of particular concern in patients with lung disease and in those undergoing one-lung ventilation, where matching of ventilation and perfusion are especially critical.

■ Circulation

The inhaled anesthetics cause circulatory depression, often manifested by hypotension. Blood pressure decreases because of vasodilation and depressed myocardial contractility and indirectly because of decreased sympathetic tone. When ventilation is controlled, these circulatory effects determine the maximum tolerated dose of an inhaled anesthetic. Overdose is manifested by hypotension, arrhythmias, bradycardia, decreased cardiac output, and cardiac arrest. Healthy patients tolerate the cardiovascular depression associated with usual doses of anesthetics, but patients in shock or those with significant ventricular dysfunction do not tolerate concentrations that are commonly used to produce anesthesia.

In a dose-dependent fashion, potent inhaled anesthetics depress left ventricular systolic function at any preload or any level of underlying sympathetic tone (Fig. 8-7), and they impair diastolic relaxation as well. The agents have minimal direct effects on left ventricular preload, but left and right ventricular end-diastolic pressures may increase during anesthesia as a consequence of impaired diastolic filling and decreased cardiac output (Fig. 8-8). Halothane and enflurane are the most potent direct myocardial depressants, followed by isoflurane, desflurane, sevoflurane, and nitrous oxide.

The impact of an individual anesthetic on cardiovascular function depends on specific effects on myocardial contractility, vascular smooth muscle tone, and sympathetic nervous system reflexes, as well as the dose of anesthetic, underlying disease states, blood loss, and underlying sympathetic tone. For example, hypotension with halothane represents decreased cardiac output due to myocardial depression, whereas with isoflurane cardiac output is changed little despite the decrease in myocardial contractility because heart rate is increased slightly and left ventricular afterload is reduced (Fig. 8-9). Sympathetic nervous system activity due to pain may mask signs of circulatory depression, whereas adrenergic antagonists exacerbate them.

Inhaled anesthetics may alter myocardial oxygen supply and demand and the potential for myocardial ischemia. Myocardial oxygen consumption usually is reduced due to afterload reduction and myocardial depression, but the increases in heart rate and sympathetic tone associated with isoflurane or desflurane may increase myocardial oxygen demand and cause ischemia in susceptible patients. Moreover, anesthetic-induced hypotension may decrease myocardial oxygen supply by reducing coronary perfusion pressure. The direct coronary artery vasodilating action of isoflurane may divert blood flow away from tissues supplied by partially obstructed coronary arteries, but isoflurane does not seem to increase the risk of myocardial ischemia except possibly in rare susceptible patients. In general, the inhaled anesthetics can be administered safely to patients with coronary artery disease when hemodynamic factors that alter myocardial oxygen supply and demand are monitored and controlled.

Inhaled anesthetics also can affect cardiac rhythm. Junctional rhythms can occur with all the inhaled anesthetics, most commonly with enflurane. Consequent loss of atrial augmentation of ventricular filling may contribute to decreased blood pressure during

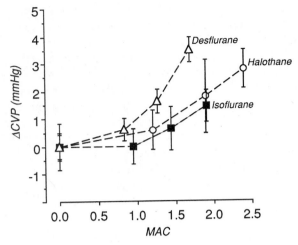

Figure 8-8

Dose-dependent changes in central venous pressure (ΔCVP) produced by halothane (**O**), isoflurane (**■**), and desflurane (Δ) in normocarbic adults.

(Data from Weiskopf RB, et al, Cardiovascular actions of desflurane in normocarbic volunteers. Anesth Analg 1991; 73:143–156).

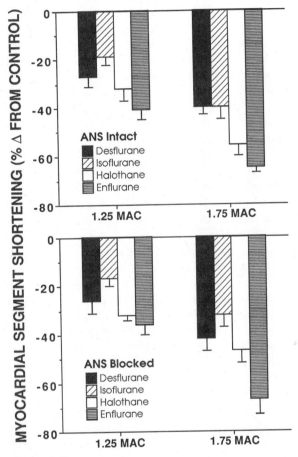

Figure 8-7

The actions of inhaled anesthetics on left ventricular myocardial segment shortening, as measured in chronically instrumented dogs with their autonomic nervous system (ANS) intact and blocked. All the inhaled anesthetics tested caused a significant decrease in segment shortening at both 1.25 and 1.75 MAC in comparison with awake animals.

(From Pagel PS, Kampine JP, Schmeling WT, Warltier DC, Comparison of the systemic and coronary hemodynamic actions of desflurane, isoflurane, and enflurane in the chronically instrumented dog. Anesthesiology 1991;74:539–551.)

anesthesia. Halothane sensitizes the myocardium to epinephrine-induced ventricular dysrhythmias. Given subcutaneously with lidocaine, 1.5 to 2.5 µg/kg of epinephrine causes ventricular premature contractions during anesthesia with halothane; four times this dose is required to produce ventricular ectopy with isoflurane, enflurane, or desflurane.

The actions of the inhaled anesthetics alter organ blood flow. In general, arterial vasodilation increases cutaneous blood flow, predisposing patients to heat loss during anesthesia. The autoregulation of blood flow in specific organs is generally blunted by the volatile anesthetics.

■ Renal Function

Anesthesia with inhaled anesthetics has little significant effect on renal function when other physiologic variables are controlled. Anesthetics, positive-pressure ventilation, and the cardiovascular depression that accompanies anesthesia result in reversible decreases in renal blood flow and glomerular filtration, but these can be corrected by fluid administration, and the changes are minor compared with those produced by blood loss and sympathetic responses. Modern anesthetics have no major effects on the function of native or transplanted kidneys, as assessed by subsequent changes in serum creatinine,

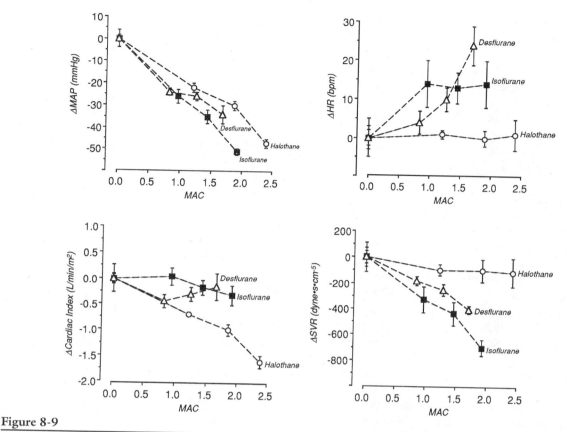

Figure 8-9

Dose-dependent changes in mean arterial pressure (ΔMAP), heart rate (ΔHR), cardiac index (ΔCardiac Index), and systemic vascular resistance (ΔSVR) produced by halothane (**O**), isoflurane (**■**), and desflurane (Δ) in normocarbic adults. Despite the myocardial depressant effects of isoflurane and desflurane, cardiac output is maintained during anesthesia with these agents in part because they decrease left ventricular afterload and increase the heart rate.
(Data from Weiskopf RB, et al, Cardiovascular actions of desflurane in normocarbic volunteers. Anesth Analg 1991;73: 143–156)

blood urea nitrogen, creatinine clearance, and urinalysis.

Methoxyflurane, which is no longer used, was nephrotoxic because it released free fluoride through biotransformation. Minor concentrations of free fluoride are detectable after the administration of the other fluorinated anesthetics, particularly sevoflurane and enflurane, but impaired renal function occurs only in unusual circumstances, such as prolonged exposure during unusually lengthy operations.

■ Gastrointestinal System

Postoperative nausea and vomiting occur less frequently after modern inhaled anesthetics than after older agents such as ether and cyclopropane. Nausea and vomiting are more common after narcotics or anticholinesterases (e.g., neostigmine) are administered or when abdominal operations are done.

Nitrous oxide distends air-filled viscera such as the stomach, small bowel, or colon. The extent of expansion depends on the concentration and duration of nitrous oxide administration; a period of approximately 100 minutes is required to double the volume of the air-filled space. This distension may contribute to postoperative nausea and vomiting and in the extreme may impede closing of the abdominal incision, but it has not been shown to impair the recovery of gastrointestinal function after abdominal operations.

Splanchnic blood flow is often reduced during inhalational anesthesia as a consequence of decreased blood pressure, decreased cardiac output, and increased sympathetic nervous system tone. In experimental studies, halothane, compared with enflurane, isoflurane, or desflurane, produces the greatest decrease in hepatic blood flow. Hepatic blood flow is generally maintained during isoflurane anesthesia. Halothane decreases hepatic blood flow by constricting hepatic arterial vessels and by decreasing visceral blood flow that subsequently enters the portal circulation. The mild decrease in splanchnic blood flow caused by the inhaled anesthetics has no clinically detectable effects except possibly in patients at risk for mesenteric or hepatic ischemia.

After operation, a few patients have experienced a reaction that is indistinguishable from viral hepatitis but is often attributed to the anesthetic exposure. The incidence of this idiosyncratic reaction is estimated to be in the range of 1 in 10,000 to 1 in 35,000 anesthetic administrations, although there remains legitimate debate about the epidemiologic evidence, given the much greater incidence of viral hepatitis in the surgical population. Reactions are usually ascribed to halothane and range from asymptomatic increases in liver enzymes to hepatic necrosis, which is often fatal and manifests itself 2 to 5 days after the anesthetic with fever, anorexia, nausea, vomiting, and increased serum concentrations of liver enzymes. Several mechanisms have been proposed to explain the association between halothane exposure and hepatotoxicity. One explanation is that halothane or its metabolites may have direct hepatotoxic effects. Experimental studies suggest that reductive metabolism of halothane leads to the production of free radicals that can cause hepatic necrosis. The conditions required for this reductive metabolism include severe hypoxia and pretreatment of animals with phenobarbital or other drugs that cause hepatic enzyme induction. The decrease in hepatic blood flow caused by halothane also may be a factor contributing to liver injury. An alternative explanation is that hepatic necrosis is caused by an immune-mediated hypersensitivity reaction to halothane or to one of its metabolites. Repeated exposure to halothane, reduced splanchnic blood flow, obesity, hypoxemia, increased levels of hepatic enzymes induced by chronic drug use, malnutrition, and underlying liver disease are believed to be predisposing factors for hepatic injury after halothane anesthesia. In the United States, halothane has given way to agents such as enflurane, isoflurane, and desflurane, which have not been implicated significantly in this process.

■ Musculoskeletal System

All the inhaled anesthetics, with the exception of nitrous oxide, cause skeletal muscle relaxation and potentiate the actions of neuromuscular blocking drugs. Enflurane produces the greatest relaxation; isoflurane, desflurane, and sevoflurane exert intermediate influences; and halothane has the least effect. Required doses of neuromuscular blocking drugs are typically reduced by half when anesthesia is maintained with a volatile anesthetic at approximately 1.3 MAC. These muscle-relaxing effects may persist after the patient awakens, because the anesthetic is eliminated from muscle much more slowly than from the brain (see Fig. 8-5). All inhaled anesthetics except nitrous oxide are capable of triggering malignant hyperthermia in susceptible patients (see Chap. 36).

■ Reproductive and Reticuloendothelial System

The effects of inhaled anesthetics on bone marrow and the issues of teratogenesis and occupational exposures are discussed in Chapter 36; effects on the gravid uterus are considered in Chapter 26.

Choice of Inhaled Anesthetic

Although it is possible to provide general anesthesia without inhaled anesthetics by using intravenous drugs, inhaled anesthetics offer significant advantages: rapid induction of anesthesia, continuous adjustment of depth, and continuous monitoring of anesthetic concentration. Elimination of the anesthetic through the lungs permits rapid emergence from anesthesia independent of drug metabolism or renal function. Inhalation can be accomplished without intravenous access, which is useful at times in children.

The varying physical characteristics and pharmacologic actions of the inhaled anesthetics may suggest choosing one drug over another in a particular clinical setting (Table 8-4). An insoluble anesthetic such as desflurane may provide rapid induction and emergence, but for an inhalation induction, halothane or sevoflurane may be chosen because they cause less airway irritation. Cardiovascular depression may weigh against the use of halothane in a

Table 8-4

Clinical Qualities of Inhaled Anesthetics

Agent	Advantages	Disadvantages
Nitrous oxide	Rapid uptake and elimination Minimal respiratory depression Minimal circulatory depression Odorless, nonpungent	Supports combustion Expansion of closed air spaces Inactivates vitamin B_{12} Lack of anesthetic potency
Halothane	Potent anesthetic Nonpungent Stable heart rate	Requires preservatives Slow uptake and elimination Undergoes biotransformation Idiosyncratic hepatic necrosis Sensitization to catecholamine-induced cardiac dysrhythmias
Enflurane	Stable heart rate Skeletal muscle relaxation	EEG seizure activity Depression of myocardial contractility
Isoflurane	Decreases cerebral metabolic rate Cardiac output maintained	Tachycardia at greater concentration
Desflurane	Rapid uptake and elimination	Airway irritation Tachycardia with rapid increase in inspired concentration Requires specialized vaporizer for administration Expensive unless low flows are used
Sevoflurane	Rapid uptake and elimination Nonpungent Less depression of myocardial contractility Stable heart rate	Reacts with CO_2 absorbents Inorganic fluoride release Expensive unless low flows are used

patient with heart failure, whereas isoflurane might be better tolerated. Despite differences among the inhaled anesthetics, clinical outcomes have not been shown to be markedly influenced by the choice of agent, either because those using them compensate for their known properties or because such studies have not been sensitive enough to detect changes. However, recognizing and understanding the unique physical and clinical properties of the agent allow the practitioner to select agents that offer specific pharmacologic advantages to offset underlying disease or pathophysiology in selected patients.

BIBLIOGRAPHY

Busy BF, Komai H. Anesthetic depression of myocardial contractility: A review of possible mechanisms. *Anesthesiology* 1987;67:745-766.

Eger EI. New inhaled anesthetics. *Anesthesiology* 1994;80:906-922.

Eger EI II, ed. *Anesthetic Uptake and Action*. Baltimore: Williams & Wilkins, 1974.

Marshall BE, Longnecker DL. General anesthetics. In Gilman AG, Rall TW, Nies AS, Taylor P, eds: *Goodman and Gilman's Pharmacological Basis of Therapeutics,* 8th ed. New York: Pergamon Press, 1990, pp 285-310.

Philip JH. *Gas Man: Understanding Anesthesia Uptake and Distribution*. Chestnut Hill, Mass: MedMan Simulations, 1990.

Quasha AL, Eger EI, Tinker JH. Determination and application of MAC. *Anesthesiology* 1980;53:315-334.

CHAPTER 9

Nonopioid Intravenous Anesthetics

Sean K. Kennedy

The components of general anesthesia include analgesia, hypnosis, blunting of reflexes, and muscle relaxation. The nonopioid intravenous anesthetic drugs principally provide hypnosis and blunting of reflexes; narcotics and neuromuscular blockers are used for analgesia and muscle relaxation.

The ideal intravenous anesthetic drug would provide all these components with rapid, nearly instantaneous onset without causing pain on injection. Induction would be smooth, without any signs of muscular twitching or excitement. The drug would be safe and cause minimal perturbation of cardiovascular or respiratory function. The drug would be short-acting, allowing the patient to awaken rapidly to full, normal central nervous system (CNS) function. Metabolism to inert substances and excretion would be rapid and complete so that accumulation would not occur, thereby allowing the drug to be used as a constant infusion over long periods of time. Amnesia for intraoperative events would be complete. No single drug meets these ideals against which we judge present intravenous anesthetics.

Barbiturates

Barbituric acid itself (Fig. 9-1) has no intrinsic CNS activity, but substitutions at the number 2 and 5 carbon atoms produce drugs with substantial CNS effects, including loss of consciousness and anticonvulsant activity. For example, at the number 5 carbon,

substituting a straight chain produces hypnotic activity, substituting a branched chain produces even greater hypnotic activity, substituting a phenyl group (phenobarbital) produces anticonvulsant activity, and substituting a methyl group (methohexital) may actually produce seizure-like muscle movement.

Barbiturates with an oxygen atom on the number 2 carbon are called *oxybarbiturates*; those with a sulfur atom are *thiobarbiturates*. Replacement of the oxygen atom with sulfur increases the lipid solubility of the drug, increasing the hypnotic potency and greatly reducing onset time and duration of action. Sulfur substitution at the number 2 carbon of pentobarbital produces thiopental, a potent hypnotic drug characterized by rapid onset and brief duration of effect. The same is true when the oxygen atom of secobarbital is replaced with sulfur, producing thiamylal.

An oxybarbiturate may be converted to a short-acting drug by adding a methyl group to the nitrogen atom of the barbiturate ring, as with methohexital. The chemical structures of several commonly used barbiturates are depicted in Figure 9-2.

Whereas the exact mechanisms of barbiturate action in the CNS are unknown, many other features are understood. The stereochemistry of barbiturates is clearly important in determining pharmacologic effects: Optical isomers can have markedly different CNS effects. This stereospecificity strongly suggests that barbiturates interact with specific membrane sites complementary to their structure, most likely particular synapses in the CNS.

Figure 9-1

Barbituric acid.

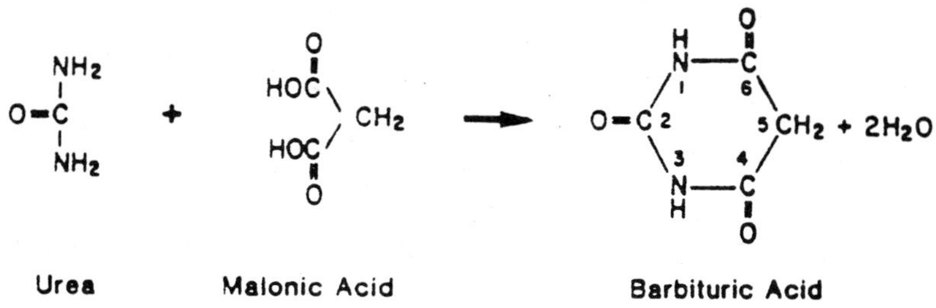

Urea   Malonic Acid   Barbituric Acid

Barbiturates can exert two types of effects at synapses in the CNS: facilitation of inhibitory transmitters, including gamma-aminobutyric acid (GABA); and blockade of excitatory transmitters, such as glutamic acid and acetylcholine. Unlike inhalation anesthetics, barbiturates do not block afferent sensory impulses very well. In fact, thiobarbiturates may actually produce an antianalgesic effect, but this is not clinically important as long as the thiobarbiturate is not the sole anesthetic agent used during a painful procedure.

■ Thiopental

In widespread clinical use for more than 50 years, thiopental remains the standard short-acting barbiturate.

Physical Properties

Like all the intravenous barbiturates, thiopental is water-soluble and stable in aqueous solution for weeks. Generally prepared as the sodium salt, thiopental in solution is quite alkaline; a 2.5% solution has

a pH of 10.5. This alkalinity makes thiopental incompatible with many other drugs that are acidic (e.g., catecholamines and some neuromuscular blockers). For example, when succinylcholine is given immediately following thiopental, a precipitate may form in the intravenous tubing, inactivating some of the drug and potentially occluding the intravenous catheter. Because extravasation of an alkaline substance such as thiopental is quite painful and may result in skin necrosis, the drug is injected only into a freely flowing intravenous system.

Inadvertent intraarterial injection is a more serious complication. This usually occurs at the antecubital space but can occur in any place where vein and artery are in close proximity. Especially in an emergency, it is easy to cannulate by mistake an anomalous radial artery at the wrist. Arterial injection produces severe pain immediately. A chemical endarteritis, which may damage even deep layers of the vessel wall, occurs rapidly, followed by thrombosis. Damage is related to the concentration of drug injected. A 5% solution (contraindicated in current practice) will readily damage vascular tissue, whereas serious injury is much less

Figure 9-2

Structures of useful barbiturate sedative-hypnotics.

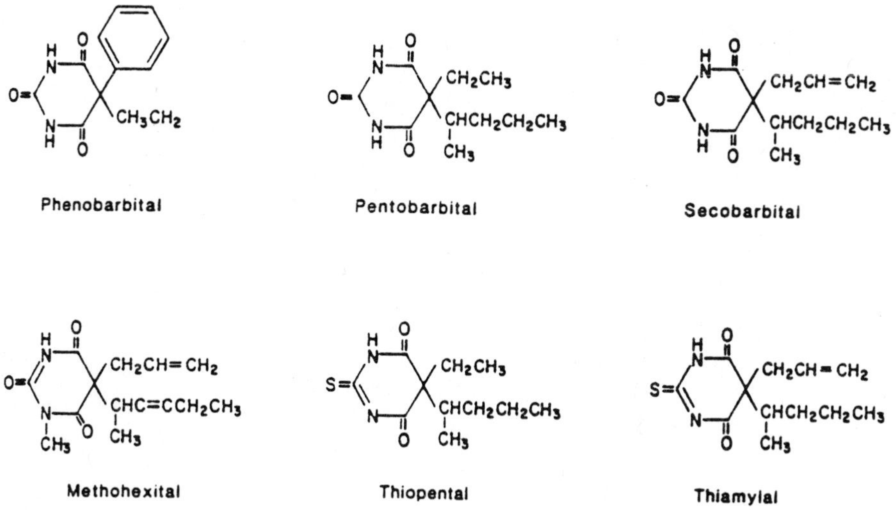

Phenobarbital   Pentobarbital   Secobarbital

Methohexital   Thiopental   Thiamylal

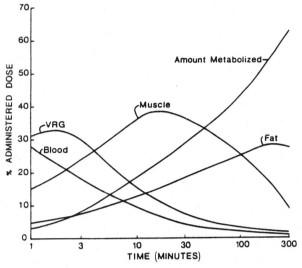

Figure 9-3

After a bolus of thiopental is given intravenously at time 0, the blood concentration decreases steadily from its maximum value as the drug is redistributed. After the first 3 minutes, the thiopental concentration in the vessel-rich group (VRG) (including the brain) decreases as well. The less well perfused muscle does not attain maximum thiopental concentration until 15 to 30 minutes after the injection, and the even less well perfused fat reaches the maximum thiopental concentration hours later.

(Reproduced with permission from Saidman LJ, Uptake, distribution and elimination of barbiturates. In Eger EI, ed: Anesthetic Uptake and Action. *Baltimore: Williams & Wilkins, 1974.)*

likely at 2.5%, the standard concentration used in clinical practice. There is no clear treatment of choice after intraarterial injection, but several reasonable measures may be applied. If the needle is still in place, 10 ml of 0.5% lidocaine may be injected to decrease the effects of alkaline extravasation. Because the mechanism of injury appears to be vasospasm, the injection of an alpha-adrenergic blocker such as phentolamine has been suggested. Heparin also has been suggested, because thrombosis is common. A subsequent stellate ganglion block also might promote vasodilatation.

Pharmacology

The physicochemical properties of thiopental determine its pharmacokinetics. Given as an intravenous bolus of 3 to 5 mg/kg, thiopental rapidly reaches its peak concentration in the central circulation. With a pK_a of 7.6, approximately 60 percent of the drug exists in the un-ionized form at the physiologic pH of

7.4, and the drug is lipid-soluble. For these reasons, there is rapid diffusion of thiopental into the vessel-rich group (VRG) of organs, namely, the heart, lungs, brain, and kidneys (Fig. 9-3). The brain concentration of thiopental increases quickly, and unconsciousness ensues within 10 to 15 seconds.

The peak concentration of drug achieved after an intravenous bolus is a function of the initial volume of distribution for thiopental, which decreases with the patient's age (Fig. 9-4). Because of this, thiopental dose requirements decrease with the patient's age also.

When first introduced, the short duration of action of thiopental was thought to result from rapid metabolism; it is now clear that the short duration of action is due to rapid redistribution of the drug (see Chap. 7). Although body fat is an important reservoir of lipid-soluble drugs like thiopental (fat:blood partition coefficient = 11), the blood supply to fat is meager compared with other organs, so entry of thiopental into fat is a slow process. Accumulation in fat occurs only after hours, and release back into the circulation is similarly slowed. In clinical practice, this reservoir phenomenon is only important after very large doses, generally given by long-term constant infusion.

The extent of plasma protein binding and tissue binding of barbiturates parallels the lipid solubility. From 70 to 85 percent of an injected dose of thiopental is bound to albumin, leaving only 15 to 30 per-

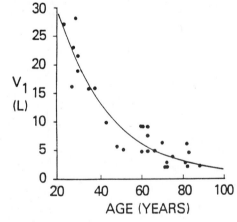

Figure 9-4

The initial volume of distribution of thiopental decreases markedly with age.

(Reproduced with permission from Homer TD, Stanski DR, The effect of increasing age on thiopental disposition and anesthetic requirement. Anesthesiology *1985;62:714.)*

cent free as the active substance. The extent of protein binding may be reduced in disease states such as cirrhosis (decreased protein concentration) or if other substances compete with thiopental and occupy some binding sites (e.g., phenylbutazone, some sulfonamides, nonsteroidal anti-inflammatory drugs including aspirin, or urea in patients with renal failure). With fewer binding sites available, more free drug enters tissue and exerts a pharmacologic effect. Acidosis also reduces protein binding. In any of these clinical situations of reduced protein binding, the dose of thiopental must be reduced.

Elimination of thiopental depends on metabolism, because less than 1 percent is excreted unchanged in the urine. All thiobarbiturates undergo a small amount of metabolism in the brain and kidneys, but for practical purposes, the liver is the site of drug biotransformation. Oxybarbiturates are metabolized exclusively in the liver. In the liver, barbiturates are converted to inactive compounds with increased water solubility to facilitate urinary excretion. Thiopental is metabolized at the rate of about 10 to 14 percent per hour, chiefly by oxidation of side chains at the number 5 carbon, desulfuration of the number 2 carbon atom, and hydrolysis of the barbituric acid ring. Thiopental has a hepatic extraction ratio of 0.1 to 0.2, implying capacity-dependent elimination (see Chap. 7).

The impact of hepatic clearance rates on elimination is clearly demonstrated when thiopental and methohexital are compared. Both these drugs have similar volumes of distribution and distribution half-times, but methohexital is cleared more rapidly, owing to its greater hepatic clearance (hepatic extraction ratio of 0.5 to 0.6).

Protein binding limits the glomerular filtration of thiopental, and its lipid solubility favors tubular reabsorption. Consequently, less than 1 percent of a thiopental dose is excreted unchanged in the urine. Of all the barbiturates, only phenobarbital, which is not greatly protein bound, is excreted in the urine in significant amounts.

For reasons that are not well understood, patients may develop acute tolerance to thiopental. Even during the course of a brief anesthetic, the dose requirement may increase.

Clinical Effects

For rapid induction of general anesthesia, thiopental has received wide acceptance among patients and clinicians alike. It is also used as an adjunct to general anesthesia. Its antianalgesic property limits its usefulness as a solitary anesthetic agent, except for brief procedures that are not painful.

As an induction agent, thiamylal is indistinguishable from thiopental. Methohexital also rapidly induces sleep, and recovery is usually quicker than with thiopental; involuntary muscle activity limits its application. Methohexital is most useful in very brief procedures such as cardioversion or electroconvulsive therapy.

The CNS effects of thiopental go beyond producing unconsciousness. Adequate concentrations of thiopental depress cortical brain activity measured on the electroencephalogram (EEG) to the point of electrical silence. Correlated with this EEG suppression is decreased brain metabolism, evidenced by decreased cerebral oxygen consumption, and a corresponding decrease in cerebral blood flow. Once enough thiopental has been given to produce electrical silence in the EEG, additional doses of thiopental produce no further reduction in brain metabolism, suggesting that the reduction in metabolism is related to the specialized electrochemical functions of neuronal tissue. The metabolism present when the EEG is isoelectric presumably represents the basal metabolic requirements of cell function (e.g., maintaining cell membrane integrity). Further reductions in brain metabolism can be achieved if the body temperature is reduced.

In patients with severe brain injury and increased intracranial pressure, an induction dose of thiopental reduces pressure in most cases. When used for this purpose, thiopental must be given carefully so as not to reduce arterial blood pressure and decrease the net cerebral perfusion pressure (see Chap. 30).

Thiopental may have a profound impact on the cardiovascular system in some patients and virtually no effect in others. Healthy patients given typical doses of 3 to 5 mg/kg may experience a transient decrease in arterial blood pressure that usually elicits a mild compensatory tachycardia and return of blood pressure toward normal. In this situation, there is little cardiac depression. Presumably, the initial decrease in pressure is due to increased venous capacitance and subsequent decreased venous return secondary to depression of the medullary vasomotor center and depression of central sympathetic nervous system activity. This is followed by a baroreceptor-mediated increase in sympathetic nervous activity, increasing contractility, heart rate, and venous return.

In isolated heart muscle preparations, thiopental

clearly has a negative inotropic effect. Large doses in otherwise healthy patients or standard doses in patients with limited ability to activate a baroreceptor reflex response produce the clinical picture of myocardial depression. Patients taking beta-adrenergic antagonists or certain antihypertensive drugs may have impaired baroreceptor compensatory ability. Hypovolemic patients are particularly likely to become hypotensive after the usual doses of thiopental, because they are dependent on intrinsic catecholamine stimulation to maintain blood pressure. Following a standard dose of thiopental, normal compensatory reflexes are blunted, and the hypovolemic patient is less able to compensate for drug-induced circulatory depression. Adequate volume repletion, slow incremental dosing (beginning with doses of 0.5 to 1.0 mg/kg), and sympathomimetic drugs all play a role in preventing and treating thiopental-induced hypotension in these patients. Because of the danger of cardiovascular collapse, it is prudent to avoid ultra-short-acting barbiturates in the presence of hypovolemia or shock. Induction drugs that have minimal cardiac depression (etomidate) or that stimulate the cardiovascular system (ketamine) are used more commonly in such circumstances.

Thiopental produces a dose-dependent depression of medullary and pontine respiratory centers. Following an induction dose, the patient typically takes a large breath and then becomes apneic for a short period. Carbon dioxide responsiveness is blunted in a dose-dependent fashion, with virtually no response at deep levels of anesthesia. Ventilatory responses to hypoxia are also blunted. As the drug redistributes, the patient resumes breathing with small tidal volumes and increased respiratory rate, resulting in a modest decrease in minute ventilation.

Apnea following induction of anesthesia is managed by administering oxygen before giving thiopental (denitrogenation, described in Chap. 13) and by manual ventilation, if necessary. Aggressive positive-pressure ventilation may lead to coughing, hiccups, or laryngospasm. It is not clear that thiopental increases airway irritability; this may result from manipulation of the airway in any lightly anesthetized patient. Thiopental is not contraindicated in asthmatic patients, but the dose of thiopental must be adequate and the airway must not be manipulated until the patient is adequately anesthetized (often with a potent vapor).

Although the recommended dose of thiopental for induction of anesthesia is 3 to 5 mg/kg, this varies among patients, mostly because of the additive effects of premedications or other drugs but also because of intercurrent disease (such as hypovolemia or cardiac disease) or old age. In addition to these anticipated instances, there remain patients who unexpectedly require less than 2.5 mg/kg or more than 6 mg/kg for induction. The first group is at risk of overdose. Some anesthesiologists routinely administer a small dose of thiopental (25 to 50 mg, the "test dose") to verify that the drug does not escape into the subcutaneous tissue and to assess the patient's response before giving additional drug; this precaution is prudent for any patient who might be sensitive to barbiturates for any reason.

Other Induction Agents

■ Ketamine

An arylcyclohexylamine related to phencyclidine (PCP), ketamine produces a unique state often called *dissociative anesthesia*, reminiscent of a cataleptic condition, as well as profound analgesia. Patients given ketamine may appear to be awake: the eyes often remain open, a slow nystagmus creates the illusion that the patient is gazing about, and muscular activity may appear purposeful. In fact, the patient is unaware and has no recollection of events under ketamine anesthesia.

Ketamine is a water-soluble molecule with an asymmetrical carbon. Its optical isomers have quite different pharmacologic effects (the positive isomer is a better analgesic and produces less delirium), suggesting specific receptor site interaction. Commercial preparations are racemic mixtures of equal amounts of each isomer. The exact mechanism of action is not known, but analgesia is thought to result from lamina-specific suppression of spinal cord activity that interrupts transmission of the affective component of pain signals to the brain.

Following intramuscular injection, bioavailability is 90 percent, and peak blood concentrations are achieved within 15 minutes. Like thiopental, its lipid solubility (5 to 10 times that of thiopental) contributes to rapid onset of the drug. About 45 to 50 percent of ketamine is bound to plasma proteins, principally alpha-1-acid glycoprotein; therefore, more free drug is available for action compared with thiopental. Neither renal failure nor hepatic enzyme induction influences the duration of the drug's effect, suggesting that redistribution plays the major role in the short duration of action of ketamine (distribution half-life is approximately 7 to 17 minutes).

Because only 5 percent of the dose is recovered unchanged in the urine, metabolism is the important route of clearance. Hepatic clearance is 18 ml/kg per minute, with a hepatic extraction ratio of 0.9. Volume of distribution is also rather large, 3 liters/kg, resulting in an elimination half-life of 2 to 3 hours. Hepatic metabolism of ketamine, mostly oxidative, is complex and produces at least eight metabolites. One of these, formed via demethylation by cytochrome P-450 enzymes, is norketamine, an active metabolite with about one-third the potency of ketamine. This substance may be responsible for prolonging the CNS effects of ketamine. Prolonged use of ketamine induces hepatic metabolic enzymes, and tolerance eventually develops.

Respiratory depression depends on dose, but at typical anesthetic doses of 2 mg/kg, only modest depression is seen. Upper airway skeletal muscle tone is well maintained with ketamine and airway reflexes are less blunted than with the usual doses of other induction agents, but the risk of aspiration and airway obstruction is still present. Ketamine relaxes bronchial smooth muscle and is a useful drug for induction of anesthesia in patients with asthma. Excess oral secretions can be a problem with ketamine; these are best prevented with an antisialagogue such as glycopyrrolate.

Emergence delirium occurs in 5 to 30 percent of patients, especially in women over age 16 and in patients with personality disorders, after doses greater than 2 mg/kg. Patients experience visual and auditory illusions and a confused state that may progress to true delirium. Vivid, unpleasant dreams, often with morbid content, may occur up to 24 hours later. Premedication with benzodiazepines helps prevent delirium but not some of the proprioceptive illusions (a "floating" sensation) or dreaming in the postoperative period. Thiopental and inhalation agents also decrease the incidence of delirium. Atropine and droperidol increase the incidence of postoperative delirium and are avoided if ketamine is to be used. In some hospitals, patients emerging from ketamine anesthesia are kept in a quiet area, but there is no evidence that this reduces the incidence or severity of emergence delirium.

Ketamine indirectly produces a dose-related increase in heart rate and arterial blood pressure secondary to central CNS stimulation. This indirect cardiovascular stimulation makes ketamine useful in patients who require rapid-sequence induction of anesthesia but who might become hypotensive with thiopental; these include trauma patients with partially corrected hypovolemia and patients with restrictive pericarditis or tamponade. The use of ketamine does not eliminate the need for appropriate monitoring and treatment with volume expansion for these patients, because the autonomic compensatory reflexes may be stimulated to maximum capacity already, allowing the direct depressant effects of the drug to predominate. Ketamine is not usually chosen for patients with hypertension or coronary artery disease, in whom hypertension or tachycardia are undesirable.

Ketamine increases cerebral blood flow and may cause a dangerous increase in intracranial pressure in patients with reduced intracranial compliance, making it unsuitable for patients with a suspected mass lesion in the brain.

The usual dose for induction of anesthesia is 0.5 to 2 mg/kg given intravenously; it can be continued as an infusion by itself to maintain ketamine anesthesia (50 to 100 μg/kg per minute) or in lesser doses (40 μg/kg per minute or less) as a supplement to nitrous oxide and narcotics in a balanced technique. Ketamine acts rapidly when given via the intramuscular route (5 mg/kg), making it useful when there is no intravenous access. Given in small intravenous increments (0.1 to 0.3 mg/kg), ketamine can provide analgesia without loss of consciousness; it is occasionally used in this manner to produce brief periods of analgesia for burn dressing changes or vaginal delivery.

■ Propofol

Propofol is a new sedative-hypnotic intravenous anesthetic agent, similar in action to thiopental, that can be used to maintain anesthesia by constant infusion. Formerly known as *disoprofol*, it is an alkyl phenol that is insoluble in water. Initially, it was dissolved in Cremophore EL, a substance that led to anaphylactic reactions. Propofol was withdrawn from clinical use and then reformulated as an aqueous emulsion of soy bean oil, glycerol, and egg phosphatide. The emulsion may produce pain on intravenous injection, especially into a small vein, but the formulation is greatly improved overall.

Unconsciousness usually follows in less than a minute after an intravenous induction dose of 2 to 2.5 mg/kg. With a three-compartment model, elimination half-life from well-perfused tissues $(t_{1/2\beta})$ is 0.5 to 1.0 hours, and terminal elimination has a half-life of 3 to 6 hours. This suggests slow return of propofol from poorly perfused tissue such as fat, especially after prolonged infusion. Clearance of propofol is reduced in the elderly but not significantly lessened by renal or hepatic disease. In the liver, the drug is metabolized to water-soluble glucuronide and sulfate conjugates and then excreted in the urine. Total clearance of propofol (30 to 60 ml/kg per minute) exceeds hepatic blood flow, implying extrahepatic sites of metabolism. Metabolites are inactive.

Propofol in the doses usually employed for induction of anesthesia reduces arterial blood pressure by about 30 percent without much effect on heart rate. This appears to result from reduced systemic vascular resistance rather than reduction of stroke volume or cardiac output. Propofol is associated with greater reductions in blood pressure than is thiopental but smaller changes in heart rate.

Compared with thiopental, the incidence of apnea on induction with propofol is similar, but the duration of apnea may be greater. A 2 to 2.5 mg/kg intravenous bolus of propofol produces 30 to 90 seconds of apnea in 60 percent of unpremedicated patients. After narcotic premedication, essentially all patients become apneic on induction with propofol. During infusion of propofol, respiratory rate may increase, but minute ventilation is reduced. Narcotics further reduce respiratory drive.

The major advantage of propofol over other induction agents is its rapid clearance and the fact that so few residual effects are seen on awakening. After short procedures under propofol anesthesia, patients awaken quickly with less likelihood of postoperative vomiting. This has made the drug particularly useful for outpatients.

Propofol may be used to begin anesthesia that is to be maintained by other general anesthetic agents, as a supplement to general anesthesia, or as a total intravenous anesthetic. Given at a rate of about 40 mg every 10 seconds to a total dose of 1 to 2.5 mg/kg, propofol rapidly induces anesthesia characterized occasionally by hiccups (15 percent) or spontaneous muscle activity (25 percent). Infusion rates of 0.05 to 0.2 mg/kg per minute, given by automated infusion pump, can be adjusted to maintain anesthesia as a supplement to nitrous oxide; infusions at half these rates suffice for sedation in the operating room and the intensive care unit setting. It also may be effective in treating nausea and vomiting in the postoperative period (10 to 20 mg) and during chemotherapy (10 to 20 µg/kg per minute). The drug is not currently approved for this purpose.

■ Etomidate

Like midazolam, etomidate contains an imidazole ring that makes it water-soluble at acid pH and lipid-soluble at physiologic pH. An induction dose of 0.3 mg/kg rapidly produces unconsciousness, followed by awakening in 3 to 12 minutes. Awakening is more rapid than with thiopental, and there is less grogginess. Etomidate has no analgesic properties.

The volume of distribution is large, consistent with substantial tissue uptake. Approximately 75 percent of etomidate is bound to albumin. Both hepatic enzymes and plasma esterases are responsible for the hydrolysis of etomidate to its carboxylic acid ester, an inactive substance. Nearly 85 percent of an administered dose is metabolized to this ester and excreted in the urine; another 10 to 13 percent appears in bile. The total clearance rate of etomidate is about five times the clearance of thiopental; its elimination half-life is 2 to 5 hours. Dose requirements are reduced in the elderly owing to a reduced volume of distribution.

Like thiopental, etomidate reduces cerebral blood flow, cerebral metabolism, and intracranial pressure. Etomidate also decreases intraocular pressure. Like methohexital, it also may stimulate seizure activity. About one-third of patients will manifest myoclonic muscle movements during induction. This is presumably caused by subcortical disinhibition of normally suppressed extrapyramidal tract motor activity. Premedication with a narcotic or benzodiazepine reduces the incidence of myoclonus.

One of the major advantages of etomidate is its minimal impact on hemodynamics. Following an induction dose of 0.3 mg/kg, there is little change in heart rate, stroke volume, or cardiac output. Arterial blood pressure may decrease 10 to 15 percent owing to a corresponding decrease in peripheral vascular resistance.

An induction dose of etomidate given rapidly may produce transient apnea, but there is generally little effect on minute ventilation once respiration resumes. In the presence of narcotics, respiratory depression may be substantial, especially if etomidate is given by infusion.

Adrenocortical suppression by etomidate was first noted in critically ill patients receiving continuous infusions of the drug. The phenomenon has been documented after a single dose, producing decreased plasma cortisol concentrations and impaired responsiveness to ACTH lasting 4 to 8 hours after the single bolus. Adrenocortical suppression could limit the normal physiologic response to stress in a critically ill patient given etomidate, although the clinical significance of this effect remains undocumented.

Induction with etomidate is associated with an increased incidence of postoperative nausea and vomiting compared with thiopental. This may be reduced with droperidol premedication.

Although myoclonic movements, adrenocortical suppression, and an increased incidence of nausea and vomiting limit its usefulness, etomidate may be a good alternative to thiopental in the patient with unstable cardiac disease. It also may be used for brief outpatient procedures, although either propofol or a short-acting barbiturate seems more appropriate. Intravenous induction requires 0.3 mg/kg; to maintain anesthesia with nitrous oxide requires about 0.01 mg/kg per minute; brief intravenous sedation can be provided with infusions at half this rate.

Choice of Intravenous Drug to Induce Anesthesia

The choice of induction drug often depends on the clinical situation and the presence of coexisting disease. For example, the ability of thiopental to reduce intracranial pressure (ICP) makes it a good induction drug prior to craniotomy for removal of a space-occupying lesion. If the lesion resulted from a motor vehicle accident with associated injuries that produced hypovolemia, thiopental might reduce the arterial pressure more than the ICP, reducing brain perfusion; etomidate might be a better choice.

In healthy patients undergoing uncomplicated operations, the choice may depend on such issues as likelihood of postoperative nausea and, increasingly, on cost. Although propofol is considerably more expensive than thiopental, outpatients who awaken rapidly with minimal residual sedation and no nausea or vomiting may be safely discharged home after only a brief stay in the recovery room. This is not only an important issue in patient satisfaction but also avoids the considerable costs involved in unplanned hospitalization due to postoperative vomiting. As new drugs are introduced, such cost issues must be considered before choosing to use expensive drugs in place of older, inexpensive alternatives.

Total Intravenous Anesthesia

Inhalation anesthesia, supplemented with narcotics and muscle relaxants, is still the mainstay of anesthetic practice. With the development of induction drugs and narcotics with rapid onset and short elimination time constants, anesthesia using only (or predominantly) intravenous agents has become practical.

Depth of anesthesia is directly related to the plasma concentration of the anesthetic, whether an inhalation or an intravenous agent. Calibrated vaporizers and end-tidal concentration monitors make it relatively easy to determine accurately desired plasma concentration. A change in the delivered concentration results in a corresponding change in the plasma concentration, the rate of change depending on such factors as solubility of the anesthetic agent, ventilation, and fresh gas flow rate (see Chap. 8). Rapid elimination of inhalation anesthetics allows the patient to awaken quickly at the end of the procedure.

Maintenance of anesthesia with intravenous agents requires repeated administration of drug because of redistribution and elimination. In practice, this usually involves giving boluses intermittently in response to signs of light anesthesia, resulting in oscillation of the plasma drug concentration around the desired target value. If the drug has a long elimination time constant, accumulation of drug and delayed awakening may occur. A drug with a short half-life may be given in very frequent, small boluses to maintain a plasma concentration appropriate for the severity of surgical stimulation. Infusion pumps, governed by an appropriately programmed computer, maintain constant concentrations but still require clinical judgment to adjust as clinical circumstances change.

Benzodiazepines as Sedatives

Benzodiazepines are used commonly as premedicants or adjuncts to regional or general anesthesia and only rarely to induce anesthesia. In some ways, these drugs are preferable to the barbiturates: they often produce amnesia; the therapeutic index is usually greater; there is less cardiovascular and respiratory depression; and tolerance is rare. However, large doses are usually required to produce unconsciousness, and the duration of effect is longer than that of the ultra-short-acting barbiturates. The most common benzodiazepines in anesthetic practice are diazepam, lorazepam, and midazolam.

■ Mechanisms of Action

The benzodiazepines exert their action at specific receptor sites, notably on postsynaptic nerves in the CNS, producing very little pharmacologic effect outside the CNS. Sedation by benzodiazepines results from facilitation of the inhibitory neurotransmitter gamma-aminobutyric acid (GABA). The benzodiazepine receptors and the GABA receptors are separate, but closely linked. When a benzodiazepine drug occupies its own site on a subunit of the GABA receptor site, the affinity of GABA and its receptor sites is increased; inhibition of nerve conduction and sedation follow. If the benzodiazepine receptor is occupied by an antagonist, GABA-mediated transmission is blocked, and the sedative effects of benzodiazepines are prevented.

Flumazenil, an imidazobenzodiazepine, binds to benzodiazepine receptors, where it competitively inhibits binding and allosteric effects of the therapeutic benzodiazepines. It is the first of the specific benzodiazepine antagonists approved for clinical use. Flumazenil may be useful in reversing the sedative effects of long-acting benzodiazepines or to treat drug overdose. Interestingly, flumazenil also may ameliorate some of the neurologic sequelae of hepatic encephalopathy that are presumably related to accumulation of endogenous benzodiazepine-like substances.

■ Diazepam

Relatively insoluble in water, diazepam is dissolved in propylene glycol and sodium benzoate for parenteral use. These organic solvents make parenteral injection painful and absorption after intramuscular (IM) injection unreliable; the IM route is not recommended. Diazepam is rapidly absorbed from the gastrointestinal tract, especially in children.

Although it is lipid-soluble and taken up rapidly in CNS tissue, the onset of action of diazepam is not rapid. The reason for this delayed onset is unclear and may relate either to the pharmacokinetics or pharmacodynamics of the drug. Like thiopental, this lipid-soluble drug distributes rapidly into well-perfused organs and then redistributes, decreasing the plasma concentration and enhancing recovery.

Lipid solubility of benzodiazepines corresponds to protein binding; thus diazepam is extensively bound. The free fraction of diazepam in blood is only about 1 to 2 percent of the total; the rest binds tightly to albumin. Anything that affects protein binding influences the amount of free drug available. Large increases in the free fraction of drug may occur in hepatic and renal disease. In hepatic disease, the increased volume of distribution and reduced drug metabolism may double the elimination half-life. In renal disease, drug metabolism is maintained, so the increased fraction of free drug leads to a two- to threefold increase in hepatic metabolism and reduces the elimination half-life. Elimination is prolonged in the elderly owing to increased volume of distribution and decreased protein binding rather than to changes in hepatic clearance.

The duration of action of diazepam is not as short as that of thiopental, partly because of the way diazepam is metabolized. Metabolism occurs principally in the liver, where oxidative metabolism produces several active metabolites, including desmethyldiazepam, 3-hydroxydiazepam, and oxazepam (itself a commercially available sedative). These active metabolites produce their own benzodiazepine effect, prolonging CNS depression, especially after multiple doses of diazepam. In addition, enterohepatic circulation may contribute to the prolonged CNS effects of diazepam. Oxidative metabolism of diazepam may be impaired by other drugs, such as cimetidine. The lipid-soluble oxidative metabolites of diazepam are conjugated in the liver to water-soluble glucuronides and then excreted in the urine. The relatively large volume of distribution (1 to 1.5 liters/kg), small clearance (0.2 to 0.5 ml/kg per minute), and small hepatic extraction ratio (0.01 to 0.025) yield a terminal elimination half-life of 20 to 40 hours.

The principal clinical uses of diazepam are as an oral premedicant (0.1 to 0.2 mg/kg), an intravenous sedating agent during regional anesthesia (0.03 to 0.07 mg/kg doses repeated as needed), and rarely as an induction agent (0.5 mg/kg). The benzodiazepines have no analgesic properties. Diazepam reduces the minimum alveolar concentration (MAC) of inhalation anesthetics; a premedication dose of 0.2 mg/kg reduces the halothane requirement by nearly 30 percent.

Although an intravenous bolus of diazepam occasionally can produce apnea, an increase in $PaCO_2$ usually is not seen until the intravenous dose reaches 0.2 mg/kg. Tidal volume is decreased. In the dose range 0.2 to 0.4 mg/kg, respiratory depression is seen within minutes after intravenous administration and typically persists for 30 minutes or more. Depression of mental status tends to correlate with the extent of respiratory depression. In combination with other respiratory depressant drugs such as opioids or with chronic lung disease, diazepam may produce substantial and prolonged respiratory depression.

Large doses of diazepam are occasionally used to induce general anesthesia for long operations, although most anesthesiologists prefer midazolam for this purpose because intravenous diazepam causes pain and subsequent phlebitis. Induction is much slower than with thiopental. At doses of 0.5 to 1.0 mg/kg, diazepam produces only a modest decrease in blood pressure, cardiac output, and vascular resistance. Because baroreceptor reflexes are blunted, compensatory tachycardia is generally not seen. Inhibition of compensatory reflexes is less with diazepam than with barbiturates and inhalation agents but may cause significant decrease in blood pressure in hypovolemic patients. Following diazepam induction, nitrous oxide does not lead to myocardial depression, as it does in the presence of narcotics.

Lorazepam

Lorazepam is 5 to 10 times as potent as diazepam but resembles it in its clinical effects on the cardiovascular and respiratory systems. Lorazepam reliably produces anterograde amnesia.

Like diazepam, lorazepam is insoluble in water, so it must be dissolved in propylene glycol or polyethylene glycol. However, it produces less pain on injection than diazepam and causes less phlebitis. Unlike diazepam, intramuscular injections as well as oral doses are absorbed reliably. Following absorption, onset of action is quite slow. Peak plasma concentrations after oral administration are achieved in 2 to 4 hours, and effects persist for up to 24 to 48 hours.

Lorazepam has a smaller volume of distribution (0.8 to 1.3 liters/kg) and greater clearance (0.75 to 1.0 ml/kg per minute) than diazepam. The elimination half-life is 10 to 20 hours. Elimination is unaffected by renal disease but is prolonged in cirrhosis.

The usual dose of lorazepam for oral premedication is 50 µg/kg to a maximum dose of 4 mg. This usually produces amnesia without excessive sedation. The slow onset and long duration of effects make it unsuitable for outpatients. Drugs with shorter onset and shorter duration are favored as adjuncts to regional anesthesia.

Midazolam

Midazolam is two to three times as potent as diazepam. Unlike other benzodiazepines, midazolam incorporates an imidazole ring that makes it stable in aqueous solutions. It is prepared in solutions buffered to a pH of 3.5; the open imidazole ring makes the drug water-soluble and painless on injection because solubilizing agents are unnecessary. Absorption after intramuscular injection is rapid and dependable. At physiologic pH, the imidazole ring closes, making the molecule lipid-soluble. Midazolam is bound to plasma albumin (95 percent).

The drug may be given orally. Absorption from the gastrointestinal tract is rapid, but a substantial first-pass effect allows only half the drug to reach the systemic circulation. After intravenous injection, peak effect is reached in 3 to 5 minutes. Peak effect after intramuscular injection occurs in 15 to 30 minutes. To a great extent, the brief action of midazolam is due to redistribution of the lipid-soluble molecule. Metabolism occurs in the liver by oxidation to metabolites that are then conjugated and excreted in the urine. Some metabolites, such as 1-hydroxymethylmidazolam, are active and contribute to the CNS effects. The volume of distribution of midazolam is similar to that of diazepam, but the clearance is nearly 10 times greater (4 to 8 ml/kg per minute), owing to the hepatic extraction ratio of 0.2 to 0.4. The elimination half-life of midazolam is 2 to 4 hours, substantially less than that of other benzodiazepines. The kinetics do not appear to be affected by advancing age. Because the drug is so extensively metabolized, elimination is not affected by renal disease.

Midazolam decreases cerebral blood flow and metabolism and does not worsen diminished intracranial compliance. Respiratory depression is similar to that produced by diazepam in equipotent doses. Just as with thiopental, doses of midazolam that induce anesthesia (0.2 mg/kg) produce cardiovascular changes, a decrease in blood pressure, and a compensatory increase in heart rate. The decrease in blood pressure is exaggerated in hypovolemic patients.

Midazolam is an anxiolytic, sedative, and amnestic drug. Amnesia is dose-related and, like respiratory depression, tends to parallel the sedative effect. An intravenous dose of 5 mg produces 20 to 30 minutes of amnesia. Intramuscular injection often produces amnesia of even longer duration. Midazolam 0.05 to 0.1 mg/kg orally or intramuscularly is an effective premedication.

One of the most popular clinical applications of midazolam is sedation during regional anesthesia or during diagnostic or therapeutic procedures. Intravenous doses of 0.5 to 2 mg are given to produce the desired effect. Patients suffer less postoperative sedation than after diazepam, but time to complete recovery is unchanged. Like other benzodiazepines, midazolam has no analgesic properties.

To induce anesthesia, midazolam can be given in doses of 0.1 to 0.3 mg/kg intravenously over 30 to 60 seconds. Induction time is prolonged compared with thiopental, so midazolam is not a popular drug for induction of anesthesia. When given by infusion at approximately 1 μg/kg per minute, it can provide unconsciousness and amnesia during general anesthesia with the combination of nitrous oxide, narcotics, and muscle relaxants.

BIBLIOGRAPHY

Dundee JW, Wyant GM. *Intravenous Anaesthesia,* 2nd ed. New York: Churchill-Livingstone, 1988.

Fragen RJ, Shanks CA, Moltgeni A, Avram MJ. Effects of etomidate on hormonal response to surgical stress. *Anesthesiology* 1984;60:652.

Hudson RJ, Stanski DR, Burch PG. Pharmacokinetics of methohexital and thiopental in surgical patients. *Anesthesiology* 1983; 59:215.

Jacobs JR, Reves JG, Glass PSA, eds. *Continuous Infusion for Maintaining Anesthesia. International Anesthesiology Clinics,* vol 29, no 4. Boston: Little, Brown, 1991.

CHAPTER **10**

Opioids in Anesthesia Practice

Thomas H. Kramer

Opiates come from the juice of the unripe seed capsule of the poppy *Papaver somniferum*. The term *opiates* refers to drugs like codeine and morphine that occur naturally in opium; *opioids* are any compounds, including natural and synthetic drugs and biologic peptides, that act on opioid receptors; the term *narcotic* is outdated and nonspecific because it includes drugs of abuse such as barbiturates, marijuana, hallucinogens, and others. Although there are significant differences among the opioids, they have many effects in common.

Opioid Pharmacology

■ Opioid Receptors

There are three distinct opioid receptors: the μ (mu), δ (delta), and κ (kappa) opioid receptors. These belong to a superfamily of pharmacologic receptors that produce their cellular effects by interacting with guanine-nucleotide binding proteins, or G-proteins. Studies using selective agonists and antagonists reveal that the receptors have diverse functions (Table 10-1). Current opioid drugs interact predominantly with μ opioid receptors (Table 10-2); most of the actions of the opioids commonly used in anesthesia can be predicted from the pharmacology of this receptor. Opioid receptors are widely distributed throughout peripheral tissues as well as the central nervous system (Table 10-3).

The rapid progress in research has left some confusion about formerly well-accepted concepts that have been revised. The initial classification scheme for multiple opioid receptors included a σ (sigma) receptor type that is now recognized as not being an opioid receptor. Also, currently popular theories describe multiple subtypes of opioid receptors (such as μ_1 and μ_2 and δ_1 and δ_2), holding out the prospect of developing drugs specific for receptor subtypes, thereby dissociating undesirable opioid effects like respiratory depression and dependence potential from opioid analgesia. This hope may prove false, since molecular biologic studies have yet to show the existence of more than one type of each receptor.

Table 10-1

Effects of Opioid Receptors

Effects	Receptor Type		
	μ	δ	κ
Analgesia, spinal cord	+++	++	++
Analgesia, brain	+++	+	+
Ventilatory depression	+++	−	+/−
Sedation	++	−	+++
Reinforcement/ dependence	+++	+/−	− −
Constipation	+++	+/−	+/−

99

Table 10-2

Agonist Activity of Available Opioids

Drug	Receptor*	
	μ	κ
Morphine	Agonist	Agonist (weak)
Fentanyl	Agonist (potent)	—
Sufentanil	Agonist (potent)	—
Alfentanil	Agonist (potent)	—
Meperidine	Agonist	Agonist (weak)
Methadone	Agonist	—
Buprenorphine	Partial agonist (potent)	Partial agonist (weak)
Nalbuphine	Partial agonist	Partial agonist (weak)
Butorphanol	Partial agonist	Agonist
Dezocine	Partial agonist	—
Naloxone	Antagonist (potent)	Antagonist (weak)

*The effect of the clinically useful opioids on the δ receptor type is minimal.

■ Endogenous Opioid Peptides

The opioid receptors, in addition to responding to morphine and related drugs, are activated by a diverse group of endogenous opioid peptides derived from three opioid precursor proteins named proopiomelanocortin (POMC), proenkephalin, and prodynorphin. POMC contains the opioid peptide beta-endorphin, along with ACTH and MSH (melanotropin); both ACTH and beta-endorphin are secreted in response to stress. Beta-endorphin is found in greatest concentrations in the pituitary, but it is not particularly selective for one opioid receptor. Proenkephalin is found in greatest abundance in the spinal cord, adrenal glands, brain, and gastrointestinal tract. This molecule contains multiple copies of the enkephalin pentapeptide sequence and produces several different peptides that activate δ and μ receptors. Prodynorphin is the precursor for the dynorphin peptides, which preferentially activate κ receptors found in the spinal cord, brain, and gastrointestinal tract. Spinal enkephalin and dynorphin modulate the perception of pain after injury; enkephalin activation of δ and μ receptors can result in decreased pain sensation (morphine administered into the spinal cord produces this effect), whereas dynorphin appears to act in an opposing fashion, causing hypersensitivity.

■ Opioid Agonists, Antagonists, and Partial Agonists

Whether it occurs by the release of endogenous opioid peptides or the administration of an opiate,

Table 10-3

Distribution of Opioid Receptors

Anatomic Location		Receptor	Effects
CNS	Cortex	μ, δ, κ	Sedation, euphoria, psychotomimetic
	Thalamus	μ, κ	Analgesia
	Ventral medulla	μ	Ventilatory depression
	Hypothalamus	μ, κ	Thermoregulatory, endocrine
	Ventral tegmental area, N. accumbens	μ, δ	Reinforcement/ addiction
	Spinal dorsal horn, postsynaptic	μ, κ	Analgesia/ hyperalgesia
Primary afferents	Spinal dorsal horn, presynaptic*	μ, δ	Analgesia
	Peripheral terminals	μ, δ, κ	Analgesia[†]
GI tract	Myenteric plexes	μ, δ, κ	Antimotility
	Mucosa	μ, δ	Antisecretory
	Smooth muscle	μ, δ	Contraction

*Opioid receptors and the central terminals of primary afferents on which they are located are within the CNS (i.e., inside the blood-brain barrier), but the primary afferent neurons are peripheral structures, with cell bodies located in the dorsal root ganglia.

[†]Opioid receptors on the peripheral terminals of the primary afferents are inactive under typical conditions, but during inflammation (and after some injuries) they may be upregulated and are able to respond to locally applied opioid drugs.

Table 10-4

Cellular Effector Mechanisms Coupled to Opioid Receptors

Mechanism	Receptor		
	μ	δ	κ
Adenylate cyclase	×	×	
Ion channel (K$^+$)	×	×	
Ion channel (Ca^{2+})			×

activation of opioid receptors usually results in cellular inhibition, mediated via a number of different biochemical pathways, depending on the particular receptor and cell type (Table 10-4). The membrane-bound opioid receptors are coupled to intracellular processes by guanine-nucleotide binding proteins (G-proteins). The conformation of the receptor determines the degree of activation of the G-protein cascade and therefore the subsequent level of effect on cellular function. Opioid ligands alter the receptor conformation to varying degrees; depending on the individual drug, the rate of activation of G-proteins is accelerated, unchanged, or even slowed.

Intrinsic efficacy may be defined as an opioid drug's ability to accelerate the activity of G-proteins. The greater the efficacy, the greater is the intensity of cellular effect that the drug may produce. Drugs with intrinsic efficacy are called *agonists* (or *full agonists*), drugs with lesser efficacy are called *partial agonists*, and those with no efficacy (or what may be termed *negative intrinsic efficacy*) are called *antagonists*. Increasing efficacy is associated with both greater potency (a lesser dose requirement) and an increased maximum possible effect (Fig. 10-1), whereas minimal or negative efficacy (as in the case of an antagonist such as naloxone) results in a competitive blockade of opioid receptors, reducing the effects of any agonist drugs present. The clinically useful opioids encompass a broad range of efficacies (see Table 10-2), although only full agonists (such as morphine or fentanyl) and the antagonist naloxone are used frequently in anesthesia.

In addition to blocking the effects of agonists, opioid antagonists such as naloxone precipitate severe abstinence (or withdrawal) symptoms in patients dependent on opioids. The dramatic decrease in G-protein activation caused by an antagonist results in effects opposite those expected of an agonist, called *abstinence* or *withdrawal*. Because antagonists have no intrinsic efficacy, it may be unclear why they

sometimes produce their own effects approximately opposite those of the opioid agonists. This phenomenon may be due to inhibition of the basal activity of the G-protein cycle, which may be present even in the absence of opioid agonists (Fig. 10-2).

Opioid Actions

■ Analgesia

Opioids act directly on spinal opioid receptors to inhibit transmission via the dorsal horn between primary afferent neurons and the central nervous system (CNS) and act on thalamic and medullary centers to cause descending inhibition of dorsal horn activity. After injury, opioid receptors on peripheral terminals of primary afferents, located in tissue, also may cause analgesia in the presence of opioid drugs or endogenous opioid peptides. Opioid analgesic effects are specific to nociceptive (injury-perceiving) neurons; nonnociceptive afferents are unaffected, and normal sensations of pressure, touch, and temperature are preserved. Some forms of pain, especially neuropathic, respond poorly to opioids; opioid relief of this sort of pain may represent sedative effects.

■ Sedation

The specific analgesic actions of opioids differ from their sedative and psychomotor effects, often seen

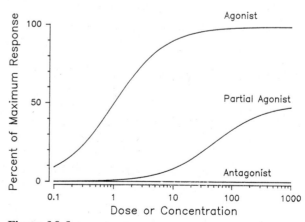

Figure 10-1

Influence of intrinsic efficacy on the opioid concentration-response relationship. Relative to full agonists (for a given receptor binding affinity), partial agonists have reduced maximal effects and potency; antagonists have no efficacy, or "negative" efficacy, and produce no response.

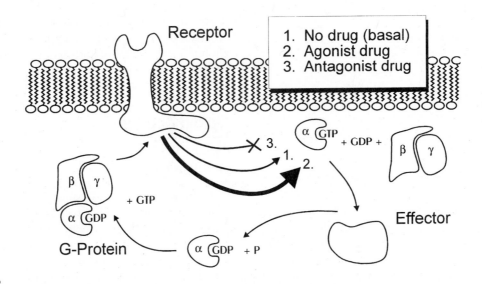

Figure 10-2

The G-protein cycle and its modulation by drug binding to receptor. The G-protein complex consists of three subunits, α, β, and γ, and binds the guanine nucleotides GDP and GTP. When GTP displaces GDP, the subunits dissociate. Cellular effectors are activated by the GTP-bound α subunit, and the cycle is completed by the spontaneous hydrolysis of bound GTP to GDP and reassociation of the three subunits. The receptor functions to facilitate the interaction of guanine nucleotides with the G-protein. A small amount of G-protein turnover occurs in the absence of receptor ligands (condition 1). Agonist drugs accelerate the cascade (condition 2), whereas antagonists slow it (condition 3).

with large doses of opioids. Large doses usually cause unconsciousness but do not produce reliably the true lack of awareness and subsequent amnesia achieved with benzodiazepines, barbiturates, and general anesthetics. Thus anesthetic techniques that rely on opioids as the primary agent usually include an additional drug to prevent awareness. The sedative effect of opioids is opposed by pain and environmental stimuli such as noise. Patients in severe pain may require very large doses of opioids while remaining alert.

■ Ventilatory Depression

Opioids act on μ receptors located in the ventral medulla, which are believed to inhibit the stimulatory input of chemosensitive neurons into the respiratory center. Thus opioids blunt, in a dose-related manner, the increase in respiratory rate and tidal volume caused by increased arterial CO_2 tension or decreased O_2 tension, the former to a greater extent than the latter. Modest increases in arterial PCO_2 are expected when analgesic doses of opioids are given, whereas larger doses such as those used in anesthesia often will induce apnea. In patients receiving opioids chronically, marked tolerance to the ventilatory depressant effects of opioids is typical.

As with the sedating effect of opioids, respiratory depression is functionally opposed by pain and stimulation from noise, movement, and touch. This is especially important in evaluating patients in the recovery room who have received opioids. The stimulation of being moved to the recovery room may arouse a patient, who may later fall asleep and become apneic after being left alone. Other factors, such as redistribution of opioids from tissues to blood by increased tissue blood flow or clearance of a previous dose of an antagonist such as naloxone, also may contribute. Close observation of respiration and oxygenation must continue until it is clear that a somnolent patient who has received opioids breathes adequately.

Opioids also depress the cough reflex. This effect can be particularly useful for awake intubation of the trachea and more generally for providing smooth induction and emergence.

■ Gastrointestinal Effects

Opioids commonly cause nausea and vomiting, which in the immediate postoperative period is inconvenient and unpleasant and can pose a risk for aspiration. This effect is mediated by opioid stimulation of the chemoreceptor trigger zone (CTZ) located in the area postrema in the floor of the fourth ventricle. Although located within the CNS, this structure has a "leaky" blood-brain barrier and is thus more exposed to the contents of the blood. Opioids, morphine in particular, and many blood-borne toxins activate the CTZ, which stimulates the vomiting center via a dopaminergic pathway; dopamine antagonists such as prochlorperazine and droperidol are useful treatments. With repeated administration, opioids exert an inhibitory effect directly on the vomiting center, counteracting the stimulatory effect on the CTZ. Nausea may worsen if the patient is moved, suggesting a vestibular component. Scopolamine or other centrally acting antimuscarinics may counteract opioid-induced nausea and vomiting.

The other major gastrointestinal effect of opioids is constipation, which results from the activation of opioid receptors in efferent pathways from the spinal cord to the gut, within the myenteric plexuses, and on the smooth muscle of the viscera. Effects include a modest decrease in gastric acid production and slowed gastric emptying, decreased small bowel motility and secretion, resulting in increased small bowel transit time, and contraction of the sphincter of Oddi and biliary tree. This can precipitate biliary colic or complicate cholangiography. The contribution of opioids to postoperative ileus remains poorly understood, but the potential for this effect is still occasionally cited as a justification for withholding opioid analgesics for postoperative pain. The constipating effects of opioids given chronically are severe, limiting their use in the management of cancer pain.

Cardiovascular Effects

Analgesic doses of opioids produce little direct effect on cardiovascular function in awake, healthy subjects. Larger doses, especially when given in combination with some drugs used in anesthesia, may depress the circulation. Stimulation (or disinhibition) of the central vagal nucleus with large, rapidly administered doses of opioids produces bradycardia. Antimuscarinics (e.g., atropine) or neuromuscular blockers with antimuscarinic properties (e.g., pancuronium) prevent this effect.

During anesthesia, opioids may produce hypotension by a number of mechanisms. Morphine in particular causes histamine release, especially with

rapid administration of large doses. This results in venodilation. Severely hemodynamically stressed patients who have become reliant on increased sympathetic tone to maintain blood pressure may suffer catastrophic hypotension after even modest doses of opioids owing to inhibition of sympathetic outflow. Intraoperative addition of an opioid analgesic to an anesthetic regimen consisting of nonanalgesic components (e.g., a volatile agent) can result in significant decreases in heart rate and blood pressure; this is not a direct effect of the opioid but rather an effect of the primary anesthetic, unmasked by the analgesic effect of the opioid.

Motor Effects

Very large doses of opioids, such as those used for patients undergoing cardiac operations, increase activity in central motor pathways, producing muscle rigidity. Chest wall rigidity can prevent adequate ventilation, and involvement of the muscles of the head and neck can cause difficulty in intubation. This effect is readily overcome by neuromuscular blockade.

Reinforcement, Tolerance, Dependence, and Addiction

Opioids present a potential for abuse for all who come in contact with them. Although opioids are now more liberally prescribed for pain, with an increased understanding that controlled use of opioids for analgesia does not result in addiction, our awareness of the diversion and abuse of opioids is similarly increased. Opioid diversion and abuse by anesthesiologists and other operating room personnel present particularly serious risks.

Much difficulty stems from misconceptions about tolerance, dependence, and addiction. Tolerance and dependence arise in patients, drug abusers, isolated tissues, or individual cells after a period of exposure to an opioid agonist. *Tolerance* is a requirement for increasing amounts of drug to achieve the original effects. With tolerance, potency decreases (the dose-response curve is displaced to the right), efficacy diminishes (reduced maximum possible effect), and slope becomes more shallow (flattening of the dose-response curve) (Fig. 10-3). *Dependence* is a state of adaptation to the drug so that the drug is required for normal function and its absence (or administration of an antagonist) causes the syndrome of abstinence or withdrawal.

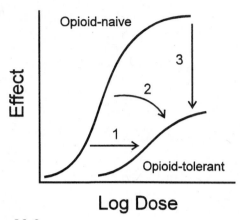

Figure 10-3

The effect of tolerance on the dose-response curve. Tolerance causes reduced potency (1), decreased slope (2), and decreased maximal effect (3).

Tolerance and dependence occur in tandem, and their magnitude is related to the duration and intensity of opioid drug use. They occur in patients receiving opioids chronically and are dealt with by providing sufficient opioid to prevent abstinence, freely administering larger doses of opioids for analgesia as the patient requires, and scrupulously avoiding the use of opioid antagonists or partial agonists, except in dire cases of respiratory depression. Tolerance and dependence resulting from appropriate medical treatment do not cause or predispose to addiction; withholding analgesics on the basis of concerns about development of addiction is inappropriate. Similarly, there is little evidence suggesting that controlled use of opioids for anesthesia or analgesia in drug abusers results in a worsening of addiction.

In contrast, *addiction* includes compulsive use of a drug, intense preoccupation with obtaining it, and a strong tendency to relapse. Uncontrolled self-administration and use of the drugs primarily for their rewarding properties are important elements. This positive reinforcement does not appear to occur in patients because the patient has reduced control over drug administration and because the patient seeks primarily relief from pain.

■ Other Effects

Miosis is a characteristic opioid effect caused by disinhibition of the Edinger-Westphal nucleus. It is not sufficiently specific for routine use as an indicator of opioid effect because many other drugs and physiologic changes associated with anesthesia result in changes in pupillary diameter.

True allergy to an opioid is exceedingly rare, but other effects are often interpreted as allergy or hypersensitivity, such as nausea and vomiting or anaphylactoid responses due to histamine release. Pruritus results from activation of central opioid receptors and possibly histamine release and usually responds to small doses of naloxone or antihistamines.

Pharmacokinetics

■ Absorption

Opioids given to surgical patients usually are administered by intravenous injection or infusion, which eliminates concerns about the rate or extent of drug absorption. Management of chronic pain involves such routes of administration as oral, subcutaneous, intramuscular, intrathecal, epidural, percutaneous, and even transnasal. An appreciation for the absorption characteristics of a drug for a given route is required for its effective use. For example, fentanyl is administered by epidural injection to selectively achieve analgesia by activating spinal opioid receptors, but owing to its lipophilic properties, it is rapidly taken up by the blood and may subsequently exert effects on the brain as well, causing sedation or even respiratory depression.

Orally administered opioids are well absorbed, but bioavailability can range from minimal to approximately 50 percent, depending on the drug, owing to metabolism of the drug on its first pass through the liver. On the other hand, drugs such as morphine or meperidine with active or toxic metabolites may yield relatively greater quantities of these substances when given orally rather than parenterally.

■ Distribution

Distribution out of the blood and into various tissues, rather than elimination by metabolism, determines the duration of action of opioids usually employed in anesthesia. Recovery is typically more rapid than would be predicted from elimination half-life but is prolonged by increased duration of drug administration. The *context-sensitive half-time* is the time required for the blood concentration of a drug to decrease to 50 percent of the steady-state value after an infusion is discontinued. For lipid-soluble drugs such as fentanyl, this measure of recovery time increases steadily as the dose and duration of the infusion increase so that this drug appears to be short-acting when given in small doses and long-acting when given in large doses (Fig. 10-4).

Onset of action is determined by the capacity of the opioids to penetrate the blood-brain barrier rapidly, determined by such factors as protein binding, ionization at physiologic pH, and lipid solubility. The equilibration half-time of alfentanil is approximately 1.5 minutes, whereas those of fentanyl and sufentanil are slightly more than 6 minutes. All three of these drugs equilibrate with the brain significantly faster than does morphine.

■ Metabolism and Excretion

All the opioids are metabolized extensively by the liver. Fentanyl, sufentanil, alfentanil, meperidine, and methadone are metabolized by the mixed-function oxidases. The opiate alkaloids morphine and codeine and the various opiate derivatives such as hydromorphone and oxycodone are metabolized by conjugation with glucuronic acid to form phenolic glucuronides, although demethylation of codeine and similar

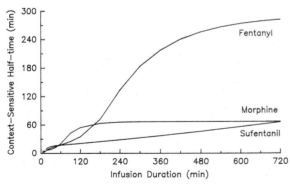

Figure 10-4

Estimated context-sensitive half-times for fentanyl, sufentanil, and morphine. Context-sensitive half-time is the time required for a 50 percent decrease in plasma concentration of the opioid after infusion to a target plasma concentration for a given period of time (the context). Pharmacokinetic parameters for fentanyl and sufentanil are those used by Shafer and Varvel (*Anesthesiology* 1991;74:53-63), as was the software used for the simulation (STANPUMP). Pharmacokinetic parameters for morphine are those of Sawe et al (*Clin Pharmacol Ther* 1981;30:629-635).

compounds is important as well. This metabolism inactivates the opioids, with two important exceptions (see individual drugs below). Patients with moderate hepatic disease may require decreased doses of opioids, but doses cannot be predicted by ordinary liver enzyme measurements.

■ Relative Potency

Particularly when comparing the potent lipophilic drugs such as fentanyl and sufentanil with morphine, widely varying estimates of relative potency are found in textbooks. This results from the variety of methods and regimens of administration used to assess potency. For example, 50 μg of fentanyl and 5 mg of morphine are roughly equivalent if the drugs are given intravenously and their effects monitored over 15 minutes; if the drugs are given intramuscularly and the desired duration of effect is 3 hours, much more fentanyl is needed to give effects equivalent to morphine. Determinations of relative potency must be based on circumstances comparable with the clinical situation at hand.

Individual Agents

Suggested doses for the most commonly used intravenous opioid preparations are given in Table 10-5

■ Morphine

Most of the general effects of opioids already listed were first described for morphine. Its major distinguishing feature is a tendency to release histamine, which causes peripheral vasodilation, hypotension, reflex tachycardia, and cutaneous flushing. Administering morphine slowly or in divided doses not only allows time to respond to the drug's cardiovascular effects but also minimizes histamine release. H_1 and H_2 blockers blunt the histamine-mediated cardiovascular effects of morphine.

Morphine is metabolized primarily to morphine-3-glucuronide and morphine-6-glucuronide. Morphine-6-glucuronide retains opioid activity, and contributes to the clinical effects of morphine, particularly after oral administration when larger amounts of the metabolite are formed due to the

Table 10-5

Intravenous Doses of Opioids for Anesthesia and Analgesia

Drug	Concentration	Analgesia	N₂O/Opioid Anesthesia	Repeat Dose	Cardiac Anesthesia
Fentanyl	50 µg/ml	0.5–1.0 µg/kg	5–15 µg/kg	0.5–1.0 µg/kg	20–100 µg/kg
Morphine	1–10 mg/ml	0.02–0.1 mg/kg	0.2–0.5 mg/kg	0.02–0.1 mg/kg	1–2 mg/kg
Sufentanil	50 µg/ml	Not recommended	1 µg/kg/h	0.1–0.3 µg/kg	5–20 µg/kg
Alfentanil	500 µg/ml	10–20 µg/kg	50–75 µg/kg + 0.5–2 µg/kg/min	10–25 µg/kg	50–75 µg/kg + 3–6 µg/kg/min

Note: These intravenous doses are suggested for typical adults and are given slowly or in divided doses. Patients with particular disease states may require smaller doses, whereas opioid-tolerant patients may require more.

first-pass effect. Both glucuronides are eliminated mainly by renal excretion, so other opioids with inactive metabolites should be considered for use in patients with renal failure, particularly when repeated doses are anticipated.

■ Fentanyl

Fentanyl is lipid-soluble and more potent than morphine. Small intravenous doses of fentanyl (1 to 4 µg/kg) can be given to produce the rapid onset of opioid effects, with rapid offset due to redistribution. In larger doses (10 to 50 µg/kg) it provides profound analgesic and sedative effects that require only minimal supplementation with sedatives or small concentrations of inhaled anesthetics to produce satisfactory general anesthesia.

Patients do not recover as rapidly from these larger doses because the time required to reduce plasma levels below the threshold for spontaneous ventilation is increased. After large doses of fentanyl, some patients experience what appears to be recurrence of effect after initial recovery, perhaps due to increased uptake of fentanyl from tissue by blood as a result of increased muscle blood flow after emergence. Other factors such as lack of stimulation, the use of other sedative drugs, and the residual effects of general anesthetics also contribute.

Large doses of fentanyl are better tolerated than large doses of morphine because fentanyl causes little or no histamine release. Direct cardiovascular depressant effects are minimal, and the only cardiovascular depression to be expected is that resulting from bradycardia or release from increased sympathetic tone. Although newer agents exhibit more rapid recovery times after long periods of administration (see Fig. 10-4), for short procedures (less than 2 hours), fentanyl remains the most useful drug for

opioid-based anesthesia for patients undergoing major operations.

■ Sufentanil

Sufentanil is an extremely potent synthetic opioid (approximately 7 times the potency of fentanyl in humans) prescribed almost exclusively by anesthesiologists. It is the most selective opioid for the µ receptor available for clinical use. When given by infusion for anesthetics of intermediate duration (2 to 6 hours), sufentanil can be expected to yield a more rapid rate of recovery than the other commonly used opioids. Otherwise, it is identical to fentanyl.

■ Alfentanil

Alfentanil is a synthetic opioid with potency in humans approximately 1/75 that of fentanyl. The pharmacokinetic profile of alfentanil differs from those of fentanyl and sufentanil in two important ways. First, alfentanil is more hydrophilic and has a correspondingly smaller volume of distribution. As a result, elimination by hepatic metabolism plays a relatively more important role in terminating the effects of alfentanil; patients with cirrhosis display prolonged elimination. Alfentanil's plasma elimination half-life is about 1.5 hours, making it the shortest-acting opioid after very prolonged infusions or very large doses. For brief administrations, it offers little advantage over fentanyl or sufentanil. Alfentanil is metabolized by the cytochrome P-450 isoenzyme 3A4, which metabolizes several other commonly used drugs. Cytochrome P-450 3A4 is inhibited by erythromycin and related macrolide antibiotics, resulting in decreased alfentanil clearance. Substantial interpatient variation in the activity of this enzyme appears to be responsible for variation in alfentanil clearance. A second distinguishing feature is alfentanil's greater un-ionized fraction at physiologic pH, giving it greater membrane permeability. Alfentanil's onset effect is the most rapid of the opioids, making it an excellent choice for administration as a single bolus dose when a brief period of intense opioid effect is required and no repeated doses or infusions are anticipated.

As with fentanyl, there have been recent reports of delayed respiratory depression (rebound) following alfentanil anesthesia. It is not clear whether these episodes were due to redistribution of the drug.

■ Meperidine

Meperidine (Demerol, known as pethidine in the United Kingdom and Australia) was the first completely synthetic opioid; its continued popularity belies its toxicity and other drawbacks. It is approximately one-tenth as potent as morphine and has a duration of action between those of morphine and fentanyl. Because the elimination half-life of meperidine is similar to that of morphine (approximately 3 hours), meperidine is often (incorrectly) prescribed on an every 3- to 4-hour as-needed basis for pain; this regimen rarely provides sustained analgesia. It is hydrolyzed and then conjugated or *n*-demethylated and conjugated in the liver. The *n*-demethylated metabolite, normeperidine, has reduced opioid agonist activity but is neurotoxic in greater concentrations. Normeperidine is eliminated by the kidney. Seizures may occur after large doses of meperidine or in patients with renal insufficiency. Given in large doses for anesthesia, meperidine has direct cardiodepressent effects and is no longer used in this fashion.

When meperidine is given to patients taking monoamine oxidase inhibitors (MAOIs), a severe, possibly fatal excitatory state results, with hypertension, tachycardia, delirium, seizures, and hyperpyrexia. This interaction seems to be specific for meperidine; other opioids appear to be safe. Meperidine is frequently given to control shivering after general anesthesia; the mechanism by which meperidine reduces shivering is unclear.

■ Heroin (Diacetylmorphine)

Heroin, a semisynthetic agonist, has no legally accepted medical use in the United States, but in England and other countries it is prescribed for treatment of chronic cancer pain. Heroin is two to three times as potent as morphine, is metabolized to morphine, and is more transient in its effect. There is no advantage to the use of heroin over morphine for pain control.

■ Methadone

In the chronic maintenance of opioid-dependent addicts, methadone replaces heroin because it has a very long duration of action and good oral bioavailability. Methadone reaches peak effect 4 hours after oral administration and 1 to 2 hours after subcutaneous or intramuscular administration. It is used for treatment of chronic cancer pain and very occasionally as an adjunct to general anesthesia.

■ Other Opioid Agonists

Hydromorphone (Dilaudid) is five times as potent as morphine, has a slightly shorter duration of action, and is otherwise similar to morphine. It is not known to have an active glucuronide metabolite comparable to morphine-6-glucuronide. Codeine, oxycodone, and hydrocodone are commonly given orally due to the improved bioavailability conferred by methylation of the phenolic hydroxyl group of the opiate molecule. Although codeine is available for injection, it is rarely used this way in contemporary practice.

■ Partial Agonists

These drugs are often referred to as *mixed agonist-antagonists* because of their ability to produce opioid agonist effects when administered alone but antagonize opioid effects of morphine and other full agonists when administered with them. Some of these drugs possess agonist effects at κ opioid receptors as well as acting as partial μ agonists.

Nalorphine was the first opioid employed as an antagonist, although it possesses significant agonist activity if not used in combination with a full agonist. After the introduction of naloxone (see p. 108), its use fell out of favor.

Attempts to produce analgesia without such undesirable opioid effects as respiratory depression, nausea, and addiction led to the development of other opioid partial agonists. Pentazocine (Talwin) produces analgesia, mild respiratory depression, and sedation in small doses but dysphoria in greater doses. This drug causes less biliary spasm than the pure agonists. It also causes an increase in catecholamine release with increased heart rate and cardiac work, which limits its application in anesthesia. It is currently prescribed for oral administration.

Partial agonist drugs used occasionally in anesthetic practice include butorphanol (Stadol), nalbuphine (Nubain), dezocine (Dalgan), and buprenorphine (Buprenex). Because the partial agonists have limited maximal effects, none have replaced the opioid full agonists in anesthetic practice.

■ Antagonists

Naloxone (Narcan) is the opioid antagonist in common clinical use. Unlike the partial agonists described above, it is a competitive antagonist for all three opioid receptors, although it is most potent at the μ receptor. Naloxone is used to reverse opioid toxicity or opioid overdose after anesthesia and to counteract some of the side effects (nausea, pruritus) of spinal opioids.

Naloxone is best given intravenously in small increments (0.1 mg or less) or by infusion to avoid the abrupt reversal of opioid effects, a dangerous syndrome that may be simply unpleasant or may include severe pain, excitation, cardiovascular stimulation, pulmonary edema, and death. The practice of giving large doses (2 mg or more) of this drug to patients with respiratory depression or coma of unknown etiology is dangerous; a safer course is to support ventilation and administer naloxone slowly. Naloxone is not given to opioid-dependent patients, either chronic pain patients or addicts, except to treat overdose, since it precipitates severe withdrawal and suffering. The elimination half-life of naloxone is 1 hour, and its duration of action is less than that of many opioids. Therefore, naloxone is often infused continuously or given intramuscularly to treat opioid overdose, and patients are observed closely for signs of returning opioid effects as naloxone is eliminated.

Naltrexone (Trexan) is a long-acting opioid antagonist given orally for the maintenance of abstinence in former opioid addicts. Patients receiving naltrexone may be temporarily resistant to opioids.

Applications of Opioids in Anesthesia

■ Opioids as Anesthetics

In 1969, Lowenstein described the use of morphine in large doses to provide anesthesia for patients undergoing open heart operations. The major benefit of this technique was hemodynamic stability for patients with severe cardiovascular disease. Newer opioids such as fentanyl that do not provoke histamine release and offer shorter recovery times have replaced morphine for this use.

For briefer operations and when the patient is expected to resume spontaneous ventilation immediately at the end of the procedure, lesser doses of opioid are used in combination with other intravenous agents, nitrous oxide, or smaller amounts of inhalation anesthetics. These "balanced techniques" seek to minimize the doses and side effects of each drug by giving synergistic combinations of agents, each chosen for a specific effect. However, adding nitrous oxide, volatile anesthetics, or intravenous agents to opioids may provoke cardiovascular depression not seen when opioids are used alone.

Opioid-based anesthetics are associated with predictable effects, including bradycardia, ventilatory depression, nausea and vomiting, and chest wall rigidity. The resulting depth of anesthesia is often light, so painful surgical stimulation may provoke hypertension, especially in patients with preexisting hypertension. The doses of fentanyl, sufentanil, and alfentanil used for major operations suppress the stress response to some extent, but "stress-free" anesthesia cannot be guaranteed for all patients.

Muscle relaxants are usually used with opioid anesthetic techniques. Should patients awaken under light anesthesia, the paralysis may keep them from making their plight known. Some clinicians intermittently allow muscle relaxation to lapse so that patients can respond to commands or to pain. Other signs of light anesthesia, such as tachycardia, hypertension, or tearing, may be absent, even though patients are aware of what is happening. Adequate doses of agents such as nitrous oxide, benzodiazepines, droperidol, or scopolamine or small doses of inhalation agents help prevent recall. Even if every effort is made to ensure adequate anesthesia, a rare patient will remember intraoperative conversations and events during light opioid-based anesthesia.

Opioids also are used as adjuncts to inhalation anesthesia: to relieve pain and decrease minimum alveolar concentration (MAC), to obtund airway reflexes at induction or emergence, to prevent tachycardia, and to slow and deepen spontaneous ventilation during inhalation anesthesia. For patients who might be sensitive to the hypotensive effects of potent inhalation agents, small doses of opioids may permit the use of lesser anesthetic concentrations, minimizing cardiovascular depression.

■ Opioids as Analgesics

Intravenously administered opioids are still the mainstay of acute postoperative pain management. The range of opioid concentrations that are effective for pain relief yet do not depress respiration is relatively narrow and varies among patients, which accounts for the failure of the practice of intermittent intramuscular injections to provide adequate analgesia. Patient-controlled analgesia (PCA) techniques have proven to be safe and permit patients to titrate opioid drugs in controlled dosages to their own level of comfort. This method, as well as the oral and spinal administration of opioids, is discussed in the chapters on pain management.

BIBLIOGRAPHY

Bartkowski RR, Goldberg ME, Larijani GE, Boerner T. Inhibition of alfentanil metabolism by erythromycin. *Clin Pharmacol Ther* 1989;46:99-102.

Bovill JG, Sebel PS, Stanley TH. Opioid analgesics in anesthesia: With special reference to their use in cardiovascular anesthesia. *Anesthesiology* 1984;61:731-755.

Cousins MJ, Mather LE. Intrathecal and epidural administration of opioids. *Anesthesiology* 1984;61:276-310.

Di Chiara G, North RA. Neurobiology of opiate abuse. *Trends Pharmacol Sci* 1992;13:185-193.

Glare PA, Walsh TD. Clinical pharmacokinetics of morphine. *Ther Drug Monit* 1991;13:1-23.

Mansour A, Khachaturian H, Lewis ME, et al. Anatomy of CNS opioid receptors. *Trends Neurosci* 1988;11:308-314.

Martin WR. Pharmacology of opioids. *Pharmacol Rev* 1984;35:283-323.

Millan MJ. κ-Opioid receptors and analgesia. *Trends Pharmacol Sci* 1990;11:70-76.

Reisine T, Bell GI. Molecular biology of opioid receptors. *Trends Neurosci* 1993;16:506-510.

Shafer SL, Varvel JR. Pharmacokinetics, pharmacodynamics, and rational opioid selection. *Anesthesiology* 1991;74:53-63.

Stein C. Peripheral mechanisms of opioid analgesia. *Anesth Analg* 1993;76:182-191.

Yun C-H, Wood M, Wood AJJ, Guengerich FP. Identification of the pharmacogenetic determinants of alfentanil metabolism: Cytochrome P-450 3A4. *Anesthesiology* 1992;77:467-474.

11

Muscle Relaxants

Dennis M. Fisher

Muscle relaxants form an important part of the armamentarium of the anesthesiologist. Whereas older anesthetic agents such as ether produced excellent skeletal muscle relaxation, current anesthetics, including both intravenous and inhaled agents, often depend on muscle relaxants to provide adequate operating conditions. Since its introduction in the 1940s, D-tubocurarine has almost disappeared from use, replaced initially by metocurine and pancuronium and more recently by atracurium and vecuronium. The development of muscle relaxants with more rapid onset, shorter and predictable duration, and minimal side effects continues.

This chapter reviews the physiology of the neuromuscular junction, the clinical pharmacology of relaxants and their antagonists, the techniques for monitoring neuromuscular blockade, and the uses of these drugs in anesthesia.

Neuromuscular Pharmacology and Physiology

Muscle relaxants produce their desired effect at the neuromuscular junction but also have nonspecific effects at many other sites. An understanding of the physiology of neuromuscular transmission aids understanding of the actions of muscle relaxants.

■ Neuromuscular Transmission

The neuromuscular junction (Fig. 11-1) consists of the terminus of the axon of a nerve, the motor endplate of a muscle, and the area between these, the synaptic cleft. In the nerve terminal of the axon are vesicles, each containing approximately 10,000 molecules of acetylcholine. The surface of the motor endplate contains invaginations called *synaptic folds.* Along the surface of the motor endplate are the nicotinic receptors, large proteins consisting of five subunits arranged in a ring to form an ion channel; the concentration of these receptors is highest at the shoulder of each synaptic fold. Molecules of the enzyme acetylcholinesterase dangle on stalks from the surface of the motor endplate, protruding into the synaptic cleft and the synaptic folds.

Normal neuromuscular transmission begins in the nerve. At rest, an active transport mechanism, the Na^+/K^+ pump, maintains a high concentration of Na^+ ions outside and K^+ ions inside the axon, producing a transmembrane potential of approximately -90 mV. When the nerve is stimulated, Na^+ channels open, permitting Na^+ ions to cross the membrane. As the transmembrane potential becomes less negative, the threshold for depolarization is reached, and an action potential is generated. This, in turn, generates local currents along the nerve surface, opening adjacent Na^+ channels and propagating the action potential along the nerve. As the action potential reaches the nerve terminal, entry of calcium into the nerve causes vesicles to move to and fuse with the cell membrane, thereby releasing acetylcholine into the synaptic cleft. These acetylcholine molecules traverse the narrow width of the synaptic cleft (50 nm), binding to one or both α subunits of the nicotinic receptor and changing its conformation. If both α subunits are occupied by acetylcholine, the channel opens, permitting rapid entry of Na^+ ions and depolarizing the motor endplate. Acetylcholine is not tightly bound to the recep-

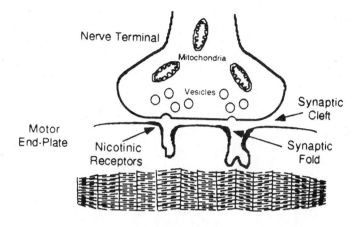

Figure 11-1

The neuromuscular junction consists of an axon of a nerve and the motor endplate, separated by the synaptic cleft. Vesicles containing acetylcholine are located in the nerve terminal. Nicotinic receptors, large proteins consisting of five subunits arranged in a ring to form an ion channel, are located in the motor endplate, near the junction of the synaptic cleft and the synaptic field.

tor and moves on and off the receptor rapidly. Within nanoseconds, unbound acetylcholine is metabolized by the enzyme acetylcholinesterase, found in the junctional cleft. The products of this enzymatic reaction, choline and acetate, return to the nerve terminal, where they are used to synthesize new acetylcholine.

When the nerve is stimulated electrically, the resulting muscle contraction is known as a *twitch*. When neuromuscular transmission is normal, the amplitude of this twitch is sustained even with rapidly repeated stimulation of the nerve.

■ Neuromuscular Blockade

Neuromuscular blockade occurs when the normal events in neuromuscular transmission are disrupted at one or more sites. Succinylcholine (Fig. 11-2), whose molecular structure resembles two acetylcholine molecules attached end to end, enters the synaptic cleft, attaches to the receptor, and depolarizes the neuromuscular junction; thus it is a depolarizing muscle relaxant. Unlike acetylcholine, whose effect is terminated rapidly by the action of acetylcholinesterase, succinylcholine is not metabolized locally at the neuromuscular junction. Consequently, the depolarizing action of succinylcholine persists longer than that of acetylcholine, and the motor endplate remains depolarized and refractory to the effects of acetylcholine. This is known as *phase I neuromuscular blockade*. With electrical stimulation, the twitch response is decreased from baseline, and repeated stimuli evoke no further decrease (Fig. 11-3). Continued exposure of the motor endplate to succinylcholine decreases the sensitivity of the neuromuscular junction to the effects of succinylcholine. Although relatively little is known about this type of neuromuscular blockade, known as *phase II*, the response to nerve stimulation has a consistent pattern: a decrease in twitch (as with phase I blockade) and fade with repeated stimuli (unlike phase I blockade).

The neuromuscular effects of nondepolarizing muscle relaxants differ greatly from those of succinylcholine: Stimulation of the nerve evokes twitches that are decreased from baseline, but repeated stimuli elicit progressively smaller twitches (see Fig. 11-3). Although these drugs act principally by binding to the same sites in the receptor as do acetylcholine and succinylcholine (a result of their similar molecular structure; see Fig. 11-2), the nondepolarizing muscle relaxants do not depolarize the motor endplate. They interfere with neuromuscular transmission by three mechanisms. First, they prevent acetylcholine from binding normally to the receptor, thereby preventing depolarization of the motor endplate. Second, if the concentration of a nondepolarizing muscle relaxant is excessive, molecules of the muscle relaxant may enter the channel of the receptor, causing channel blockade. Finally, nondepolarizing muscle relaxants act at presynaptic sites, blocking Na^+ channels and preventing movement of acetylcholine from synthesis sites to release sites, although the clinical importance of this mechanism has been questioned.

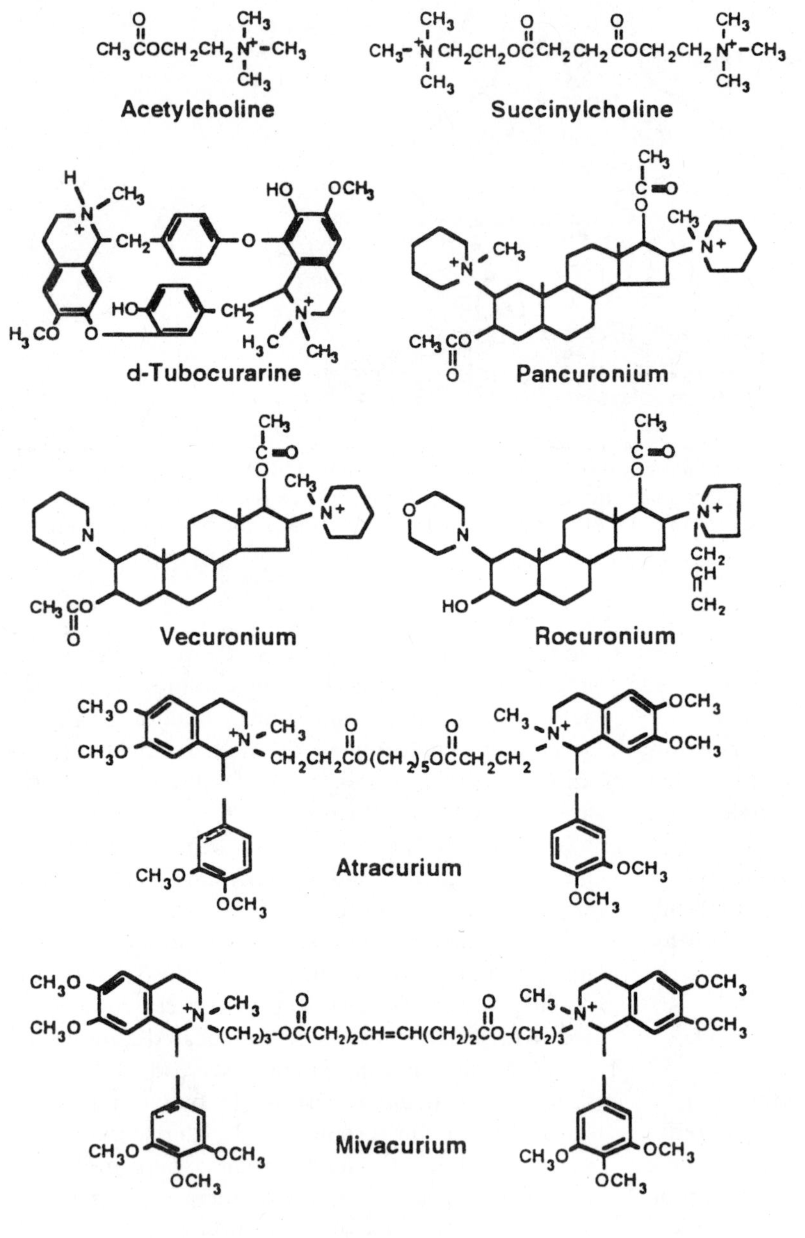

Figure 11-2

The molecular structures of acetylcholine, succinylcholine, and eight nondepolarizing muscle relaxants are shown. Succinylcholine consists of two molecules of acetylcholine; the nondepolarizing muscle relaxants each contain some portion of the acetylcholine molecule.

Because the motor endplate is depolarized only when both α subunits of the receptor are occupied by acetylcholine, and because neither acetylcholine nor the muscle relaxants in clinical use are tightly bound to the α subunits, the neuromuscular response to nondepolarizing muscle relaxants depends on the relative concentrations of acetylcholine and muscle relaxant at the receptor (*competitive inhibition*). If the concentration of muscle relaxant is great relative to that of acetylcholine, it is unlikely that acetylcholine will occupy both α subunits, and thus neuromuscular transmission will be compromised. As the ratio of the concentration of nondepolarizing muscle relaxant to the concentration of acetylcholine decreases, it is more likely that both α subunits will be occupied by acetylcholine and that neuromuscular transmission will be normal. This competitive relationship is exploited to speed recovery from nondepolarizing muscle relaxants. Drugs such as neostigmine increase the local concentration of acetylcholine in the synaptic cleft (either by slowing normal destruction of acetylcholine or by increasing its release from the nerve terminal), thereby increasing the ratio of acetylcholine to the nondepolarizing muscle relaxant and favoring normal neuromuscular transmission. Although the physiology is not well understood, increasing the local concentration of acetylcholine also improves neuromuscular transmission when succinylcholine-induced phase II blockade has occurred; succinylcholine-induced phase I blockade is not antagonized by this mechanism.

Blood flow to a muscle also influences its response to muscle relaxants. Following administration of bolus doses of muscle relaxants, well-perfused muscles such as the diaphragm may develop neuromuscular blockade before muscles with less blood flow such as those in the hand. In addition, various muscles respond differently to muscle relaxants. For example, the diaphragm is resistant to the effects of nondepolarizing muscle relaxants compared with in-

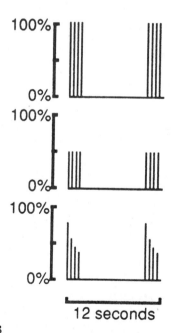

Figure 11-3

The motor response (twitch) in response to a 2-Hz stimulus is shown in three different circumstances. In the absence of muscle relaxants (*above*), all responses are similar in amplitude. After a subparalyzing dose of succinylcholine, all responses are similar in amplitude but smaller than the baseline value (*center*). After a subparalyzing dose of a nondepolarizing muscle relaxant, the first response is smaller than baseline, and subsequent responses demonstrate fade (*below*); a similar response is seen during succinylcholine-induced phase II block.

tercostal and abdominal muscles or the adductor pollicis (the muscle typically monitored during clinical anesthesia).

Clinical Pharmacology of Depolarizing and Nondepolarizing Relaxants

■ Depolarizing Relaxants: Succinylcholine

Pharmacokinetics

Succinylcholine (and mivacurium, a nondepolarizing muscle relaxant described later) differs from other muscle relaxants in that the acute offset of its effects is due not only to redistribution of the drug but also to metabolism by pseudocholinesterase (plasma cholinesterase). Because pseudocholinesterase exists in plasma but not at the neuromuscular junction (unlike acetylcholinesterase, the enzyme that degrades acetylcholine), succinylcholine is not metabolized at the neuromuscular junction. Thus the action of succinylcholine terminates as its plasma concentration decreases and it diffuses from the neuromuscular junction into plasma.

This process of enzymatic destruction provides for succinylcholine a much more rapid offset of effect than does the redistribution, hepatic metabolism, and renal excretion typical of other muscle relaxants. This uniquely rapid recovery is especially advantageous if airway or intubation difficulties make it important for a patient to recover from neuromuscular blockade as soon as possible. Likewise, the rapid destruction of succinylcholine permits the use of very large doses, accounting for its quick onset (30 to 60 seconds from intravenous administration to adequate relaxation for intubation), faster than the onset of the nondepolarizers. Although similar overdoses (8 times the dose producing 95 percent twitch depression, ED_{95}) of nondepolarizing drugs likely produce similarly rapid onsets, the prolonged recovery limits the use of this technique.

Recovery of ventilatory effort following succinylcholine-induced neuromuscular blockade occurs in most patients within 5 to 10 minutes but may be prolonged in those who have decreased pseudocholinesterase activity, either drug-induced or associated with liver disease or pregnancy. More significant prolongation results from genetically abnormal pseudocholinesterase, most commonly atypical pseudocholinesterase. Patients who have heterozygous atypical pseudo-cholinesterase abnormality (1 in 480) have slightly prolonged blockade (recovery to 90 percent of baseline twitch in 15 minutes following succinylcholine 1 mg/kg), whereas patients with the homozygous abnormality (1 in 3200) show marked prolongation (160 minutes to 90 percent recovery). A history of prolonged blockade following succinylcholine in the patient or family suggests this enzymatic abnormality. Laboratory evaluation includes measurement of cholinesterase activity and the dibucaine number, which represents the extent of inhibition of the enzyme by dibucaine. The normal enzyme is inhibited to the extent of 80 percent and the abnormal by 20 percent (dibucaine numbers of 80 and 20 percent, respectively).

Side Effects

Malignant Hyperthermia. The massive, sustained depolarization of the muscle membrane caused by succinylcholine probably accounts for the fact that the drug readily precipitates malignant hyperthermia syndrome (see Chap. 36). The drug is contraindicated in patients susceptible to this syndrome.

Masseter Spasm. On occasion (approximately 1 percent of children given halothane for induction of anesthesia), after succinylcholine has been administered for tracheal intubation, the jaw muscles become rigid rather than relaxed; this limits but usually does not prevent tracheal intubation. This spasm of the masseter muscles sometimes progresses to malignant hyperthermia, although increased jaw tone and decreased mouth opening occur far more frequently after succinylcholine than does malignant hyperthermia.

Cardiovascular. Succinylcholine, because of its similarity to acetylcholine, exerts many of its side effects via the autonomic nervous system. Ganglionic stimulation may either increase or decrease both heart rate and blood pressure depending on the prior state of the patient's autonomic nervous system. Cardiac slowing occurs more frequently following a second dose (particularly if atropine has not been administered) and more frequently in children than in adults. Rarely, asystole may occur, even following single doses or brief infusions.

Hyperkalemia. Serum potassium concentration usually increases 0.5 to 1.0 mEq/liter following succinylcholine, but in some instances the increase may exceed 5 mEq/liter, as in patients with acute upper motor neuron lesions, spinal cord injury, extensive burns, massive trauma, or closed head injury. The period of vulnerability, although variable, usually begins a few days after the insult and persists for 6 months or longer. Such patients may suffer lethal hyperkalemia if given succinylcholine.

Myalgias. After succinylcholine, many patients report postoperative muscle pain, typically worse in the shoulders and back and sometimes exceeding the discomfort produced by the operation. This is most prevalent in young, muscular men, especially those who are physically active after minor operations. Assuming this pain to be related to fasciculations, efforts at prevention have focused on minimizing fasciculations (described below).

Increased Intraocular, Intragastric, and Intracranial Pressure. Because the initial effect of succinylcholine is depolarization, the tone of various muscles increases briefly when the drug is given, probably explaining increases in intraocular and intragastric pressure. The etiology of increased intracranial pressure is less well understood. These pressure increases provoke concern: increased intraocular pressure might force vitreous fluid from a ruptured globe; increased intragastric pressure might cause a patient with residual gastric contents to regurgitate and, possibly, aspirate; and increased intracranial pressure might compromise the patient with limited intracranial compliance. Whether to avoid succinylcholine because of these potential problems is controversial. In one study, patients with ruptured globes given succinylcholine did not extrude vitreous fluid. Although intragastric pressure increases after succinylcholine, distal esophageal pressure increases as well, maintaining the normal gradient. It seems likely that the magnitude of the clinical problem depends on the occurrence of fasciculations as well as predisposing factors such as hiatal hernia. Maneuvers that decrease the incidence and magnitude of fasciculations may minimize increases in pressure and resulting complications.

Clinical Use

Bolus Administration. The most common use of succinylcholine is to facilitate tracheal intubation, particularly if rapid control of the airway is necessary, as in the patient at risk for aspiration. The onset of relaxation is sufficiently rapid (60 seconds in adults given 1.5 mg/kg) that most patients can be left apneic from the time succinylcholine is administered until intubation is completed. Additional relaxation for the remainder of the operation is provided by additional doses of succinylcholine or nondepolarizing relaxants.

Defasciculation. The most popular technique to prevent fasciculations is to administer a small dose of a nondepolarizing muscle relaxant several minutes before succinylcholine. Presumably, the nondepolarizing relaxant occupies enough receptors to prevent the usual sustained depolarization. Such "defasciculating doses" are approximately one-tenth the dose required for intubation and usually do not produce symptoms of weakness in awake patients. The dose of succinylcholine is increased 50 percent to ensure adequate paralysis. A small number of patients (1 to 5 percent) experience significant weakness after defasciculating doses of any nondepolarizing blocker, in which case prompt induction of anesthesia and controlled ventilation are required. This constitutes the chief hazard of this technique. Attempts also have been made to prevent fasciculations by administering small doses of succinylcholine (e.g., 10 mg/70 kg, not in awake patients), followed 3 to 5 minutes later by a usual dose. This technique, known as *self-taming*, was briefly popular, but it now appears to be ineffective.

Continuous Infusion. Rapid elimination by pseudocholinesterase makes succinylcholine an ideal candidate for administration by infusion. However, with repeated administration, the effect of the drug changes from phase I to phase II blockade, accompanied by increases in dose requirement (tachyphylaxis) and fade with repeated stimuli. Some signs of phase II blockade may be apparent even following a single dose. The occurrence of phase II blockade has limited the popularity of continuous infusions.

Antagonism of Phase II Blockade. Recovery from phase I succinylcholine-induced neuromuscular blockade typically is quite rapid and is not hastened by drugs such as neostigmine or edrophonium. In contrast, recovery from phase II blockade frequently is prolonged. Cholinesterase inhibitors such as neostigmine promote recovery from succinylcholine-induced phase II block, but inhibition of pseudocholinesterase by neostigmine delays clearance of any remaining succinylcholine, impeding the patient's recovery. This risk makes it wise to withhold neostigmine in most cases and to await spontaneous recovery, usually a matter of 20 to 30 minutes.

■ Nondepolarizing Relaxants

The nine nondepolarizing relaxants now available include those of brief duration (mivacurium), intermediate duration (atracurium, vecuronium, and rocuronium), and prolonged duration (D-tubocurarine, metocurine, pancuronium, doxacurium, and pipecuronium). One additional relaxant, gallamine, is no longer in common use, since it causes pronounced tachycardia.

Pharmacokinetics and Pharmacodynamics

Because nondepolarizing muscle relaxants are charged polar molecules, they do not penetrate cell membranes well. Consequently, the volume of distribution at steady state for all muscle relaxants is approximately the volume of the extracellular fluid space. All require minimal time to move on and off the receptor, so the factors limiting onset of effect and recovery are blood flow to the muscle, partitioning between the plasma and the neuromuscular junction, and changes in the plasma concentration of the muscle relaxant.

These pharmacokinetic and pharmacodynamic characteristics determine the onset of paralysis. Time to peak effect for doses of most nondepolarizing muscle relaxants producing less than 90 percent blockade is similar, approximately 4 to 6 minutes. However, the greater amounts usually employed in practice produce greater than 99 percent blockade and cause twitch to decrease to less than 1 percent of baseline in less than 2 minutes.

Pharmacokinetic and pharmacodynamic characteristics also influence the recovery of neuromuscular function. Following a single dose, neuromuscular recovery begins during redistribution of the drug, whereas recovery from repeated doses depends on elimination of the muscle relaxant. Thus recovery from initial doses is rapid compared with that from subsequent doses, a phenomenon known as *cumulation*. In addition, even when failure of the metabolizing organ results in almost no elimination of the muscle relaxant, neuromuscular function may recover after a single dose through redistribution alone. However, with repeated doses, the decline in plasma concentration of the muscle relaxant is slowed by organ failure, and cumulation is pronounced. Most nondepolarizing relaxants are eliminated by the kidney (D-tubocurarine, pancuronium, metocurine, gallamine, doxacurium, and pancuronium) or the liver (vecuronium, D-tubocurarine). While it is wise to select muscle relaxants for patients with liver or kidney failure accordingly, the effects of even marked degrees of organ failure on the pharmacokinetics of muscle relaxants are unpredictable in the individual patient.

Atracurium was synthesized specifically to undergo Hofmann elimination (spontaneous degradation at physiologic pH and temperature); it also undergoes ester hydrolysis and hepatic and renal elimination. Since its elimination does not depend exclusively on organ function, it is a good choice for patients with renal or hepatic failure.

Mivacurium is eliminated via pseudocholinesterase, the same enzyme responsible for the elimination of succinylcholine. Although the clearance of mivacurium varies as a function of plasma cholinesterase activity, the range of enzyme activities in normal patients is sufficiently small and the rate of recovery sufficiently rapid that infusion requirements need not be adjusted for most patients. However, the same patients who fail to metabolize succinylcholine require markedly less mivacurium and recover slowly from its effects. Neuromuscular monitoring is needed to avoid overdose and prolonged paralysis.

Pediatric Patients. The volume of distribution at steady state of nondepolarizing muscle relaxants changes with age just as does the volume of the extracellular fluid space, being greatest at birth and decreasing during the first year of life. Plasma clearance also changes with age; clearance of D-tubocurarine improves as glomerular filtration increases during the first year of life. Compared with the changes in volume of distribution, these changes in clearance are minimal. The larger volumes of distribution found in younger patients produce longer pharmacologic half-lives and slower recovery from nondepolarizing blockers. Although atracurium is similar to other nondepolarizing muscle relaxants in having a larger volume of distribution in young patients, atracurium is eliminated by hydrolysis from both plasma and tissue compartments, resulting in minimal changes in duration of action with age. Another factor that changes with maturation is sensitivity to the nondepolarizing muscle relaxants. For both D-tubocurarine and vecuronium, neuromuscular blockade occurs at lower concentrations in neonates and infants than in children and adults. Age-related changes in neuromuscular junction sensitivity to atracurium appear to be minimal.

Elderly Patients. The durations of action of D-tubocurarine, metocurine, pancuronium, and ve-

curonium (but not atracurium) are prolonged in the elderly. The prolonged action of the former drugs likely results from pharmacokinetic changes associated with aging, particularly decreased hepatic and renal function, rather than from changes in neuromuscular junction sensitivity. The absence of age-related changes for atracurium may be due to its multiple elimination pathways.

Drug Interaction

The effect of the nondepolarizing muscle relaxants depends on other drugs administered to the patient, including inhaled anesthetics and some antibiotics, which can prolong neuromuscular blockade.

Inhaled Anesthetics. Although most inhaled anesthetics do not produce measurable decreases in twitch, they depress the response of the motor endplate to acetylcholine, thereby potentiating the effects of nondepolarizing muscle relaxants. The degree of potentiation varies for each inhaled agent and each muscle relaxant. For example, atracurium is least affected by inhaled anesthetics, whereas both D-tubocurarine and pancuronium are potentiated markedly by both isoflurane and enflurane. This potentiation requires clinicians to administer lesser doses of the muscle relaxant, resulting in smaller plasma concentrations of the muscle relaxant. At the end of anesthesia, potentiation of muscle relaxants by inhaled anesthetics may persist because of relatively slow washout of anesthetics from muscles.

Magnesium. Magnesium reduces the release of acetylcholine from the nerve terminal, presumably by competing with calcium, as well as decreasing the depolarizing action of acetylcholine on the motor endplate and the excitability of muscle fibers. When magnesium sulfate is used to treat preeclampsia and eclampsia, serum magnesium concentrations are sufficient to potentiate neuromuscular blockade caused by both succinylcholine and nondepolarizing muscle relaxants. Although calcium enhances release of acetylcholine from the nerve terminal and should antagonize magnesium's effects, calcium also stabilizes the postjunctional membrane, which may explain why calcium only partially antagonizes a combined magnesium-nondepolarizing muscle relaxant blockade and may augment combined magnesium-succinylcholine blockade.

Antibiotics. Numerous antibiotics potentiate muscle relaxants, acting variously at both prejunctional and postjunctional sites. The prejunctional mechanism appears to be similar to that of magnesium. Neostigmine antagonizes the increased blockade produced by many antibiotics. Calcium may antagonize this effect, but it also may antagonize the antibacterial effects of some antibiotics.

Other Drugs. Numerous drugs potentiate or antagonize the effects of nondepolarizing muscle relaxants. Those which potentiate include furosemide, local anesthetics, quinidine, and calcium channel blockers, while phenytoin, carbamazepine, and theophylline appear to antagonize neuromuscular blockade.

Adverse Effects

The adverse effects of nondepolarizing muscle relaxants are generally of less consequence than those of succinylcholine.

Cardiovascular. Some muscle relaxants release histamine, producing hypotension and tachycardia. D-Tubocurarine is most likely to release histamine; histamine release due to atracurium and mivacurium rarely results in significant effects. Administering the drugs in divided doses over several minutes eliminates the risk of histamine release.

In contrast, pancuronium produces hypertension and tachycardia, owing to release of norepinephrine and blockade of cardiac vagal receptors. These effects are dose-dependent and can be minimized by slow administration of pancuronium over 1 to 2 minutes. Metocurine has few cardiovascular effects but is used only rarely now. Vecuronium has minimal cardiovascular effects, even with large doses, making it a good choice when cardiovascular changes must be avoided. Doxacurium and pipecuronium produce minimal cardiovascular effects also.

Pulmonary. Some nondepolarizing muscle relaxants produce wheezing in susceptible patients. This problem has been well documented for D-tubocurarine. Although atracurium and mivacurium release histamine, wheezing rarely has been reported.

Time Course of Nondepolarizing Muscle Relaxants

A critical factor in the use of muscle relaxants is management of the time course of their action, including both the onset and duration of neuromuscular blockade.

Onset of Neuromuscular Blockade. The speed of the onset of neuromuscular blockade depends primarily on the time it takes a muscle relaxant to reach the neuromuscular junction and the magnitude of the dose administered. Onset is faster in younger patients, presumably because of their greater cardiac outputs and more rapid circulation times. Greater doses of vecuronium eliminate all responses to a train-of-four stimuli more rapidly than do lesser ones (Fig. 11-4), so large doses approach the rapidity of succinylcholine, at the expense of a markedly prolonged duration of action. Some muscle relaxants do not demonstrate a faster onset with larger doses; most likely, cardiovascular changes produced by these muscle relaxants delay their delivery to the neuromuscular junction.

The onset of neuromuscular blockade varies; it is faster in certain central muscles such as the laryngeal adductors, the diaphragm, and the orbicularis oculi than at the adductor pollicis, the muscle typically monitored during anesthesia. Assuming that conditions for tracheal intubation correlate with relaxation of the laryngeal muscles and the diaphragm, tracheal intubation can be performed before complete paralysis is achieved at the adductor pollicis, possibly at 80 to 90 percent twitch depression.

None of the available nondepolarizing muscle relaxants has a time profile identical to that of succinylcholine. The onset of rocuronium is fastest, but its duration is comparable with that of atracurium and vecuronium rather than that of succinylcholine. No

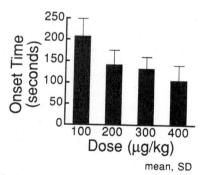

Figure 11-4

Onset time (defined as time from administration of vecuronium to disappearance of all four responses to a train-of-four stimulus) following varying doses of vecuronium in adults. As the dose increases, onset time decreases.

(Redrawn with permission from Ginsberg B, Glass PS, Quill T, et al: Onset and duration of neuromuscular blockade following high-dose vecuronium administration. Anesthesiology *1989;71:201-205.)*

nondepolarizing muscle relaxant has a duration of action as brief as that of succinylcholine.

Duration of Neuromuscular Blockade. Because nondepolarizing muscle relaxants are not metabolized at the neuromuscular junction, their effects terminate as the plasma concentration decreases, causing the muscle relaxant to diffuse from the neuromuscular junction to plasma. Consequently, the duration of action of nondepolarizing muscle relaxants is influenced predominantly by factors affecting the plasma concentration of the drug. With usual single doses of nondepolarizing muscle relaxants, recovery occurs late in the redistribution phase or early in the elimination phase. As a result, differences in duration of action of the nondepolarizing muscle relaxants do not correlate well with their elimination half-lives. For example, the elimination half-life of atracurium is 20 minutes, while that of vecuronium is 70 minutes (Table 11-1). Despite this marked difference between the two drugs, the time course of paralysis following single doses used for tracheal intubation is similar.

Methods of Administration

Cumulation, interpatient variability, the potentiating effects of anesthetics and other medications, and the inconsistent effects of organ failure make it impractical to give muscle relaxants according to a fixed dosage schedule. Although suggested doses are given in Table 11-2, successive doses must be judged according to the patient's response. Infusion rates, the size of bolus doses, or the intervals between doses must be adjusted to give the minimum degree of relaxation required at any given stage of the operation and the anesthetic. This scheme of titration to effect usually allows even patients with severely compromised organ function or those with unusual sensitivity to the drugs to be managed without unwanted postoperative weakness. When extreme prolongation of relaxant effect is anticipated, atracurium is a rational choice because of its multiple elimination pathways and minimal cumulative effects.

Bolus Administration. The initial dose of a nondepolarizing muscle relaxant depends on whether succinylcholine has been administered for tracheal intubation. If the nondepolarizing muscle relaxant is given for tracheal intubation, then a large dose, twice the ED_{95}, hastens the onset of relaxation. If succinylcholine is used for tracheal intubation, then the subsequent dose of the nondepolarizing muscle relaxant may be small (the ED_{50}), in which case additional doses may be required to produce the adequate relaxation. Rocuronium has an onset nearly identical to that of succinylcholine.

Table 11-1

Pharmacokinetic Characteristics of Muscle Relaxants

	Plasma Clearance (ml/kg/min)	Volume of Distribution at Steady State (ml/kg)	Elimination Half-Life (min)
Atracurium	5	100	20
Doxacurium	3	250	100
Mivacurium			
cis-trans stereoisomer	105	300*	2
trans-trans stereoisomer	60	150*	2
cis-cis stereoisomer	5	340*	50
Pancuronium	2	250	140
Pipecuronium	2.5	300	150
Rocuronium	3	200	70
Succinylcholine	Unknown	Unknown	Unknown
D-Tubocurarine	3	300	90
Vecuronium	5	270	70

Note: These values are for healthy adults and are rounded to facilitate their use in clinical practice; variation among patients exceeds the rounding errors. Mivacurium consists of three stereoisomers, two of which (cis-trans and trans-trans) are believed to be equipotent to the chiral mixture and compromise 94 percent of that mixture; the third stereoisomer, cis-cis, comprises 6 percent of the mixture and is believed, based on studies in animals, to be less than one-tenth as potent as the mixture.

* $V\beta$.

Table 11-2

Suggested Doses of Muscle Relaxants

	Initial Dose for Tracheal Intubation (mg/kg)	Initial Dose Not for Intubation (mg/kg)	Supplemental Doses (mg/kg)	Dosing Interval (min)
Atracurium	0.5	0.3	0.1	15
Doxacurium	0.05	0.025	0.01	40
Mivacurium	0.2	0.1	See below	See below
Pancuronium	0.1	0.05	0.015	40
Pipecuronium	0.1	0.05	0.015	40
Rocuronium	0.6	0.3	0.2	40
Succinylcholine	1.0	0.3	0.3	5
D-Tubocurarine	0.6	0.3	0.1	30
Vecuronium	0.1	0.05	0.02	20

Note: These doses are for healthy adults and children (not infants) and are rounded to facilitate their use in clinical practice. Supplemental doses should be administered based on clinical signs such as recovery of twitch response rather than by a predetermined schedule. It may be appropriate to administer doses smaller than those shown, giving additional muscle relaxant depending on the response to the initial dose. For rapid-sequence induction, larger doses (e.g., double those shown) will speed onset but may cause additional side effects and prolonged neuromuscular blockade. When potent inhaled anesthetics are administered, reduce supplemental doses of the nondepolarizing muscle relaxants (i.e., all but succinylcholine) by 30 to 50 percent. Data for supplemental doses of mivacurium are omitted—its brief duration of action suggests that infusion at 2 to 10 µg/kg/min is probably more appropriate.

Priming Doses. The slow onset of the effect of nondepolarizing muscle relaxants has limited their use for rapid tracheal intubation. One solution has been to administer a small dose of the muscle relaxant, a "priming dose," several minutes before the usual dose. The initial dose (10 to 20 percent of the dose for intubation) occupies many of the receptors at the neuromuscular junction but usually does not produce weakness. The patient breathes spontaneously, maintains a patent airway, and avoids aspiration. Following an interval of about 4 minutes, a large bolus of the muscle relaxant produces paralysis markedly faster than if the two doses were administered together. This technique is of limited value in clinical practice, because some patients become profoundly weak following the initial dose, and the benefits of priming vary from patient to patient.

Continuous Infusions. A small volume of distribution, rapid clearance, and rapid equilibration between plasma and the neuromuscular junction would make a muscle relaxant ideal for administration by continuous infusion. Of the available nondepolarizing muscle relaxants, only mivacurium meets these criteria. Atracurium and vecuronium are sometimes given by continuous infusion, but the advantages of continuous infusion remain to be demonstrated for these drugs.

Combinations of Muscle Relaxants. Combinations of pancuronium with either D-tubocurarine or metocurine appear to be synergistic. Administration of one-half the ED$_{50}$ of each drug results in more than 50 percent neuromuscular blockade. Synergy may result from combined prejunctional and postjunctional effects specific to each drug or from their different affinities to the α subunit of the postjunctional receptor. Either of these mechanisms would explain why other combinations of muscle relaxants (metocurine with D-tubocurarine or pancuronium with vecuronium) are not synergistic. An advantage of combining muscle relaxants is that cardiovascular effects are minimized compared with the effects of the drugs used individually. The development of muscle relaxants having minimal cardiovascular effects (vecuronium) has diminished this advantage.

Choice of Nondepolarizing Relaxant

Many factors influence the choice of muscle relaxant for a given patient. First, consider that patients with liver or kidney failure may suffer prolonged weakness if given neuromuscular blockers metabolized primarily by the diseased organ. Second, consider the operation. For brief procedures, administration of a long-acting muscle relaxant may result in postoperative paralysis. However, when operations last several hours, repeated administration of an intermediate-duration muscle relaxant may result in fluctuating levels of neuromuscular blockade. Third, consider the cardiovascular effects of the muscle relaxants. For example, pancuronium may produce tachycardia that is undesirable in an elderly patient with heart disease but advantageous in pediatric patients. Fourth, patients with asthma might not be given agents that release histamine, such as D-tubocurarine, atracurium, or mivacurium. A final consideration is cost: generic muscle relaxants are less expensive than those under patent. Single doses of vecuronium or atracurium cost 10 times as much as equivalent doses of pancuronium. The newer drugs are shorter-acting as well, making them even more expensive for longer procedures.

Antagonism of Neuromuscular Blockade

After receiving nondepolarizing relaxant, patients recover neuromuscular function spontaneously, provided enough time passes. Except for mivacurium, waiting for spontaneous recovery is usually impractical, particularly if paralysis is continued to the end of the operation. Usually, recovery of neuromuscular function is hastened by giving an antagonist drug

(*reversal*) that increases the concentration of acetylcholine in the synaptic cleft. Neostigmine, edrophonium, and pyridostigmine inhibit acetylcholinesterase, thereby increasing the local concentration of acetylcholine, whereas 4-aminopyridine increases acetylcholine release from the nerve terminal. Undesirable side effects limit the clinical use of 4-aminopyridine.

These cholinesterase antagonists share one problem: Because the increase in acetylcholine concentration is not limited to the neuromuscular junction, these drugs produce multiple side effects, including profound cardiac slowing, nodal rhythms, increased intestinal tone, and oral secretions. These effects can be minimized or prevented by an anticholinergic drug, typically atropine or glycopyrrolate (Table 11-3).

Several characteristics distinguish edrophonium, neostigmine, and pyridostigmine. The greatest differences relate to onset time, edrophonium being the fastest and pyridostigmine the slowest. The durations of action of edrophonium and neostigmine are similar; pyridostigmine is slightly longer-acting. The antagonists differ in their abilities to antagonize profound neuromuscular blockade, such as 95 to 99 percent twitch depression. Usual doses of edrophonium (i.e., 0.5 mg/kg) do not antagonize adequately profound blockade, although larger doses (e.g., 1.0 mg/kg) reportedly are effective; neostigmine is the pre-

---

Table 11-3

Drugs for Antagonizing Nondepolarizing Neuromuscular Blockade

Anticholinesterases		
	Time to Peak Clinical Effect (min)	Dose (mg/kg)
Edrophonium	1–2	0.5–1.0
Neostigmine	3–5	0.04–0.07
Pyridostigmine	10–20	0.2–0.3

Anticholinergics			
	Dose (mg/kg)	Dose for Typical Adult (mg)	Use With
Atropine	0.015	1.0–1.5	Edrophonium, neostigmine
Glycopyrrolate	0.008	0.5–0.6	Neostigmine, pyridostigmine

Note: For best results, allow spontaneous recovery to three of four twitches in response to a train-of-four stimulus. For patients with more profound neuromuscular blockade, greater doses of anticholinesterase may be needed. If additional neostigmine is administered, doses in excess of 0.14 mg/kg are unlikely to produce additional improvement.

ferred antagonist in this setting. The cardiovascular effects of the antagonists differ markedly. When given without an anticholinergic drug, edrophonium produces rapid and profound bradycardia, whereas the effects of neostigmine and pyridostigmine are slower in onset. For neostigmine or pyridostigmine, either atropine or glycopyrrolate can be given as the anticholinergic. However, edrophonium-induced bradycardia occurs more quickly and is more profound than glycopyrrolate-induced tachycardia, making this combination of drugs undesirable.

Monitoring Neuromuscular Function

Decades of clinical experience with muscle relaxants have demonstrated their effectiveness, the risks associated with their administration, and interpatient variability in the dose-response relationship and duration of action. Accordingly, close monitoring of neuromuscular function, both during and after administration of relaxants, has become the standard of practice. Monitoring assesses blockade during the operation so that additional relaxant can be administered as indicated and demonstrates recovery afterwards to ensure patient safety.

During anesthesia and operation, the desired degree of neuromuscular blockade varies. For example, during tracheal intubation, complete paralysis of the diaphragm is required, but during most operations, significant but less intensive blockade is needed. Immediately after operation, usually the patient must regain full strength promptly.

The intensity of neuromuscular blockade is estimated by assessing the response of various muscles to electrical stimulation of the innervating nerve. For example, stimulation of the ulnar nerve, either at the wrist or at the elbow, produces contraction of the adductor pollicis, a muscle supplied solely by the ulnar nerve. When access to an extremity is limited, the facial nerve can be stimulated, but the relationship between facial muscle twitch and ventilatory function has not been investigated well. Inadvertent direct muscle stimulation must be avoided because it bypasses the neuromuscular junction. When fade is expected after administering a nondepolarizing muscle relaxant but is not present, direct muscle stimulation may be the cause. More confusing is mixed direct and indirect muscle stimulation: fade may be present initially but absent with more intense blockade. Direct muscle stimulation is common when

the facial nerve is used, probably because of the superficial position of the facial muscles.

To stimulate the nerve, a square-wave pulse is administered for 0.1 to 0.3 ms through either surface electrodes or needles placed subcutaneously near the nerve. The stimulus must be supramaximal so that further increases in stimulus strength produce no increase in response. The strength of contraction is quantified using either a mechanical strain gauge or an electromyogram (EMG). An acceptable method in clinical practice is to feel the strength of thumb contraction. To observe, but not feel, thumb movement is less accurate, since visual observation tends to underestimate the intensity of neuromuscular blockade.

A single stimulus is administered no more frequently than every 10 seconds, since more frequent stimulation results in smaller evoked responses due to fade. Each response is compared with the initial response preceding paralysis, the control or baseline twitch. This method may be impractical in the operating room because it requires measuring neuromuscular response before drug administration, which is not always feasible. Alternatively, stimuli can be administered rapidly, at 50 to 100 Hz. This rapid tetanic stimulation provokes fade if any receptors are occupied by muscle relaxants and is valuable in detecting subtle neuromuscular blockade during recovery.

A third approach, train-of-four stimulation, consists of a burst of four stimuli administered at 2 Hz every 10 to 15 seconds. The response to 2-Hz stimuli declines maximally by the fourth twitch. The ratio of the fourth to the first twitches (the train-of-four ratio) is similar to the ratio of the first to the baseline response. Thus the train-of-four ratio can be used to estimate neuromuscular blockade without obtaining a baseline value. This similarity of train-of-four and first-to-baseline response ratios is valid only during recovery; during onset, the train-of-four ratio is not depressed as much as is the first-to-baseline ratio.

A final form of stimulation, specifically designed to assess profound neuromuscular blockade when there is no response to other modes of stimulation, is to administer a 50-Hz tetanic stimulus for 5 seconds, wait 3 seconds, and then administer a single stimulus at 1 Hz; the number of twitches present is known as the *posttetanic count*. During the tetanus, all available acetylcholine is recruited from storage sites in the nerve terminal to the vesicles. With profound neuromuscular blockade, vesicular reserves of acetylcholine are insufficient to produce neuromuscular transmission in response to the tetanus; however, when stimulation decreases to 1 Hz, newly recruited acetylcholine will produce evidence of neuromuscular function. This is known as *posttetanic facilitation.*

Many nerve stimulators are offered commercially. Although differing in appearance and certain characteristics, they generally offer single, train-of-four, and tetanic stimuli (50 or 100 Hz). The output of these devices, whether constant voltage or constant current, can be adjusted to ensure supramaximal stimuli.

Numerous clinical signs are associated with various degrees of neuromuscular recovery and can be used to assess recovery of neuromuscular function. Spontaneous breathing provides little assurance of adequate recovery, because the diaphragm is resistant to the effects of muscle relaxants. A patient may be able to breathe spontaneously yet develop airway obstruction when the endotracheal tube is removed. The ability of a supine adult to lift the head free of the pillow for 5 seconds or a supine child to lift the leg is a sign of adequate recovery. Another well-accepted standard has been a patient's ability to generate negative inspiratory airway pressures of at least 25 cmH$_2$O when the endotracheal tube is occluded and the

maximal inspiratory pressure is measured. Recent evidence suggests that a value of −40 cmH$_2$O is more appropriate. This maneuver may carry the risk of pulmonary edema with sustained negative intrathoracic pressure. Table 11-4 correlates the depths of neuromuscular blockade as measured by nerve stimulator and as observed in the patient.

The rapid spontaneous recovery of function possible with intermediate-acting relaxants such as vecuronium and atracurium suggests the possibility that anticholinesterases might be avoided. However, even patients who appear strong may have up to half their cholinergic receptors occupied by neuromuscular blockers (see Table 11-4); studies show that patients often have residual weakness after neuromuscular blockade despite passing superficial tests of strength. These facts suggest that anticholinesterases are appropriate for almost any patient who has received neuromuscular blockers, especially when extubation of the trachea is planned.

A probable exception to this approach is the patient with normal pseudocholinesterase activity who has been given mivacurium. The rapid elimination of mivacurium from plasma permits prompt neuromus-

Table 11-4

Hierarchy of Neuromuscular Blockade

Approximate Fraction of Receptors Occupied by Nondepolarizing Relaxants (%)	Response to Nerve Stimulator	Whole-Body Signs
99-100	No response, even with posttetanic facilitation (PTF)	Flaccid: extreme relaxation needed only rarely to guarantee immobility
95	PTF present	Diaphragm moves; hiccough possible
90	One of four twitch of TOF* present	Abdominal relaxation adequate for most procedures
75	Twitch tension 100%	Tidal volume and vital capacity normal
	Four twitches of TOF present TOF ratio 0.7 50-Hz tetanus sustained	
50	100-Hz tetanus sustained	Passes inspiratory pressure test
30	200-Hz tetanus sustained	Head-lift and hand-grip sustained

Note: Receptor occupancies are approximate. There are some differences in results among various studies. Note that while much of normal function returns between 90 and 70 percent occupancy, subtle but important weakness persists until fewer than half the receptors are occupied by relaxant molecules.

*TOF: train-of-four stimuli.

cular recovery in most patients, provided the dose was not excessive. Indeed, neostigmine both antagonizes the neuromuscular effects of mivacurium and impairs elimination. Additional clinical experience is needed to guide the administration of anticholinesterase drugs following mivacurium.

Despite the availability of information about proper doses of muscle relaxants, antagonists, and the use of nerve stimulators, patients often arrive in the recovery room with significant residual neuromuscular blockade. This may be less common following atracurium and vecuronium than after longer-acting drugs such as pancuronium and D-tubocurarine. The potentially devastating consequences of persistent neuromuscular blockade, airway obstruction, and hypoventilation make it mandatory that clinicians demonstrate and document the presence of adequate neuromuscular function in their patients at the end of the anesthetic, unless postoperative mechanical ventilation is planned.

To demonstrate full recovery of the patient's strength at the end of the procedure, one may use any of the more stringent tests such as leg lift, head lift, negative inspiratory pressure, or response to tetanic nerve stimuli, provided the response is sustained for a period of 5 seconds. This approach tests the adequacy of acetylcholine reserves and often reveals weakness not demonstrated by briefer challenges. When the patient's strength seems inadequate or the result of the testing is equivocal, a few minutes delay for additional recovery, or additional antagonist followed by retesting, is best.

BIBLIOGRAPHY

Baurain MJ, d'Hollander AA, Melot C, et al. Effects of residual concentrations of isoflurane on the reversal of vecuronium-induced neuromuscular blockade. *Anesthesiology* 1991;74:474-478.

Bevan DR, Smith CE, Donati F. Postoperative neuromuscular blockade: A comparison between atracurium, vecuronium, and pancuronium. *Anesthesiology* 1988;69:272-276.

Donati F, Meistelman C, Plaud B. Vecuronium neuromuscular blockade at the adductor muscles of the larynx and adductor pollicis. *Anesthesiology* 1991;74:833-837.

Donati F, Meistelman C, Plaud B. Vecuronium neuromuscular blockade at the diaphragm, the orbicularis oculi, and adductor pollicis muscles. *Anesthesiology* 1990;73:870-875.

Fisher DM, Rosen JI. A pharmacokinetic explanation for increasing recovery time following larger or repeated doses of nondepolarizing muscle relaxants. *Anesthesiology* 1986;65:286-291.

Ginsberg B, Glass PS, Quill T, et al. Onset and duration of neuromuscular blockade following high-dose vecuronium administration. *Anesthesiology* 1989;71:201-205.

Libonati MM, Leahy JJ, Ellison N. The use of succinylcholine in open eye surgery. *Anesthesiology* 1985;62:637-640.

Pavlin EG, Holle RH, Schoene RB. Recovery of airway protection compared with ventilation in humans after paralysis with D-tubocurarine. *Anesthesiology* 1989;70:381-385.

Viby-Morgensen J. Correlation of succinylcholine duration of action with plasma cholinesterase activity in subjects with the genotypically normal enzyme. *Anesthesiology* 1980;53:517-520.

Viby-Morgensen J, Jorgensen BC, Ording H. Residual curarization in the recovery room. *Anesthesiology* 1979;50:539-541.

Wright PMC, Hart P, Lau M, et al. Cumulative characteristics of atracurium and vecuronium: A simultaneous clinical and pharmacokinetic study. *Anesthesiology* 1994;81:59-68.

Wright PMC, Hart P, Lau M, et al. The magnitude and time course of vecuronium potentiation by desflurane versus isoflurane. *Anesthesiology* 1995; 82: 404-411.

CHAPTER **12**

The Medical Gases

Roderic G. Eckenhoff

This chapter concerns the simple gases that are important for medical practice, including oxygen, carbon dioxide, carbon monoxide, nitrogen, helium, water vapor, and nitric oxide. Anesthesia gases and vapors and respiratory pathophysiology are covered elsewhere (especially Chaps. 8 and 22).

Oxygen

Gaseous oxygen derives from hydrolysis by photosynthetic organisms. The production of medical oxygen begins with air that is compressed and cooled to a liquid and then distilled into its major fractions: nitrogen (78 percent), oxygen (21 percent), and argon (1 percent) (Table 12-1). Oxygen in large quantities is supplied as the liquid, the safest and most economical form, requiring only low-pressure insulated flasks (Dewars) and a minimum of space: 1 liter of liquid oxygen yields about 850 liters of oxygen gas at standard temperature and pressure. Compressed gaseous oxygen needs no insulated containers but at 2250 lb/in^2 yields only 150 liters of gas per liter of storage space. Further, compressed oxygen is more dangerous to store than the liquid. Oxygen gas containers and piping are color-coded green in the United States and white in the United Kingdom.

Oxygen analyzers measure either partial pressure (activity, tension) or fraction (concentration, percentage) of oxygen in a gas mixture. Most operating room oxygen analyzers (fuel cell, paramagnetic, polarographic) measure oxygen partial pressure (PO_2) and not percentage but display the result as the fraction of 1 atm pressure. For example, a typical operating room oxygen analyzer calibrated for sea-level operation reads 42 percent, not 21 percent, when exposed to air at 2 atm. Mass spectrometry measures true fractional concentrations. Although fractional units (FIO_2) are convenient, partial pressure is the biologically important unit. Oxygen toxicity can ensue at an FIO_2 of 0.2 and hypoxia at an FIO_2 of 1.0 depending on the barometric pressure (P_B). Thus it is necessary to convert fractional concentration to partial pressure by multiplying by P_B. Neglected variations in P_B can be a significant source of error in calculations of arterial-alveolar oxygen gradients.

■ Oxygen Administration

Oxygen is administered by inhalation, except when extracorporeal oxygenators dissolve it directly in the exteriorized blood. Oxygen inhalational devices include nasal cannulas, masks, tents or hoods, and tracheal tubes.

Nasal Cannulas

Plastic tubing is used to deliver 2 to 5 liters/min of oxygen into one or both nostrils. The nasopharynx serves as an oxygen reservoir, the contents of which are diluted with room air during inspiration. The resulting inspired oxygen concentration of less than 35 percent is unpredictable and depends on the patient's ventilatory pattern.

Face Masks

A wide variety of masks that cover both the mouth and nose is available for oxygen administration. Masks supplied with flow rates insufficient to meet peak

Table 12-1

Composition of Air (by Volume)	
Component	Percent
Nitrogen	78.08
Oxygen	20.95
Argon	0.93
Water vapor*	0–7.0
Carbon dioxide	0.03
Neon	0.002
Helium	0.0005

*Depending on temperature and relative humidity.

inspiratory demand either entrain room air through ports or include reservoir bags that fill with fresh gas during exhalation. One-way valves in the bag and sides of the mask encourage escape of exhaled gas, but a small amount of rebreathing occurs. Such masks require a close fit to the face and must be monitored for proper operation of the valves and reservoir bag. Oxygen flow rates must be sufficient to prevent bag collapse during inhalation.

Demand valve masks require negative pressure during inspiration to trigger oxygen flow, making it mandatory that the mask fit tightly. These demand-type masks can deliver the greatest oxygen concentration, but they are probably the least comfortable for extended use. A tight-fitting seal to the face is less important for masks that deliver gas flows that are sufficient to meet peak inspiratory demands, such as masks using Venturi orifices. However, because these masks provide adequate inspiratory flows by diluting oxygen with room air, oxygen concentrations are limited to 50 percent or less.

Hoods, Tents

Consistent oxygen concentrations can be administered by enlarging the inspiratory reservoir to encompass the entire head (hood) or body (tent) of the patient. These devices are comfortable and require little cooperation from the patient, but they are not suitable during anesthesia or critical care. Fresh gas flow rates must be great enough to prevent carbon dioxide accumulation.

Tracheal Tubes

A cuffed tracheal tube reliably delivers inspired gas mixtures of known oxygen concentration. Such tubes are used commonly during anesthesia or in the care of the critically ill, usually in combination with mechani-

cal ventilation. Further details are provided in the chapters on airway management (Chap. 13) and critical care (Chap. 33).

■ Oxygen Uptake and Distribution

Oxygen Uptake

Oxygen moves down a partial pressure gradient from the inspired air to the mitochondria (Fig. 12-1). Oxygen partial pressure decreases as the air is delivered to the distal airways and alveoli by inspiration because of dilution with carbon dioxide and water vapor and oxygen uptake into the blood. If ventilation and perfusion are well matched (see Chap. 22), the partial pressure of oxygen in the alveoli can be calculated to be approximately 110 mmHg in persons breathing air at 1 atm. Diffusion of oxygen into the pulmonary capillary blood is driven by the gradient in oxygen tension between alveolar gas and mixed venous blood. Because of the extremely thin diffusion barrier between the alveolar space and pulmonary capillary blood, the difference between the PO_2 of end-capillary blood and that in the alveoli is small. Mismatching of ventilation and perfusion influences the size of this difference and thus the rate of equilibration and end-capillary PO_2.

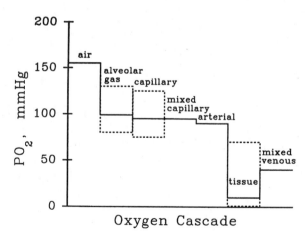

Figure 12-1

Normal partial pressure cascade for oxygen as it passes from the inspired air to the tissues and venous blood. The steps are created by normal physiologic processes, such as ventilation-perfusion inequality, shunt, and metabolic use. Ultimately, metabolic consumption of oxygen is the driving force for oxygen movement through this cascade. The boxes indicate regions where a range of oxygen partial pressures is normally encountered, and the size of the box is an estimation of this range under normal conditions.

The partial pressure of oxygen in arterial blood (PaO_2) is less than that of mixed pulmonary capillary blood because of the addition of a small fraction of venous blood (shunt fraction). Together, the diffusional barrier, ventilation/perfusion inhomogeneity, and shunt fraction are the major components of the alveolar to arterial oxygen difference (A-a difference), normally 10 to 12 mmHg when breathing air and 30 to 50 mmHg when breathing 100% oxygen.

In tissue capillary beds, oxygen again follows a partial pressure gradient out of the blood and into the cells and ultimately to mitochondria. As a result of the loss to the tissues, the PO_2 of mixed venous blood is less than that of arterial blood by about 40 mmHg. Mean tissue PO_2 is even less than the mixed venous value because of diffusional barriers and oxygen consumption in the tissues. At rest, approximately 3 ml of oxygen is consumed per kilogram of body weight per minute.

Blood Oxygen Content

The majority of blood oxygen is carried in chemical combination with hemoglobin; lesser amounts are dissolved directly in plasma. The relationship between hemoglobin oxygen content and PO_2 is described by the sigmoid-shaped oxyhemoglobin dissociation curve (Fig. 12-2). When fully saturated, each gram of hemoglobin binds about 1.3 ml of oxygen. In healthy subjects breathing air, hemoglobin is about 98 percent saturated; further increases in PO_2 produced by breathing oxygen increase blood oxygen content largely by increasing the amount dissolved in plasma. The solubility of oxygen in plasma is only 0.003 ml/dl/mmHg. Even in a healthy patient who achieves an arterial PO_2 of 500 mmHg by breathing 100% oxygen, each 100 ml of plasma carries only 1.5 ml of oxygen in solution, the amount carried by slightly more than 1g of saturated hemoglobin. Although seemingly trivial, this constitutes 25 percent of normal oxygen consumption when viewed as a fraction of the arteriovenous oxygen content difference (5 to 6 ml/dl).

■ Uses for Oxygen

Oxygen is administered primarily to correct for its deficiency in the blood (hypoxemia) or tissues (tissue

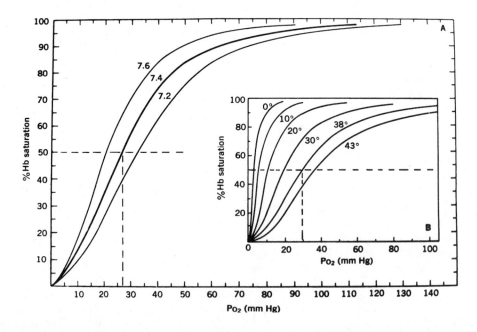

Figure 12-2

Oxyhemoglobin dissociation curves for whole blood. Large curve demonstrates the influence of hydrogen ion concentration on hemoglobin affinity for oxygen; the inset shows the effect of temperature on this affinity. In a working muscle, the increase in carbon dioxide and metabolic acid, combined with the increase in temperature, cooperates to increase oxygen unloading from hemoglobin.

(Reproduced with permission from Lambertsen CT, Transport of oxygen, carbon dioxide and inert gases by the blood. In Montcastle VB, ed: Medical Physiology, 14th ed, vol 2. St Louis: Mosby, 1980.)

hypoxia). It is also used to dilute other gases, to enhance the elimination of an inert gas, and in hyperbaric chambers to treat specific diseases or intoxications.

Treatment of Hypoxia

Hypoxemia and tissue hypoxia rarely are due to a primary deficiency of oxygen in the inspired gas but usually reflect underlying pathophysiology for which oxygen is a temporizing therapy. In the practice of anesthesiology and critical care medicine, the goals are to reduce the patient's need for supplemental oxygen by treating the pathophysiology responsible for hypoxia and to ensure that blood flow is adequate to supply the various tissues.

Oxygen as a Diluent

Oxygen is also used as a carrier gas for the administration of other vapors and gases, such as inhaled anesthetics. Patients undergoing operation and anesthesia also often require oxygen supplementation to prevent hypoxemia.

Oxygen to Reduce Inert Gas Partial Pressure

The predominant gas in the body is nitrogen. Because nitrogen is relatively insoluble, reducing the inspired nitrogen concentration by oxygen inhalation rapidly decreases the blood and tissue nitrogen tension, speeding the removal of nitrogen from gas spaces. Closed spaces with free gas include the middle ear, sinuses, and bowel, especially an obstructed or atonic bowel. Acquired gas spaces include pneumothorax and pneumomediastinum or result from pneumoencephalography, air embolism, or microembolism (decompression sickness).

Hyperbaric Oxygen Therapy

Hyperbaric oxygen (HBO) therapy has two inseparable components: increased hydrostatic pressure and increased oxygen tension. For gas bubble disease (decompression sickness, air embolism), both factors are therapeutic; hydrostatic pressure reduces bubble volume, and oxygen increases the gradient for nitrogen elimination while reducing hypoxia in downstream tissues. Increased tissue oxygen tension is the therapeutic goal for most other indications for HBO therapy. For example, even a small increase in PO_2 in previously ischemic areas may permit leukocyte bactericidal activity, fibroblast function, and angiogenesis. Thus HBO is a useful adjunct in chronic osteomyelitis, osteoradionecrosis, crush injury, or compromised skin/tissue grafts or flaps. Further, increased oxygen tension alone can be bacteriostatic; spread of organisms and toxin production by *Clostridium* species are slowed by tissue oxygen tensions greater than about 250 mmHg, justifying the early use of HBO in clostridial myonecrosis (gas gangrene).

Hyperbaric oxygen therapy also has found use in selected instances of generalized hypoxia. Carbon monoxide (see later) and cyanide intoxication both produce defects in oxygen utilization that are partially reversible by increased oxygen partial pressures. Hyperbaric oxygen therapy also may be useful in severe acute anemia because sufficient oxygen can be dissolved in plasma at 3 atm to meet metabolic needs.

■ Oxygen Toxicity

Oxygen therapy is limited by pulmonary oxygen toxicity resulting from an increased PO_2 despite a normal or below-normal oxygen content. Defenses against oxidative injury evolved along with mechanisms for using oxygen in energy production. These defenses consist of enzymes (superoxide dismutase, glutathione peroxidase, catalase) and reducing agents (glutathione, ascorbate, iron), as well as systems designed to eliminate damaged cellular constituents. Evolved in an atmosphere of less than 150 mmHg oxygen, these defenses fail at increased oxygen tensions. Oxidative injury probably begins with increased concentrations of reactive oxidants such as superoxide anion, singlet oxygen, hydroxyl radical, and hydrogen peroxide. The damage can be propagated and exaggerated by lipid peroxidation to finally involve the whole cell. Although oxygen is toxic to all cells, the effects of hyperoxia vary among tissues because of inherent differences in the tissues and differences in tissue PO_2.

Pulmonary Oxygen Toxicity

The lungs are continuously exposed to the greatest PO_2 of any organ system, and they are the first to demonstrate toxicity at 1 atm of oxygen pressure. Oxygen inhalation for as little as 6 to 8 hours decreases tracheal mucus velocity, and symptoms of tracheobronchial irritation and chest tightness begin in as little as 12 hours in normal subjects. Changes in pulmonary function begin after 12 to 24 hours of exposure. Nausea, vomiting, anorexia, and occasionally orthostatic hypotension are prominent symptoms resulting from exposures of greater than 24 hours. The development of pulmonary oxygen toxicity is directly related to the P_IO_2, so that substantial signs and symptoms are apparent after only 3 to 6 hours of exposure to 2.0 atm of oxygen. Survival times of otherwise normal primates in 1 atm of oxygen exceed 1 week, with death the result of pulmonary edema and, ironically, hypoxia.

The influence of concurrent disease on oxygen tolerance is unpredictable and poorly understood; individual susceptibility to oxygen toxicity varies substantially. The maximum safe P_IO_2 has not been established, but prolonged exposure to 0.5 atm of oxygen produces few symptoms in normal subjects and even allows recovery from acute lung injury in animals and humans. Although sometimes occurring with oxygen therapy, absorption atelectasis is not an important contributor to pulmonary oxygen toxicity.

The therapy for oxygen toxicity relies on decreasing the P_IO_2 and providing supportive measures. There are no specific pharmacologic approaches. Some amelioration in animals has been obtained by the parenteral administration of antioxidant enzymes in forms designed to gain access to the intracellular space. Dramatic improvements in oxygen tolerance have been produced with prior exposure to sublethal hyperoxia in some species; paradoxically, hypoxic exposure also can result in increased resistance to pulmonary oxygen toxicity. Similarly, human oxygen tolerance has been shown to increase with brief interruptions of oxygen inhalation, a technique commonly employed in HBO therapy. In animals, adaptation is associated with increased cellular antioxidant enzyme levels, proliferation of alveolar type II cells, and increased alveolar surfactant levels.

Central Nervous System Oxygen Toxicity

Central nervous system (CNS) oxygen toxicity does not usually occur at less than 2.0 atm of oxygen pressure. It usually precedes pulmonary toxicity at pressures above 3.0 atm, and as with pulmonary toxicity, there is wide variation in individual sensitivity. The major manifestation of toxicity is convulsion, which may be preceded by visual symptoms or muscular twitching. Exercise and hypercarbia speed the onset of symptoms, probably due to cerebral vasodilatation and increased delivery of oxygen to the brain. Central nervous system oxygen toxicity is reversed rapidly by decreases in P_IO_2, and sequelae have not been reported. In fact, it has been proposed as an

alternative to electroconvulsive therapy for depression.

Retinal Oxygen Toxicity

Exposure of infants younger than 44 weeks' gestational age to increased alveolar oxygen tensions may be associated with retrolental fibroplasia, thought to be the result of aberrant angiogenesis in the developing eye. The fibroplastic changes may regress or may progress to blindness. The syndrome may be largely prevented by titration of oxygen therapy to achieve defined hemoglobin saturation levels as detected by oximetry. Oxygen-induced retinopathy in adults is rare, even in hyperbaric exposures. Hyperbaric oxygen has been associated, however, with reversible alterations in vision due to a poorly understood effect on corneal shape.

Carbon Dioxide

Carbon dioxide (CO_2) is a product of oxidative respiration; its concentration is less than 0.1 percent in air. At rest, normal human metabolic processes produce about 2.5 ml of carbon dioxide per kilogram of body weight each minute. Having a diffusion coefficient 20 times that of oxygen, CO_2 readily diffuses out of mitochondria and cells with only a small gradient. It is then carried in the blood in three forms: dissolved carbon dioxide, carbamino compounds, and bicarbonate. The bicarbonate form predominates, while the dissolved form is the second largest pool in plasma. In red blood cells, carbamino forms constitute the second largest carbon dioxide pool because of the large concentration of amino groups in deoxygenated hemoglobin (Table 12-2).

Blood carbon dioxide content is substantially greater than blood oxygen content and (in contrast to oxygen) changes little across the lungs. The arterial to alveolar carbon dioxide difference is normally close to zero and occasionally negative. This small arteriovenous carbon dioxide content change keeps to a minimum pH fluctuations at the tissue and cellular levels.

Inspired carbon dioxide concentrations greater than 7 percent produce dyspnea and headache owing to increased cerebral blood flow. Concentrations of 10 to 20 percent can cause significant CNS depression, while slightly greater concentrations (25 to 30 percent) can produce CNS excitability and con-

Table 12-2

Distribution of Carbon Dioxide Content in Blood			
1 Liter of Blood	Arterial	Venous	A-V
PCO_2 (mmHg)	41.0	46.0	5.0
pH	7.40	7.37	
Plasma carbon dioxide (ml)			
Dissolved	0.7	0.8	0.1
Bicarbonate	13.8	14.7	0.9
Carbamino compounds	0.2	0.2	0.0
RBC carbon dioxide (ml)			
Dissolved	0.5	0.5	0.0
Bicarbonate	6.0	6.4	0.4
Carbamino compounds	0.8	1.2	0.4
Total carbon dioxide (ml)	22.0	23.9	1.9

vulsions. Even greater concentrations produce an anesthetic-like CNS depression once again. These concentrations are accompanied by significant acidosis.

Carbon dioxide has opposing direct and indirect cardiovascular effects. Inhalation of moderate concentrations (7 to 10 percent) produces activation of the sympathetic nervous system and marked increases in circulating catecholamine concentrations. These effects are offset somewhat by a direct depressant effect on cardiac and vascular muscle. Cerebral vessels, having no important sympathetic innervation, dilate at increased carbon dioxide tensions. Carbon dioxide is also a coronary vasodilator but has little effect on the renal or splanchnic circulations. The thresholds for convulsions are increased by CO_2. Arrhythmias during hypercarbia result from a decreased threshold for catechol-induced arrhythmias, combined with a general sympathetic activation. Hyperventilation-induced hypocarbia also can produce arrhythmias, due to hypokalemia.

Carbon dioxide has few therapeutic applications, the most common being to stimulate ventilation. Administered to a spontaneously breathing patient from an anesthesia machine, 5% to 7% carbon dioxide markedly increases minute ventilation, thereby decreasing the time constants of volatile anesthetic uptake or elimination from the lung. This kinetic benefit is further aided by the increase in cerebral blood flow produced by carbon dioxide inhalation. However, because anesthetics and narcotics depress the CO_2 ventilatory response, and because of the effects of neuromuscular blockers, the minute ventilation of anesthetized patients may not respond ad-

equately to CO_2 inhalation, causing respiratory acidosis. Similarly, carbon dioxide is not used to stimulate ventilation in patients with respiratory depression because of the possibility of further CNS depression and acidosis. Cerebral vasodilation and a rightward shift of the oxyhemoglobin dissociation curve during carbon dioxide inhalation increase tolerance of hypoxic atmospheres. Although carbon dioxide inhalation has been suggested for the treatment of carbon monoxide intoxication, the risk of further CNS depression and acidosis make it less desirable than the current standard of care, hyperbaric oxygenation.

Because it is absorbed rapidly, does not burn or support combustion, and conducts heat poorly, carbon dioxide is also used to inflate body cavities during endoscopic procedures requiring electrocautery.

Carbon dioxide is stored in compressed-gas cylinders for medical use and in the solid form (dry ice) for refrigeration. Like nitrous oxide, carbon dioxide in cylinders at room temperature has a liquid phase. The room temperature vapor pressure is about 900 lb/in^2 (Table 12-3).

Carbon Monoxide

A toxic product of combustion, carbon monoxide (CO) plays a small role in respiratory diagnostics. It is found in the smoke or exhaust of almost any form of combustion (fires, internal combustion engines, cigarettes) and in cities may reach levels of 50 parts per million (ppm) in the atmosphere. It has no therapeutic indications but is stored for diagnostic use in a

Table 12-3

Physical Constants for Medical Gases

Gas	MW (g/mol)	Density* (g/liter)	Viscosity* (μP)	Solubility* (blood/gas)	Thermal Conductivity* (cal/s · cm · °C)	Specific Heat (cal/g · °C)
Oxygen	32	1.43	202	0.024†	64	0.22
Nitrogen	28	1.25	175	0.013	62	0.25
Nitrous oxide	44	1.98	145	0.45	41	—
Argon	40	1.78	222	0.026	43	0.12
Carbon dioxide	44	1.98	148	0.60	40	—
Helium	4	0.18	194	0.008	360	1.24

*Density and viscosity at about 20°C; solubility in ml gas/ml solvent with 100 percent gas and at 17°C.
†Not including that bound to hemoglobin.

premixed form (0.3%) with oxygen and helium in compressed-gas cylinders.

Carbon monoxide can be detected readily by infrared absorption, but because concentrations are usually small, detectors must be very sensitive. Carbon monoxide concentration in inspired gas is generally monitored only in specific high-risk industrial situations.

■ Carbon Monoxide Poisoning

Highly toxic, carbon monoxide is a leading cause of poisoning deaths in the United States. It interferes with oxygen delivery and utilization because of its interactions with heme-containing proteins (hemoglobin, cytochromes), especially under hypoxic conditions. The result is tissue hypoxia, manifest usually as neurologic depression, coma, and perhaps hemodynamic instability, rhabdomyolysis, and myoglobin-induced renal failure. Patients who recover from significant CO exposures are at risk for delayed (2 to 20 days) neurologic symptoms, such as confusion, ataxia, and depression.

Normal persons have carboxyhemoglobin concentrations (HbCO) of from 1 to 2 percent, owing to endogenously generated carbon monoxide and the small amounts normally present in the atmosphere. Continuous inhalation of only 0.1% (1000 ppm) carbon monoxide produces HbCO levels in excess of 40 percent and severe symptoms. Although the concentration of carboxyhemoglobin correlates poorly with symptoms and prognosis, it remains the most useful practical measure of CO exposure.

The treatment of acute CO poisoning relies on administering 100% oxygen or hyperbaric oxygen (HBO). Oxygen competes with carbon monoxide for

binding sites on heme proteins; displaced CO becomes available for elimination. For patients experiencing unconsciousness or hemodynamic instability or who are at the extremes of age, hyperbaric oxygen given up to 6 hours after CO exposure, regardless of HbCO levels, reduces the incidence of delayed neurologic sequelae.

Because cigarette smoke contains 1 to 5 percent CO, smokers have HbCO levels of 5 to 12 percent, usually with no symptoms. Cessation of smoking before operation reduces HbCO levels and increases oxygen-carrying capacity. Longer periods of abstention improve lung function and pulmonary symptoms, although a transient increase in airway secretions and cough may occur due to recovery of mucociliary function.

Recent case reports and in vitro studies have raised the fear that patients breathing desflurane from a closed system may be exposed to CO generated by a reaction between the anesthetic and the CO_2 absorbent. The few case reports involve CO_2 absorbents that were exceptionally dry because of dry gas flow for several days; the laboratory conditions required to liberate CO from desflurane were similarly extreme. Such reports do not negate the extensive history of the safe use of closed and low-flow breathing systems for delivery of inhalational anesthetics.

■ Diagnostic Use

Carbon monoxide is used as a tracer gas for the measurement of pulmonary diffusing capacity because its high binding affinity for hemoglobin (200-fold that of oxygen) results in a negligible CO tension in capillary blood and simplifies the calculations necessary to derive diffusing capacity. The diffusing capacity for oxygen is calculated as 1.23 times that for carbon monoxide.

Helium

Although the second most common element in the universe, helium is uncommon on earth, constituting only about 0.003 percent of the atmosphere. Primarily the product of radioactive decay, it is obtained in limited quantities from underground wells in the Midwest. It is stored as high-pressure gas in cylinders or in the liquid form (a few degrees above absolute zero). The low density, insolubility, and thermal conductivity of helium form the basis for its medical and diagnostic applications.

Although mass spectrometry can be used to measure helium, monitoring normally consists of measuring other inspired gases (usually oxygen) and subtracting from the ambient pressure. Helium is mixed with the desired concentration of oxygen and administered by mask, mouthpiece, or tracheal tube. In certain hyperbaric applications, the entire surrounding atmosphere consists of a helium-oxygen or helium-nitrogen-oxygen mixture.

■ Pulmonary Diagnostic Tests

Determinations of residual lung volume and functional residual capacity and derived measures require a highly diffusible gas carried away by the pulmonary circulation only in negligible amounts so that dilution into the lung gas can be measured. Of the inert gases, helium bests meets these criteria. In practice, a single large breath of known helium concentration is administered, and the concentration of helium is then measured in the mixed expired gas; lung volumes are then derived by appropriate calculations.

■ Respiratory Obstruction

Most gas flow in the lungs is laminar, especially in the distal airways, but increased flow rates or airway obstruction favor turbulent flow. Resistance to turbulent flow is proportional to gas density. Because the density of helium is substantially less than that of air, helium-oxygen mixtures may be useful in cases of respiratory obstruction. Three factors reduce the practicality of this approach. First, oxygenation is often the principal concern in airway obstruction, and

the increase in flow rates with helium-oxygen mixtures may not improve oxygenation as well as 100% oxygen would. Second, the addition of oxygen to helium increases the density of the mixture. Third, the viscosity of helium exceeds that of air, which reduces gas flow in regions where laminar flow predominates (small airways). One predicts that helium breathing may be most helpful with large airway obstruction and perhaps even detrimental in asthma, where small airway obstruction is the primary problem.

■ Laser Airway Surgery

Helium neither burns nor supports combustion, making it valuable during laser operations on the airway. It conducts heat well, lessening not only the spread of tissue damage but also the chance of igniting flammable materials in the airway. Helium also improves the flow of gas through the small endotracheal tubes commonly used for such operations.

Although the thermal conductivity of helium is known to increase heat loss in subjects surrounded by a helium atmosphere in a hyperbaric chamber or diving suit, the respiratory component of heat loss is not increased with helium as compared with air or oxygen. This is because respiratory gas is fully equilibrated with body temperature by the time of exhalation, regardless of composition; thus the heat capacity of the gas mixture, not its conductivity, is the relevant property. The heat capacity of helium per unit volume is less than that of air, so helium-oxygen mixtures may actually reduce the respiratory component of overall heat loss.

■ Hyperbaric Applications

Diving or hyperbaric chamber activity can be limited by oxygen toxicity, by nitrogen narcosis, and by tissue inert gas content on decompression (occasionally producing decompression sickness, or the "bends"). Helium is used as a diluent inert gas for diving because it lacks narcotic potential and because its minimal solubility in body tissues and fluids reduces the volume of dissolved helium, thereby reducing decompression time and the risk of microembolism (bubbles) after decompression. The lesser density of helium also reduces the work of breathing in otherwise dense hyperbaric atmospheres.

There is no specific toxicity of helium at atmospheric pressure. Under hyperbaric conditions, its thermal conductivity can result in hypothermia, and the absence of any narcotic potential unmasks the direct CNS excitatory effect of hydrostatic pressure (high-pressure neurologic syndrome).

Water Vapor

Normal biologic humidification of inspired gases maintains a moist and mobile mucociliary blanket, as well as a liquid layer in the respiratory regions that provides elasticity at larger lung volumes, permits a substrate layer on which pulmonary surfactant can function, and generally promotes effective gas exchange. The administration of inspired gases other than atmospheric air is the principal indication for supplementary humidification, especially when a tracheal tube is in place or in patients at increased risk of hypothermia (infants) or of pulmonary complications.

The fully humidified air in the alveoli at 37°C contains 50 mg of water per liter, of which the person at rest contributes about half, or approximately 200 ml per day. Dry inspired gas mixtures increase this requirement, and placement of a tracheal tube shifts the humidification site into the tracheobronchial tree, thereby increasing the heat lost to vaporization and decreasing mobility of the mucociliary blanket. External warming and humidification of the inspired gas reduce respiratory heat loss and promote mucociliary mobility.

Supplemental water vapor can be delivered through any of the devices listed previously for inhalation of oxygen or by bubbling the inhaled gas through water that is heated to increase its vapor pressure. Alternatively, water or saline solution may be nebulized ultrasonically to deliver both water vapor and water droplets, which may carry bronchodilators, mucolytic drugs, or steroids to the respiratory system.

Adverse effects from simple humidification of inspired gases are rare. Adverse reactions to aerosols include infection, airway irritation, bronchospasm, overhydration, and thermal injury.

Nitrogen

Nitrogen is the most common gas in our atmosphere. Its principal medical use is as a diluent for oxygen to avoid oxygen toxicity. It is provided in either compressed or liquid form.

Nitrogen is a weak anesthetic (minimal alveolar concentration about 10 atm). Although a few studies have purported to demonstrate its anesthetic effects under normobaric conditions (suggesting that we are all slightly anesthetized!), the effect is only significant above 3 atm. Therefore, this psychomotor impairment is a hazard for undersea divers, caisson workers, and workers in hyperbaric chambers. The anesthetic effect is reduced by diluting the inspired gas with other inert gases, such as helium.

Although nitrogen is not very soluble, sufficient amounts can be dissolved in blood and tissue at increased pressure so that on decompression it is released in the form of nitrogen bubbles. This is the etiology of the decompression sickness syndromes, which range in severity from pruritus to paraplegia to death. These syndromes are prevented by gradual decompression or by increasing the gradient for nitrogen elimination by breathing oxygen prior to or during decompression. The treatment for decompression sickness is hyperbaric oxygen, as discussed earlier.

Nitric Oxide

Recent studies have shown that nitric oxide, a reactive oxidation product of arginine, possesses biologic functions ranging from vasodilation to neurotransmission. The current therapeutic role for NO is based on its vasodilatory properties combined with a very short half-life. It also produces bronchodilation. Inhaled NO (60 ppb to 60 ppm) produces selective pulmonary vasodilation, owing to both the route of administration and its rapid deactivation by hemoglobin in the pulmonary blood. The inhaled route is especially attractive because it is preferentially delivered to well-ventilated lung regions, presumably resulting in improved matching of perfusion to ventilation. Although its current therapeutic use is experimental, inhaled NO has been used successfully in patients with persistent fetal circulation, pulmonary hypertension due to cardiac dysfunction or surgery, and the adult respiratory distress syndrome.

Nitric oxide is also toxic and can lead to pulmonary damage with concentrations greater than 50 to 100 ppm. Part of its toxicity may be related to further oxidation to nitrogen dioxide in the presence of increased oxygen concentrations. This reaction is sufficiently rapid to require bedside mixing of the gases in the inspiratory limb of the breathing circuit.

Nitric oxide is available as various dilutions in compressed nitrogen, and inspired concentrations may be monitored with chemiluminescent detectors.

BIBLIOGRAPHY

Deneke SM, Fanburg BL. Normobaric oxygen toxicity of the lung. *N Engl J Med* 1980;303:76-86.

Eckenhoff RG, Longnecker DE. The therapeutic gases: Oxygen, carbon dioxide, helium and water vapor. In Gilman AG, Rall TW, Nies AS, Taylor P, eds: *The Pharmacologic Basis of Therapeutics,* 8th ed. New York: Pergamon Press, 1990, pp 332-334.

Klocke RA. Carbon dioxide transport. In *Handbook of Physiology,* sec 3, vol 4. Bethesda, Md: American Physiologic Society, 1987, pp 173-198.

Nunn JF. *Applied Respiratory Physiology,* 3d ed. Boston: Butterworth, 1987.

Rossaint R, Pison U, Gerlach H, Falke KJ. Inhaled nitric oxide: Its effects on pulmonary circulation and airway smooth muscle cells. *Eur Heart J* 1993;14(suppl 1):133-140.

Thom SR. Hyperbaric oxygen therapy. *J Intensive Care Med* 1989;4:58-74.

Thom SR, Kiem LW. Carbon monoxide poisoning: A review. Epidemiology, pathophysiology, clinical findings and treatment options including hyperbaric oxygen therapy. *Clin Toxicol* 1989; 27:141-156.

Weibel ER. *The Pathway for Oxygen.* Cambridge, Mass: Harvard University Press, 1984.

SECTION **4**

Administering Anesthesia

CHAPTER **13**

Airway Management

Andranik Ovassapian and Ronald M. Meyer

Airway obstruction and ventilatory depression occur frequently in unconscious patients; the most serious perianesthetic mishaps evolve from inadequate ventilation and oxygenation. Thus careful airway management is essential in caring for patients in the operating room, the postanesthesia care unit, and/or the intensive care unit.

Applied Anatomy of the Airway

Large and mobile despite its attachments to the mandible, hyoid bone, and epiglottis, the tongue is the major cause of airway obstruction in anesthetized patients. Though subject to obstruction by polyps or septal deformity, the nasal passages provide an alternate route for ventilation, and they help stabilize tracheal tubes. Epistaxis results from lacerating the mucosal coverings of the three bony turbinates that project from each lateral wall.

The pharynx extends from the base of the skull to join the esophagus at the level of the sixth cervical vertebra. There, the lower portion (cricopharyngeus) of the inferior constrictor muscle attaches to the cricoid cartilage, forming the upper esophageal sphincter. External pressure on the cricoid ring against the vertebral bodies while the neck is extended (Sellick's maneuver) occludes the esophagus, deterring regurgitation of gastroesophageal contents. Anteriorly, the pharynx communicates with the nasal cavity, the oral cavity, and the larynx (Fig. 13-1).

The nasopharyngeal tonsil (or adenoids) overlies the sphenoid bone. Although it atrophies after childhood, it may be the site of obstruction or hemorrhage during nasotracheal intubation. The soft palate

can block exhalation through the nose during anesthesia.

Inferior to the nasopharynx, at the level of the second and third cervical vertebrae, the oropharynx communicates with the mouth via a passage called the *fauces*. At the level of the fourth to sixth cervical vertebrae, the hypopharynx provides access to the

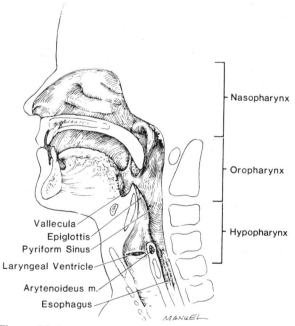

Figure 13-1

A sagittal section of the pharynx showing three subdivisions of the pharynx.

Reproduced with permission from Ovassapian A. Fiberoptic airway endoscopy in anesthesia and critical care. *New York: Raven Press, 1990.*

137

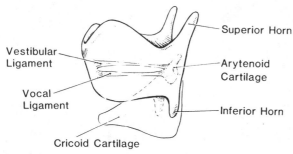

Figure 13-2

Demonstrates the relationship of thyroid, cricoid, and arytenoid cartilages.

Reproduced with permission from Smith C, Ramsey RG. Xeroradiography of the lateral neck. Radio Graphics 1982;2: 306-328.)

larynx and esophagus and laterally includes the two piriform fossae.

Three single cartilages (thyroid, cricoid, and epiglottic) and three paired cartilages (arytenoid, corniculate, and cuneiform) shape the larynx (Fig. 13-2). Abduction of the vocal cords during inspiration imparts a triangular shape to the glottic opening (rima glottidis), the narrowest portion of the airway in patients older than 8 years (Fig. 13-3). In younger children, the cricoid ring is narrowest. The true and false vocal cords insert anteriorly on the thyroid cartilage and posteriorly on the arytenoid cartilages. The pyramid-shaped arytenoids articulate with the posterosuperior aspect of the cricoid cartilage; movement of the cricoid and arytenoids controls the position and tension of the vocal cords. Atop the arytenoids and embedded in the aryepiglottic folds, the corniculate and cuneiform cartilages form medial and lateral prominences that may be the sole landmarks to guide difficult tracheal intubation.

Viewed perpendicular to its longitudinal axis, the adult epiglottis has a crescent-shaped cross section; in infants and a few adults, this cross section assumes more of a U shape that combines with greater relative length to hinder glottic exposure. The valleculae are depressions between a median and two lateral glossoepiglottic ligaments. The ligaments allow indirect elevation of the epiglottis with a curved laryngoscope to expose the glottis.

Though often subtle in women and children, the superior thyroid notch is the most distinctive landmark on the anterior surface of the neck. Identified as the depression between the thyroid and cricoid cartilages, the cricothyroid ligament is a site for transla-

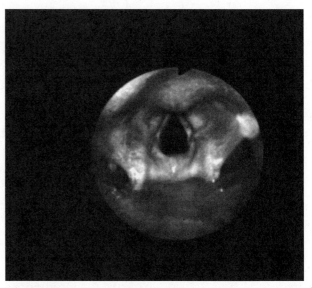

Figure 13-3

Endoscopic view of the larynx. Black triangle at 12 o'clock indicates the tubercle of epiglottis, below which true and false vocal cords with laryngeal ventricle appear. Pyriform sinuses represented by deepest part of hypopharynx lateral to aryepiglottic folds bilaterally.

ryngeal injection of local anesthetics or emergency needle or surgical cricothyrotomy (Fig. 13-4). The essential landmarks for a superior laryngeal nerve block are the lateral horns of the thyroid cartilage, found at the level of the third cervical vertebra.

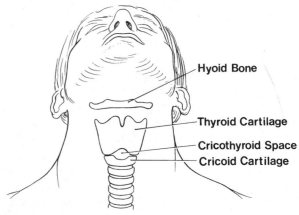

Figure 13-4

Front view of neck. Demonstrates the cricothyroid membrane and relation of hyoid bone to the thyroid cartilage.

(Reproduced with permission from Smith C, Ramsey RG. Xeroradiography of the lateral neck. Radio Graphics 1982;2: 306-328.)

Growing from a length of 4 cm in the neonate to 10 to 14 cm in the adult, the trachea extends from the lower border of the cricoid cartilage to the carina, where it divides into the right and left mainstem bronchi at the level of the fifth thoracic vertebra. Horseshoe-shaped tracheal cartilages, linked posteriorly by the trachealis muscle, lend a D shape to the cross section and confirm that a fiberscopic view is of the trachea instead of a bronchus. A prominent aortic arch, congenital vascular anomalies, anterior mediastinal masses, and enlarged lymph nodes can compress the trachea and interfere with ventilation.

In adults, the right mainstem bronchus is 1.8 cm long and deviates less from the axis of the trachea than does the 5-cm-long left bronchus. In infants, the angles formed by the two main bronchi are nearly equal, so there is less certainty that an accidental bronchial intubation will be right-sided.

Assessment of the Airway

Because difficulties in management are easier to surmount when they are anticipated, preoperative evaluation of patients' airways demands the utmost care. Difficult airway management results from anatomic extremes, specific pathologic states, and/or technical problems (Table 13-1). These factors may prevent a snug fit between mask and face, interfere with positioning of the head and neck, limit opening of the mouth, narrow the airway, or distort and immobilize tissues. Information obtained from the history may be suggestive (Table 13-2), but most problems are identified by a thorough examination that begins with the patient's posture and habitus and then examines the face, mouth, jaw, and neck (Table 13-3). The examination begins from the front and then from the side, while the patient sits looking forward, opens the mouth, protrudes the tongue, closes the mouth, and then extends the neck. In the oral cavity, the view of the fauces is noted, as is the appearance of dental appliances or loose, missing, or damaged teeth (dental claims are commonly the basis of lawsuits). The mouth opening with the head in neutral position is assessed, as is the distance from the mandibular mentum to the superior thyroid notch during neck extension. The hyoid bone, superior thyroid notch, and cricothyroid ligament are each palpated, and the size, firmness, and mobility of any masses are evaluated. Listening to the patient's breathing reveals worrisome upper airway sounds.

Table 13-1

Some Causes of Difficult Airway Management

Anatomic features
  Short, muscular neck
  Limited neck mobility
  Prominent maxillary incisors
  Awkwardly placed, incomplete dentition
  Long, high-arched palate with narrow mouth
  Small mouth opening
  Receding chin
Pathologic states
  Anaphylactic airway edema
  Arthritis and ankylosis
    Cervical spine
    Temporomandibular joint
    Laryngeal arthritis
  Congenital syndromes
    Klippel-Feil (short, fused neck)
    Pierre Robin (micrognathia, cleft palate, glossoptosis)
    Treacher Collins (mandibulofacial dysostosis)
  Endocrinopathies
    Obesity
    Acromegaly
    Hypothyroid macroglossia
    Goiter
  Infections
    Ludwig's angina (floor of the mouth)
    Peritonsillar abscess
    Retropharyngeal abscess
    Epiglottitis
  Mediastinal masses
  Myopathies with myotonia or trismus
  Scarring from burns or radiation
  Trauma and hematomas
  Tumors and cysts
Technical and mechanical factors
  Body cast
  Halo fixation or cervical collar
  Foreign bodies in the airway
  Leaks around a face mask
    Edentulous
    Flat bridge of nose
    Large face and head
    Whiskers
    Nasogastric tubes
  Poor technique, inexperience, or haste

Radiologic studies are indicated when anatomy is distorted by trauma or tumors. Lateral cervical spine films, computed tomography, or magnetic resonance imaging confirms vertebral damage and reveals the degree of airway compression. When doubt remains about the ability to intubate, inspection of the airway using topical anesthesia, sedation, and rigid or fiberoptic laryngoscopy determines the choice of con-

Table 13-2

Clues from the History that Suggest Difficult Airway Management

Finding	Implication
Dry cough	Possible tracheobronchial compression
Easy bleeding	Epistaxis
Gastroesophageal reflux	Aspiration
Long-standing diabetes mellitus	Limited cervical mobility
Loud snoring	Soft tissue obstruction
Major trauma	Unstable neck, swelling, or hematoma
Radiation to the neck	Fibrosis, immobility
Recent temporal craniotomy	Limited mandibular mobility
Smoking	Salivation, cough, laryngospasm
Undigested food returning to the mouth	Aspiration risk from pharyngeal pouch

Table 13-3

Physical Findings that Suggest Difficult Airway Management

Finding	Implication
Obesity	Easily obstructed airway; aspiration risk; diminished chest wall compliance; difficult laryngoscopy because of macroglossia and immobile head
Pregnancy	All the problems associated with obesity, especially aspiration risk; large breasts impair laryngoscope insertion; swollen mucosae bleed easily
Ascites	Aspiration risk; diminished chest wall compliance
Whiskers, flat nasal bridge, large face	Difficult mask seal
Mouth opens less than 40 mm	Glottic exposure blocked by maxillary teeth
Cervico-occipital extension limited to an angle at the hyoid less than 160 degrees	Difficult to align mouth and pharynx for glottic exposure
Short, thick, muscular neck	Prone to soft tissue obstruction; difficult to extend neck for intubation or mask ventilation
Thyromental distance less than 60 mm; receding chin	Difficult to mobilize tongue for glottic exposure; glottis too anterior to see
Maxillary gap from missing incisors with other teeth present to the right	Laryngoscope fits into gap, while adjacent teeth, lip, or gum block view of glottis and passage of tracheal tube
Edentulous, with atrophic mandible	Small face and furrowed cheeks impair mask fit; tongue and soft palate block exhalation
Prominent or protruding maxillary incisors	Teeth block view of glottis
Advanced caries, loose teeth, caps, bridges	Damage to teeth; risk of aspiration of dislodged teeth; can tear cuff
Stridor, retractions	Airway obstruction
Hoarseness	Vocal cord malfunction or airway masses
"Underwater" voice	Vallecular or epiglottic cysts
Nasogastric tube in situ	Difficult to seal mask
Poorly visualized soft palate and fauces in upright patient with mouth fully open (Mallampati's sign)	Difficult to expose glottis with rigid laryngoscopy
Large goiter or immobile tumor displacing trachea	Difficult to expose glottis; airway obstruction or tracheal collapse
Tracheostomy scar	Possible tracheal stenosis

scious intubation or conventional induction of anesthesia.

Hypoventilation, Apnea, and Denitrogenation

Airway obstruction causes hypoventilation, resulting in hypercapnia and hypoxemia. During apnea, $PaCO_2$ increases 6 to 8 mmHg in the first minute and 2 to 3 mmHg each minute thereafter. Although hypoventilation while breathing room air leads to hypoxemia if the alveolar ventilation decreases to about 1.5 liters/min, supplemental oxygen is an effective remedy. At an inspired oxygen concentration of 50 percent, a healthy patient can maintain an oxyhemoglobin saturation above 95 percent with an alveolar ventilation of 0.5 liter/min. At 100 percent FIO_2, the oxyhemoglobin saturation may remain near 100 percent even during apnea, as long as a patent airway provides a path from the oxygen source to the alveoli. This apneic oxygenation technique is used occasionally during airway surgery.

Denitrogenation and preoxygenation increase the margin of safety in the event of prolonged apnea (Table 13-4). A typical adult consumes 250 ml/min of oxygen and has a functional residual capacity (FRC) of 2500 ml. When the inspired oxygen concentration is 21 percent, the FRC contains less than 500 ml of oxygen, enough to meet the patient's metabolic requirements for less than 2 minutes. After denitrogenation with 100% oxygen, the FRC contains 8 to 10 minutes of oxygen supply. Routine analysis of end-expired gas confirms that denitrogenation has increased the alveolar oxygen concentration above 90 percent. In a patient whose FRC contains 90 percent oxygen when airway obstruction supervenes, the $PaCO_2$ increases to about 70 mmHg in the 8 minutes before profound hypoxemia occurs. Excepting patients with specific diseases (intracranial or pulmonary hypertension), hypercarbia is less likely to cause serious morbidity than is hypoxia. Infants, gravidas, and the obese fare worse because of their greater oxygen consumptions and smaller FRCs.

Airway Management without Tracheal Intubation

Airway management without endotracheal intubation employs a face mask, laryngeal mask airway, or Combitube.

■ Face Mask Ventilation

The skillful use of a face mask is a challenging technique that can be divided into six steps beginning with assessing ventilation.

Assessing Adequacy of Ventilation

In the absence of arterial blood gas analysis, the assessment of ventilation relies on many observations, each of which may be difficult to interpret (Table 13-5). Capnography may be unreliable during mask ventilation because reduced tidal volumes and increased deadspace under the mask may cause measured end-expiratory PCO_2 to underestimate the alveolar PCO_2. Pulse oximetry is not a sensitive indicator of airway obstruction because hypoxemia is a late sign of hypoventilation. Nevertheless, pulse oximetry increases the safety of mask airway management because other signs of hypoxemia are even less sensitive and reliable. The detection of cyanosis requires 5 g/dl of deoxygenated hemoglobin (arterial hemoglobin oxygen saturation of 50 to 60 percent in patients with hemoglobin concentrations of 10 to 15 g/dl). The cardiorespiratory signs of hypercarbia and hypoxemia are nonspecific and are blunted by anesthetics, opioids, or beta-adrenergic antagonists.

Once recognized, airway obstruction must be relieved promptly for three reasons. First, even after denitrogenation, hypoxemia is a threat. Second, attempts at positive-pressure ventilation in the presence of an obstructed airway may fill the stomach, decreasing the FRC and increasing the gastric pressure. The latter, combined with spontaneous inspiratory efforts, increases the gastroesophageal pressure gradient, predisposing to regurgitation. Finally,

Table 13-4

Steps for Effective Denitrogenation

Pressure relief valve fully open to avoid excessive airway pressure

Oxygen flow at 8 to 10 liters/min

Leak-free mask fit to prevent room air entrainment (a moving reservoir bag and normal capnographic tracing indicate a snug fit)

Two to three minutes of tidal breathing or four vital capacity breaths

Table 13-5

Assessment of Ventilation

Suggest Adequate Ventilation	Suggest Inadequate Ventilation
Normal breath sounds	Stridor, phonation, snoring
Sequential rise and fall of the subcostal region	Motionless subcostal region or progressive subcostal expansion
Upper chest expansion before or during subcostal expansion	Upper chest retraction during subcostal expansion; intercostal or supraclavicular retraction; tracheal tug; flaring nasal alae
Prompt refilling of the reservoir bag during exhalation	Depleted reservoir bag
Appropriate measured tidal volume with each breath	Reduced tidal volume measured
Square-shaped capnogram with normal end-expiratory CO_2	Capnogram without a plateau; large or small end-expiratory CO_2
$SpO_2 \geq 97\%$	$SpO_2 < 95\%$
Normal vital signs and ECG	Tachycardia, bradycardia, dysrhythmias, hypotension, hypertension, tachypnea

the negative airway pressure that results from unsuccessful efforts to inhale can precipitate pulmonary edema.

Positioning to Facilitate Ventilation

Upper airway obstruction during anesthesia is caused by the epiglottis and by the base of the tongue dropping posteriorly as the genioglossus and geniohyoid muscles relax. The sniffing position, achieved by resting the adult occiput on a firm 8- to 10-cm support while extending the cervico-occipital joints, opens the airway; the large occiputs of small children eliminate the need for head support. Displacing the mandible anteriorly (jaw thrust) improves the airway by mobilizing the hyoid bone, epiglottis, and tongue. Paradoxically, this anterosuperior force on the mandible can compact the tongue and adjacent soft tissues enough to compromise ventilation, especially in the edentulous patient. In some cases, positive-pressure mask ventilation pushes gas into the lungs, but exhalation is blocked. This unidirectional obstruction can be relieved by an artificial airway.

When airway patency cannot be achieved with the patient's chin in the midline, turning the head to one side may prove effective. Roentgenographic and fiberoptic examinations have shown that the epiglottis itself may produce airway obstruction unrelieved by any maneuver short of tracheal intubation.

To decrease upper abdominal pressure, improve thoracic compliance, and maintain the FRC, tilting the table head up is advantageous. However, the patient who regurgitates is rapidly repositioned head down, with the head turned to the side, to drain the pharynx, even before a suction catheter is applied to the pharynx.

Sealing Mask to Face

When the seal between the mask and the face is inadequate, positive-pressure ventilation is difficult, anesthetics pollute the workspace, and room air may dilute inspired gases. With the reusable black anatomic mask, the first requirement for ensuring a good fit is an air-filled cushion that does not leak (Fig. 13-5). After spreading the body of the mask, its superior angle is fitted into the lowest point of the bridge of the nose while the left hand lifts the mandible anteriorly until the chin meets the cushion. The hypothenar eminence is used to draw the soft tissue of the left cheek to meet the cushion; a mask strap may perform the same function on the right if needed. With the ulnar three fingers of the left hand gripping the mandible to displace it anteriorly, the mask is held on the face by the thumb and index finger, one above and one below the connector. Fatigue of the hand is reduced by exerting the majority of force upward through the arm and ulnar three fingers rather than by gripping. If mask straps are used, one must remain alert to their complications, such as pressure injury to facial skin and nerves and retention of vomitus.

Disposable clear masks reveal secretions, vomitus, cyanosis, and the sequential fogging and clearing that accompany ventilation. Their large, soft cushions fit patients with flat noses, but the routine use of such disposable items is increasingly difficult to justify. In small children, molded, cushion-free masks (Rendell-Baker Soucek) minimize apparatus deadspace. The thumb and forefinger are used as in the conventional grip, but only the third finger is needed to lift the chin.

For edentulous patients with buccal furrowing, an oral airway stretches the cheeks and facilitates a mask fit. Other tactics include filling the buccal cavities with gauze sponges, inserting the inferior rim of the

cushion between the inferior alveolar ridge and the inside of the lower lip, and cautiously leaving dentures in place.

In some patients, a patent airway and mask seal may be achieved only with a two-handed jaw thrust. Both thumbs press down on the mask, while all fingers apply anterior traction to the mandibular rami and angles. An assistant must squeeze the reservoir bag.

Positive-Pressure Ventilation

During face mask ventilation, positive airway pressure exceeding 20 cmH$_2$O (15 mmHg) can fill the stomach with gas. Gentle, shallow breaths minimize this risk and are less likely than abrupt, large breaths to precipitate coughing in lightly anesthetized patients. Continuous positive airway pressure of 5 to 10 cmH$_2$O by itself is sufficient in many spontaneously ventilating patients to open the airway by separating the pharyngeal soft tissues, thereby obviating the need for an artificial airway.

When assessment of the airway indicates that positive-pressure ventilation by mask will be easily accomplished, it is acceptable practice to administer hypnotics, opioids, or muscle relaxants so that controlled ventilation is required immediately. In case of doubt, or as a matter of routine for some practitioners, positive-pressure ventilation may be started gradually as anesthesia is induced and deepened, progressing from spontaneous ventilation during denitrogenation to assisted ventilation (synchronized with the patient's own breaths) and eventually to controlled ventilation. These steps are retraceable if ventilatory problems supervene. Doses of hypnotics, sedatives, or relaxants that produce apnea are avoided until ventilation is certain.

Neuromuscular Blockers

Although often beneficial, neuromuscular blockers can add risks to airway management. Along with relaxing the powerful muscles of mastication to permit opening the mouth, they reduce the potentially traumatic force with which a rigid laryngoscope contacts the delicate lingual mucosa. They eliminate untoward responses, such as coughing, laryngospasm, and rigidity of strap and chest wall muscles. Administration of 10 to 20 mg of intravenous succinylcholine immediately relaxes upper airway muscles to permit ventilation in cases of laryngospasm. Yet, in patients with trauma, tumors, edema, abscesses, or extrinsic compression, airway patency can vanish irretrievably when muscle tone is lost. Neuromuscular

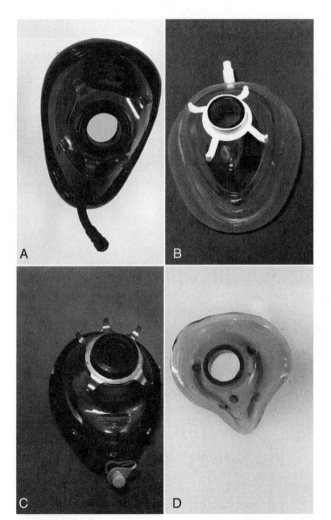

Figure 13-5

Selection of face masks: (*A*) deformable, padded mask; (*B*) universal disposable mask; (*C*) Ambu transparent mask; (*D*) Rendell-Baker Soucek pediatric mask.

blockers are used with caution when ventilation by mask will be difficult.

■ Mechanical Airways

An oropharyngeal airway is inserted when obstruction occurs and the mandibular muscles have relaxed, suggesting that the patient will tolerate stimulation at the base of the tongue (Fig. 13-6). Using a scissoring action of the right thumb and index or middle finger, the operator opens the patient's mouth and lifts the base of the tongue forward with a tongue blade held in the left hand, permitting insertion of the airway between the tongue and the posterior pharyngeal wall. If the patient reacts to the tongue blade, airway insertion is deferred, but the stimulus itself may improve airway patency. Inspired anesthetic concentrations may then be increased to deepen anesthesia. Alternatively, the airway responses may be depressed by using intravenous opioids, hypnotics, or relaxants.

The nasopharyngeal airway is used when patients with clenched jaws require relief of soft tissue obstruction or if obstruction coexists with a preserved gag reflex (see Fig. 13-6). The likelihood of epistaxis is reduced by applying a topical mucosal vasoconstrictor before warming, lubricating, and gently inserting the airway with its bevel facing laterally.

In caring for the patient whose airway is obstructed due to anesthesia, trauma, or other causes, tracheal intubation is often necessary. If it is impossible, or if a skilled intubator is not present, other techniques are applied, such as the use of a laryngeal mask airway or blind esophageal intubation with a Combitube. Intended to restore airway patency by separating the tongue, soft palate, and epiglottis from the posterior pharyngeal wall, these devices entail the risk of trauma, coughing, laryngospasm, regurgitation, and vomiting. Lubrication, gentleness, and obtunded gag reflexes minimize such complications.

■ Laryngeal Mask Airway

The laryngeal mask airway (LMA) gained popularity in the United Kingdom before its introduction to the United States in 1992. Conceived as a mask positioned over the larynx, it provides an alternative to the face mask without tracheal intubation, allowing airway patency without using one hand constantly to support the mandible. The LMA consists of a tube that opens into an elliptical mask with an inflatable rim. Two flexible bars at the junction between the tube and the mask keep the epiglottis from obstructing the tube. The LMA is made of reusable, autoclavable silicone rubber and is available in sizes applicable to patients from neonates to large adults.

With the patient's head in the sniffing position, one hand opens the patient's mouth, while the other hand presses the lubricated LMA against the hard palate

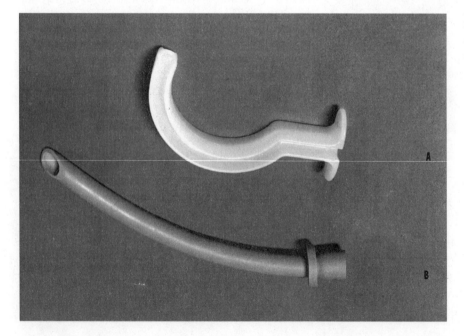

Figure 13-6

Artificial airways: (*A*) oropharyngeal; (*B*) nasopharyngeal.

A

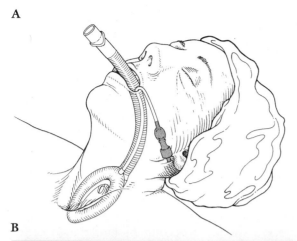

B

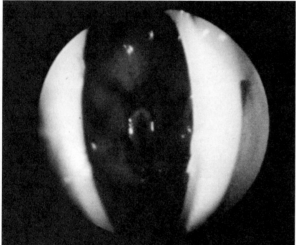

Figure 13-7

(*A*) Schematic presentation of perfectly positioned laryngeal mask airway (Courtesy of Gensia Pharmaceutcals). (*B*) Endoscopic view of perfectly positioned laryngeal mask airway. The epiglottis is out of view. Glottis is in view through the two bars of the LMA.

just behind the incisors and guides it posteroinferiorly until resistance arises to further advancement. Cuff inflation effects a seal around the laryngeal inlet, permitting positive-pressure as well as spontaneous ventilation. Although gas usually leaks at airway pressures exceeding 15 cm H_2O (Fig. 13-7), the seal may improve over time. Despite its limitations, the laryngeal mask airway may be replacing the tracheal tube in some settings (Table 13-6).

The LMA has given rise to new strategies for airway management. The ease and speed of insertion of the LMA, requiring no muscle relaxants or glottic visualization, have prompted its use in managing patients in whom tracheal intubation has failed and ventilating

by face mask is difficult. The LMA can be used as a conduit for blind or fiberoptic-guided tracheal intubation and provides excellent conditions for diagnostic fiberoptic bronchoscopy in anesthetized and sedated children and adults. In the latter application, the LMA accommodates a large bronchoscope while minimizing the required ventilating pressures and permitting inspection of the larynx and upper trachea.

■ The Esophageal Tracheal Combitube

The esophageal tracheal Combitube is a disposable double-lumen device with two proximal 15-mm connectors, either of which can be attached to a standard breathing circuit. One lumen connects to a series of ventilating ports between a proximal pharyngeal cuff and the distal cuff. The second lumen continues to the distal tip of the Combitube (Fig. 13-8).

The Combitube is inserted blindly, with a 90 to 95 percent chance that its tip will enter the esophagus. After the distal cuff is inflated with 15 ml of air, the pharyngeal cuff, which should be in contact with the soft palate, is filled to its capacity of 110 ml. The pharynx remains continuous with the trachea, but is isolated from both the esophagus and the atmosphere; the lungs can be ventilated through the pharyngeal ports. If the tube enters the trachea, ventilation is still possible, but through the lumen that connects to the distal tip.

Indicated for managing trauma, resuscitation, and failed intubation, rapid Combitube placement demands less skill than tracheal intubation, protects against pulmonary aspiration better than a face mask,

Table 13-6

Benefits and Limitations of Laryngeal Mask Airway (LMA)
Benefits of the LMA
Permits ventilation when face mask and intubation have failed
Permits lighter depth of anesthesia and faster emergence
Facilitates blind or fiberoptic tracheal intubation
Provides better airway for fiberoptic bronchoscopy
Easier to learn than tracheal intubation
Limitations of the LMA
Proper position of the LMA may be difficult to achieve
Probable gas leak when airway pressure exceeds 20 cmH_2O
Primarily useful in spontaneously ventilating patient
No protection against aspiration
No protection against laryngospasm

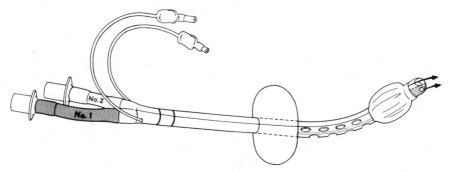

Figure 13-8

The esophageal tracheal Combi-tube.

and can be achieved with the head and neck in neutral position. Disadvantages include the risk of esophageal damage, the inability to clear the trachea by suction, and difficulty in using the device in awake patients.

Tracheal Intubation

Although general anesthesia without a tracheal tube is safe and effective for many patients, intubation is indicated in a variety of situations and has become accepted as a part of routine anesthesia management (Table 13-7). Until 1992 when the laryngeal mask airway was introduced in the United States, the prevalence of tracheal intubation during anesthesia increased steadily, reflecting an appreciation of the consequences of hypoventilation, hypoxia, and aspiration and the need for two free hands for other tasks.

■ Equipment

Laryngoscopes

The laryngoscope consists of a handle and a blade. The handle contains batteries for the light, which may be at the blade's tip or in the handle. The latter style uses a fiberoptic bundle to transmit light to the tip of the blade. A number of different blades attach to any handle (Fig. 13-9). Despite the range of blade styles and sizes, a Macintosh 3 (curved) and Miller 3 (straight) blade suffice for the vast majority of adults.

Because they may lacerate mucous membranes, blades are disinfected after each use, killing all vegetative microorganisms. Preliminary removal of blood, mucus, and other residues by soaking and scrubbing blades in an enzyme detergent is necessary before the application of glutaraldehyde or ethylene oxide. The disinfection process must not impair the intensity or reliability of the light or leave toxic residues.

Tracheal Tubes

In the United States, most tracheal tubes are disposable and are made of clear, bioinert polyvinyl chloride that molds to the contour of the airway upon softening at body temperature. Lengths are marked in centimeters, and internal diameters are indicated in millimeters. Tracheal tubes for oral placement can be trimmed to 26 cm in length. For women of average size, a 7.0- or 7.5-mm (internal diameter) tube is commonly chosen; an 8.0-mm tube is popular for men. Adapters ensure that all tubes present a 15-mm male fitting to the breathing circuit. Moistening an

Table 13-7

Indications for Tracheal Intubation
During anesthesia
To ensure ventilation or oxygenation
Critical illness (sepsis, cardiopulmonary disease, trauma)
Procedures that compress the diaphragm and chest wall (laparoscopy)
Positions that compromise thoracic compliance (steep lithotomy)
Effects of surgical trespass (massive transfusion)
Intrathoracic operations
To ensure airway patency
Airway operation
Prolonged anesthesia
Abnormal airway anatomy
Positions that limit access to the airway
To protect against pulmonary aspiration
"Full stomach"
Hiatal hernia
Intraabdominal surgery
Positions, such as head down
To provide separate ventilation to each lung
To free one's hands for other tasks
Postanesthesia or critical care
To provide ventilation or other airway pressure therapy
To maintain patency of the airway
To protect the airway from contamination
To facilitate bronchopulmonary toilet

Figure 13-9

Laryngoscope set. (*A*) the Miller straight blade; (*B*) Macintosh curved blade; (*C*) laryngoscope handle.

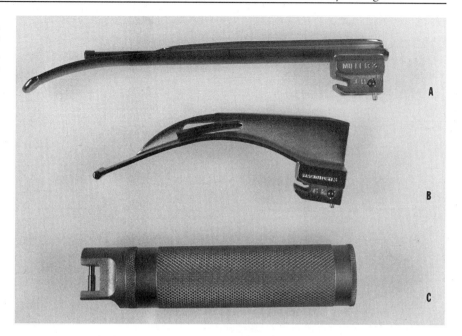

adapter with alcohol allows it to be twisted snugly into the tube.

Cuffed tubes, used in patients older than 8 years, produce an airtight seal to guard against aspiration and facilitate positive-pressure ventilation. Inflating the cuff beforehand with 10 ml of air ensures that the cuff is leak-free.

Styles (Figs. 13-10 and 13-11) include standard single-lumen tubes, wire-reinforced tubes that prevent kinking and compression, preformed tubes to avoid kinking and displacement during nasal, oral, or tracheostomy insertion, and double-lumen tubes or

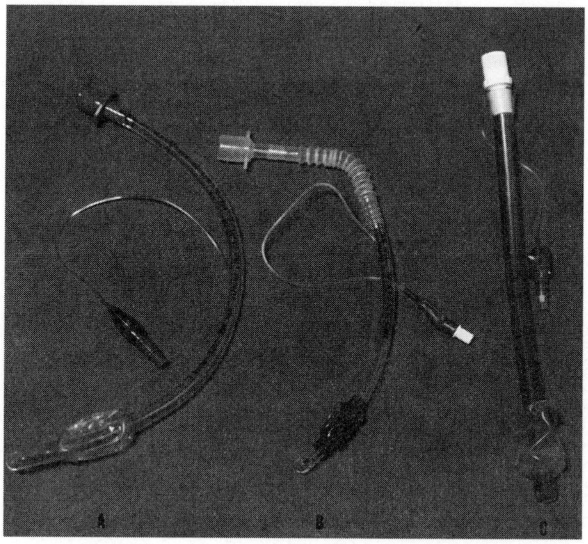

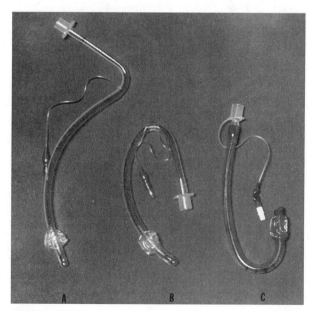

Figure 13-10

Tracheal tubes: (*A*) cuffed oral/nasal tracheal tube; (*B*) cuffed oral tracheal tube with flexible connector; (*C*) armored (anode) cuffed tube with imbedded wire to prevent kinking.

Figure 13-11

Preformed tracheal tubes: (*A*) RAE (right angle) cuffed nasal tracheal tube; (*B*) RAE (right angle) cuffed oral tracheal tube; (*C*) armored (anode) cuffed tracheostomy tube shaped to prevent bronchial intubation.

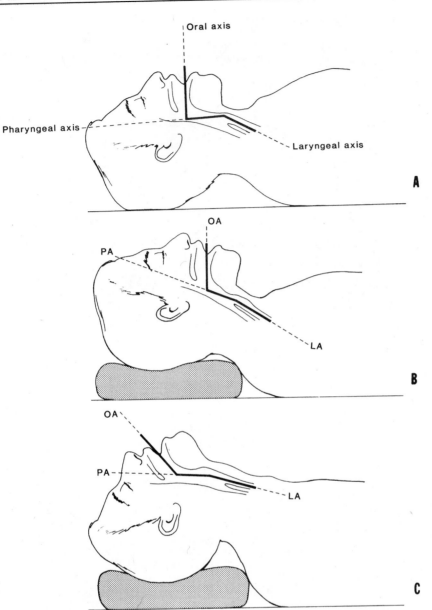

Figure 13-12

Intubating position during rigid laryngoscopy; (*A*) Supine patient without head rest; (*B*) Head elevation and neck flexes bring the pharyngeal and laryngeal axes into line. Head rest 8-10 (3-4) inches cm high is usually optimal; (*C*) Extension of head at occipitocervical joint aligns the oral axis with the other two.

tubes with bronchial blockers to allow separate ventilation of the lungs.

Stylets and Introducers

A wire stylet is placed inside the endotracheal tube to control its shape or confer rigidity. If bent 5 cm from its tip to resemble a hockey stick, a styletted tracheal tube can be guided into an unseen or difficult-to-reach glottis. Lubrication eases the stylet's removal. Excessively stiff or carelessly used stylets can cause serious lacerations or perforations in the oral cavities or hypopharynx.

Introducers may be placed into the trachea as guides for tubes that are then passed over them. They may be firm with a bent tip to facilitate placement during rigid laryngoscopy or soft and flexible to serve as tracheal tube exchangers after insertion through an existing tracheal tube. Some have even been adapted for jet ventilation if reintubation is doubtful.

■ Techniques of Tracheal Intubation

Except in emergencies, intubation is undertaken only after assembling all monitors, equipment, and

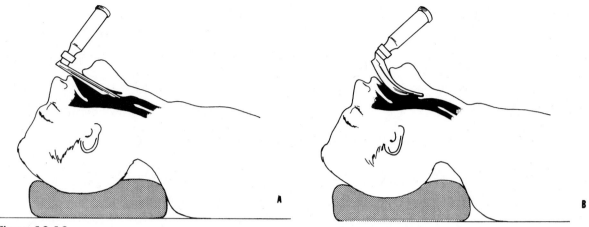

Figure 13-13

Demonstrates the different placements of straight (*A*) and curved (*B*) blades in relation to the epiglottis during laryngoscopy.

Table 13-8

Steps in Rigid Laryngoscopic Intubation

Using an 8- to 10-cm occipital rest, provide sniffing position and neck flexion with cervico-occipital extension to align the oral, pharyngeal, and laryngeal axes (see Fig. 13-12).

Elevate the table to avoid bending over.

With the scissored thumb and index finger of the gloved right hand contacting the right mandibular and maxillary premolars, respectively, pry open the mouth. To avoid lacerations, sweep the lips away from the teeth.

Fully open the mouth.

Holding the laryngoscope in the left hand with the fifth finger close to the hinge and the handle pointing right of the sagittal plane, carefully introduce the blade along the right margin of the tongue. Rotate the laryngoscope into a parasagittal plane to displace the tongue to the left.

Advance the blade until the right tonsillar fossa is identified. Medial to the tonsillar fossa, locate the epiglottis. Advance a curved blade to the midline glossoepiglottic reflection (see Figure 13-13). Slip the tip of straight blade beneath the epiglottis.

Maintaining wrist rigidity to avoid using the maxillary teeth as a fulcrum, expose the glottis by displacing the tongue and epiglottis in an anteroinferior direction.

If necessary, bring the glottis into better view using the right hand to apply backward, upward, and rightward pressure on the thyroid cartilage. An assistant can replicate this maneuver and retract the upper lip out of the line of sight.

Insert the tracheal tube from the right, keeping it from blocking the view of the glottis until the last moment possible. Advance the tube until the proximal margin of its cuff lies 3 to 4 cm beyond the vocal cords.

drugs for airway management, general anesthesia, and resuscitation. After denitrogenation, patients may be sedated or anesthetized, as permitted by their medical problems.

Rigid Laryngoscopic Intubation

In patients undergoing general anesthesia, tracheal intubation is usually performed using rigid laryngoscopy (Figs. 13-12 and 13-13) to insert the tube under direct vision (Table 13-8). A few technical lapses commonly make laryngoscopy more difficult (Table 13-9). Though skill with both curved and straight blades is important, certain patients may benefit from one style or another. Because it reveals the relationship of the epiglottis to other anatomic features, the Macintosh curved blade is recommended when learning intubation. It also features a flange that is very effective at retracting a large tongue or the prominent lips of an edentulous patient. Because a curved blade avoids contacting the sensitive laryngeal surface of the epiglottis, it is well suited for conscious intubation.

In a patient with micrognathia, a floppy epiglottis, or an anterior larynx, a straight blade often affords a superior view of the glottis by directly lifting the stubbornly overlaying epiglottis. The Miller straight blade, with its small cross section, is especially useful in patients with prominent maxillary teeth or limited temporomandibular mobility.

Nasotracheal intubation guided by oral rigid laryngoscopy is undertaken for some head and neck

Table 13-9

Technical Lapses Common during Rigid Laryngoscopy

Improper "sniffing" position
    Insufficient neck flexion: glottis appears anterior
    Excessive flexion: interferes with opening the mouth
Sacrificing binocular vision by bending too close to the patient
Insufficient muscle relaxation
Scissoring open the mouth with fingers too far leftward, leaving insufficient room for the blade
Failing to open the mouth widely
Introducing the blade too far to the left
Failing to identify the epiglottis
Allowing the tongue or tube tip to obscure the glottic view
Inserting the laryngoscope blade to an incorrect depth
    Curved blade: tip not in far enough
    Straight blade: tip in too far
Neglecting to request assistance or to direct the assistant
    Using cricoid pressure (Sellick's maneuver) instead of laryngeal pressure to facilitate laryngoscopy
    Excessively forceful cricoid pressure that immobilizes the larynx
    Failure to retract the right upper lip

operations or for prolonged intubation outside the operating room (Table 13-10) but must be avoided in patients with coagulopathies, nasal obstruction, retropharyngeal abscesses, or fractures of the base of the skull. It is facilitated by applying a vasoconstricting local anesthetic preparation such as 3% lidocaine with 0.25% phenylephrine to the larger nasal passage and by selecting a 0.5-mm smaller diameter tube than usual. Magill intubating forceps are used on the right side of the mouth to direct the distal tip of the

Table 13-10

Advantages and Disadvantages of Nasotracheal Intubation

Advantages
    The tube is more secure with less possibility for spontaneous extubation
    An awake patient is more comfortable
    Eliminates biting tube
    Oral feeding is possible during long-term intubation
    Superior oral hygiene
Disadvantages
    Need for smaller-size tube, rendering suctioning and fiberoptic bronchoscopy difficult
    Higher incidence of bacteremia
    Epistaxis
    Sinusitis

Table 13-11

Indications for Conscious Intubation

Patients at risk for aspiration
Patients in whom ventilation by face mask is expected to be difficult
Patients unlikely to need or tolerate anesthetic drugs
To confirm intact neurologic function after intubation
To allow patients to position themselves after intubation

nasotracheal tube through the glottis without blocking the view provided by laryngoscopy. Rigid laryngoscopic intubation is applicable in patients who are awake, sedated, or under general anesthesia.

Managing Intubation in the Conscious Patient

Although endotracheal intubation may be accomplished without sedation in the moribund patient (i.e., "awake intubation"), the administration of conscious sedation plus topical anesthesia ("conscious intubation") is more common (Table 13-11). A combination of verbal support and explanation of the rationale with sedation and topical anesthesia improves conditions for both the patient and the operator. Sedatives, opioids, and topical anesthetics are used with caution because somnolence or unconsciousness can result in loss of muscle tone, protective reflexes, or respiratory drive, leading to airway obstruction, aspiration, or hypoventilation.

Typical intravenous sedatives include midazolam in 0.5- to 1-mg increments and fentanyl in 25- to 50-μg increments, chosen because specific antagonists exist. To ensure that these synergistic drugs have reached their peak effect, 3 to 5 minutes is allowed to elapse between doses. Repeatedly commanding the patient to inhale and protrude the tongue avoids oversedation.

Table 13-12

Routes for Anesthetizing the Airway

Spray during rigid laryngoscopic or fiberoptic visualization
Gargling
Nebulization
Ointment on a laryngoscope blade
Pledgets applied to the nasal passage
Superior laryngeal nerve block
Lingual nerve block
Translaryngeal injection

Table 13-13

Miscellaneous Applications for the Fiberoptic Bronchoscope

Evaluate upper airway obstruction or pathology
Evaluate vocal cord motion
Assess laryngotracheal injury after burns or prolonged intubation
Position endotracheal or endobronchial tubes
Change from orotracheal to nasotracheal tube while maintaining a path into the trachea

Topical or local anesthesia of the upper airway can be applied to improve comfort and lessen hemodynamic responses (Table 13-12). Antisialagogues such as glycopyrrolate (0.2 to 0.4 mg intravenously) ensure maximal efficacy for topical anesthetics while minimizing secretions.

Fiberoptic Laryngoscopy

The skillful fiberoptic laryngoscopist may use this instrument for routine as well as challenging intubations and in the presence of airway tumors or infections or cervical spine instability. A number of other applications exist (Table 13-13).

Oral or nasal fiberoptic intubations are easier in the conscious than in the unconscious patient; the tongue and epiglottis are less likely to obscure the vocal cords, and the patient can assist by phonating or protruding the tongue. Haste is unnecessary while the patient is breathing. Viewed through the fiberscope, the distance to the vocal cords is exaggerated, and the true cords may not be seen until the false cords have been passed. Small amounts of secretions and blood, contact with tissues, or fogging of the lens completely obscure the view (Table 13-14).

Fiberoptic intubation via the mouth begins with applying topical anesthetic to the tongue and oropharynx. A special oropharyngeal airway prevents biting on the fiberscope, keeps it in the midline, and restrains the tongue. The operator then clears the pharynx of secretions by suction, inserts a tracheal tube into the airway, and passes the well-lubricated fiberscope through the tube and the oropharynx to view the vocal cords. Spraying 4 ml of 4% lidocaine through the suction channel facilitates passage of the fiberscope into the trachea, whereupon it is used to guide the tube into final position. Alternatively, transtracheal injection of 3 ml of 4% lidocaine prior to laryngoscopy avoids coughing and laryngospasm.

In the conscious patient, fiberoptic nasotracheal intubation is often easier than the orotracheal approach because the patient gags less and cannot bite the tube. Advancing the fiberscope from the nasopharynx facilitates visualization of the glottis and passage of the tube through the cords. The tube is placed through the larger nasal passage and into the oropharynx as described for nasotracheal intubation. The tube then serves as a channel to clear the pharynx by suction and to seek the glottis with a well-lubricated fiberscope. Laryngeal anesthesia and intubation proceed as described for the oral approach.

Fiberoptic oral or nasal intubation in the anesthetized patient requires an assistant to monitor the patient and apply jaw thrust. Intubation attempts are interrupted to ventilate the patient as needed.

Blind Nasotracheal Intubation

Blind nasotracheal intubation is indicated for emergency situations or as an alternative to fiberoptic-assisted nasotracheal intubations. Care is required so that epistaxis will not jeopardize alternative techniques should blind intubation fail.

For blind nasotracheal intubation, the patient's head is placed in exaggerated sniffing position. The lubricated tube is advanced posteriorly along the floor of the nasal passage slowly and gently; when resistance is met, the tube is withdrawn and twisted before it is advanced again. Guiding the tracheal tube into the oropharynx over a soft 14 French suction catheter decreases trauma to the mucosa covering the turbinates, occipital bone, and atlas. Haste, large, rigid tubes, an upward course, and abrupt force precipitate epistaxis.

The operator listens at the proximal end of the

Table 13-14

Practical Suggestions for Fiberoptic Intubation

Practice the techniques on a model and in elective cases before applying them in a difficult situation.
When possible, administer an antisialagogue.
Adjust the diopter ring by focusing on a fine test pattern before working on a patient.
Prevent fogging by immersing the tip of the fiberscope for a few minutes in warm water.
Use only water-soluble lubricants.
Avoid smearing the objective lens with lubricant.
If passage of the tracheal tube is obstructed by the epiglottis and aryepiglottic folds, withdraw the tube, twist it 90 degrees, and advance it again.

endotracheal tube for breath sounds while using one hand to advance the tube during inspiration and the other to palpate the thyrohyoid membrane. Clues to position include intensity of breath sounds, lateral bulging produced by the tip of the tube in the piriform fossae, resistance to passage if the tube enters the valleculae, and disappearance of breath sounds with passage into the esophagus. Twisting the tube sweeps its tip from side to side; extending or flexing the neck moves the tip anteroposteriorly. Entry into the trachea is signaled by coughing, aphonia, and a normal capnograph tracing.

Bullard Laryngoscope

The Bullard laryngoscope is useful for patients confined to the neutral position or with limited mandibular movement. It is loaded with a tracheal tube over a stylet and has a tongue retractor shaped much like an oropharyngeal airway that fits into the valleculae; fiberoptics allow the tube to be inserted while visualizing the glottis. As with flexible fiberscopic scopes, pharyngeal blood or secretions obscure the view.

Light-Wand Technique

Light wands are flexible, battery-powered stylets with lighted tips. Placed inside the tracheal tube and then bent into a hockey stick shape, the light wand is passed in the midline over the tongue, which must be pulled forward. With the room lights darkened, tracheal entry is signaled by a beam of light appearing in the midline of the neck inferior to the thyroid notch. Light appears above the thyroid cartilage if the tip of the tube enters the valleculae or laterally on entry into a piriform fossa, and it disappears if the tube passes into the esophagus. The light wand permits oral intubation in the presence of limited temporomandibular motion and unstable neck fractures.

Augustine Guide

This instrument was designed for blind oral intubation in the neutral position because of cervical instability, limited temporomandibular mobility, or blood, vomitus, or edema in the pharynx. The tongue-retracting guide is loaded with a tracheal tube that in turn contains a special hollow stylet with distal perforations and an anteriorly directed curve. The guide passes over the tongue until it engages the glossoepiglottic ligament, as demonstrated by transmission of side-to-side movements from the guide to the larynx. The stylet is advanced into the trachea; this position is confirmed by free aspiration of air into a large syringe. The stylet then guides the tracheal tube into position.

Retrograde Intubation

If necessary, blind intubation is possible using a retrograde guidewire technique. The cricothyroid ligament is punctured with a needle and a flexible wire is advanced superiorly through the trachea, vocal cords and pharynx, exiting through the mouth. The tracheal tube is passed into the proximal trachea over the guidewire, which is then removed. Special kits for this procedure include a J-tipped guidewire and an introducer to facilitate passage of the tracheal tube over the guidewire.

■ Intubation in Patients at High Risk for Aspiration

Induction of anesthesia in patients who do not have empty stomachs or in those with poorly functioning gastroesophageal sphincters may result in regurgitation and pulmonary aspiration. Histamine 2 (H_2) blockers, metoclopramide, and nasogastric suction reduce the risks but may still leave the patient with stomach contents of sufficient volume and acidity to cause severe bronchospasm, hypoxemia, and pneumonitis. In these patients, intubation may precede the induction of anesthesia ("awake intubation").

Alternatively, anesthesia may begin with a "rapid sequence" of an intravenous hypnotic plus a rapid-acting muscle relaxant (e.g., 1 to 1.5mg/kg of succinylcholine or 1.2mg/kg of rocuronium) and intubation as soon as muscle relaxation is confirmed. An assistant maintains cricoid pressure from the onset of anesthesia through cuff inflation and verification of tube position. If intubation is delayed, gentle ventilation at airway pressures of less than $30cmH_2O$ while maintaining cricoid pressure avoids gastric distension and regurgitation. Coexisting diseases in patients at risk for aspiration pose dilemmas that challenge ingenuity and skill (Table 13-15).

The Difficult Intubation

Even among experts, 0.5 to 2 percent of rigid laryngoscopic intubations prove difficult. The American Society of Anesthesiologists Task Force on the

Table 13-15

Intubation When Complicating Conditions Coexist with an Increased Risk of Aspiration

Complicating Condition	Drugs or Techniques to Consider
Anticipated difficult intubation or ventilation	Conscious intubation
Asthma	Conscious intubation with good topical anesthesia and opioid sedation, or deep anesthesia with mask induction while maintaining cricoid pressure intubation, or beta-2-adrenergic agonists, theophylline, lidocaine, opioids, ketamine induction, and rapid-sequence intubation
Contraindication to succinylcholine	Rapid-acting nondepolarizing relaxant, or conscious intubation
Ischemic heart disease	Conscious intubation with generous sedation and good topical anesthesia, or opioid, beta-adrenergic antagonist, nitroglycerin, and rapid-sequence intubation, or unhurried induction while maintaining cricoid pressure
Open eye injury	Rapid-sequence intubation using a rapid-onset, nondepolarizing relaxant
Pharyngeal pouch	Conscious intubation
Moribund condition or shock	Conscious intubation, or muscle relaxant alone, possibly with small dose of scopolamine, etomidate, or ketamine
Small bowel obstruction	Conscious intubation or rapid-sequence intubation if stomach is not distended
Upper gastrointestinal bleeding	Conscious intubation or rapid-sequence intubation

Management of the Difficult Airway (ASA Task Force) defines *difficult laryngoscopy* as occurring when no portion of the vocal cords is visible using conventional rigid laryngoscopy. *Difficult endotracheal intubation* exists if more than three attempts at conventional laryngoscopy are needed or if the process takes more than 10 minutes.

■ Understanding Difficult Intubation

Tracheal intubation by direct laryngoscopy requires viewing and reaching the glottis via a curved course, anterior to a near obstacle (the maxillary teeth) and posterior to a distant barrier (the tongue). It is accomplished by attempting to align the mouth, pharynx, and larynx while displacing the tongue anteriorly into the mandibular space, a sequence that can be confounded by a number of subtle factors (Table 13-16). Though at times difficult intubation comes as a surprise (Table 13-17), it is important to attempt to anticipate problems so as to avoid panic

Table 13-16

Factors that Confound Laryngoscopy

Inability to straighten the path
   Cervico-occipital pathology
   Poor muscle relaxation
Near obstacles
   Full set of prominent teeth
   Overbite
   Isolated teeth that end up to the right of the laryngoscope blade as it rests on the gum
   Long, narrow maxilla
   Large upper lip in edentulous patient
Distant barriers
   Limited temporomandibular mobility
   Micrognathia (limits mandibular space and pulls larynx into an anterior position)
   Obesity
   Macroglossia
   Large lingual tonsil or thyroid
   Noncompressible tongue (e.g., tumor, inflammation, amyloidosis)
   Floppy epiglottis
   Anteriorly situated larynx

Table 13-17

Unpredictable Difficult Intubation
Sudden anaphylactic airway edema
Severe masseter muscle rigidity
Lingual tonsil or lingual thyroid
Floppy epiglottis
Epiglottic mucoid cyst
Tracheobronchial obstruction or compression

and allow a broad range of alternate techniques, many of which preserve spontaneous ventilation.

■ Prediction

Numerous series published over the past 10 years have failed to identify predictors of difficult intubation that are both sensitive and specific; a fundamental confounding factor is the low prevalence of difficult intubation. Also, most investigators examine only a few hundred patients and artificially increase the incidence of the problem by using difficult laryngoscopy as their endpoint instead of difficult intubation (Table 13-18). Often, though it may be done blindly and require a stylet, an experienced person can intubate the trachea even when layrngoscopy and direct visualization of the glottis are difficult.

Mallampati's classification illustrates some of the problems with predicting difficult intubation. The evaluation is based on visualization of progressively more remote structures (hard palate, soft palate, tip of the epiglottis and tonsillar pillars) in a sitting patient who protrudes the tongue. The airway is described as "class I" if all the structures are visible, or "class IV" if only the hard palate is visible. The test has been applied too broadly by novices in anesthesiology, who often describe an airway simply as "class I" even though no account is taken of other essential factors

Table 13-18

Popular Scheme for Classifying Difficulty of Laryngoscopy	
Grade I:	Entire glottis seen
Grade II:	Only posterior structures of glottis seen
Grade III:	Only the epiglottis seen
Grade IV:	Even the epiglottis not seen

Source: From Cormack RS, Lehane J. Difficult tracheal intubation in obstetrics. *Anaesthesia* 1984;39:1105.

such as suppleness and mobility of the neck or the state of dentition. Interpreting the Mallampati score is uncertain in those who cannot sit, individuals who arch their tongues upward when protruding it, and patients who approximate their soft palate and tongue by nose breathing. Further, there are conflicting opinions regarding whether the patient should phonate during the examination.

The prediction of difficult intubation remains an art of recognizing subtle signs and combinations thereof (see Tables 13-1, 13-2, and 13-3), with a tendency for the experienced practitioner to err on the side of overdiagnosis because of the difficulty of managing an unanticipated failed intubation.

■ Managing the Difficult Airway

Often the lungs can be ventilated by mask or laryngeal mask airway when endotracheal intubation is difficult. Except for those at high risk for aspiration, injury will be avoided in most patients simply by maintaining ventilation and oxygenation. When intubation has failed but ventilation is adequate, careful management ensures that each new maneuver represents a logical, substantive change from steps that have failed. Repeated rigid laryngoscopy rapidly provokes airway edema and hemorrhage that confound subsequent attempts and may even prevent adequate gas exchange. Often, a return to spontaneous ventilation may be the wisest course. Experienced assistance is invaluable.

Responding to the severe consequences of failed airway management, the ASA Task Force has developed a management algorithm (Fig. 13-14).

■ Percutaneous Transtracheal Jet Ventilation

When both mask ventilation and tracheal intubation are impossible, ventilation via a 14- or 12-gauge venous catheter passed through the cricothyroid ligament into the trachea may be lifesaving. To avoid pneumomediastinum, the intratracheal position of the catheter is ensured by the ability to aspirate air freely. Effective ventilation is possible using a source of intermittent oxygen at 18 to 30 lb/in^2, but exhalation requires a patent larynx.

Because of the rapid and severe consequences of airway obstruction, anesthetizing locations must have a preassembled hose, adapted to fit a venous catheter

Figure 13-14

ASA difficult airway algorithm.

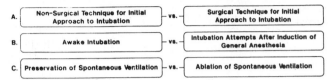

1. **Assess the likelihood and clinical impact of basic management problems:**

   A. Difficult Intubation

   B. Difficult Ventilation

   C. Difficulty with Patient Cooperation or Consent

2. **Consider the relative merits and feasibility of basic management choices:**

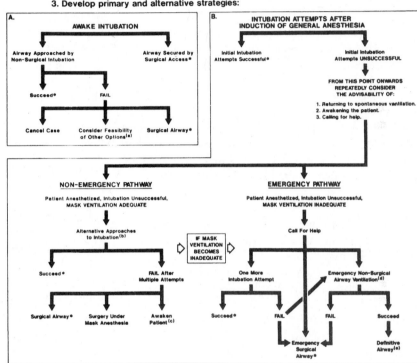

on one end and a jet injector or the common gas outlet of the anesthesia machine on the other. The flush valve activates the latter.

■ Tracheostomy and Cricothyrotomy

Tracheostomy is best performed unhurriedly, even by an experienced surgeon. Cricothyrotomy is the preferred approach when attempts at intubation of the trachea or mask ventilations have failed or if exhaled gases (from a jet ventilator) cannot pass through the glottis. To accomplish cricothyrotomy, the cricothyroid ligament is palpated on the hyperextended neck. Transverse incisions through the skin,

subcutaneous tissue, and the ligament allow insertion of a narrow tracheal tube or a specially designed airway.

Care after Tracheal Intubation

■ Confirming Tracheal Intubation

Immediately after intubation, it is vital to inflate the cuff and observe the sequential rise and fall of the chest while listening with a stethoscope over each midaxillary line and the epigastrium to ensure that the trachea, not the esophagus or a mainstem bronchus,

Table 13-19

Reliable Indicators of Tracheal Tube Position
Repeated detection of at least 15 mmHg (2 percent) exhaled carbon dioxide
Confirming by laryngoscopy the passage of the tracheal tube between the vocal cords
Seeing tracheal rings through a fiberscope passed through the ETT (assuming tube tip has passed the larynx)
Aspiration of 50 ml of air abruptly from the tube with a suction bulb

has been intubated. Because breath sounds have misled even skilled clinicians, the American Society of Anesthesiologists' intraoperative monitoring standards mandate confirming tracheal intubation by detecting consistent levels of exhaled carbon dioxide in successive breaths. Carbon dioxide can enter the esophagus and stomach during mask ventilation, but its exhaled concentration decreases rapidly during esophageal "ventilation." During shock, little carbon dioxide may appear in the exhaled gas despite proper tracheal tube position. Among numerous methods for confirming tracheal tube position, only a few are highly reliable (Table 13-19). When in doubt, the tracheal tube should be removed and the lungs ventilated by mask and airway.

For average-sized women and men, securing orotracheal tubes with the 21- and 23-cm marks, respectively, at the gum or central incisors usually results in a satisfactory position of the tip. Nasotracheal tubes are inserted 3 cm deeper. A note is made in the anesthesia record to document the procedure (Table 13-20).

■ Maintaining the Tracheal Tube

Tracheal tube cuffs must be maintained with care to prevent tracheal mucosal ischemia from chronic

Table 13-20

Documenting Intubation in the Anesthesia Record
Size and type of laryngoscope blade used
Size of tube
Ease and number of attempts at intubation
Reason for difficulty and maneuvers that worked well
Depth of insertion at teeth 8 and 9 or gums
Inflation of cuff, milliliters of air
Method of confirmation of tracheal position
Method of fixation

overinflation. During long procedures, nitrous oxide can diffuse into a cuff and increase its pressure. In the absence of a gauge to ensure that the cuff pressure is in the proper range (25 to 34 cmH$_2$O), most clinicians use a low-pressure, high-volume cuff filled so that there is a small audible leak at peak airway pressure and assure that the pilot balloon is full but not tense.

Tracheal tubes are usually fixed in position with adhesive tape. Tincture of benzoin or other skin preparation solutions may improve stability. An oropharyngeal airway or roll of gauze sponges placed between the teeth keeps the patient from biting the tube. Nasotracheal tubes must be taped securely while avoiding pressure on the nares. The position of the tube is verified each time the patient's position changes.

■ Removing Tracheal Tubes

After verifying that the criteria for safe removal of the tube have been met (Table 13-21), the lungs are inflated with oxygen at 10 to 20 cmH$_2$O pressure and the cuff is deflated just before removing the tube. This ensures that the patient will exhale immediately upon extubation of the trachea, lifting the epiglottis away

Table 13-21

Checklist for Extubation at the Conclusion of Anesthesia
There is no medical indication for continued intubation, such as impending ventilatory failure or circulatory instability.
Muscle relaxants are fully reversed.
Spontaneous ventilation is adequate.
Desired level of consciousness has been achieved.
Anesthetized, to prevent coughing: Patient does not respond to cuff deflation or wiggling the tracheal tube.
Awake, to prevent aspiration and airway obstruction: Patient follows commands or moves purposefully.
All equipment for airway management is present.
Denitrogenate with high-flow oxygen.
Clear the pharynx by suction.
Deflate the cuff.
Apply positive pressure to the breathing system and gently remove the tracheal tube.
Clear the pharynx by suction again only if required, only to avoid hypoxemia.
Reassess airway patency and ventilation; correct as needed.
Apply mask with high-flow oxygen, and check vital signs.

from the glottis and forcing any secretions upward into the mouth. The patient is observed to determine patency of the airway, adequacy of ventilation and oxygenation, and the likelihood of regurgitation, vomiting, or laryngospasm. Supplemental oxygen is usually administered, and the patient is encouraged to take deep breaths.

Complications of Intubation

During airway management for anesthetized patients, minor trauma such as lacerated lips, chipped, loosened, or displaced teeth, and epistaxis are common. More serious complications include perforations of the hypopharynx, esophagus, or trachea, which may result in pneumothorax, pneumomediastinum, or mediastinitis. Only immediate recognition and therapy in such cases can prevent serious morbidity or death. Attention to careful technique minimizes the incidence of complications from intubation (Table 13-22).

Inability to ventilate immediately following extubation can result from obstructing supraglottic soft tissues, laryngospasm, bronchospasm, tracheobronchial compression, chest wall rigidity, and even problems with anesthesia machines (e.g., attempting to use the reservoir bag with the selector valve still set for mechanical ventilation). Assessment and treatment are carried out as during induction of anesthesia, including jaw thrust, positive airway pressure by mask, and reintubation if necessary.

Uncontrolled autonomic responses result from laryngoscopy and intubation in lightly anesthetized patients at the beginning of anesthesia or at the end of operation during emergence from anesthesia with an endotracheal tube still present. Depending on the patient's condition and the setting, these responses may be controlled with deep anesthesia, adrenergic blocking drugs, topical anesthesia, intravenous lidocaine, or opioids.

Spinal cord injury may result from attempts at intubation in patients with unstable neck fractures or severe rheumatoid arthritis. Neurosurgeons, orthopedists, or trauma surgeons may render valuable assistance by providing axial stabilization of the neck during intubation. Sore throat is a frequent complication of tracheal intubation but also can follow anesthesia without intubation. Nasogastric tubes compound the problem. If there is hoarseness, the patient should be followed to exclude a

Table 13-22

Complications of Tracheal Intubation

During intubation
 Trauma to lips, teeth, tongue, nasal passage, pharynx, larynx, trachea, esophagus
 Cardiovascular
  Hypertension and tachycardia
  Arrhythmias
  Reflex bradycardia or asystole
  Cardiac ischemia
 Respiratory
  Coughing and chest wall spasm
  Laryngospasm
  Bronchospasm
  Aspiration
 Central nervous system
  Increased intracranial pressure
  Spinal cord injury with unstable neck
 Unrecognized improper intubation
  Esophageal
  Endobronchial
  Cuff between cords
While tracheal tube is in place
 Obstruction from kinking, secretions, compression, biting
 Endobronchial intubation or extubation
 Barotrauma
 Cuff leak
 Disconnection from breathing circuit
 Nosocomial infections
Immediately following extubation
 Laryngospasm
 Aspiration
 Acute laryngotracheal edema
 Trauma during extubation
 Vocal cord palsy
Late complications
 Sore throat and hoarseness
 Tracheal stenosis
 Vocal cord polyps

persistent vocal cord paralysis or injury. Preanesthetic teaching and sympathetic postanesthetic visits will help patients keep this condition in perspective. Warm fluids and throat lozenges minimize symptoms until the expected resolution in 1 to 2 days.

BIBLIOGRAPHY

ASA Task Force on Management of the Difficult Airway. Practice guidelines for management of the difficult airway. *Anesthesiology* 1993;78:597-602.

Asai T, Morris S. The laryngeal mask airway: Its features, effects, and role. *Can J Anaesth* 1994;41:930-960.

Bellhouse CP, Dore C. Criteria for estimating likelihood of difficulty of endotracheal intubation with the Macintosh laryngoscope. *Anaesth Intens Care* 1988;16:329-337.

Benumof JL. Management of the difficult adult airway: With special emphasis on awake tracheal intubation. *Anesthesiology* 1991;75:1087-1110.

Birmingham PK, Cheney FW, Ward RJ. Esophageal intubation: A review of detection techniques. *Anesth Analg* 1986;65:886-891.

Caplan RA, Posner KL, Ward RJ, Cheney FW. Adverse respiratory events in anesthesia: A closed claims analysis. *Anesthesiology* 1990;72:828-833.

Cormack RS, Lehane J. Difficult tracheal intubation in obstetrics. *Anaesthesia* 1984;39:1105-1111.

Dorsch JA, Dorsch SE. *Understanding Anesthesia Equipment: Construction, Care and Complications.* Baltimore: Williams and Wilkins, 1994.

Finucane BT, Santora AH. *Principles of Airway Management.* Philadelphia: F. A. Davis, 1988.

Frass M, Rodler S, Frenzer R, et al. Esophageal tracheal Combitube, endotracheal airway, and mask: Comparison of ventilatory pressure curves. *J Trauma* 1989;29:1476-1479.

Latto IP, Rosen M. *Difficulties in Tracheal Intubation.* Philadelphia: Bailliere Tindall, 1985.

Mallampati SR, Gatt SP, Gugino LD, et al. A clinical sign to predict difficult intubation: A prospective study. *Can Anaesth Soc J* 1985; 32:429-434.

Ovassapian A. *Fiberoptic Endoscopy and the Difficult Airway.* Philadelphia: Lippincott-Raven Press, 1996.

Wilson ME. Predicting difficult intubation (editorial). *Br J Anaesth* 1993;71:333-334.

CHAPTER 14

Conduct of General Anesthesia

Frank L. Murphy

Skilled anesthesiologists are recognized by patients, surgeons, and colleagues for providing "good anesthesia." This concept has different meanings to different observers, but it includes making the patient comfortable, avoiding complications and "near misses," managing the anesthetic so that it harmonizes with the surgical procedure, reacting calmly and decisively in emergencies, using resources efficiently, working quickly but not in haste, performing technical procedures skillfully, and maintaining pleasant, professional relationships with coworkers. Ease and familiarity are important components of skilled practice, but those beginning training can adopt good habits with the first anesthetics they administer.

In relating the scientific foundations of anesthesia to the principles of safe practice, textbooks leave unwritten folklore, routines, and advice for the management of anesthesia that are handed down orally from instructors to students. These elements of good practice are the subject of this chapter.

Planning Anesthesia

A well-managed anesthetic begins with a good plan. Indeed, in discussions with colleagues and in the oral examination of the American Board of Anesthesiology (ABA), an anesthesiologist's medical judgment is tested by the quality of the anesthesia plan, the extent to which it is based on scientific principles, its consideration of changing circum-stances, and the clarity with which the anesthesiologist can explain it. There is no rigid format for planning anesthesia. Rather, each plan is adapted to the patient at hand.

■ Goals

The goals of anesthetic management are unchanging: safety, comfort, convenience, and efficiency first for the patient and second for those caring for the patient. Rarely can one satisfy all these perfectly; compromise is common. Other goals may include teaching, research, containing costs, or reducing malpractice exposure, but the patient's interests remain paramount.

Consider the goals for the management of the patient described in the accompanying boxed preoperative note. The major safety-related goal is to reduce blood loss. Beyond the usual effort to avoid the use of banked blood, special efforts may be required to avoid postoperative anemia in a patient who refuses all blood products. A related safety goal is to avoid myocardial ischemia, achieved primarily by avoiding extremes in blood pressure and heart rate, important in this untreated hypertensive patient, especially if anemia becomes severe. Achieving the goal of patient comfort by relieving her anxiety may help reduce tachycardia and hypertension in the preoperative period. Avoiding blood products and spinal or epidural anesthesia serves the goal of patient convenience.

Anesthesia Preoperative Note   5/19/96

A 64-year-old woman for revision total hip arthroplasty

Dentition:	normal
Airway:	uvula visible, neck and jaw mobile, no snoring
Meds:	none
Allergies:	none
Prior anesthetic:	GA elsewhere, no complications
Problems, plans:	

1. Obesity: 5'4", 180 pounds, no airway compromise, no snoring. Plan: cimetidine, metoclopramide, no rapid sequence needed.
2. Mild hypertension, × 5 years, bp 150/95, normal ECG changes, no history of stroke, angina, MI; BUN/Cr normal.
   Plan: avoid hypertension, tachycardia, hypothermia, use beta blockers.
3. Pt refuses all blood products, risks discussed, Hb 12.4.
   Plan: deliberate hypotension; isoflurane + beta blocker + nitroprusside if needed; MAP = 65; A-line; CVP; blood scavenging.
4. Pt says, "I'm very anxious. Knock me out before I go in the OR."
   Plan: oral diazepam at bedtime, A.M.
5. Refuses spinal or epidural: fears needle in spine.
   Plan: no spinal or epidural.

ASA PS II (obesity, hypertension)
I have reviewed the database, discussed the plan with the patient, who agrees, and answered all questions.

J. L. Doe, M.D.
beep 555-2222

(This preoperative note describes the patient discussed throughout this chapter. Preoperative notes must be written quickly but also must document fully the anesthesia plan and the reasons for it; the telegraphic style used here represents a compromise between a checklist and a complete narrative.)

■ Types of Plans for Anesthesia

Many kinds of thinking go into planning anesthesia management:

1. Formal algorithms for planning the management of specific problems have begun to appear. These schemes can be thought out prospectively and offer the advantages of careful analysis; they are useful for emergencies, for managing unfamiliar problems, and for careful analysis of costs. Disadvantages include rigidity and lack of understanding of the medical concepts that underlie the algorithm.
2. A list of problems and a method for managing each often provides a valuable summary and can serve to point out conflicting goals and approaches. An example appears in the accompanying preoperative note.
3. Chronological planning involves imagining the course of the anesthetic and the problems that might arise in sequence, such as preoperative evaluation, premedication, monitoring, induction, airway management, maintenance of anesthesia, management of surgical stress, emergence, and postoperative care. This approach serves well as a checklist, but it relies on experience and is not oriented to physiologic problems.
4. Target planning requires that the anesthesiologist imagine the state to be achieved for the patient at the end of the case and work back in time to plan the needed steps to achieve that state. As with chronological planning, this relies on experience, but it may alert one to conflicts and inconsistencies in elements of the plan. This approach is most valuable when the major goal is to achieve a specific postoperative state. For example, if a patient must awaken promptly at the end of an anesthetic to allow evaluation of the results of neurosurgery, this goal must be paramount in the anesthetic plan.
5. Conflicting goals can require the plan to focus on one issue, even at the expense of others. For example, the goals of reducing blood loss and myocardial ischemia would both be well served by using an epidural anesthetic; combining the epidural with a general anesthetic would help manage the anxiety; but the patient's overriding goal of avoiding a needle in her back requires compromise in managing blood loss.
6. Planning by routine is an appropriate choice when patients and cases are similar; it is likely that laparoscopy in a healthy patient can be accomplished successfully using an anesthetic that has worked well in healthy patients previously. The benefit of following a routine is the opportunity to refine the technique based on prior experience. The danger is that by following routines one may overlook the needs of the unusual patient.

Skilled practitioners use all these schemes at one time or another, depending on what seems most appropriate for the case at hand. Often, it is appropriate to use several methods for planning a single case. A problem-oriented description of the plan for this woman's management was added to the preoperative note. Adding the planned therapy for each problem completes a problem-oriented description of an anesthesia plan for the preoperative note.

Although this plan was formulated as a list of problems and solutions, it was backward planning that reminded the anesthesiologist of the need for special attention to warming the patient to avoid hypertension and tachycardia in the postanesthesia care unit (PACU). The choice of general anesthesia was based on the patient's refusal of regional anesthesia but also ensures ventilation and oxygenation in an obese patient undergoing a potentially prolonged procedure (revisions of total hip arthroplasties may be lengthy). Isoflurane is a popular choice for induced hypotension because hypotension with this agent is characterized by decreased peripheral vascular resistance and maintained cardiac output.

■ Characteristics of a Good Plan

Good anesthesia plans share certain characteristics. First, they take into account interpatient variability. For example, a nitroprusside infusion of 1 mg/kg per minute might give the needed hypotension, but this is not the planned starting dose, which would be less. Alternatively, nitroprusside might be required in doses that risk cyanide toxicity; in this case, adding propranolol will reduce the required dose of nitroprusside by blunting compensatory tachycardia and renin release. Thus good anesthesia plans anticipate extreme responses, not just average responses.

Second, good anesthesia plans do not assign the same importance to various goals. For example, our anxious patient asked to be made unconscious before leaving her room. Though she does not have a history suggestive of sleep apnea, the goals of avoiding somnolence and airway obstruction in an obese patient dictate that she will receive only moderate doses of diazepam in her room. Midazolam can be given intravenously once she reaches the holding area outside the operating room, where the anesthesiologist can observe the effect of the drug and monitor oxygen saturation.

Third, planning involves weighing the magnitude of risks and benefits to be expected. An example in our patient might be the decision to use an arterial cannula to monitor blood pressure. In all likelihood, her blood pressure can be managed without such monitoring, but the consequences of inadvertent hypotension may be severe; her large, tapered upper arm will not accept a blood pressure cuff readily; and the risks of the invasive monitoring are small.

Fourth, a plan for anesthesia recognizes that the various elements interact, even in a simple anesthetic plan. In our patient, the decision to use H_2 blockers preoperatively was a response to the decision not to use a rapid-sequence induction and intubation, which in turn resulted from the fear of myocardial ischemia in this patient. It is often necessary to make reasonable compromises in the management of one problem in order to allow successful management of another.

Fifth, a good anesthesia plan is practical; it does no good to frame a plan that cannot be accomplished with the people and equipment at hand. For example, this patient's blood could be conserved by reinfusing her own blood that is salvaged during the operation (if she agreed); without the necessary equipment, this plan would be impractical.

Preparing for Anesthesia

After a good plan, a good anesthetic requires adequate preparation. For our patient, adequate preparation includes all the routine measures listed in the checklist given in Chapter 5, as well as these special steps:

1. Verify that the equipment and technicians are available for intraoperative recovery of shed blood.
2. Prepare the nitroprusside and esmolol infusions, calculate appropriate pump settings for various dose rates, and post a table of doses with the pumps.
3. Have ready the monitors, transducers, and insertion kits for the arterial and central venous cannulas.

Such preparations help ensure patient safety because minor problems may become major ones if one is not ready to deal with them; on the other hand, there is waste and delay in overpreparation. Thus neither a nitroglycerine infusion nor trimethaphan is prepared ahead of time, despite the possibility that signs of myocardial ischemia might prompt the use of the one (NTG), and hypoxemia associated with nitroprusside might require an alternative hypotensive technique. Rare but life-threatening complications may require advance preparations; an example is the availability in the operating suite of a defibrillator for this patient.

All preparations are completed before the patient enters the room, thereby keeping to a minimum the time during which the awake, anxious person must lie on the operating table. This also allows the anesthesiologist to focus attention on the patient rather than on technical preparations.

Bringing the Patient into the Operating Room

Before bringing the patient into the operating room, it is important to verify the patient's identity and the planned operation. Greeting this patient by name and asking her to point to the site of the operation achieve these goals. At this time, another review of the chart reveals any overnight events, new laboratory data, or consultants' reports. Also, the patient is questioned as to the time of the last meal and any medications received. This potentially repetitive questioning may puzzle or even annoy some patients, especially if it appears that the data recorded in a preoperative visit have been ignored. Limiting questions to the essentials and an explanation of the need to avoid errors are steps that reassure patients.

Depending on staffing and available space, the intravenous catheter and electrocardiograph (ECG) pads or other monitoring devices can be placed (and some regional anesthetics performed) before bringing the patient into the operating room. This can improve operating room efficiency if it can be accomplished during the preceding operation or while the operating room is being cleaned. In the holding area, our patient receives 2-mg increments of drug to a total of 6 mg, until she responds to her name but appears indifferent to her surroundings. Had this patient been an elderly, less robust woman with a fractured hip, the same drugs might have been used for the same purpose, but almost surely in markedly reduced amounts (e.g., 0.5 mg midazolam, 10 to 20 µg fentanyl).

Our patient for hip repair comes to the operating room in some discomfort and is unable to move herself to the operating table. Rather than induce anesthesia with the patient in bed (sometimes done for patients with fractures), this patient's anesthesiologist administers oxygen by nasal prongs and 50 µg fentanyl intravenously before moving the patient to the operating table with the help of five people; the anesthesiologist stands at the head, another person holds the feet, and two people on each side lift the sheet on which the patient lies.

Once the patient is in the room, the remaining monitoring equipment is attached as quickly and deftly as possible. Not all the monitoring devices that will be used intraoperatively need be attached or inserted before inducing anesthesia. Invasive monitors not needed for induction are often inserted after anesthesia has begun. For our patient for a hip operation, the arterial catheter, the central venous pressure (CVP) catheter, and the urinary bladder catheter can be placed after anesthesia begins, because they are needed primarily to monitor the effects of blood loss and deliberate hypotension; a smooth induction can be managed without invasive cardiovascular monitoring.

Before proceeding with induction, the immediate preoperative vital signs are recorded and evaluated in light of what is known about the patient. For example, this woman might be found to have a peripheral oxygen saturation of 94 percent while breathing room air, not unexpected in view of her obesity, especially if she has become somnolent due to sedatives. Her blood pressure might be 180/105 just before induction. This is greater than her preoperative blood pressure but understandable in the circumstances. Because leads II and V_5, properly calibrated for voltage, appear to be identical to the preoperative ECG and the patient has no complaints of chest pain, anesthesia begins. During this time, the patient breathes oxygen, to provide denitrogenation, which is especially important in obese patients with compromised functional residual capacity (FRC).

Induction of Anesthesia

The induction of general anesthesia is a topic that recurs throughout this text; it is a crucial maneuver in managing an anesthetic. Because of unpredictable responses, it seems appropriate to give incremental doses of anesthetics until the proper depth of anesthesia is reached. Ordinarily, such titration is good practice, but prolonged induction of anesthesia can be as dangerous as proceeding too quickly. Patients in very light stages of anesthesia (stage II) are hyperreflexic and may be harmed by catecholamine excess, violent movement, vomiting, or laryngospasm.

While breathing oxygen, our patient receives an additional 50 μg fentanyl intravenously to blunt the hypertensive and tachycardic responses to intubation of the trachea. Because she is somnolent from the midazolam, she receives coaching to remind her to breathe.

After denitrogenation, thiopental is injected into a free-running intravenous infusion at about 100 mg/min. (The induction could be completed with midazolam, but the anesthesiologist fears postoperative somnolence with large doses of this drug.) The slow infusion of thiopental allows the anesthesiologist to stop short of the usual dose (4 mg/kg, or 300 mg for this patient) if the patient loses consciousness (because of the midazolam) or becomes hypotensive or apneic (because of her hypertension or the other intravenous drugs she has received). After 125 mg thiopental, the patient stops breathing and fails to respond to commands to open her eyes; at this point, she is lightly anesthetized. By cautious efforts at controlled ventilation, the anesthesiologist verifies that the patient's airway is patent and that she accepts controlled ventilation without coughing or breath holding. For several minutes, manual ventilation continues with a mixture of 50% nitrous oxide, 48% oxygen, and 2% isoflurane; the goal is to deepen anesthesia so that the patient will not respond to tracheal intubation with excessive hypertension or tachycardia and to deepen anesthesia gradually so as to avert abrupt and severe hypotension.

Intubation might be accomplished without the aid of a muscle relaxant, but experience has taught that it will be difficult to achieve deep enough anesthesia for intubation without hypotension in a patient such as this. D-Tubocurarine is chosen to facilitate endotracheal intubation because it is the relaxant to be used for the remainder of the procedure. (For a prolonged operation, D-tubocurarine or pancuronium are better choices than the shorter-acting relaxants; for deliberate hypotension, D-tubocurarine is a better choice than pancuronium because of the tachycardia induced by the latter.) To prevent histamine release and hypotension, the D-tubocurarine is given in divided doses (0.1 to 0.2 mg/kg each) a minute or two apart. After the response to the nerve stimulator has de-

creased to posttetanic facilitation (PTF) only and 6 minutes of isoflurane administration has decreased the blood pressure to 90/50, the depth of anesthesia is sufficient to permit intubation (intravenous lidocaine may be administered to blunt the hypertension associated with laryngoscopy).

Three minutes after endotracheal intubation, the blood pressure is 70/40 and the heart rate 52; this is treated with ephedrine, which corrects both the hypotension and the bradycardia. Soon thereafter, induction is complete and maintenance begins.

Working with the Surgeon

Anesthetics are not conducted in isolation; the anesthetic and the operation must be coordinated for best results. The anesthesiologist must be fully informed about the operation: the anatomy, the duration, the expected blood loss, and the physiologic effects that can be expected. If these matters are not clear, consultation between anesthesiologist and surgeon before the patient comes into the operating room is in order. Ignorance of the surgical procedure not only leads to a clumsy anesthetic but also impairs the relationship between surgeon and anesthesiologist.

For our patient undergoing a hip operation, even though the surgeon and the anesthesiologist have worked together before on similar cases, they confer preoperatively about measures to reduce and treat blood loss and about plans to use cement to secure the femoral component (which can lead to severe hypotension). During the operation, it is important for the anesthesiologist to keep the surgeon advised of this patient's condition, especially the hemoglobin concentration and the patient's tolerance of anemia, so that together they can consider whether the procedure can be completed safely.

Maintenance of Anesthesia

■ Maintaining Vigilance

Although maintenance of anesthesia often appears uneventful, profound changes may occur in the patient's condition. In studies of critical incidents in anesthesia, it was found that significant problems with patients went unrecognized during maintenance and were not detected until another individual replaced the dulled observer. The antidote to this problem is vigilance, the motto of the American Society of Anesthesiologists; unfortunately, vigilance is the very quality that is lost to boredom.

To overcome this effect, skilled anesthesiologists manage the maintenance of anesthesia aggressively. The first element in this approach is to make vigilance an active process. Instead of waiting for alarms to sound, one surveys at regular intervals the monitoring data (see Chap. 6), recording the results and seeking to interpret any changes. A valuable approach is to establish a systematic pattern of reviewing the data, beginning at the patient (operative site, chest excursion, intravenous site, nerve stimulator), progressing to the airway (endotracheal tube, breathing circuit, valves, airway pressure), and then moving to the various monitors and the anesthesia machine (ECG, oxygen saturation, blood pressure, gas flows).

The intervals between observations and the attention given to each item vary according to circumstances. Selection of monitoring for a procedure entails not only choosing the devices to be used but also directing one's attention to the most important data of the moment during the procedure. During this patient's hip operation, such moments might occur with intubation; when changes in heart rate, rhythm, ST-segment elevation, and blood pressure might be expected; or during placement of the cement for the femoral component of the new prosthesis, when pulmonary embolization, hypoxemia, and hypotension may occur.

The second element of active vigilance is to approach the anesthetic as a scientific experiment, framing hypotheses to explain observed changes and taking steps to confirm them. For example, during our patient's hip operation, the amount of nitroprusside needed to maintain the mean arterial pressure at 70 mmHg might increase from 0.5 to 3.0 µg/kg per minute over the course of 45 minutes. Several explanations are possible. If it has been an hour since the initial dose of fentanyl was given, perhaps the loss of analgesia is responsible; a favorable response to a second dose of fentanyl might support this hypothesis. On the other hand, perhaps intact barostatic reflexes have produced increases in heart rate and renin release. If a review of the record shows that the heart rate has increased from 68 to 107 over the same 45 minutes and there is a positive response to esmolol, this is a likely explanation. Perhaps cyanide toxicity has resulted from nitroprusside infusion; a review of the total dose given and the $PaCO_2$ and pH values can help identify this possibility.

A third element of active vigilance is to change the anesthetic periodically to verify requirements and responses, even if all is going smoothly. When a system remains unchanged for a time, it can be helpful to introduce a change to verify the accuracy of the monitoring and the efficacy of the treatment. For example, if our patient undergoing a hip operation has experienced no change in her blood pressure for an hour, it may be appropriate to reduce the rate of administration of nitroprusside to verify that the present dose is needed.

■ Controlling Depth of Anesthesia

In modern practice, the depth of anesthesia is best thought of as corresponding to the degree of depression of reflex responses to surgical stimuli. At light depths of anesthesia, patients develop tachycardia and hypertension in response to surgical stimuli and may even move; at deeper levels of anesthesia, responses are less vigorous and movement is absent. Cardiovascular responses are monitored as indicators of depth of anesthesia, but these can be deceptive when there are reasons other than deep anesthesia to explain decreased blood pressure or when a narcotic-based anesthetic blunts hypertensive responses without rendering the patient fully unconscious.

Because stimulation varies throughout an operation, and because blood concentration of infused or inhaled anesthetics changes with time, it is wise to test periodically the depth of anesthesia by decreasing the concentration of an inhaled anesthetic or the infusion rate of the intravenous agent. When a reflex response signifying light anesthesia (changes in heart rate, blood pressure, respiratory rate or depth, or even movement) appears, the amount of anesthetic can be increased, with the assurance that the patient is not anesthetized too deeply. The measurement of the concentration of anesthetic in end-tidal gas is an effective means of quantifying the dose but is not a direct measure of the depth of anesthesia, which represents a pattern of patient responses and not a drug concentration.

In a skillfully administered anesthetic, the depth of anesthesia varies throughout the operation to meet the needs of the moment and in anticipation of the planned emergence. For our hypertensive patient undergoing a hip operation with general anesthesia and deliberate hypotension, anesthesia begins with the intravenous sedation administered outside the operating room.

After intubation, the arterial catheter, CVP catheter, extra intravenous cannula, and urinary bladder catheter are placed. Anesthesia of adequate depth to deal with these mild stimuli may not require isoflurane, which is reduced in concentration or turned off to prevent hypotension. Amnesia and analgesia are provided by the combination of nitrous oxide, midazolam, fentanyl, and thiopental. When the cannulas have been inserted, the same light depth of anesthesia may prove sufficient for turning the patient to the lateral position and for the surgical preparations.

Just before the incision, the alveolar isoflurane concentration is again increased in anticipation of the patient's response to this painful stimulus. If the patient has shown no tendencies to hypotension, alveolar concentrations of as much as 1.5 times minimum alveolar concentration (MAC) may be required; more likely, lesser concentrations will suffice. During the majority of the procedure, the fresh gases added to the breathing circuit consist of 0.5 liter/min of nitrous oxide, 0.5 liter/min of oxygen, and enough isoflurane to maintain an end-tidal concentration of about 0.8 percent. Less isoflurane is not used because when it is decreased, the patient's blood pressure increases, requiring that more nitroprusside be given. Just before the surgeon closes the wound, the nitroprusside is discontinued and the inspired concentration of isoflurane is decreased to allow the blood pressure to return to preoperative values. This helps the surgeon to ensure adequate hemostasis.

About 15 minutes before the anticipated time of applying the dressing, the fresh gas flows are increased to a total of 6 liters/min, and the isoflurane vaporizer is turned off. Beginning the emergence from anesthesia this early may require that small amounts of isoflurane be administered again later, but it also helps ensure against delayed awakening at the end of the procedure. D-Tubocurarine administration has been discontinued earlier, and the response to the train-of-four impulses from the nerve stimulator has increased to three or four twitches; administering conventional doses of neostigmine and atropine restores full strength. No muscle relaxation is needed for this portion of the procedure, but dislocation of the hip is possible if the patient moves violently, so the surgeon

is warned to control the leg as the patient awakens. Well before the end of the operation, after neuromuscular function returns and as the blood concentration of isoflurane decreases, the patient is allowed to regain spontaneous or assisted ventilation. To control the anticipated pain on awakening, morphine is given intravenously in doses of 1 to 5 mg, guided by the respiratory rate.

This patient's anesthesia might be managed in many ways; a supplemental regional anesthetic might have been quite helpful if the patient had permitted it. However, no matter what drugs or overall plan is chosen, management of the depth of anesthesia will resemble the pattern described here. During most of the procedure, even during maintenance, the depth of anesthesia and the rates of administration of the drugs producing anesthesia are changed to meet circumstances. The management of emergence, removal of the endotracheal tube, and transport to the recovery room are described in Chapter 35.

■ Transferring the Patient's Care to Another During the Anesthetic

Ideally, it might seem that the patient's best interests are served when the same individual attends to the anesthetic throughout the operation. In prac-

---

Checklist for Relieving Another Anesthesiologist

1. A summary of the preoperative evaluation of the patient
2. The anesthesia plan
3. The course of the anesthetic and any changes that have been made in the plan, including any unresolved problems
4. The current state of the operation and its anticipated course
5. Every item being monitored, including the findings and their interpretation
6. An examination of the patient, including at least breath sounds and the position of the endotracheal tube
7. Introduce the new anesthesiologist to the patient if the patient is awake
8. A review of the accounting of the narcotics
9. A note in the anesthesia record documenting the transfer of care

tice, it is often desirable to have another person take over the anesthetic during a lunch break or at the end of the day. There is no doubt that fatigue impairs performance, and the new person often sees problems and solutions overlooked by a tired predecessor. To make this transfer of care safe, a systematic review of the case is needed, including all the information the new anesthesiologist needs to manage the complete anesthetic. A checklist is given in the accompanying boxed text.

Error, Chaos, and Emergencies

The testimony of experienced anesthesiologists, case presentations at departmental conferences, analyses of closed malpractice claims, Cooper's studies of critical incidents in anesthesia, and experience in high-technology industries all provide insight into accidents and near misses.

First, error is unremitting. Something is always going wrong, but usually nothing comes of it. These background errors do not propagate themselves, either because they are of little consequence in the first place (0.5 mg atropine is given instead of 0.3 mg), or because the problem is noticed and corrected (the endotracheal tube becomes disconnected and is immediately reattached). These problems occur continually during even the most routine cases.

Second, healthy patients undergoing usual operations may withstand many such errors without harm, but sick patients are more vulnerable.

Third, catastrophes tend to occur when errors summate. For example, if the endotracheal tube becomes disconnected from the breathing circuit while at the same time the airway pressure alarm fails and the anesthesiologist is distracted by a phone call from the blood bank, hypoxia may occur. If the pulse oximeter also fails, the patient might suffer a cardiac arrest.

Fourth, most problems are due to human error, not mechanical malfunctions or patient aberrations.

Fifth, complex, highly interlinked processes are more vulnerable to disruption than are less complex ones. When the plan calls for a rapid succession of linked treatments, then a minor occurrence has serious consequences. For example, unexpected infiltration of an intravenous infusion, of no consequence in a healthy young patient undergoing arthroscopy of the knee, might have led to disaster in our patient

undergoing hip reconstruction. Loss of intravenous access might have meant loss of nitroprusside effect and inability to give fluids, with hypertension, hemorrhage, and inability to replace lost blood. One of the reasons for using a second peripheral intravenous cannula as well as a CVP catheter was to prevent this sort of occurrence. These insights suggest several remedies.

When something goes wrong, it is best to focus directly on the patient's welfare and not on correcting the problem. If a problem is simple, for example the hose from the ventilator falls off the connector, then it is possible to correct it immediately. If the origin of the problem is not obvious immediately, as in a mysterious ventilator malfunction, do not focus on the problem, but focus instead on preventing harm to the patient by instituting manual ventilation. Later, it is important to find an explanation for what happened. No malfunction and no abnormal finding can be left unexplained, lest a minor problem grow into a major one. For example, if our patient's arterial pressure were to decrease suddenly to 50/30, the first steps would be to discontinue the anesthetics and the nitroprusside, administer fluids, and possibly give vasopressors, not to seek causes. Later, investigation might reveal unmeasured blood loss.

Sick patients require more precautions because the consequences of misadventure are more grave for them. For example, if our patient for the hip operation had been healthier and had been willing to accept blood if needed, then invasive monitoring might not have been required.

When several things go wrong at once, take definitive steps to break the chain of events and ensure the patient's safety. For example, if one undertook a rapid-sequence induction in our patient and misjudged the dose of thiopental, she might become hypotensive. If at the same time a novice anesthesiologist could not see the glottis, the right course of action would be to have an experienced person intubate the trachea immediately to ensure adequate oxygenation and interrupt a chain of events leading to cardiac arrest.

Because prompt action often prevents maloccurrences from summating, anesthesiologists mentally rehearse their responses to some common problems. It is a good idea for all anesthetists to rehearse and know a management plan for abrupt disasters such as severe hypoxemia, hypotension, or cardiac arrest (see accompanying boxed text). Therapy and diagnosis

Immediate Action in Anesthesia Emergencies

1. Abrupt decrease in peripheral oxygen saturation
   Check: position of pulse oximeter probe
   F_{IO_2}
   ventilation of lungs: listen/measure
   capnogram
   blood pressure
   Treat: increase F_{IO_2}, ventilation
   correct any hypotension
   PEEP if appropriate
2. Abrupt onset of hypotension
   Check: heart rate, rhythm
   F_{IO_2} and ventilation
   repeat blood pressure
   anesthetic concentrations
   fluid balance, blood loss
   surgical field: compression of heart,
   vena cava
   Treat: discontinue anesthetics
   give 100% oxygen
   increase fluids
   discontinue vasodilators
   vasopressors, inotropes as indicated
3. Loss of breath sounds
   Check: capnogram
   placement, integrity, patency of airway
   ventilator
   breathing circuit
   pneumothorax
   Treat: switch to manual ventilation
   100% O_2
   intubate, reintubate, or ventilate by mask
4. Increased airway pressures or wheezing
   Check: measure PIP, plateau pressures
   capnogram
   oxygen saturation
   breath sounds

patency of airway
retractors, packs, elevating diaphragm
   Treat: switch to manual ventilation
   allow adequate time for exhalation
   100% F_{IO_2}
   consider deepening anesthesia, bronchodilators
5. Cardiac arrest
   Discontinue anesthetics, give 100% O_2
   Diagnosis and treatment according to
   CPR and ACLS protocols
6. High fever
   Check: CO_2 production
   cardiac rate, rhythm
   ABG
   drapes
   Treat: increase flows of gases
   if malignant hyperthermia (see
   Chap. 36), cooling measures
7. Bradycardia
   Check: hypoxemia
   F_{IO_2}
   vagal stimuli (peritoneum, carotids, eyes,
   others)
   Treat: atropine
   ACLS protocols
8. Tachyarrhythmias
   Check: depth of anesthesia
   blood pressure
   IV infusions (epinephrine?)
   temperature
   oxygenation
   capnogram
   electrolytes
   Treat: lighten or deepen anesthetic as required
   ACLS protocols

usually proceed together, a process facilitated by thoughtful consideration ahead of time.

Although attention to detail, checklists, alarms, and other compulsive steps are important, active use of the imagination has its place as well. The habit of anticipating events, imagining what will happen next or what might happen next, sometimes allows one to avoid disaster or at least be more prepared when it occurs. Because the hypotension following intubation had been imagined ahead of time, the automated blood pressure cuff had been set to take frequent measurements, and the ephedrine was ready when needed.

If at all possible, avoid management schemes in which a single misstep or unanticipated event can disrupt the whole plan. Good anesthesia plans should offer easy alternatives for unexpected contingencies. Rapid-sequence induction and intubation were not chosen for our patient because this plan is vulnerable to disruption (wrong thiopental dose, failed intubation) and offers her no appreciable benefits in compensation for the increased risk. The plan chosen offered more alternatives: the chance to limit the dose of thiopental or the dose of isoflurane and the chance to abort the induction if airway difficulties occurred.

Complex Cases

Anesthesia for some operations and for some patients cannot be managed by simple means. Many cardiac procedures, large-scale abdominal procedures, liver transplants, some trauma or other emergency cases, some operations on the great vessels, and any patient whose condition deteriorates rapidly or who is near death may require more anesthesia care than a single person can give. Some anesthesiologists who perform well while alone do poorly when teamwork is required. Likewise, analysis of cockpit tapes recorded during airline disasters has shown that capable pilots often do not use effectively the help available to them from copilots, flight engineers, and air traffic controllers. Experience with complex cases has shown how an anesthesia team can function most effectively.

First, the effort must be organized; an uncontrolled group of well-intentioned assistants will not be effective. Just as is practiced in acute management of trauma patients, someone is assigned to each of the important jobs: watching the patient, administering drugs, adjusting the anesthesia machine and ventilator, keeping an accurate record, providing intravenous access, administering blood and intravenous fluids, running errands, planning overall care of the patient, communicating with surgeons, and directing the anesthesia team. In most instances, one person will fulfill several of these functions; in truly massive cases, the anesthesia team may number four or more and include anesthesia technicians, perfusionists, and respiratory care technicians, as well as physicians and nurses.

Second, members of the anesthesia team must communicate effectively with each other and with the surgeons so that their efforts are coordinated. Extraneous chatter must be suppressed, but everyone must be able to share data and ideas. Surgeons and anesthesiologists must understand each other's thinking and plans. The blood bank must receive advance notice of the blood products needed. Speaking slowly and calmly can help control the atmosphere in the room, reducing the ill effects of anger, frustration, and anxiety on the group's performance. From time to time, someone must summarize the case, as for example: "We have a healthy 22-year-old man with a gunshot wound to the upper abdomen. The aorta is clamped, and the heart is full but not contracting.

There is something wrong besides hypovolemia. What?"

Despite a calm, orderly approach, a massive case sometimes becomes confusing. If the situation can be salvaged at all, attention to simple measures is usually effective:

1. Adequate ventilation with oxygen
2. Support of the circulation with fluids, pressors, inotropes, or cardiac massage as required
3. Correction of acidemia and hyperkalemia
4. Consideration of possible myocardial ischemia, pneumothorax, or cardiac tamponade as the explanation of failure to resuscitate

Costs

Traditionally, anesthesiologists and nurse anesthetists, like others in health care, have felt that their primary responsibility is to the patient and not to the hospital or third-party payer. Older drugs such as halothane, enflurane, D-tubocurarine, pancuronium, thiopental, fentanyl, and morphine lose out to newer (patented) drugs such as desflurane, vecuronium, atracurium, propofol, alfentanil, and sufentanil. The more modern drugs may offer important advantages, but in most clinical settings, the older and less expensive drugs yield satisfactory results.

Money can be saved in the conduct of anesthesia without compromising results by reserving the more expensive drugs for those situations in which their special advantages justify their use. As an example, our woman received the cheaper muscle relaxant D-tubocurarine, whereas another patient with renal failure and electrolyte abnormalities and taking gentamicin might require atracurium. It is also important to remember that the cost of drugs does not represent the entire cost of care. If the use of an inexpensive drug should prolong the patient's stay in the recovery room, the total cost may be greater than if a more rapidly metabolized but expensive drug were used.

Anesthesia Record

A properly conducted anesthetic includes a good record, a necessary tool for keeping track of what has been done and of the patient's responses. Good records improve the conduct of anesthesia in the same way that accurate laboratory notebooks improve experiments: they focus attention and oblige one to confront data objectively. An adequate record meets these criteria:

1. Every space or box is completed, legibly.
2. All significant findings and therapies are recorded with no gaps in monitoring.
3. Any anesthesiologist can reconstruct the case from the record.
4. The record gives the rationale for various actions. For example, the record not only records that the endotracheal tube was removed, but also that the patient responded to command, supported his head for 5 seconds, and breathed freely through an open airway when the tube was removed.

The Conduct of Those Who Provide Anesthesia

Some who provide technically excellent anesthesia do not inspire confidence in patients, surgeons, or coworkers, perhaps because of behavior. The sympathetic relations with patients and collegial communication with surgeons already described do a great deal to inspire confidence. Other behaviors are more subtle.

Dealing with the awake patient in the operating room requires a different approach than that used during the preoperative visit. The patient is at a marked disadvantage: unclothed, supine, drugged, frightened, and helpless when everyone else in the room is dressed, upright, alert, at ease, and in control of events. The anesthesiologist must speak gently and reassuringly, informing the patient of each step in preparing for induction of anesthesia, projecting at least an air of calm confidence and avoiding frightening exclamations (e.g., "Oops").

A neat and orderly approach to the work also improves one's professional standing. A long litany of advice could follow this general injunction without enlarging on the basic concept: neatness and organization count. Speed and efficiency are also valuable attributes for an anesthesiologist, given the increasing economic pressures for more efficient use of operating room time. While a calm, orderly approach and attention to patient safety are mandatory, much can be done to work quickly.

Varying one's speed according to the task is efficient so that one opens a spinal anesthesia kit quickly but mixes the drugs and places the needle with deliberation. By performing tasks in parallel, not in series, the anesthetist can do two things at once. For example, while the patient breathes oxygen, the automated blood pressure cuff can obtain the first blood pressure reading and one can enter data in the record. Anticipation likewise saves time. Drawing up the neostigmine and atropine ahead of time saves minutes at the end of the procedure. Keeping surgeons informed of the progress of the anesthetic allows them to keep pace and work efficiently. For example, often preparation of the skin can begin before the induction of anesthesia is complete.

In all, the efficient and safe conduct of anesthesia is a complex undertaking. The person who does it well must strive to perfect the practices described here, as well as the ordinary technical and intellectual skills of anesthesia.

BIBLIOGRAPHY

Cooper J, Long CD, Newbower RS, Philip JH. Critical incidents associated with intraoperative exchanges of anesthesia personnel. *Anesthesiology* 1982;56:456.

Muravchick S. *The Anesthetic Plan: From Physiologic Principles to Clinical Strategies.* St Louis: Mosby-Year Book, 1991.

Perrow C. *Normal Accidents.* New York: Basic Books, 1984.

Managing Fluids, Electrolytes, and Blood Loss

David R. Jobes

Before and after operations, patients receive fluids containing electrolytes, glucose, macromolecules such as starch or albumin, and blood products to meet normal needs, correct preexisting abnormalities, and compensate for intraoperative changes such as evaporative losses, tissue edema, bleeding, consumption of clotting factors, and sometimes fluid absorption from the operative field. Fluid management is complicated by the effects of anesthetics on the endocrine, renal, and cardiovascular systems and the special requirements of intracranial and some other operations. This chapter reviews the basic information needed to manage these problems in the average adult; advice about specific procedures and pediatric patients is contained in the relevant chapters elsewhere. Basic information on the size and composition of fluid compartments and disorders of electrolyte balance is summarized in Fig. 15-1 and Tables 15-1 to 15-5

Volume Deficiency and Excess

Management of fluid therapy begins with determining whether the patient suffers from a deficiency or excess (i.e., *volume status*) of overall volume of body water or any of its components. Although healthy patients scheduled for elective operations have no such disorders, many sick patients who require anesthesia are hypovolemic, and some may have fluid overload (Table 15-6). Beginning anesthesia without treating hypovolemia risks catastrophic hypotension, because anesthetics depress the circulation and obtund the sympathetic reflexes that sustain these patients. By comparison, moderate volume overload is well tolerated in anesthetized patients, perhaps because anesthetics promote vasodilation, the depressed myocardium benefits from generous diastolic filling, and positive-pressure ventilation obviates the tendency to pulmonary edema.

Extracellular Fluid (ECF) Anions

The major ECF anions are chloride and bicarbonate, frequently referred to as *exchangeable anions*. When renal reabsorption of one anion is increased, renal excretion of the other is enhanced. For example, patients with chronic obstructive lung disease and carbon dioxide retention may have bicarbonate values between 35 and 40mEq/liter and chloride values between 85 and 95mEq/liter. The major intracellular (ICF) anions include phosphates, organic acids, and the negatively charged intracellular proteins. Because proteins cannot move freely between compartments, they play a major role in determining the distribution of water.

Normally, the sum of plasma sodium and potassium concentrations does not exceed the sum of chloride and bicarbonate concentrations by more than 15 mEq/liter.

Should a larger difference exist, increased amounts of other unmeasured anions, such as lactate, ketones, or anions from an exogenous source (i.e., salicylate or ethylene glycol), are suspected. This anion gap is a reflection of the differences in unmeasured cations and anions:

$$\text{Anion gap} = (NA^+ + K^+) - (HCO_3^- + Cl^-)$$
$$\text{Normally} < 15 \text{ mEq/liter.}$$

■ Assessing Volume Status

In anesthesia practice, assessment of the patient's volume state begins by considering the adequacy of intravascular volume and thus of left ventricular diastolic filling and cardiac output. In patients suffering from hypotension, tachycardia, and oliguria, the diagnosis of hypovolemia can be made almost immediately after ruling out cardiac failure. In patients with less severe hypovolemia, compensatory vasoconstriction may be so effective that the patient's vital signs (including a single measurement of central venous pressure) do not reveal the problem. Yet these patients with well-compensated hypovolemia may suffer severe hypotension when administered spinal, epidural, or general anesthesia.

When hypovolemia is suspected but not evident, a test for orthostatic hypotension can be performed by placing the patient in a steep head-up position for 1 minute by tilting the operating table. An increase in heart rate of more than 10 beats per minute or a decrease in systolic blood pressure of more than 10 mmHg indicates hypovolemia or a deficiency in the sympathetic mechanisms that defend against postural hypotension, as with diabetes, sympathoplegic drugs, or dysautonomia. Signs of volume overload, except outright pulmonary edema, are more subtle and sometimes more equivocal than those of hypovolemia and include polyuria, edema, signs of excess lung water such as rales at the lung bases or impaired arterial oxygenation, jugular venous distension, and increased pressures in the right atrium or pulmonary artery.

Disorders in the volumes of the interstitial and intracellular compartments are of less immediate importance than abnormalities of intravascular volume. Assessment is less direct and depends on recognizing edema, poor skin turgor, dry mouth, and acute changes in weight. In conditions such as ascites and some forms of edema, the total-body stores of water and sodium may be increased, although the intravascular volume remains deficient.

■ Treating Volume Deficiency

Once volume deficiencies are recognized, intravenous (IV) fluid therapy is prescribed. In the hypotensive, dehydrated patient with adequate cardiac function, the extracellular fluid can be replenished with isotonic saline or lactated Ringer's solution. Fluid deficiencies are usually underestimated; water and sodium distribute themselves rapidly from the intravascular space, and intact kidneys easily dispose of excess water and salt. For these reasons, when it is urgent to begin anesthesia, it is both necessary and safe to give patients saline solutions rapidly and in large quantities: a liter every 10 to 15 minutes, to a total of 3 to 5 liters in severe cases. In less urgent cases, slower infusions over several hours are preferred.

The endpoint for fluid resuscitation is simple to describe but requires judgment to detect. Intravenous fluids are stopped after the signs of hypovolemia remit and before signs of fluid overload appear. This may involve monitoring cardiac output, venous filling pressures, urine output, orthostatic hypotension, or simple bedside signs of dehydration and hypovolemia, depending on the clinical situation. For otherwise healthy patients with good cardiac and renal function, simple clinical signs suffice. In patients with renal, cardiac, or pulmonary dysfunction, there may be only a narrow margin between adequate and inadequate intravascular volume, so invasive cardiovascular monitoring and slow stepwise titration (100 to 200 ml at a

Figure 15-1

Distribution of total-body water for a normal 70-kg man with 60 percent water (range can be 40 to 68 percent).

TOTAL BODY WATER = 60% OF BODY WT (kG) = 42L IN 70kG MAN		
INTRACELLULAR WATER = 40% OF WT - 28L	EXTRACELLULAR FLUID = 20% OF WT = 14L	
	INTERSTITIAL SPACE = 15.7% = 11L	PLASMA VOLUME = 4.3% = 3L

Table 15-1

Average Fluid Volumes

Measurement	Common Adult Value		ml/kg	
	Men	Women	Men	Women
Weight	70 kg	60 kg		
Hematocrit, whole blood	42%	37%	—	—
Plasma volume	3200 ml	2700 ml	45	45
Red blood cell volume	2000 ml	1500 ml	33	25
Blood volume*	5200 ml	4200 ml	74	70
Extracellular water	16.4 liters	14.2 liters	240	230
Total-body water	42 liters	30 liters	600	500

*Blood volume may be as little as 60 ml/kg in obese, older patients or as great as 80 ml/kg in robust infants. Estimated blood volume for adults as a function of body habitus (ml/kg of body weight):

Adult	Male	Female
Obese	60	55
Thin	65	60
Normal	70	65
Muscular	75	70

time) of fluid administration are needed. In severe cardiac disease, fluid administration sometimes produces signs of fluid overload, such as increases in venous filling pressures, without correction of depressed cardiac output or oliguria. In these patients, an inotrope or other measures to improve cardiac performance may be required.

■Fluid Overload

Excessive intravascular volume found in patients preoperatively is usually due to renal failure or exces-

sive fluid administration; these patients rarely require treatment before beginning anesthesia, but attention must be given to avoiding depressed myocardial contractility. Volume overload sometimes appears in patients immediately after emergence from anesthesia as the vasodilation associated with general or regional anesthesia resolves and as positive-pressure ventilation is discontinued. Manifestations range from dyspnea, tachycardia, and mild hypoxemia or other early signs of increased lung water to the appearance of pink froth in the endotracheal tube. The problem becomes evident postoperatively because patients under anes-

Table 15-2

Representative Values of the Major Solutes in the Respective Fluid Compartment (mEq/liter)

Solute	Plasma	Fluid Compartment	
		Interstitial Fluid	Intracellular Fluid
Na^+	142	142	10
K^+	4	4	140
Ca^{2+}	5	5	<1
Mg^{2+}	3	3	58
Cl^-	103	106	4
HCO_3^-	27	27	10
$(HPO_4^-, H_2PO_4^-)$	4	4	75
SO_4^{2-}	1	1	2
Organic acid$^-$	7	7	25
Proteins (g/dl)	17	2	66

Table 15-3

Extracellular Cation Abnormalities and Their Treatment

Abnormality	$\uparrow K^+$	$\downarrow K^+$	$\downarrow Ca^{2+}$	$\downarrow Mg^{2+}$
Major clinical problems	Cardiac arrhythmias: ultimately sinus arrest	Cardiac arrhythmias: ultimately ventricular fibrillation Muscle weakness or loss of reflexes	Inotropic cardiac failure Hyperreflexia and tetany	Hyperreflexia and tetany Psychiatric symptoms Neuromuscular weakness Increased arrhythmias with digitalis, inability to defibrillate ventricular fibrillation
Most common causes	Renal failure Acidosis, iatrogenic	Diuretic therapy; steroid therapy Treatment of acidosis; nasogastric suction Alkalosis Dehydration	Alkalosis Hypoparathyroidism Massive transfusion (rare)	Alcoholism Diuretic therapy Chronic renal disease GI losses
Laboratory values*	>5 mEq/liter	<3.0 mEq/liter	<4.5 mEq/liter >9 mg/100 ml	<1.5 mEq/liter <1.8 mg/100 ml
ECG changes	Peaked T waves Loss of P wave Loss of peaked T wave Bradycardia Spread of QRS	ST-segment depression T-wave inversion U-wave (may be a positive or negative wave)	Prolonged QT interval	Prolonged QT interval; nonspecific ST-T wave changes
Acute therapy in 70-kg adult (life-threatening situations only)	100 mEq NaHCO$_3$, IV over 2 min 50 g glucose, 20 units regular insulin IV	K$^+$ IV at 1 mEq/min until symptoms reverse	CaCl$_2$ 250 mg IV every 5 min; if calcium gluconate, multiply dose by 3	MgSO$_4$ 5 g/h IM or IV

*These are threshold values; the severe forms of the syndromes appear only at more abnormal values.

Table 15-4

Comparison of Extracellular Fluid and Various Replacement Solutions

Total	Na$^+$ (mEq/liter)	K$^+$ (mEq/liter)	Cl$^-$ (mEq/liter)	Base (mEq/liter)	pH	Ca^{2+} (mEq/liter)	Mg^{2+} (mEq/liter)	Calories per liter
Extracellular fluid	142	5	03	27	7.4	5	3	12
5% Dextrose and water	0	0	0	0	4.5	0	0	200
Normal saline	154	0	154	0	6.0	0	0	0
Lactated Ringer's	130	4	109	28	6.5	3	0	9
Normosol	140	5	98	50	7.4	0	3	24
5% Albumin	145	0			7.4	0	0	—
Hetastarch	154	0	154	0	5.5	0	0	—

Table 15-5

Effect of Administering Too Little or Too Much Water and Certain Solutes

Substance	Too Little	Too Much
Water	Hyperosmolar hypernatremia Concentrated, sparse urine Thirst Oliguria Fever Circulatory failure	Hypoosmolar hyponatremia Very dilute urine Polyuria Intracranial hypertension Headache, confusion, nausea, and vomiting Weakness Muscle twitching and cramps Convulsions Coma
Sodium	Extracellular fluid volume decreased Hemoconcentration Lost tissue elasticity Hypotension Circulatory failure Uremia	Extracellular fluid volume increased Edema formation and congestive heart failure Tendency to potassium deficiency
Phosphorus	Hypophosphatemia Other effects	Hyperphosphatemia Hypocalcemia
Carbohydrate	Ketosis Protoplasmic catabolism augmented Tendency to greater water and electrolyte losses	Hyperglycemia Glycosuria Hepatic failure

Source: Adapted from Talbot NB, Kerrigan GA, Crawford JD, et al. Application of homeostatic principles of parenteral fluid therapy. *N Engl J Med* 1955;252:856–862.

Table 15-6

Common Preoperative Conditions Associated with Volume Disorders

Hypovolemia	Fluid Overload
Prolonged fasting	
Impaired thirst in the elderly	
Fever	Congestive heart failure
Shock	Excessive fluid therapy
Malnutrition	
Vomiting, diarrhea, gastric drainage	
Burns	
Diabetes with hyperglycemia	
Bleeding	
Peritonitis, other inflammations	
Bowel obstruction, infarction	
Ascites (intravascular volume)	Ascites (total water)
Polyuric nephropathies	Renal failure

thesia tolerate volume overload well and give little sign of the condition until it is severe. For most patients, this problem can be avoided by limiting fluid therapy during operation to only that needed to correct signs of hypovolemia (usually hypotension or oliguria) and by avoiding the administration of prescribed volumes of fluid dictated by protocol.

Treatment of volume overload is straightforward and includes fluid restriction, diuretics, oxygen, and positive-pressure ventilation if needed.

■ Conflicting Goals in Fluid Therapy

Volume management in the perioperative period is complicated by the conflicting requirements imposed by treatment of various organ systems. When increases in ECF volume must be avoided, as in patients threatened by cerebral or pulmonary edema, it is best to limit fluids to the minimum required to ensure acceptable cardiac output. These and other complex problems are considered in the appropriate chapters elsewhere in this book, but the process of adjusting the patient's circulating blood volume (and, secondarily, the extravascular volumes) to a carefully considered endpoint is fundamental to the management of all anesthetics.

Routine Perioperative Fluid Management

Routine perioperative fluid management for healthy patients undergoing ordinary operations is summarized in Table 15-7. For those undergoing minimally invasive operations, perhaps in a day surgery setting, intravenous fluids may be limited to those required to maintain intravenous access.

Once the intravenous catheter is in place, the patient is promptly given enough water to account for the period during which nothing was taken by mouth; this fluid may contain glucose, salts, or both. During the procedure, a fluid infusion of 2 ml/kg

---

Table 15-7

Intravenous Fluid Management

For urgent or emergency procedures
1. Diagnose any abnormalities of volume, electrolytes, or acid-base balance.
2. Establish required monitoring.
3. Correct abnormalities as rapidly as dictated by urgency of operation.
4. Then proceed as below.

For elective procedures in healthy patients
1. Over the first half hour, give water the patient has not taken while NPO; may be given as glucose, saline, or saline-glucose solution.
2. Give free water over the range of none to no more than that required to meet insensible losses (about 2500 ml/day in adults), unless indicated by hypernatremia.
3. Administer isotonic saline at 2 ml/kg per hour.
4. Administer additional isotonic saline from 2 to 8 ml/kg per hour, depending on extent and severity of operation, in response to signs of hypovolemia not due to blood loss ("third space losses").
5. Replace blood loss 3:1 with isotonic saline until anemia dictates use of red blood cells.
6. Maintain urine output greater than 0.5 to 1 ml/kg per hour.
7. Treat oliguria, hypotension, or other signs thought to represent decreased cardiac output or hypovolemia with rapid infusions of isotonic saline, 2 to 6 ml/kg.
8. Administer albumin only as indicated for specific deficiencies.

---

per hour is maintained to account for insensible losses. Total free water is limited to one day's requirement (2500 ml in adults) to avoid water intoxication; other fluids contain physiologic quantities of salts. Wide deviations from this suggested protocol are without consequences in healthy patients with functioning kidneys who begin taking oral fluids within hours after operation.

■ Oral Fluids

The simplest maneuver to promote normal water balance is to allow patients to drink until just hours before anesthesia. Unless gastric emptying is abnormally delayed, feedings of clear liquids up to a few hours before operation do not increase the volume in the stomach or the risk of pulmonary aspiration. For adults scheduled for afternoon operations, an early morning clear-liquid breakfast is safe and appropriate. However, if delayed gastric emptying is likely, a longer interval (up to 8 hours) of complete fasting is appropriate. Infants and young children, in whom prolonged fasting may result in severe dehydration, are encouraged to drink clear fluids 2 or 3 hours prior to elective operation.

■ Balanced Salt Solutions versus Simple Sodium Chloride

Some physicians prefer to administer balanced salt solutions rather than simple isotonic saline. These more costly formulations contain ions other than sodium and chloride and more nearly mimic the chemical composition of the ECF (see Table 15-4). There is no reason to use these solutions routinely; the small amounts of divalent cations and potassium they contain are inconsequential, and the available base does not obviate the need for acid-base evaluation in patients receiving major fluid therapy.

■ Glucose-Containing Solutions

Most patients coming to operation have fasted for a period of time; this argues for adding glucose to the intravenous fluids. In addition, the use of a limited amount of 5% glucose solution provides free water to replace insensible losses once the glucose is metabolized. On the other hand, hormonal responses to stress produce increases in blood glucose in most patients undergoing operation, and excess glucose administration might contribute to unwanted hyperosmolality. Thus a suitable compromise for patients who do not have diabetes is to give either no glucose or only that required to allow the administration of required free water.

Special Perioperative Problems

Normally, fluid and electrolyte balance is maintained by a complex neuroendocrine control system (see Fig. 15-2). Healthy patients undergoing limited surgical procedures are remarkably tolerant of a wide variety of fluid regimens, but careful management is required in patients with compromised organ function or in those who are undergoing more severe operations. Listed here are the major areas within which problems arise.

■ Water Toxicity

Antidiuretic hormone (ADH) is released in response to stress, general anesthesia, opioids, pain,

blood loss, and positive-pressure ventilation, despite normal or decreased ECF tonicity. This inappropriate release of ADH, combined with administration of excess free water, can result in dilutional hyponatremia and expansion of intracellular volume, including neuronal swelling. Cerebral symptoms may begin on the first to the third day after operation and range from mild lethargy and disorientation to delirium, coma, convulsions, and death. The condition may be worsened by opioids given in an effort to treat delirium.

The syndrome is more common in patients over 60 years of age and is rarely seen in adults with normal renal function if they receive less than 2 liters of free water per day (including water absorbed during transurethral resection of the prostate, for example). Although serum sodium concentrations at the on-set of symptoms are usually less than 125 mEq/liter, the rapidity of the change is more relevant than the absolute sodium concentration. Urine osmolarity is inappropriately increased (>500 mOsmol/liter), while serum osmolarity is decreased (<240 mOsmol/liter).

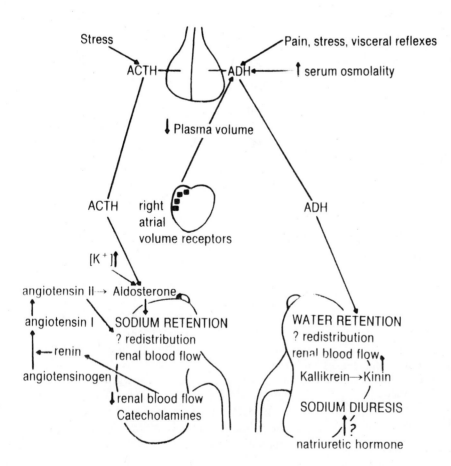

Figure 15-2

Schematic overview of hormonal and central nervous system interaction in the control of fluid and electrolyte balance. ACTH is secreted from the anterior pituitary and ADH from the posterior pituitary gland.

(Reproduced with permission from Twigley AJ, Hillman KA, The end of the crystalloid era? Anaesthesia 1983;40:800-871.)

Treatment includes restricting fluids to less than 1000 ml of isotonic saline per day, with no free water intake. Serum osmolarity can be increased more quickly by the use of diuretics or hypertonic saline. Since the fundamental problem is an excess of water, not a deficiency of sodium, this controversial and potentially dangerous therapy is not used except in extreme situations, in the hope of shifting water from the intracellular to the extracellular space at the expense of increasing the total burden of water. Symptoms may persist for several days despite restoration of normal serum sodium concentrations. This complication accounts for the usual practice of limiting sodium-free water (such as D_5W) to that needed to replace losses, including those caused by overnight fluid restriction.

■ Third Space Losses

Even when shed blood is meticulously replaced and insensible water losses are restored, some patients undergoing more invasive operations experience hypovolemia, losing ECF to a "third space." The magnitude of these losses varies from negligible for noninvasive operations (e.g., cataract removal) to many liters for massive procedures (e.g., resection of inflamed or ischemic bowel). This third space includes the interstitial spaces swollen by the local responses to the trauma of the operation and by the systemic hormonal responses to surgical stress. This third space fluid accumulates during and immediately after operation, when the process produces hypovolemia unless the patient receives generous fluid therapy. Subsequently, third space fluids return to the circulation several days after operation, when fluid overload is likely if IV fluids are administered to increase urine output.

Protocols that replace third space losses according to a schedule (in the range of 3 to 10 ml/kg per hour) that depends on an estimate of the severity of the operation are not very useful in clinical practice. They fail to account for individual variation and amount to little more than an admonition to be generous with fluids. Further, it is impossible to distinguish third space loss from blood loss in clinical practice. Measurements of blood loss made in the operating room are inaccurate estimates at best, so much of the fluid given for "third space loss" in reality replaces unrecognized blood loss. The recommendations in Table 15–7 call for replacing blood loss and third space loss separately, but in practice, one treats hypovolemia

from whatever cause with fluid infusions, adding red blood cells as needed to prevent anemia.

■ Overdose of Salt-Containing Solutions

Just as ADH secretion may be increased postoperatively despite decreased extracellular tonicity, adrenocorticoid production may increase in spite of increased ECF volume. As with ADH, increases in circulating glucocorticoids and aldosterone are related to stress. In part, these increases are provoked by response to a functional decrease in ECF due to loss of fluid to sites from which it cannot be mobilized rapidly (third space losses). Such functional decreases in ECF and the tendency toward renal salt conservation can be overcome by giving saline solutions that exceed basal fluid volume requirements.

Administration of large amounts of saline solutions is not without hazard. Previously healthy adults given large quantities of isotonic salt solution (3000 ml or more) rapidly for the treatment of shock can develop pulmonary edema. Lesser quantities may cause deterioration in pulmonary gas exchange even in the absence of overt edema. Pulmonary symptoms may not occur until several days postoperatively when sequestered third space fluid is mobilized. Although most patients tolerate excess saline better than excess free water, indiscriminate use of salt solutions without indication is inappropriate.

■ Colloid versus Crystalloid

Intraoperatively, fluids are given to maintain intravascular volume despite losses to bleeding and edema. Unless red blood cells are needed to treat anemia, simple salt solutions can be used to replace both losses. Because sodium is distributed throughout the ECF, to increase the intravascular volume by 1 liter requires the administration of 3 or more liters of saline so that the extravascular ECF increases in volume by 2 liters, accounting for the increases in lung water and generalized edema seen in patients who receive large amounts of saline for these purposes.

Because macromolecules such as albumin and starch ("colloid") are confined to the intravascular space by their size, these colloid solutions have been used in the hope of reducing the total volume needed for volume resuscitation and avoiding the complications of ECF expansion. Unfortunately, these macromolecules equilibrate with the extravascular ECF over a matter of hours; even less time is required for equilibration when capillaries are rendered more permeable by injury. In most instances, solutions containing only glucose and various salts ("crystalloid") are as useful as colloid solutions, as well as being less expensive. In certain circumstances, the use of albumin may be justified, when it is lost rapidly as in peritonitis, burns, or removal of ascites or when short-term benefits in reducing the extravascular ECF volume are desirable, as with brain swelling.

■ Renal Protection

Fluid administration beyond replacement of measured losses is used commonly to protect the kidneys during an operation. An intraoperative diuresis of 50 ml/hr or more decreases the risk of postoperative renal failure, especially in adults with major trauma or those undergoing resection of an aortic aneurysm, where renal perfusion is especially at risk. Usually, crystalloid solutions are used to increase urine output, although diuretics such as mannitol or furosemide may be used as well.

The safe limits for fluid volume administration in excess of measured losses are not available. Clinicians estimate fluid replacement by considering what is known about each patient's renal, pulmonary, and cardiac function, by monitoring cardiovascular and pulmonary function, and by plans for postoperative mechanical ventilation.

■ Fluids for Managing Spinal or Epidural Anesthesia

Volume expansion is used commonly as prophylaxis for treatment of hypotension due to spinal or epidural anesthesia. Certainly, any deficits must be replaced before such profound sympathectomy can be permitted, but it is less clear that volume expansion is the best treatment for patients who are not hypovolemic before anesthesia. If no bladder catheter is in place, the resulting diuresis may produce bladder distension before recovery from the anesthetic allows the patient to void. Also, simple volume expansion does nothing to treat the bradycardia and decreased contractility that may result from sympathetic denervation of the heart. Treatment with small doses of vasopressors that have vasoconstrictor, inotropic, and chronotropic effects (ephedrine, epinephrine), combined with adequate volumes of fluid, may be better

than fluids alone for maintaining cardiac output with spinal or epidural anesthesia.

■ Potassium

Abnormalities of electrolytes and other solutes are assessed by direct measurement of their concentrations in a blood sample. By considering the distribution of the various ions throughout the body fluid compartments other than blood (see Tables 15-1 and 15-2), overall deficits can be estimated and treatment prescribed. For example, only a small decrease in plasma potassium is associated with a large total-body potassium deficit, because potassium occurs predominantly in the much greater volume of the intracellular water. Perioperatively, hyperkalemia may occur with diabetic ketoacidosis or renal failure; the diagnosis and treatment follow conventional lines. Two unique sources of hyperkalemia occur in surgical patients. First, solutions used for cardioplegia or to preserve organs for transplantation may contain large quantities of potassium; inadvertent administration of these solutions has caused hyperkalemic cardiac arrest. Second, reperfusion of ischemic tissue, as with correction of aortic occlusion, bowel ischemia, or profound hemorrhagic shock, is associated with washout of fixed acid and potassium, sometimes in lethal quantities. Treatment requires frequent measurement of blood potassium levels and aggressive treatment with insulin, glucose, bicarbonate, and calcium.

Perioperative hypokalemia is seen most often in older patients taking diuretics, who may present for elective operation with potassium concentrations of 3.0 mEq/liter or less. Although there is a fear of arrhythmias in these patients, especially since the hyperventilation used during anesthesia decreases serum potassium concentration further, the risks seem small, and studies to document their magnitude have been inconclusive. Blood samples taken from these patients just before operation consistently show lesser potassium concentrations than those taken several days previously, suggesting that epinephrine-induced hypokalemia may be part of the cause. Even overnight treatment is unlikely to correct the large total-body potassium deficits in these patients. It seems appropriate to proceed with operation in patients with diuretic-associated hypokalemia unless arrhythmias are evident already, the hypokalemia is acute, the patient takes digoxin, or the serum potassium level is less than 2.8 mEq/liter.

Managing Blood Loss

Well over half the blood collected in the United States is administered to surgical patients in the perioperative period, much of it intraoperatively. Administration of blood products requires careful consideration of risks and vigilance to prevent error. Modern practice limits transfusion of blood from the blood bank to the minimum required for safe care by permitting moderate anemia when possible, by using blood component therapy, by employing autologous blood transfusion, and by substituting other products for blood when appropriate.

■ Allowable Blood Loss

In the past, many anesthesiologists insisted that patients have hemoglobin concentrations of 10 g/dl or greater before the beginning anesthesia. The rigid adherence to any prescribed value is illogical, in that no one value can be applied to all patients or settings. However, the safe lower limit for most patients is now thought to be in the range of 7.0 g/dl. Patients with compromised blood flow to critical organs, as in some cases of coronary artery disease, may be exceptions. Two groups of patients, Jehovah's Witnesses (with acute blood loss) and those with end-stage renal failure (chronic anemia), have demonstrated clearly that hemoglobin concentrations of 5 g/dl or less can be tolerated when necessary, although the chronic condition is tolerated better than acute anemia.

It is a common practice in otherwise healthy patients to replace blood loss with either crystalloid (at a volume ratio of 3:1) or colloid solution (volume ratio of 1:1) until red blood cell transfusion is required by the anemia that results from this hemodilution. An approximation of the allowable loss is given by

$$\text{Allowable loss} = \text{EBV} \times (\text{Hb}_{\text{initial}} - \text{Hb}_{\text{target}})/(\text{Hb}_{\text{initial}})$$

where $\text{Hb}_{\text{initial}}$ is the hemoglobin concentration at the start of blood loss, $\text{Hb}_{\text{target}}$ is the target hemoglobin concentration, and EBV is the estimated blood volume (see Table 15-1).

For example, in a 65-kg woman with an EBV of 4500 ml (see Table 15-1) and a hemoglobin concentration of 12.0 g/dl, the target hemoglobin concentration of 7.0 g/dl would be achieved by replacing the first 1800 ml of blood loss with colloid or crystal-

loid solutions, that is, $4500 \text{ ml} \times (12 - 7)/12 = 1800 \text{ ml}$. This estimate errs on the conservative side in that blood lost is further diluted by the crystalloid or colloid administered to maintain normal blood volume.

■ Blood Component Therapy versus Whole Blood

Over 80 percent of blood collected in the United States is fractionated before use. Each donor unit provides components for several patients, thus promoting goal-directed specific therapy in lieu of whole-blood administration and permitting the available blood supply to serve a larger population. For modest bleeding, transfusion with red blood cells suffices, since the moderate dilution of platelets, albumin, and soluble clotting factors is well tolerated. However, when rapid replacement of large amounts of blood is required, then all the components of whole blood are required. Thus the scarcity of whole blood resulting from the fractionation of donated units has complicated the treatment of massive hemorrhage because component therapy exposes these patients to a greater number of donor units and slows the process of transfusion.

■ Autologous Blood Transfusion

Autologous transfusion offers several advantages. Not only does this practice save banked blood, but compatibility and disease transmission are not issues, unless errors result in giving the wrong blood. There are several variants of autologous blood transfusion.

Preoperative collection and storage of blood before elective operations can produce a store of 4 units of autologous blood; by freezing the stored cells, even greater reserves can be accumulated. In some patients with rare blood types this may be the only way to provide compatible blood. To avoid anemia, these patients receive iron supplements; erythropoietin also increases the volume of blood that can be collected. To ensure against clerical errors, at least ABO and Rh matching of patients and their autologous units is required.

Acute isovolemic hemodilution is a form of autologous transfusion unique to the operating room and to the practice of anesthesia. At the start of the operation, some portion of the allowable loss is removed through the arterial catheter or a large-bore venous cannula, while intravenous fluids are infused to maintain blood volume. The dilution of the blood that is to be lost during operation reduces somewhat the total loss of red cells, but the major benefit comes from reinfusion of the stored blood near the end of the operation to provide fresh platelets stored for only a few hours.

Intraoperative scavenging of blood shed during operation is especially valuable in trauma patients and other emergency cases where there is no time to crossmatch homologous units. Available commercial devices use various anticoagulants and provide either washed red blood cells (RBCs) or all the blood collected. The risk of collecting bacteria or tumor cells with the shed blood rules out intraoperative blood scavenging in operations involving open bowel or malignancies. Salvage of blood collected from chest tubes and other wound drains also decreases use of homologous blood.

■ The Safety of the Blood Supply

Infection

Although bacterial and parasitic infections such as malaria can be transmitted via transfusion, the commonly occurring transmissible infections are viral in origin. Commercial blood collected from paid donors, as compared with that collected from volunteer donors, carries an increased risk of hepatitis and is rarely used today. All units collected are tested for markers of hepatitis A, B, and C as well as human immunodeficiency virus (HIV). Unfortunately, blood collected from an infected donor during the incubation period before development of antibodies may transmit one of these diseases. HIV is transmitted with an estimated incidence of between 1 in 40,000 and 1 in 400,000 units, depending on the population of donors. Lawsuits have been brought following such infections, so some institutions demand specific written informed consent prior to elective blood transfusion or elective procedures where transfusion is likely.

Fear of HIV has led some patients to select the donors who provide blood for their operations. Many blood banks resisted this practice, contending that any given population of relatives, neighbors, or co-workers provides blood that is no safer than the nation's volunteer blood donor population. In a study of 12,000 donors, the incidence of serologic markers of infection among "directed donors" was identical to that in the donor pool at large. Despite these

arguments, and in the face of considerable public pressure and even legislation, most blood banks have developed a system to designate donors when requested.

Incompatibility

The first step in ensuring against incompatible transfusions is to identify carefully the intended recipient and then collect a blood sample that is clearly marked with the name, hospital number, and date of collection. The final step, when the unit of blood is administered to the patient, requires equally careful patient identification and matching of patient name and hospital number to that on the unit to be transfused. These procedures prevent the most common cause of fatal transfusion reactions, the administration of ABO-incompatible blood resulting from clerical error.

Typing and crossmatching is a procedure in which a patient's serum and a potential donor's cells are incubated together (major crossmatch) for 30 minutes with Coombs' reagent to detect gamma G immunoglobulin (IgG) antibody coating of the red cell surface. Agglutination is a sign that the patient's antibodies react to donor antigens and are therefore incompatible. The mixing of the patient's cells and the donor's serum (minor crossmatch) is no longer performed routinely.

Type and screen, used when a need for blood is unlikely, is performed by incubating the patient's serum with RBCs carrying known antigens to detect recipient antibodies. Units of compatible blood are then made available in case a need for blood occurs, but these units are not reserved for the exclusive use of one patient, because the likelihood of use is small. In some centers, type and screen is the only compatibility testing done if the antibody screen is negative. A full crossmatch offers little additional safety over simple testing for ABO-Rh compatibility when the antibody screen is negative.

Immunologic Consequences of Transfusion

Renal transplant recipients are less likely to reject a donor kidney if they have received a homologous transfusion. This effect of transfusion on the immune system benefits these patients. Conversely, transfusion has been correlated with early recurrence and poor prognosis in several forms of malignancy, as well as increased risk of bacterial infection. The logical suggestion that the need for blood is correlated with more advanced disease has been refuted by other detailed studies. This effect is more marked following whole blood transfusion than after RBCs and has been attributed to an unidentified component of stored plasma or associated cellular debris.

■ Emergency Transfusion

When an emergency precludes even an antibody screen, O-negative whole blood ("universal donor") can be administered without any testing. If time permits, uncrossmatched ABO-Rh type-specific blood is superior. The use of O-negative RBCs instead of whole blood decreases the administered volume of plasma containing anti-A and anti-B antibodies that would hemolyze recipient A, B, or AB cells. Prior to administration of type-specific blood to patients who have received O-negative blood as an emergency measure, the concentrations of anti-A and anti-B must be demonstrated to have decreased so that they will not produce hemolytic transfusion reactions.

■ Blood Substitutes

The use of electrolyte or colloid solutions to replace initial blood loss is the first step in blood substitution. Plasma protein fraction (PPF), 5% albumin, dextran, and starch solutions are colloidal solutions commonly used. Plasma protein fraction and 5% albumin have the same oncotic pressure as plasma, whereas dextran and starch have a slightly greater oncotic effect. None of these products provides coagulation proteins or transports oxygen efficiently, but they may be stored at room temperature, transmit no diseases, and require no compatibility testing.

Potential acellular carriers of oxygen, often referred to as *artificial blood*, include stroma-free hemoglobin, recombinant hemoglobin, and perfluorocarbon compounds. Stroma-free hemoglobin, from which all red cell membranes have been removed, delivers oxygen to tissues and also supports oncotic pressure. The preparation is not antigenic, and compatibility testing is not required prior to infusion. However, the hemoglobin is excreted by the kidneys within hours and colors plasma and urine red, potentially masking pathologic conditions associated with hemoglobinemia or hemoglobinuria. Experimental recombinant hemoglobin is a promising alternative because it is retained in the intravascular compartment for considerably longer intervals (at least in

animals) and the molecule can be altered to influence its oxygen dissociation characteristics.

Perfluorocarbon compounds do not carry sufficient oxygen to justify their clinical use currently. They are rapidly exhaled by the lungs, must be stored frozen, and may cause pulmonary insufficiency and complement activation. They do not provide oncotic or coagulation effects.

Recombinant erythropoietin has been used to stimulate red cell production in anemic patients with end-stage renal failure. The hormone is now approved for use in such patients; its use in surgical patients may further decrease the demand for homologous blood.

■ Hemolytic Transfusion Reaction

The various transfusion reactions are listed in Table 15-8. Acute hemolytic reactions are usually the result of incompatible RBC transfusion (most often clerical error), incompatible fluids infused with RBCs, and gram-negative sepsis from contaminated blood. Unexplained bleeding at an operative site is an important clinical sign of acute disseminated intravascular coagulopathy (DIC) due to a hemolytic transfusion reaction. Table 15-9 outlines the treatment of a hemolytic transfusion reaction.

Delayed hemolytic reactions derive from incompatibility involving non-ABO antigens and require only monitoring of the hematocrit, renal function, and coagulation profile. Febrile and allergic reactions are elicited by antibodies to white blood cells (WBCs), platelets, and plasma proteins, including gamma A immunoglobulin (IgA). Treatment consists of antipyretics, antihistamines, vasopressors if needed, and use of washed RBCs in future transfusion.

Hemostatic Disorders

■ Diagnosis

The best means of detecting an important deficiency of hemostasis preoperatively is to review the history, especially the hemostatic response to prior operations or dental extractions. In the absence of a positive history or physical findings such as petechiae or ecchymosis, routine screening tests usually are not indicated, because they yield few true-positive results and the false-positive tests produce further dilemmas (see Chap. 2 for an example of the statistics for the PTT).

Table 15-8

Signs and Symptoms of Transfusion Reactions

Type of Reaction	Awake Patient	Anesthetized Patient
Acute hemolytic	Pain at infusion site, anxiety, chest pain, dyspnea, chills, headache, flank pain	Fever, hemoglobinemia, hemoglobinuria, shock, DIC*
Febrile	Chills, faintness	Fever, shock (rare)
Hypervolemic	Dyspnea, headaches, palpitations	Pulmonary edema, hypertension, arrhythmias
Allergic	Pruritus, hoarseness, faintness, urticaria	Urticaria, stridor, hypotension
Delayed hemolytic	Fever, malaise, decreasing hematocrit, increased indirect bilirubin, increased urine urobilinogen	Not applicable

*DIC = disseminated intravascular coagulation.

When the history is suggestive, when large blood losses are anticipated, or when bleeding during operation appears excessive, the tests outlined in Table 15-10 permit a specific diagnosis and rational therapy. Repeating the tests after treatment ensures that the abnormality has been corrected.

■ Management of Hemostatic Disorders

Table 15-11 lists the blood products available to treat specific hemostatic deficiencies. The first step in treatment is meticulous surgical hemostasis.

Fresh frozen plasma (FFP) is the acellular portion of blood that has been separated and frozen within 6 hours of collection. Fresh frozen plasma differs from single-donor plasma (which has not been frozen) in that it contains adequate quantities of factor V and

Table 15-9

Management of a Suspected Hemolytic Transfusion Reaction

1. Discontinue the blood transfusion, but do not remove the intravenous catheter.
2. Maintain intravenous catheter flow with normal saline.
3. Notify the blood bank.
4. Send a newly collected and labeled blood specimen to the blood bank.
5. Send the blood unit and administration set to the blood bank.
6. Recheck any other units set up for this patient.
7. Send a urine specimen to the laboratory for hemoglobin analysis.

VIII, which decay with storage at room temperature. Fresh frozen plasma also replaces factors II (prothrombin), V, VII, IX, X, and XI to reverse the effects of warfarin and to provide antithrombin III. In massive blood transfusion, especially when red cells are used in lieu of whole blood, FFP is also required to replace these soluble factors lost to dilution. To replace clotting factors, 15 to 20 ml of plasma per kilogram of body weight is required to provide a 25 percent increase, which suffices for all factors except factor VIII. Attempts to increase concentrations of clotting factors more than 25 percent by infusion usually result in fluid overload, a problem that may be overcome by exchange transfusion.

Platelet concentrates are indicated for the treatment of bleeding due to thrombocytopenia or abnormal platelet function but are relatively ineffective in idiopathic autoimmune thrombocytopenic purpura (ITP), septicemia, and hypersplenism. One unit of platelets usually provides an increase of 5000 to 10,000 platelets/mm^3 in adults not actively consuming platelets. The usual adult dose is 6 to 8 units. In patients who have received multiple platelet transfusions, platelet alloimmunization requires HLA-matched platelets. In Rh-negative girls and women with childbearing potential, ABO-Rh compatible platelets are transfused to prevent Rh immunization.

Cryoprecipitate is the residual that remains when FFP is thawed at 4°C and is rich in factor VIII/von Willebrand factor and fibrinogen. One unit of plasma generally will yield 100 units of factor VIII and 300 mg fibrinogen. Ten such units provide a 25 percent increment in the factor VIII plasma concentra-

Table 15-10

Tests of Hemostasis Used to Confirm the Presence of a Disorder of Hemostasis

Primary (screening) tests:

1. Activated coagulation time (ACT)	Can be done in OR; observe for clot retraction and lysis (similar to a PTT but much less sensitive).
2. Fibrinogen	Depressed in DIC.
3. Prothrombin time (PT)	Prolonged in liver disease, vitamin K deficiency, warfarin anticoagulation, DIC
4. Partial thromboplastin time (PTT)	Prolonged in factors V and VIII deficiency (massive transfusion), the hemophilias, or the presence of heparin.
5. Platelet count	Decreased in thrombocytopenia and DIC.

Secondary tests:

1. Bleeding time	Widely accepted clinical test of platelet function.
2. Platelet aggregation	A more refined test of platelet function using various agents to determine the responsiveness of the platelets.
3. Protamine titration	Definitive test used to confirm heparin effect.
4. Individual factor	Used to diagnose and follow therapy with hemophilia.
5. Fibrin split products	Confirmatory test for DIC.

Table 15-11

Blood Products for Hemostatic Disorders

Hemostatic Factor	Minimal Needed for Surgical Hemostasis (% Normal)	In Vivo Half-Life	Therapeutic Agent
I	50–100	3–6 days	Cryoprecipitate
II	20–40	3–4 days	Plasma
V	5–20	12 hours	Fresh plasma Fresh frozen plasma
VII	10–20	4–6 hours	Plasma
VIII	30	10–18 hours	Cryoprecipitate Antihemophilic factor
von Willebrand's	30		Desmopressin Plasma
IX	20–25	18–24 hours	Plasma Prothrombin complex concentrate
X	10–20	2–4 days	Plasma
XI	20–30	2–3 days	Plasma
XII	0		Plasma
XIII	1–3	5+ days	Plasma
Platelets	50,000–100,000	Variable	Platelet concentrates

tion in a 70-kg patient and increase the fibrinogen by 100 mg/dl.

Antihemophilic factor (AHF) concentrates used to treat factor VIII-deficient hemophiliacs are prepared by plasma fractionation and lyophilized for storage.

The large pool of donors from which the product is derived considerably increases the risk of disease transmission, especially hepatitis or HIV.

Prothrombin complex concentrate (PCC) is available to treat the deficiencies of factors II (prothrom-

Table 15-12

Peripheral Intravenous Technique

Veins
  Choose upper extremity veins before lower extremity veins in adults (more prone to develop phlebitis and thrombosis).
  Choose more distal sites first, moving up the arm as necessary if difficulty is encountered.
  Choose the flat portion of the dorsum of the hand or the forearm for stability and security.
  Choose a straight segment of vein the length of the catheter.
  Avoid segments of vein that bridge a joint.
Catheter
  Choose a size consistent with the anticipated use. If rapid flow is needed, shorter catheters are better than longer catheters of the same diameter.
  Consider a guidewire exchange system (Seldinger technique) if very large catheters are needed (see Chap. 6).
  Before venipuncture, inspect the catheter and needle, and move the catheter slightly to ensure free separation from the needle.
  Use a small catheter for drug administration at the beginning of the procedure if only small veins are present and rapid infusion of fluids is not needed, and seek a larger vein after induction of anesthesia.
  Use longer catheters when veins are deep below the skin surface and where the overlying skin is very mobile (e.g., antecubital veins in obese patients, femoral, internal and external jugular veins).
Technique
  Use a wide tourniquet applied without pinching the skin or pulling on hair to provide adequate venous engorgement but not occlusion of arterial flow.
  Lower the arm below the shoulder. Gravity will increase vein distension.
  Cleanse the skin with antiseptic.
  Create a skin weal with local anesthetic via a 27-gauge needle.
  Stretch the skin distally to inhibit vein movement during cannulation, but do so gently to avoid compressing the vein.
  Use a 10- to 20-degree angle of approach. If the vein is very mobile, increase the angle for puncture of the anterior wall and then reduce the angle for insertion to avoid posterior wall.
  Aim to enter the vein with the tip of the needle just after it passes through the skin. This improves the likelihood of entering the vein cleanly and increases the length of catheter in the vein.
  Allow the venous pressure to cause blood to appear at the needle hub to indicate entry of the needle tip. Aspirating blood with a syringe may collapse the vein.
  Insert both needle tip *and* catheter tip into vein (1 to 3 mm additional) before sliding catheter off the needle further into the vein.
  Secure IV catheter to tubing from infusion set with a locking connector.
  Do not place tape completely around an extremity.
Previously placed catheters
  Completely inspect and replace tubing and tape of an existing catheter before judging that it is suitable for what you are anticipating.
  Do not rely on a catheter distal to a recent venous puncture site for administering large volume of fluids.
  Do not rely on catheters when evidence of phlebitis is present at the site.
  When in doubt, place a new IV catheter.

bin), VII, IX, and X. This product could be used for neutralization of warfarin, but because it is a pooled product that carries a great risk of disease transmission, PCC is reserved almost exclusively for patients with severe factor IX deficiency.

Desmopressin (DDAVP) is a vasopressin analogue that acts by releasing factor VIII/von Willebrand factor from endothelial cells; it increases concentrations of that factor acutely and transiently, which can be effective in patients with von Willebrand's disease. It has been given to other bleeding patients thought to have impaired platelet function but has not proved to be uniformly effective.

Establishing Vascular Access

An essential technical skill for management of fluids is the ability to establish and maintain intravascular access for fluid and drug administration and monitoring. An intravenous catheter is part of good management even for minor operations in healthy patients, if only for emergency administration of drugs. Catheters inserted over a needle into a peripheral vein are standard. A 24-gauge catheter may suffice for medication, whereas multiple no. 8 French catheters may be indicated for massive blood transfusion. The major complications of catheters are sepsis and thrombophlebitis, which become more likely the longer the catheter is left in place. Catheters are changed or discontinued if possible within 48 to 72 hours of insertion. The choice of site and catheter are often dictated by positioning of the patient for the operation, the operation itself, and occasionally by the abnormal anatomy of individual patients. It is essential to be certain of the integrity of the system created. Commonly observed guidelines for peripheral venous access are listed in Table 15-12.

The combination of adequate vascular access and hemodynamic, hemoglobin, electrolyte, and urine flow monitoring allows the anesthesiologist to diagnose and treat fluid and electrolyte abnormalities and to ensure adequate oxygen delivery even during life-threatening conditions such as prolonged operations, major blood loss, massive trauma, or major translocations of fluids.

BIBLIOGRAPHY

Consensus Conference. Perioperative red blood cell transfusion. *JAMA* 1988;260:2700-2703.

Moore FD. *Metabolic Care of the Surgical Patient.* Philadelphia: WB Saunders, 1959, p 146.

Roberts JP, Roberts JD, Skinner C, et al. Extracellular fluid deficit following operation and its correction with Ringer's lactate: A reassessment. *Ann Surg* 1985;202:1-8.

Toy PTCY, Strauss RG, Sterling LG, et al. Predeposit autologous blood for elective surgery, a national multicenter study. *N Engl J Med* 1987;316:517-520.

Twigley AJ, Hillman KA. The end of the crystalloid era? *Anaesthesia* 1985;40:800-871.

CHAPTER 16

Positioning the Surgical Patient

Christian M. Alexander

The patient's position during an operation is chosen to provide the optimal exposure of the anatomic target. Unfortunately, a single position is unlikely to be ideal for surgeon, patient, and anesthesiologist. The absence of pain under anesthesia allows patients to assume positions that they would not tolerate when awake; many surgical positions produce potentially deleterious cardiovascular and respiratory effects, as well as complications such as backache, alopecia, or peripheral nerve injury. The anesthesiologist and the surgeon must work together to position the patient in a way that will do the least harm yet allow the operation to proceed.

Safe positioning of patients requires a knowledge of the advantages and disadvantages of various surgical positions and an understanding of the physiologic consequences of each. Positioning problems anticipated during the preanesthetic visit, as well as measures undertaken in the operating room (OR), must be documented on the medical record. A sufficient number of trained people must help with positioning to minimize risk to patients and OR personnel. Last, all necessary positioning equipment must be present at the start of the procedure.

Patients are positioned just after the induction of anesthesia, before surgical stimulation begins. At this time, postural changes often produce hypotension owing to vasodilation and peripheral pooling of blood in dependent areas, while compensatory reflexes are obtunded by anesthesia. Deficits in circulating volume, preexisting illnesses, autonomic nervous system

insufficiency, and rapid alterations in posture make hypotension more severe. Frequent determination of blood pressure allows the anesthesiologist to detect any changes and to judge whether the new posture is acceptable. If hypotension occurs, further changes in posture are postponed until the blood pressure is corrected by fluid infusions, vasopressors, or decreasing concentrations of anesthetic drugs. When these measures fail, the position must be adjusted to one that achieves cardiovascular stability.

At the end of operation, when patients are again moved, intravascular volume deficits or electrolyte abnormalities acquired during operation may again produce hypotension, especially when venous return is compromised by return to the supine position from the Trendelenburg or lithotomy position. Conversely, lightly anesthetized patients may become hypertensive from airway stimulation or pain with movement, requiring appropriate treatment with anesthetics, opioids, or vasodilators.

The Supine Position

People spend the majority of their lives upright; changes in cardiopulmonary function occur within minutes of assuming the supine position. External forces acting on the lungs change; in the supine position, the abdominal contents limit movement of the diaphragm and force it cephalad, reducing functional residual capacity (FRC) by 20 percent. An additional 20 percent loss of FRC occurs after induction of anesthesia, probably because of changes in diaphragmatic and abdominal muscle tone.

This decreased lung volume produces small airway closure. In the anesthetized, supine patient, the FRC is markedly less than in the sitting position, whereas the closing volume (the lung volume at which airway closure begins in dependent regions of lung) remains the same. Therefore, closing volume may exceed FRC in the supine position, producing small airway closure during tidal breathing (Fig. 16-1). Airway closure leads to hypoxemia from venous admixture. This is particularly likely in elderly patients because closing volume increases with age. These adverse effects on lung volume are partially offset by positive-pressure ventilation.

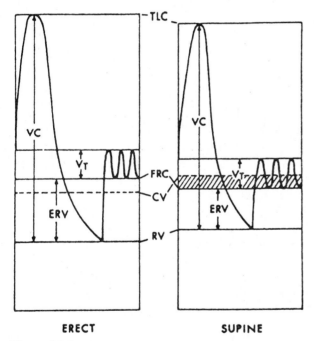

ERECT   **SUPINE**

Figure 16-1

Spirometric tracing imposed on lung volumes in erect and supine positions. The ordinate represents lung volume and the abscissa, time. In the supine position, the closing volume is greater than functional residual capacity so that tidal volume and closing volume overlap. Abbreviations: TLC, total lung capacity; VC, vital capacity; VT, tidal volume; ERV, expiratory reserve volume; RV, residual volume; FRC, functional residual capacity; CV, closing volume.

(Reproduced with permission from Martin JT, Positioning in Anesthesia and Surgery, 2nd ed. Philadelphia: WB Saunders, 1987.)

Gravitational effects on pulmonary arterial pressure, described in Chapter 22, are less severe in the supine position, so pulmonary blood flow is more homogeneous than when the patient is upright. The distribution of ventilation (see Chap. 22) is also affected by position. Pleural pressure is more uniform in the supine position, so variation in ventilation-perfusion ratios is less than when the patient is erect. In the erect position, the base-to-apex ratio is 1.5:1 for ventilation and 3:1 for perfusion. In the supine position, the base-to-apex ratio is 0.9:1 for ventilation and 1.3:1 for perfusion.

The circulatory effects of the supine position are unremarkable except when an obese abdomen, abdominal mass, ascites, or a gravid uterus compresses the inferior vena cava, impedes venous return, and decreases cardiac output. Rolling the patient with an abdominal mass into a 10-degree left lateral position by tilting the operating room table or using a pelvic wedge shifts the abdominal weight from the vena cava, relieving the obstruction.

In the supine position, when the head is poorly padded or in the presence of hypotension, pressure on the occipital scalp can cause pain, swelling, and alopecia, which may last for months or be permanent. Skin biopsies in these areas show obliterative vasculitis. Appropriate padding and frequent turning of the head (every 30 minutes) can prevent this complication. This condition is to be differentiated from the generalized hair loss that rarely follows anesthesia and operation, for which the etiology is unknown.

The lithotomy position (Fig. 16-2) is a variation of the supine position; the patient is supine with the legs flexed at the knees and elevated so that the perineum and rectum are accessible to the surgeon. The principal hazards of the lithotomy position are peripheral nerve injury (see "Peripheral Nerve Injury" below), compartment syndrome, and iliac artery thrombosis. Circulatory and respiratory effects are similar to those of the supine position. Vital capacity and FRC are further decreased by restriction of diaphragmatic movement if the patient's knees are flexed onto the abdomen or if the patient is placed head down. Circulatory effects are minimal unless a mass or abdominal obesity obstructs the inferior vena cava. Hypotension can occur when the patient's legs are lowered at the conclusion of operation as the venous capacitance vessels of the lower extremities refill with blood. This relative hypovolemia is accentuated by untreated surgical blood loss or cardiac disease.

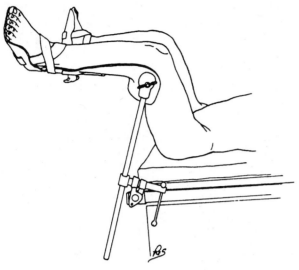

Figure 16-2

Proper lithotomy position: minimal external rotation of legs, thighs minimally flexed toward abdomen, symmetrical position of legs. Protective padding not shown.

(Reproduced with permission from Martin JT, Positioning in Anesthesia and Surgery, 2nd ed. Philadelphia: WB Saunders, 1987.)

Prone Position

The prone position (Fig. 16-3) is used for operations on the rectum, spine, or dorsum of the body. Respiratory effects of this position may be severe if the patient is not positioned appropriately, since compression of the abdominal viscera against the operating table causes several ill effects. Inspiratory movement of the diaphragm is restricted by the abdominal contents, so the thoracic weight must be raised to expand the chest, increasing the work of breathing. Increased airway pressures are required to accomplish positive-pressure ventilation. Atelectasis can occur, and there can be excessive movement of the patient's back in the surgical field. Compression of the inferior vena cava decreases cardiac output and increases central venous pressures (Fig. 16-4). Venous return from the extremities is diverted into pathways offering less resistance, such as the venous plexus of the vertebral column (Batson's plexus). During spinal operations, this may be a source of increased intraoperative bleeding.

A wide variety of devices and frames are used to redistribute body weight to the shoulders and hips so that the abdomen hangs free and can descend with expansion of the chest. These include rolls placed longitudinally from clavicle to pelvis along the lateral edges of the torso, rolls that support the patient at the clavicles and iliac crests, or kneeling arrangements using the patient's buttocks and thighs as supports for the pelvis (Fig. 16-5). All these devices require adequate padding of pressure points, free abdominal and chest expansion, no greater than 90-degree abduction of the arms, and protection of the ulnar nerve at the elbows.

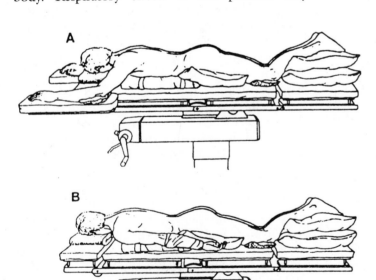

Figure 16-3

Classic prone position with arms extended next to head (*A*) or alongside torso (*B*). Chest roll placed below clavicle and pillow under iliac crest to allow abdomen to hang free. The table is flexed to a variable degree depending on the lumbar lordosis and the needs of the surgeon. With flexion, a subgluteal anchor is needed to prevent caudal slippage of the patient.

(Modified with permission from Martin JT, Positioning in Anesthesia and Surgery, 2nd ed. Philadelphia: WB Saunders, 1987.)

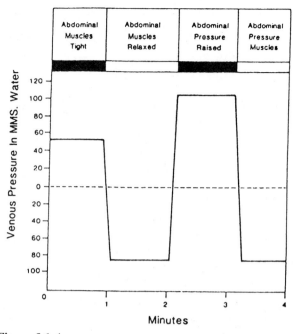

Figure 16-4

Venous pressure changes in the prone, supported position. When abdominal muscles are tight or abdominal pressure is increased, there is an increase in central venous pressure. *(Reproduced with permission from Pearce DJ, The role of posture in laminectomy. Proc R Soc Med 1957;50:109.)*

With proper positioning, the weight of the freed abdomen draws the diaphragm downward, so the FRC is greater in these prone positions than in either the supine or the lateral position. Pulmonary blood flow is as homogeneous as in the supine position.

Studies of pulmonary shunting show no change when anesthetized patients are turned from supine to prone.

Other circulatory effects depend on the positioning device in use. If the legs are horizontal, there is no pressure gradient between the legs and the torso. When the patient is kneeling, significant venous pooling is likely in the legs, producing relative central hypovolemia. In addition, there is a considerable gravitational gradient between the right side of the heart and the vertebrae in the prone position. This gradient, combined with a contracted blood volume or inadequate fluid replacement and a position that enhances negative caval pressures, favors air entrainment into the venous circulation. Thus positioning that favors respiratory compliance and decreases bleeding may increase the risk of venous air embolism.

Positioning the patient's head is a challenge in the prone position (Fig. 16-6). Rotation of the head and neck may produce cerebral ischemia by occluding the carotid or vertebral arteries; turning the head 80 degrees may completely obstruct the contralateral vertebral artery. Patients with intact vascular anatomy compensate by increased flow through the opposite vertebral artery or the circle of Willis, but those with vessels partially obstructed by atherosclerosis may suffer ischemia, thrombosis, or an embolic stroke. In most cases, the patient's head should not be turned from the sagittal plane. This is usually accomplished by using a foam support or a horseshoe-shaped pad that supports the periphery of the face without pressing on the eyes.

Figure 16-5

The Andrews frame, which supports the chest and buttocks, with the knees padded. The knees are never flexed more than 90 degrees on the thighs.

(Reproduced with permission from Martin JT, Positioning in Anesthesia and Surgery, 2nd ed. Philadelphia: WB Saunders, 1987.)

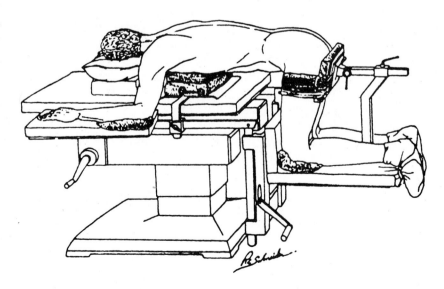

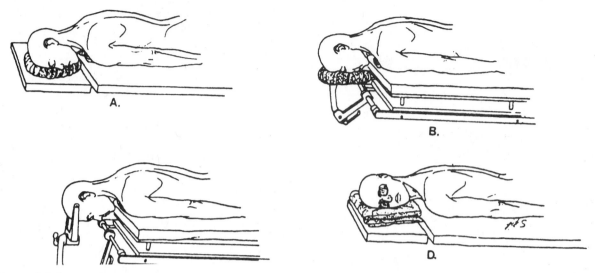

Figure 16-6

Methods of avoiding excessive turning of the head in the prone position. *A, B,* and *C* are acceptable. Extreme rotation of the neck (*D*) may be dangerous in patients with cervical spine disease or cerebrovascular disease. The eyes themselves must be free from pressure, since pressure on the globe may reduce flow in the retinal vessels enough to produce permanent retinal blindness.

(Reproduced with permission from Martin JT, Positioning in Anesthesia and Surgery, *2nd ed. Philadelphia: WB Saunders, 1987.)*

The Head-Down (Trendelenburg) Position

Tilting the supine patient head down results in a cephalad shift of large and small bowels and improves exposure of pelvic organs. The classic Trendelenburg position, with 30- to 40-degree tilt, necessitated some means of preventing patients from sliding cephalad. Historically, wrist cuffs or shoulder braces were used, but both can stretch or compress the brachial plexus. At present, the tilt is usually limited to 10 to 15 degrees, which does not require patient restraints.

The head-down position causes decreased arterial pressure in the legs and relative engorgement of the vessels of the mediastinum. In healthy patients, baroreceptor reflexes keep this increase small; volunteers placed 15 degrees head down show only a 2 percent increase in central blood volume and no significant hemodynamic changes. Although cardiac output and central venous pressure are increased transiently, vasodilation and bradycardia soon follow.

Although the head-down position is used widely to treat hypotension and shock, studies of patients with acute cardiac disease, hypotension, sepsis, or shock do not show a consistent beneficial effect. In hypotensive patients in shock (placed head down), there was either no effect or a decrease in mean arterial pressure; left-sided heart filling pressures (PCWP) and cardiac output did not change. When hypovolemia is present, the Trendelenburg position does not improve blood pressure but may improve cardiac output slightly. Many clinicians elevate the patient's legs while keeping the body level to increase venous return without triggering harmful baroreceptor changes or risking cerebral venous congestion.

Patients with coronary artery disease placed head down for subclavian or internal jugular vein cannulation experience significant increases in mean arterial pressure and pulmonary capillary wedge pressures (PCWP), implying increased myocardial oxygen demand. In patients with significantly decreased cardiac reserve, increased PCWP resulting from the head-down position can cause acute congestive heart failure or myocardial ischemia.

The head-down position is harmful when intracranial compliance is decreased, since the increased jugular venous pressure caused by this maneuver increases intracranial pressure. Increased cerebral venous pressures also may decrease cerebral perfusion pressure, which is the difference between mean arterial pressure and either venous pressure or intracranial pressure, whichever is greater.

In the head-down position, abdominal contents compress the lung bases so that, compared with the supine position, FRC and pulmonary compliance are decreased and the work of breathing is increased. Since left atrial pressure increases in relation to alveolar pressure, pulmonary edema, congestion, and atelectasis are more likely in this position. This tendency to develop atelectasis and hypoxemia is greatest in obese or elderly patients or when surgical retractors are placed in the upper abdomen.

Endotracheal tube position must be verified after any change in the patient's position, but particularly after patients are placed head down. Gravity displaces the lungs and carina cephalad, causing the tip of the endotracheal tube to lie more distally in the trachea. Even a tube that is appropriately anchored at the mouth can enter the right mainstem bronchus due to the shift in intrathoracic contents.

The Sitting Position

The sitting position (Fig. 16-7) is used during posterior fossa craniotomy or operations on the cervical spine, face, neck, and shoulders to facilitate exposure and enhance venous drainage. The full sitting position is uncommon; patients are usually semireclining with the head flexed and legs elevated.

In the anesthetized patient, hemodynamic changes can be significant even at head-up angles of less than 60 degrees; cardiovascular changes progress for an hour after the position is established. Gravity impedes venous drainage from the legs, shifting blood from the upper body to the lower extremities; atrial filling diminishes, decreasing cardiac output by 20 to 40 percent. In healthy unanesthetized subjects, these changes are opposed by increases in sympathetic tone, tachycardia, and increases in systemic vascular resistance. With these protective reflexes obtunded by anesthesia, postural hypotension can be sudden and severe, especially in elderly or hypertensive patients or in the presence of dehydration or cardiac disease. Mean arterial pressure may be measured at the level of the circle of Willis instead of the right atrium to more accurately assess cerebral perfusion.

Respiratory effects of the sitting position are often advantageous. Compared with the supine position, inspiratory movement of the diaphragm is less impeded by abdominal viscera. The work of breathing is

decreased for spontaneous ventilation, and inflating pressures are decreased during positive-pressure ventilation. The functional residual capacity increases, and age-related increases in closing capacity are minimized.

The risk of air embolism via open veins above the heart increases with the height of the operative site above the right atrium. Unappreciated or "silent" air embolism occurs frequently in head-elevated positions. Usually, the volume of air is small and detectable only by sophisticated means. Larger volumes of air are potentially lethal because they create compressible foam in the right side of the heart, making ventricular contractions inefficient. Small bubbles also obstruct the peripheral pulmonary vasculature. Air embolism is recognized by changes in the tones produced by a Doppler probe directed at the heart from the second right interspace, decreases in expired carbon dioxide, increases in expired nitrogen, arrhythmias, hypotension, or a characteristic "mill-wheel" murmur.

Air embolism can be particularly dangerous in the 20 to 35 percent of the population having a patent

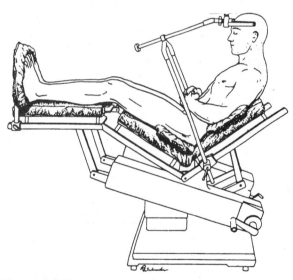

Figure 16-7

Neurosurgical sitting position. The legs are slightly flexed and raised to the level of the heart. The feet are padded to maintain a dorsiflexed position. The sciatic nerve is protected by gluteal padding. The frame of the head holder is clamped to the back section of the table so that the patient's head can be lowered in case of air embolization.

(Modified with permission from Martin JT, Positioning in Anesthesia and Surgery, 2nd ed. Philadelphia: WB Saunders, 1987.)

foramen ovale. In these patients, the foramen ovale is closed only when pressures in the left atrium are greater than in the right. This is usually the case, but this pressure gradient can be reversed in the sitting position. Air in the right side of the heart may then pass through the foramen ovale and enter the coronary or cerebral circulations, causing ischemia and permanent injury. The treatment of air embolism is discussed in Chapter 30.

The Lateral Decubitus Position

The lateral position (Fig. 16-8) is used for thoracotomy or renal or orthopedic surgery. It is designated right or left, denoting the dependent side; for example, in the right lateral decubitus position, the patient lies on the right side.

Blood pressure values in the lateral position depend on the position of the blood pressure cuff or arterial pressure transducer in relation to the heart. Because the distance between the arms of an adult patient may be as great as 40 cm, blood pressures measured in the two arms may differ by as much as 32 mmHg. When measuring arterial pressure directly, this effect is avoided by opening the transducer system to air at the level of the heart while zeroing the amplifier.

Respiratory effects of the lateral position are significant. The weight of the chest and restriction of the movement of the dependent ribs, combined with the pressure of the abdominal viscera, decrease the vital capacity and the FRC of the dependent lung. However, in awake patients breathing spontaneously in this position, the cephalad displacement of the dome of the dependent diaphragm enhances its contractions, increasing ventilation in the dependent lung. Because the dependent lung also receives the majority of the pulmonary blood flow, ventilation-perfusion relationships remain normal in awake patients in the lateral position.

In contrast, with controlled ventilation under anesthesia, the majority of the tidal volume is distributed to the nondependent lung, because the decreased FRC in the dependent lung makes it less compliant, and positive-pressure ventilation eliminates any mechanical advantage the dependent diaphragm enjoys during spontaneous ventilation. After the pleura or chest wall is opened, the upper lung becomes even more compliant and receives an even larger fraction of the tidal volume. Gravitational gradients in pulmonary artery pressure shunt blood to the dependent lung, which receives the larger fraction of pulmonary blood flow. Decreased cardiac output and compromised hypoxic pulmonary vasoconstriction under anesthesia serve to reduce further the blood flow to the upper lung (see Chap. 22). Thus, in the patient receiving controlled ventilation under anesthesia, the majority of the blood flow goes to the dependent lung, and the majority of the ventilation goes to the

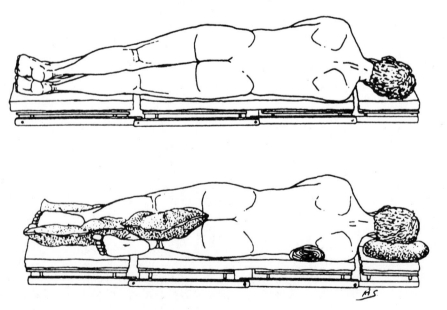

Figure 16-8

The right lateral decubitus position. (*Above*) Inadequate padding and improper head position. (*Below*) Padding over bony prominences, chest roll to protect neurovascular bundle in the axilla, and proper alignment of the cervical spine. The lower leg is flexed to stabilize the patient.

(*Reproduced with permission from Martin JT*, Positioning in Anesthesia and Surgery, *2nd ed. Philadelphia: WB Saunders, 1987.*)

Figure 16-9

Flexed lateral decubitus position. The point of flexion lies beneath the dependent iliac crest to minimize interference with the dependent lung and diaphragm.

(Modified with permission from Martin JT, Positioning in Anesthesia and Surgery, 2nd ed. Philadelphia: WB Saunders, 1987.)

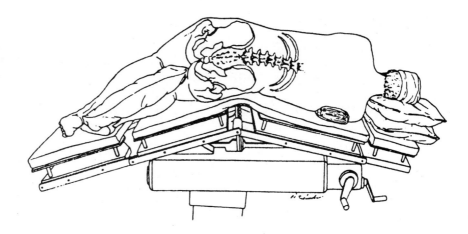

nondependent lung. This mismatch can produce severe arterial hypoxemia.

In the lateral position, the upper arm is positioned on an elevated board suspended from a metal frame or supported on pillows. A small pad (axillary roll) is placed under the chest just below the axilla to support the upper part of the rib cage, to avoid compression of the axillary neurovascular bundle, and to remove pressure from the deltoid muscle and the head of the humerus. The axillary roll may itself cause compression of the contents of the axilla if placed too cephalad.

A modified form of the lateral position is used for renal operations (Fig. 16-9). The upper leg is straight, and the lower leg flexed at the hip and knee. The iliac crest is positioned at the midpoint of the operating table, over a retractable fulcrum called a *kidney rest*. With the table flexed and the kidney rest elevated, the costal margin is separated from the iliac crest, improving surgical exposure of the kidney.

This position impairs inflation of the dependent lung, predisposing it to atelectasis. Pooling of blood occurs in the two dependent parts of the body, the legs and the head and upper torso. If abdominal flexion partially obstructs the inferior vena cava, further pooling of blood in the lower extremities occurs. These pulmonary and circulatory effects are minimized by avoiding extreme flexion, controlling ventilation, and positioning the patient properly over the kidney rest, with the fulcrum at the iliac crest. If the flexion point is placed improperly at the flank or costal margin, ventilation of the dependent lung or venous return is further compromised.

Nonneural Injury

■ Back Pain

Low back pain is frequent after either spinal or general anesthesia, occurring in as many as 37 percent of patients. It is unrelated to the type of anesthesia but is correlated with the duration of operation and with the position used. The lithotomy, supine, and prone positions are most likely to produce backache. Anesthesia and neuromuscular blockers relax paraspinal muscles so that the lordosis of the lumbar spine is flattened and tension is applied to the posterior ligaments and muscles. Postoperatively, patients complain of back pain, sometimes with radiation in the sciatic nerve distribution, lasting from a few days to several months. To avoid this injury, the hips and knees are flexed slightly in the supine position with padding to reinforce the lumbar lordosis (Fig. 16-10). This also increases venous return from the extremities and decreases anterior abdominal wall tension. While placing patients in the lithotomy position, the legs are raised and lowered simultaneously to avoid lumbar torsion.

■ Skin Necrosis

Prolonged pressure on skin can result in ischemia and even ulceration. Skin over bony prominences where pressure is exerted (heels, malleoli, sacrum, or supraorbital ridge) is vulnerable to ischemic damage and must be carefully padded or moved from time to time to relieve pressure. Tape tightly applied to skin,

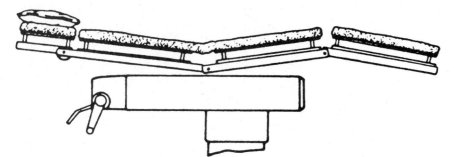

Figure 16-10

The lawn chair position with flexion of the hips, minimal knee flexion, and trunk section level. *(Modified with permission from Martin JT,* Positioning in Anesthesia and Surgery, *2nd ed. Philadelphia: WB Saunders, 1987.)*

ears, or the nose also can lead to necrosis of skin or cartilage.

■ Injury to the Eye

Eye injuries in the anesthetized patient are usually of two types. Pressure on the globe while patients are in the prone or lateral position may cause thrombosis of the retinal artery or retinal ischemia when pressure transmitted through the eye is sufficient to occlude the retinal artery. Intraoperative hypotension or a history of glaucoma make this complication more likely. Irreversible blindness results, but this complication is avoidable; the anesthesiologist must ensure that patients' eyes are free from pressure.

Corneal abrasion is the most common intraoperative ocular injury. Its etiology is not completely understood but is probably related to drying of the exposed cornea, exacerbated by reduced lacrimation during general anesthesia or direct trauma from the anesthesia mask or other equipment. Its symptoms include a foreign-body sensation, lacrimation, and eye pain aggravated by movement. Taping the eyelids to prevent exposure of the cornea, eye shields, and the use of ophthalmic lubricant in the conjunctival sac help prevent this injury.

■ Crush Injury

Whenever parts of the operating table are moved, the patient may be injured. When the foot of the surgical table is returned to the horizontal position after a procedure in the lithotomy position, the patient's fingers may be crushed between the two sections of the operating table. When the surgical table is raised, overhanging equipment such as an instrument stand may harm the patient.

■ Compartment Syndrome

Prolonged pressure on body parts can produce compartment syndrome. The etiology of this syndrome is ischemia (either from vascular compromise or direct local muscle pressure) causing loss of capillary integrity and massive edema within a closed fascial compartment, eventually leading to increased pressure and tissue necrosis. In the perioperative period, compartment syndrome most commonly results from prolonged lithotomy positioning and involves the lower extremities. Thigh flexion not only can compress femoral vessels but places the legs above the heart, decreasing perfusion pressure. The most severe cases have occurred where the legs were supported for more than 4 hours by devices that compress the popliteal fossa and posterior calf. Patients who are undergoing perineal prostatectomy in the extreme lithotomy position are also at increased risk for this complication.

Compartment syndrome usually becomes manifest several hours postoperatively. In the recovery room, examination of the lower extremities for muscle pain on stretch, edema, or color changes is important. Distal pulses and capillary refill may remain intact at first. Compartment syndrome is best prevented by limiting the time patients spend in the lithotomy position to less than 4 hours. During combined abdominal and perineal procedures, the legs can be returned to the supine position when the lithotomy position is not mandatory.

Peripheral Nerve Injury

Nerve damage is the second most common complication related to anesthesia that results in malpractice litigation. It represented 16 percent of malpractice claims in the American Society of Anesthesiologists Closed Claims Study. The overall reported incidence lies between 0.1 and 13 percent. Ulnar and brachial plexus injuries usually occurred during general anesthesia, but lumbosacral neuropathies usually followed regional anesthesia (Fig. 16-11). Examination of the pattern of malpractice claims over the past 15 years has shown that claims related to death, brain damage, or respiratory events have declined, so nerve injury may become a relatively more prominent cause of anesthetic-related injury in the future.

Peripheral nerve injuries are presumed to occur during anesthesia because the patient is placed in a distorted position and cannot feel the discomfort or move to relieve pressure or stretch. Injury occurs as a result of direct trauma from operation or nerve blocks, nerve compression by surgical retractors or hard operating room table surfaces, or pressure from tourniquets or from stretching of nerves around bony prominences (e.g., the head of the humerus displaces the brachial plexus when the arm is abducted). Mechanisms of nerve damage include mechanical injury to the nerves or their myelin sheaths and ischemia from direct compression or stretch-related rupture of small capillaries. Other factors contribut-

ing to nerve injury include congenital anomalies (such as anomalous derivation of the brachial plexus), diabetes, compression by hematomas, hypothermia, and use of a tourniquet. Thin patients and those who smoke cigarettes are at greatly increased risk of developing a lower extremity motor neuropathy after the lithotomy position.

The differential diagnosis of postoperative nerve damage includes preexisting neuropathy, central nervous system damage such as stroke, misplaced needles, or surgical manipulation (femoral nerve injury from self-retaining retractors). When a patient suffers a nerve palsy after an operation, a neurologic examination is performed and documented, and a neurologist is consulted so that nerve conduction studies can be obtained and the patient can receive follow-up care. An accurate recording in the preanesthesia note of any neurologic deficiencies that may exist is essential for appropriate diagnosis and postoperative management.

Peripheral nerve injuries are grouped into three classifications. Least severe is transient ischemic nerve block, the temporary paralysis that follows compression of a nerve, as from a blood pressure cuff. This is commonly described by patients as the extremity "going to sleep," usually lasts 20 minutes or less, and

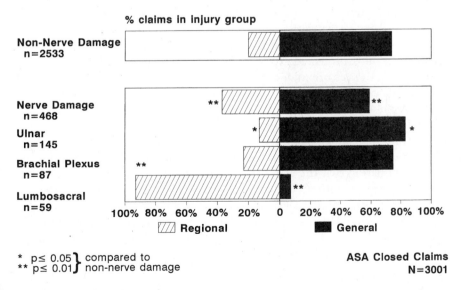

Figure 16-11

Incidence of regional and general anesthesia in each category of injury. Nonnerve damage includes all other claims for injury. **p <0.01 compared with nonnerve injury.

(Modified with permission from Kroll DA, Caplan RA, Ward RJ, Cheney FW. Nerve injury associated with anesthesia. Anesthesiology 1990;73:202.)

is not associated with structural damage. More persistent is neuropraxia, which also constitutes temporary paralysis or sensory loss, although recovery takes 4 to 6 weeks or longer. Pathologically, nerve fibers become demyelinated near the periphery of the nerve trunk, but continuity of the nerve trunk and the endoneurial sheath is preserved. Remyelinization parallels clinical recovery. Most grave are severe stretch injuries or laceration of a nerve, entailing complete disruption of the axons within an intact sheath (axonotmesis) or of the entire nerve trunk (neurotmesis). Wallerian degeneration of the peripheral nerve distal to the site of injury follows. Complete recovery is unlikely in injuries that disrupt the axon and its connective tissue structure.

The ulnar nerve is the peripheral nerve most commonly injured in patients undergoing anesthesia and operation. Damage occurs when the nerve is compressed at the elbow against the posterior aspect of the medial epicondyle of the humerus. This can happen when the patient's elbow slips off the operating table mattress, encountering the edge of the table. The ulnar nerve also can be compressed in the cubital tunnel when the elbow is fully flexed as the arm is secured across the abdomen or chest. When placing the patient's arm on an arm board, it is best to supinate the hand rather than to place it with the palm down; this maneuver rolls the ulnar nerve into a more protected position. In 20 percent of individuals, the ulnar nerve has a more medial course than is described in anatomy texts, passing behind the tip of the epicondyle rather than in the more protected groove, rendering it more susceptible to pressure injury.

Results from the ASA Closed Claims Study shed new light on postoperative ulnar nerve injury. Ulnar injury accounted for 34 percent of the nerve injury claims, but the mechanism of damage was apparent in only 6 percent. For 18 percent of cases, the file contained the specific information that the arm was padded over the ulnar nerve. Symptoms of ulnar nerve injury also occurred late, suggesting that injury sometimes occurred during the postoperative rather than the intraoperative period. Patients with postanesthetic ulnar nerve lesions frequently have abnormalities of nerve conduction testing in both the affected and the unaffected arms, perhaps owing to a chronic neural disorder exacerbated by positioning or the blood pressure cuff. Patients who experience ulnar paresthesia or dysesthesia preoperatively must be warned that a surgical procedure may aggravate this condition. Although more women than men appear

in the closed claims database, in several studies three to five times as many men as women suffered ulnar nerve damage, suggesting an anatomic predisposition among men.

Although ulnar nerve palsy may result in litigation because of the assumption that an error occurred during patient positioning, in fact the mechanism of this injury is unclear; it may not be a preventable complication. It is prudent to avoid any obvious causes of injury by padding the elbow, avoiding prolonged flexion, and positioning the arm so that external compression is unlikely. These maneuvers as well as any preexisting symptoms such as numbness or paresthesias should be documented in the medical record.

After the ulnar nerve, the second most common neurologic injury is to the brachial plexus, which is susceptible because of its long course between two firm points of fixation, the vertebral fascia above and the axillary fascia below. In addition, the clavicle and the humerus serve as fulcrums to further stretch the plexus. Stretching of the brachial plexus occurs when the neck is extended, the head is turned or flexed to the contralateral side, or the arm is abducted to greater than 90 degrees (Fig. 16-12). Sternal retraction during cardiac surgery can compress the brachial plexus between the clavicle and the first rib, causing a persistent neurologic deficit that most commonly affects the lower roots of the plexus and may mimic an injury of the ulnar nerve.

Patients with stretch injuries to the brachial plexus may complain of mild shoulder pain in the supraclavicular area, but usually there is a nearly painless motor deficit. Any combination of roots can be affected; the upper roots are involved more frequently than the lower.

The radial nerve may be injured as it passes laterally around the humerus by pressure against operating table hardware. Injury is followed by wrist drop, weakness of abduction of the thumb, and inability to extend the metacarpophalangeal joints.

The median nerve in the antecubital fossa is close to the medial cubital and basilic veins. It may be injured by intravenous catheters or the extravasation of drugs such as sodium thiopental. Median nerve injury causes decreased sensation on the palmar surface of the first three and one-half fingers, inability to oppose the thumb and little finger, and weakness of thumb abduction.

The common peroneal nerve is the most frequently injured nerve in the lower extremity. Injuries usually

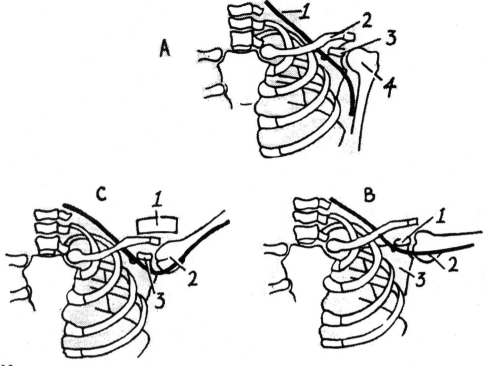

Figure 16-12

Brachial plexus in relation to surrounding structures. (A) Arm at side: (1) brachial plexus, (2) clavicle, (3) coracoid process, and (4) head of humerus. (B) Arm at right angle. (C) Arm hyperextended by shoulder brace, which depresses scapula, stretching brachial plexus beneath coracoid process and around humeral head.

occur when patients are in the lithotomy position; the nerve is compressed between the head of the fibula and the stirrup that suspends the leg. Proper padding of the head of the fibula avoids this complication. Nerve damage causes foot drop and loss of extension of the toes. Injury also can occur in a thin patient in the lateral position after prolonged pressure against a poorly padded operating room table.

The femoral nerve can be injured by excessive angulation of the thigh on the abdomen in the lithotomy position or by the blade of a self-retaining retractor during a laparotomy. This injury results in loss of hip flexion and extension of the knee; sensation is diminished over the anterior thigh and anteromedial calf.

If the ankles are plantar flexed during anesthesia in the sitting or prone position, the anterior tibial nerve in the ankle is vulnerable to stretch injury. Plantar flexion increases the distance the nerve travels over the anterior ankle joint. To prevent this injury, a foot support or ankle roll maintains a neutral, slightly dorsiflexed position.

The sciatic nerve can be injured in patients in the lithotomy position if the thighs and legs are externally rotated or if the knees remain extended. Both maneuvers increase the distance between the sciatic notch and the neck of the fibula, stretching the nerve. Patients in the sitting position must have their knees slightly flexed for the same reason. Sciatic nerve damage causes weakness of all the muscles below the knee and numbness of the lateral calf and entire foot except the inner arch.

Airway equipment and the anesthesiologist's hand also may cause nerve injury to the face. Excessive pressure from the mask or head strap results in paralysis of the buccal branch of the facial nerve with loss of function of the orbicularis oris muscle. If forward pressure on the ascending ramus of the mandible is required to maintain a patent airway, the facial nerve may be compressed, resulting in loss of muscle tone on the affected side of the face. The supraorbital nerve can be compressed medial to the eyebrow by an endotracheal tube connector, producing eye pain, photophobia, and forehead numbness.

Although complications from positioning have been described since the early days of anesthesia, they still constitute a large portion of anesthetic complications. Many positioning injuries are preventable by padding bony prominences, moving patients slowly and gently, avoiding positions that strain ligaments or nerves, and proper attention to the physiologic effects of positioning. However, for ulnar and possibly brachial plexus injuries, our incomplete understanding of the mechanisms of nerve damage limits our ability to prevent these lesions completely.

BIBLIOGRAPHY

Britt BA, Gordon RA. Peripheral nerve injuries associated with anesthesia. *Can Anaesth Soc J* 1964;11:514-536.

Coonan TJ, Hope CE. Cardiorespiratory effects of changes of body position. *Can Anaesth Soc J* 1983;30:424-437.

Dawson DM, Krarup C. Perioperative nerve lesions. *Arch Neurol* 989;46:1355-1360.

Kroll DA, Caplan RA, Posner K, et al. Nerve injury associated with anesthesia. *Anesthesiology* 1990;73:202-207.

Lincoln JR, Sawyer HP. Complications related to body positions during surgery. *Anesthesiology* 1961;22:800-809.

Martin JT. Compartment syndromes: Concepts and perspectives for the anesthesiologist. *Anesth Analg* 1992;75:275-283.

Martin JT. *Positioning in Anesthesia and Surgery,* 2nd ed. Philadelphia: WB Saunders, 1987.

Perreault L, Drolet P, Farny J. Ulnar palsy at the elbow after general anesthesia. *Can J Anaesth* 1992;39:499-503.

Stoelting RK. Post-operative ulnar palsy: Is it a preventable complication? *Anesth Analg* 1993;76:7-9.

SECTION 5

Conduction Anesthesia

17

Pharmacology of Local Anesthetics

Robert R. Gaiser

Local anesthetics produce reversible blockade of neural conduction by their actions on the sodium channels of neurons. The first recognized anesthetic was cocaine, a natural alkaloid introduced into use in 1880. The first synthetic ester, procaine, followed in 1905 and the first synthetic amide, lidocaine, in 1943.

Mechanism of Nerve Conduction

When a stimulus reduces the resting membrane potential of a nerve from approximately −90 to −60 mV, a spontaneous rapid phase of depolarization is generated that propagates down the nerve axon and constitutes a neural impulse. Depolarization results from the inward movement of sodium ions from the extracellular to the intracellular space via specific sodium channels in the membrane. The flow of potassium ions from the interior to the exterior of the nerve causes repolarization, returning the nerve membrane potential to the original resting level. At the completion of the action potential, ionic equilibrium is reestablished by the membrane sodium-potassium pump. Local anesthetics block neural conduction by inhibiting the inflow of sodium ions (Fig. 17-1). They do not affect the ionic gradient nor the resting membrane potential; rather, they inhibit the increase in sodium permeability that causes depolarization.

■ Sodium Channel Blockade

The sodium channel at which local anesthetics act is a complex structure consisting of three subunits: α, β, and β_2. The α subunit contains the transmembrane pore. The transmembrane voltage controls the conformation of the α subunit and its permeability to sodium. The channel assumes three conformations. Between impulses, the channel is closed (resting) so that neither sodium nor drugs can enter; with stimulation, the channel becomes open (activated); the transition from open to closed (inactivated) follows (Fig. 17-2). Local anesthetic molecules first diffuse through the cell wall of the neuron. Inside the axon, where the hydrogen ion concentration is greater than in the extracellular space, local anesthetic molecules are protonated, enter the sodium channel, and bind to the transmembrane pore (Fig. 17-3). Local anesthetics bind with the sodium channel only when it is open or inactive; resting channels do not bind drug. Once the channel contains local anesthetic, it is closed, rendering it unable to propagate conduction. As the frequency of stimulation increases, more sodium channels remain open for longer periods of time, with more opportunity for local anesthetic to enter the channel. This explains frequency-dependent blockade. Rapid repetitive depolarization opens sodium channels, promoting access for the local anesthetic and enhancing neural block.

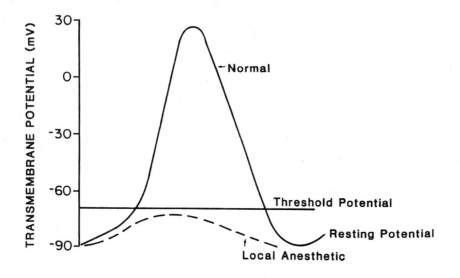

Figure 17-1

Local anesthetics prevent the nerve from reaching the threshold potential, thus preventing propagation of the action potential.

(Reprinted by permission from Stoelting RK, Pharmacology and Physiology in Anesthetic Practice. *Philadelphia: JB Lippincott, 1987.) 265-270.*

■ Membrane Expansion

Other mechanisms also account for conduction blockade. Benzocaine and benzyl alcohol are unionized compounds possessing local anesthetic activity. The blockade they produce is reversible by increased atmospheric pressures, whereas the block produced by conventional local anesthetics is only partially reversed. Benzocaine and benzyl alcohol appear to act like general anesthetics, inhibiting sodium influx and blocking nerve conduction by expanding or altering the configuration of the nerve membrane, thus decreasing the diameter of the sodium channel.

■ Differential Neural Blockade

Dilute local anesthetic solutions may produce differential neural blockade, characterized by partial sensory blockade but retained motor function. Differential effects may be evident during the onset of blockade, usually progressing in the following order:

Figure 17-2

The sodium channel in the nerve. The channel probably traverses a protein structure that spans the entire thickness of the axonal membrane. A single receptor on the inner aspect of the channel binds all types of local anesthetics.

(Reprinted by permission from Savarese JJ, Covino BG, Basic and clinical pharmacology of local anesthetic drugs. In Miller RD, ed: Anesthesia, *2nd ed. New York: Churchill-Livingstone, 1986.)*

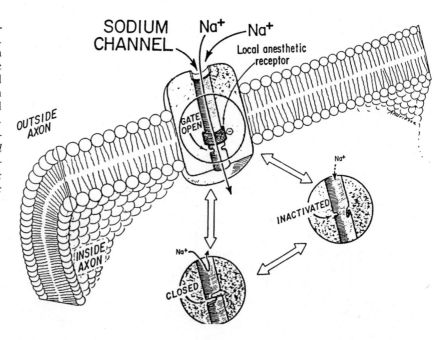

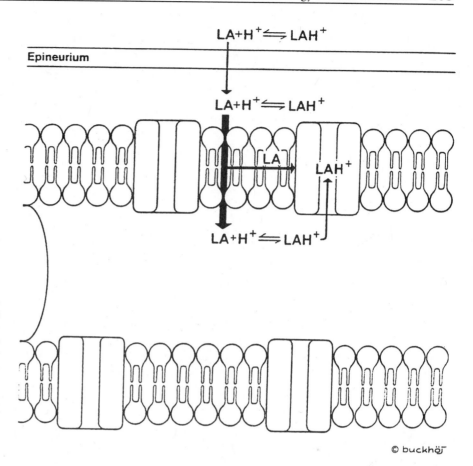

$$LA + H^+ \rightleftharpoons LAH^+$$

Epineurium

$$LA + H^+ \rightleftharpoons LAH^+$$

$$LA \rightarrow LAH^+$$

$$LA + H^+ \rightleftharpoons LAH^+$$

© buckhöj

Figure 17-3

Local anesthetics diffuse across the nerve membrane in the uncharged form. Once inside the nerve, they become positively charged and attach themselves to the outer part of the sodium channel.

(Reprinted by permission from Scott DB, Techniques of Regional Anaesthesia. *Norwalk, Conn: Appleton & Lange, 1989.)*

loss of pain and temperature sensation, loss of proprioception, loss of touch and pressure sensation, and finally motor paralysis. The sensitivity of nerve fibers to local anesthetics depends on size, location within the nerve, and myelination. Of the sensory nerve fibers, the small A∂ and unmyelinated C fibers (which are nociceptors responding to injurious stimuli only) are most sensitive to local anesthetics, whereas the sensory Aβ (nonnociceptors) and the large myelinated motor fibers are most resistant. The anatomy of the nerve also affects the apparent sensitivities of the nerve fibers. Those fibers which are located close to the nerve surface and exposed to the solution of local anesthetic (sensory nerve fibers) are more easily and promptly blocked. Myelination confers resistance to the effects of local anesthetics.

Pharmacology of Local Anesthetics

Local anesthetic molecules consist of an aromatic ring and a carbon chain bearing an amino group; these two components are joined by an ester or an amide link (Table 17-1). The esters include procaine, cocaine, 2-chloroprocaine, and tetracaine; the amides are lidocaine, mepivacaine, prilocaine, bupivacaine, etidocaine, and ropivacaine. The two classes of local anesthetics differ with regard to metabolism, allergic potential, and stability (Table 17-2), but the primary pharmacologic characteristics of each drug is determined by lipid solubility, protein binding, pK_a, and vasodilation.

■ Lipid Solubility

The more lipid-soluble local anesthetic molecules penetrate the nerve membrane more easily and have greater intrinsic anesthetic potency (Fig. 17-4). There is a direct correlation between the lipid:water partition coefficient of a local anesthetic and the minimum concentration required for conduction blockade. Agents with partition coefficients of less than 1 require concentrations of 2% to 3% for conduction blockade; those with coefficients of 1 to 3 require

Table 17-1

The Local Anesthetics

Agent	Chemical Configuration — Aromatic Lipophilic	Intermediate Chain	Amine Hydrophilic	Molecular Weight (Base)	PK_a (25°C)	Partition Coefficient	Percent Protein Binding	Onset	Relative Potency	Duration
ESTERS										
Procaine				236	8.9	0.02	6	Slow	1	Short
Tetracaine				264	8.5	4.1	76	Slow	8	Long
Chloroprocaine				271	8.7	0.14	—	Fast	1	Short
AMIDES										
Prilocaine				220	7.9	0.9	55	Fast	2	Moderate
Lidocaine				234	7.9	2.9	64	Fast	2	Moderate
Mepivacaine				246	7.6	0.8	78	Fast	2	Moderate
Bupivacaine				288	8.1	27.5	96	Slow	8	Long
Etidocaine				276	7.7	14.1	94	Fast	6	Long
Ropivacaine				274	8.1	6.1	92	Slow	8	Long

Procaine:
H_2N—(benzene ring)—$\overset{O}{\underset{}{C}}$—O—$(CH_2)_2$—N$\begin{cases} C_2H_5 \\ C_2H_5 \end{cases}$

Tetracaine:
$\overset{H}{\underset{C_4H_9}{N}}$—(benzene ring)—$\overset{O}{\underset{}{C}}$—O—$(CH_2)_2$—N$\begin{cases} CH_3 \\ CH_3 \end{cases}$

Chloroprocaine:
H_2N—(benzene ring with Cl)—$\overset{O}{\underset{}{C}}$—O—$(CH_2)_2$—N$\begin{cases} C_2H_5 \\ C_2H_5 \end{cases}$

Prilocaine:
(benzene ring with CH_3)—NH—$\overset{O}{\underset{}{C}}$—CH($CH_3$)—N$\begin{cases} C_3H_7 \\ H \end{cases}$

Lidocaine:
(benzene ring with two CH_3)—NH—$\overset{O}{\underset{}{C}}$—$CH_2$—N$\begin{cases} C_2H_5 \\ C_2H_5 \end{cases}$

Mepivacaine:
(benzene ring with two CH_3)—NH—CO—(piperidine ring with N—CH_3)

Bupivacaine:
(benzene ring with two CH_3)—NH—CO—(piperidine ring with N—C_4H_9)

Etidocaine:
(benzene ring with two CH_3)—NH—$\overset{O}{\underset{}{C}}$—CH($C_2H_5$)—N$\begin{cases} C_2H_5 \\ C_3H_7 \end{cases}$

Ropivacaine:
(benzene ring with two CH_3)—NH—CO—(piperidine ring with N—C_3H_7, H)

Table 17-2

	Metabolism	Stability in Solution	Allergic Reaction
Characteristics of Ester and Amide Local Anesthetics			
Esters	Plasma esterase	Unstable	Rare
Amides	Hepatic enzymatic	Stable	Very rare

concentrations of 1% to 2%; lipid-soluble agents with partition coefficients of greater than 4 are effective at concentrations of 0.25% to 0.5%.

■ Protein Binding

The duration of action of a local anesthetic depends on binding to the protein components of the nerve membrane. Agents of short duration, such as procaine, bind poorly. Tetracaine, bupivacaine, and etidocaine avidly bind to membrane proteins and are effective for long periods. Local anesthetics also bind to two principal sites in the plasma: alpha-glycoprotein and albumin.

■ pK_a

In solution, some local anesthetic molecules are unionized free base (B), while others accept a hydrogen ion and carry a positive charge:

$$B + H^+ \leftrightarrow BH^+$$

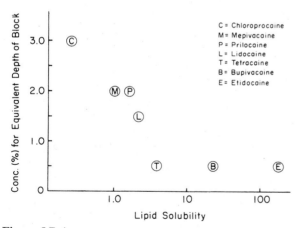

Figure 17-4

Relation between lipid solubility and inherent potency of local anesthetics.

(Reprinted by permission from Covino BG, Clinical pharmacology of local anesthetics. In Cousins MJ, Bridenbaugh PO, eds: Neural Blockade, *2nd ed. Philadelphia: JB Lippincott, 1988.)*

Since conduction blockade depends on the diffusion of local anesthetic molecules through lipid cell membranes to reach the inside of the neurons, the greater the fraction of the drug that is in the more lipid-soluble uncharged free base form, the faster is the onset of anesthesia. The relationship between the concentrations of the uncharged and charged forms depends on the hydrogen ion concentration:

$$\log([B]/[BH^+]) = pH - pK_a$$

When the pH of the solution is the same as the pK_a of the drug, the ionized and un-ionized forms are present in equal amounts. As one would expect, local anesthetics of lesser pK_a, such as lidocaine at 7.9, act more quickly than those of greater pK_a, such as bupivacaine at 8.1 (Fig. 17-5).

The onset of anesthesia can be hastened by administering a greater mass of drug, thereby increasing the concentration gradient that drives diffusion. Chloroprocaine has a pK_a of 8.7 and should be slow in onset. However, when given in concentrations of 3%, it produces rapid onset of blockade.

■ Intrinsic Vascular Activity

Local anesthetics alter vascular tone in a dose-dependent manner; the usual clinical concentration causes local vasodilation. The vasodilator actions of local anesthetics influence efficacy and duration of action. After injection of a local anesthetic agent, some is taken up by neural tissue, and some is carried away by the blood that perfuses the area in which the drug is injected. Although the intrinsic anesthetic potency of lidocaine is greater than that of mepivacaine, it also produces more vasodilation, so in clinical use lidocaine is no more potent than mepivacaine and has a shorter duration of action. Cocaine provides an exception to the rule and is associated with vasoconstriction (due to blockade of neural uptake of norepinephrine).

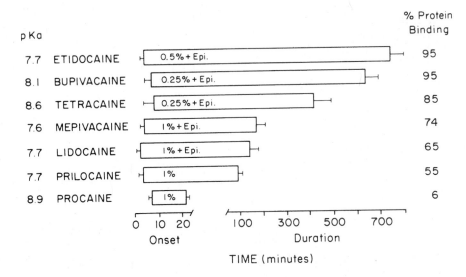

Figure 17-5

Relation between pK_a and onset of anesthesia *(left)* and relation between protein binding and duration of anesthesia *(right)*.

(Reprinted by permission from Covino BG, Clinical pharmacology of local anesthetic agents. In Cousins MJ, Bridenbaugh PO, eds: Neural Blockade, 2nd ed. Philadelphia: JB Lippincott, 1988.)

Specific Local Anesthetics

Although many local anesthetics have been developed, a relatively small number provide the com-plete range of effects useful in clinical practice (Table 17-3).

■ Ester-Derived Local Anesthetics

Cocaine

Because of the risks of systemic toxicity and addiction, cocaine is not used for regional anesthetic techniques. Applied as a topical anesthetic, it produces vasoconstriction, making it useful for anesthetizing the nasal mucosa prior to nasotracheal intubation and for nasal sinus operations. Solutions of other local anesthetics to which vasoconstrictors such as phenylephrine have been added mimic this effect.

Procaine

Procaine penetrates tissues poorly, produces anesthesia slowly, and dissipates rapidly. Because of rapid hydrolysis by plasma pseudocholinesterase, it can be used safely in large amounts with little fear of systemic toxicity. Its primary uses are infiltration anesthesia, differential spinal blockade, and occasionally, spinal anesthesia.

Chloroprocaine

Chloroprocaine is short-acting, not very potent, and not likely to cause systemic toxicity. Several case reports have described permanent paraplegia from the inadvertent subarachnoid administration of chloroprocaine during epidural anesthesia owing to its low pH and the use of sodium bisulfite preservative. Replacing the bisulfite with EDTA has led to reports of severe spasmodic back pain after large epidural doses of chloroprocaine; binding of calcium by EDTA results in hypocalcemic tetany in the paraspinous muscles. Chloroprocaine shortens the duration of the effect of bupivacaine when the two are administered as a mixture into the epidural space, and epidural chloroprocaine antagonizes the analgesic effect of subsequently administered epidural opioids.

Table 17-3

Classification of Local Anesthetics Based on Potency and Duration

Based on differences in anesthetic potency (lipid solubility) and duration of action (protein binding), the local anesthetic compounds fall into three categories:

1. Agents of weak anesthetic potency and short duration of action:
   Procaine
   Chloroprocaine
2. Agents of intermediate anesthetic potency and duration of action:
   Lidocaine
   Mepivacaine
   Prilocaine
3. Agents of great anesthetic potency and long duration of action:
   Tetracaine
   Bupivacaine
   Etidocaine
   Ropivacaine

Tetracaine

Tetracaine is a long-acting, potent anesthetic. It is used primarily for spinal anesthesia in isobaric, hypobaric, or hyperbaric solutions, providing rapid onset, good sensory anesthesia, and profound motor blockade that is of longer duration than the sensory blockade. Isobaric solutions of tetracaine produce 2 to 3 hours of spinal anesthesia; the addition of epinephrine can extend the duration to 4 to 6 hours. Tetracaine is an excellent topical anesthetic also and is useful for corneal and endotracheal topical anesthesia. Rapid absorption of this drug from the tracheobronchial tree can produce toxicity.

■ Amide Agents

Lidocaine

Lidocaine was the first drug of the amide class to be introduced into clinical practice. Its potency, rapid onset, moderate duration of action, and topical anesthetic activity make it the most versatile and commonly used local anesthetic. Solutions of lidocaine are available for infiltration, peripheral nerve block, and spinal or epidural anesthesia; ointment, jelly, and aerosol forms are applied topically. Intravenous lidocaine is of value as an antiarrhythmic, an antiepileptic, an analgesic, a cough suppressant, and a supplement to general anesthesia.

Mepivacaine

The effects of mepivacaine are similar to those of lidocaine, although its metabolism is markedly prolonged in the fetus and the newborn, so it is not employed for obstetric anesthesia. In adults, mepivacaine is apparently less toxic than lidocaine. The duration of its effect is longer than that of lidocaine due to less marked vasodilation.

Prilocaine

Prilocaine is similar to lidocaine, rapidly producing profound block of moderate duration. It causes significantly less vasodilation than does lidocaine, so prilocaine without epinephrine has a duration of effect similar to that of lidocaine with epinephrine, making prilocaine particularly useful in patients in whom epinephrine is contraindicated. It is the least toxic of the amide local anesthetics, making it particularly useful for intravenous regional anesthesia, since central nervous system toxicity rarely occurs after tourniquet release. Methemoglobinemia may follow the use of large doses (more than 600 mg) in adults; the risk of methemoglobinemia in the newborn rules out its use in obstetric anesthesia.

Bupivacaine

Bupivacaine provides anesthesia of slow onset and long duration; it is both potent and toxic. In lesser concentrations, it produces excellent sensory analgesia with little or no motor impairment, unlike most local anesthetics. This may be due to the alkaline pK_a of this agent: At physiologic pH, few uncharged molecules are available to penetrate the diffusion barriers surrounding large motor fibers. Such differential blockade is important in the use of this drug for obstetric and postoperative analgesia.

Bupivacaine is more cardiotoxic than lidocaine. Both bupivacaine and lidocaine block the sodium channels in the heart and depress conduction. However, bupivacaine binds to the open sodium channel for a much longer time than does lidocaine, making bupivacaine 16 times more potent than lidocaine in reducing cardiac contractility.

Etidocaine

Etidocaine produces conduction blockade of rapid onset and long duration, with the depth and duration of motor blockade exceeding those of sensory block. Because of this, it is used primarily for operations where muscle relaxation is especially important.

Ropivacaine

Ropivacaine is a new amide local anesthetic structurally similar to mepivacaine and bupivacaine but prepared as the (S)-isomer rather than as a racemic mixture, as is common for other local anesthetic solutions. Its pK_a and plasma protein binding are similar to those of bupivacaine, but it is less lipid-soluble. At a concentration of 0.5%, it produces less motor blockade than does bupivacaine. Ropivacaine is eliminated more rapidly than bupivacaine, resulting in less myocardial toxicity.

Pharmacokinetics of Local Anesthetic Agents

Absorption from the site of injection, redistribution of the drug, and metabolism and excretion determine the concentration in the blood that results from the injection of a given dose of local anesthetic.

Patient-related factors such as age and hepatic function also influence the physiologic disposition of local anesthetics. Because effective regional anesthesia may require using nearly the maximum safe dose of local anesthetic, it is important to consider these factors in each patient before selecting the technique, the drug concentration, and the total dose to be administered.

■ Absorption

The site of injection, dose, addition of vasoconstrictor agents, and the vasoactive properties of the local anesthetic control the systemic absorption of the drug. The most rapid absorption and greatest peak blood concentrations are seen after intercostal nerve block, followed by caudal block, lumbar epidural block, brachial plexus block, subcutaneous tissue infiltration, and subarachnoid block (Fig. 17-6). A quantity of local anesthetic agent may be safe when given at one site but toxic when given at another. For example, 400 mg of lidocaine without epinephrine administered for intercostal blockade results in greater blood concentrations than when administered for brachial plexus blockade.

Local anesthetic solutions often include a vasoconstrictor to retard absorption, usually epinephrine in a concentration of 5 µg/ml. The addition of a vasoconstrictor prolongs the duration of anesthesia, decreases peak blood concentrations, and permits the use of larger amounts of local anesthetic without increased risk of systemic toxicity.

The physical and chemical characteristics of the specific local anesthetic drug also influence the rate and degree of vascular absorption. After epidural administration, etidocaine produces lesser peak blood concentrations than does bupivacaine, although both have similar vasodilator activity. The greater lipid solubility of etidocaine may result in sequestration by the epidural fat, slowing vascular absorption and decreasing peak blood concentration.

■ Distribution

Like other drugs used in anesthesia, the distribution of local anesthetics can be described by a two- or three-compartment model (Fig. 17-7). Blood concentrations decrease rapidly as the drug is redistributed to well-perfused tissue and more slowly as the drug is taken up elsewhere, metabolized, and excreted. Prilocaine redistributes more rapidly from blood to tissues than does lidocaine or mepivacaine and also has a more rapid rate of metabolism. Etidocaine shows a more rapid rate of tissue redistribution and metabolism than does bupivacaine.

■ Metabolism and Excretion

The metabolism of local anesthetics depends on their chemical structures. Esters are hydrolyzed in the plasma by pseudocholinesterase, but the rate of metabolism varies markedly among drugs. Chloroprocaine undergoes the most rapid hydrolysis, 4.7 µmol/ml per hour, compared with 1.1 µmol/ml per hour for procaine and 0.3 µmol/ml per hour for tetracaine.

Amides are broken down in the liver by N-dealkylation of the tertiary amine and then hydroxylation of the aromatic nucleus. Prilocaine is metabolized the most rapidly, lidocaine at an intermediate

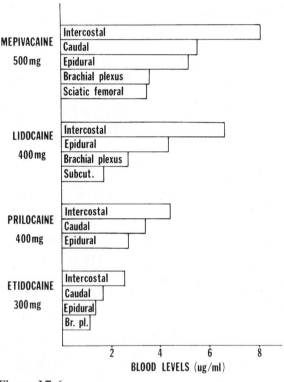

Figure 17-6

Comparative peak blood concentrations of several local anesthetic agents following various blocks.

(Reprinted by permission from Covino BG, Vassallo HG, Local Anesthetics: Mechanism of Action and Clinical Use. *New York: Grune & Stratton, 1976.)*

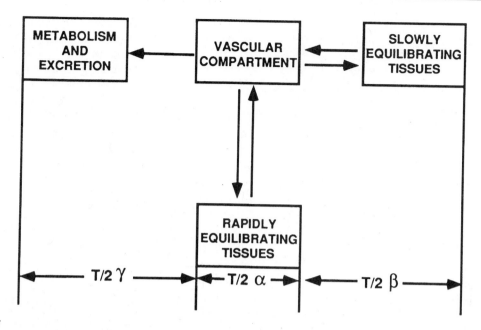

Figure 17-7

Pharmacokinetic phases according to a three-compartment model.
(Reprinted by permission from Covino BG, Vassalo HG, Local Anesthetics: Mechanism of Action and Clinical Use. *New York: Grune & Stratton, 1976, p 110.)*

rate, and mepivacaine somewhat more slowly. Clearance rates of amide local anesthetics are identical to their rates of hepatic metabolism, since direct renal elimination is negligible.

The disposition of local anesthetics depends on the patient's age and health. The elimination half-life of lidocaine in patients 22 to 26 years of age is 81 minutes, compared with 139 minutes in patients 61 to 71 years of age. The elimination of lidocaine may be slowed several-fold in patients with liver disease. Although single-injection techniques tend to be safe in these patients, the administration of additional local anesthetic must be curtailed to account for the slow disposition of the drug.

Choosing a Local Anesthetic Mixture

Table 17-4 lists the local anesthetics and their primary uses (injection sites). As a rule, the actions of the many available local anesthetics are more alike than they are different; almost any local anesthetic can be made to work for any kind of regional anesthesia. In practice, it is best to employ a small number of drugs whose pharmacologic properties are well understood. When there are special advantages to particular local anesthetics, the choice depends on the planned nerve block, duration of anesthesia, speed of onset, and potential toxicity.

■Local Anesthetics for Specific Nerve Blocks

Neurologic complications after spinal anesthesia are rare but devastating. For this reason, practitioners use only a small number of drugs with well-established records for safe use in spinal anesthesia. These include tetracaine, lidocaine, and bupivacaine in hyperbaric, isobaric, and hypobaric formulations. Additives are limited to preservative-free opioids and epinephrine, which is added to prolong duration. The dose of epinephrine (200 µg) is chosen to yield an expected concentration of 5 µg/ml when diluted in the 40 ml of cerebrospinal fluid (CSF) in the lumbosacral region of an adult. There is no need to add sodium bicarbonate to increase the pH of the solution because the small amount of drug is effectively buffered by the CSF into which it is injected.

Table 17-4

Uses of Common Local Anesthetics	
Agent	**Uses**
Cocaine	Topical
Procaine	Infiltration
	Differential spinal
	Spinal
Chloroprocaine	Brachial plexus
	Epidural
Lidocaine	Topical
	Infiltration
	IV regional
	Brachial plexus
	Spinal
	Epidural
Mepivacaine	Infiltration
	Brachial plexus
	Spinal
	Epidural
Prilocaine	Infiltration
	IV regional
	Brachial plexus
	Epidural
Bupivacaine	Infiltration
	Brachial plexus
	Epidural
	Spinal
Etidocaine	Infiltration
	Epidural
Tetracaine	Topical
	Spinal
Ropivacaine	Infiltration
	Brachial plexus
	Epidural
	Spinal

For epidural anesthesia, bupivacaine and lidocaine are most popular, although chloroprocaine and etidocaine are used occasionally. Additives include preservative-free opioids and epinephrine, usually in the amount of 5 μg/ml of local anesthetic solution. In contrast to the small doses employed in spinal anesthesia, epidural anesthesia requires much greater quantities of local anesthetics, whose actions are improved by the addition of sodium bicarbonate (see below).

For peripheral neural blocks, lidocaine, bupivacaine, and mepivacaine are popular. Additives include vasoconstrictors and sodium bicarbonate.

■ Duration of Blockade

On first consideration, it might seem best to choose local anesthetics to provide the longest pos-

sible duration of effect so as to delay as long as possible the onset of postoperative pain. There are significant disadvantages to this practice. First, the molecular properties that confer long action on local anesthetics (protein binding) also imply slow onset of action, which is a major obstacle to the practical use of regional anesthesia. Second, prolonged anesthesia with paralysis may delay recovery and discharge from the recovery room when a patient undergoes an outpatient operation. Third, delayed recovery from the anesthetic hinders prompt postoperative evaluation of possible neurologic damage (from the operation or the anesthetic), compartment syndromes, or tight plaster casts. Fourth, bladder distension and failure to void are common complications exacerbated by prolonged spinal or epidural anesthesia. Thus most practitioners choose a local anesthetic drug with the goal of providing surgical anesthesia that exceeds the duration of the operation only by enough time to allow for reasonable operative delays. A catheter, such as used in continuous spinal, epidural, or brachial plexus anesthesia, permits reinjecting local anesthetic and controlling the duration of the anesthesia.

■ Improving Onset of Anesthesia: Carbonation and Bicarbonate

The slow onset of anesthesia with bupivacaine and other long-acting drugs (30 minutes or longer to full effect) may require that the block be performed outside the operating room in a patient holding area. Although such holding areas are convenient, they are not always available. Choosing a faster-acting drug such as lidocaine or mepivacaine is the most direct approach to this problem. When this is not possible, other methods can be used to speed the onset of regional anesthesia.

Because diffusion of the local anesthetic into the interior of the axon depends on the unionized lipophilic base, the onset of anesthesia can be hastened by adding CO_2 to the local anesthetic (carbonating) or by increasing its pH with sodium bicarbonate. CO_2 from carbonated solutions diffuses across the nerve membrane, thereby increasing the intracellular hydrogen ion concentration. This in turn increases the fraction of intracellular local anesthetic that is protonated, or charged, and is unable to diffuse back out of the neuron. This "ion trapping" produces a more profound block more rapidly, as compared with that produced by uncarbonated formulations of local

Table 17-5

Amount of Sodium Bicarbonate for Alkalinization of Local Anesthetic Solutions

Local Anesthetic (pK_a)	HCO$_3^-$ Required (mEq/20 ml)
Chloroprocaine 3% (8.7)	1.92
Mepivacaine 1.5% (7.6)	1.92
Etidocaine 1% to 1.5% (7.7)	0.048
Bupivacaine 0.25% (8.1)	0.024
Lidocaine 1% to 2% (7.9)	1.92

anesthetic. Carbonated local anesthetics are only available commercially in Canada and some European countries.

The usual anesthetic solution is manufactured to have a pH of 3.5 to 6.5 to enhance shelf life and solubility. Adding sodium bicarbonate brings the pH of the solution closer to the pK_a of the local anesthetic, thereby increasing the relative concentration of the uncharged form of the molecule and shortening latency. Increasing the pH too much causes precipitation of the relatively insoluble free base. Solutions of chloroprocaine and lidocaine can be brought to near physiologic pH without precipitation. Delayed precipitation occurs in mepivacaine solutions above neutral pH. Bupivacaine and etidocaine solutions form precipitates after the addition of small amounts of sodium bicarbonate and cannot be alkalinized to physiologic pH. These more alkaline solutions of local anesthetics also cause less pain when used for local infiltration (Table 17-5).

Local anesthetic solutions manufactured with epinephrine are supplied at a pH of 3.5 to prevent oxidation of the epinephrine. The speed of onset of anesthesia is greatly improved by increasing the pH of these solutions. An alternative is to purchase local anesthetic solutions manufactured without added epinephrine, which are typically less acid, and adding the epinephrine just before injection, but objective clinical studies demonstrate that premixed solutions can result in rapid onset of analgesia when sodium bicarbonate is added prior to injection.

Toxicity of Local Anesthetic Agents

Local anesthetics produce few side effects when given in an appropriate dose at the proper site. Most

toxic reactions occur after the accidental intravascular injection of a large dose of local anesthetic, although an excessive dose given into an appropriate anatomic location can lead to systemic toxicity.

■ Systemic Toxicity

Systemic effects of local anesthetics occur when the drugs reach the circulation from the site of injection. When they are mistakenly injected in large doses into an artery or vein and the anesthetic appears in the blood as a bolus, a catastrophic combination of seizures, coma, arrhythmias, and cardiac arrest can occur. When the blood concentration of local anesthetic increases more slowly due to uptake from tissue, there appears gradually a characteristic spectrum of effects, each representing a specific concentration of anesthetic. Aside from methemoglobinemia and other minor effects specific to individual drugs, these systemic effects all result from interference with sodium channels in electrically excitable membranes in the heart and the nervous system.

Central Nervous System Toxicity

Toxic effects of local anesthetics occur in the central nervous system (CNS) at lesser blood concentrations than are required to produce cardiovascular toxicity; therefore, CNS toxicity appears earlier than cardiovascular toxicity in the typical clinical course of a toxic reaction that follows slow uptake of drug. In the order of appearance, these CNS signs and symptoms consist of lightheadedness, dizziness, a metallic taste in the mouth, numbness of the tongue or lips, slurred speech, tinnitus, agitation, seizures, sedation, and coma (Table 17-6). The seizures appear to be due

Table 17-6

Signs and Symptoms of Local Anesthetic-Induced CNS Toxicity

Initial events
  Tinnitus
  Lightheadedness
  Confusion
  Circumoral numbness
Excitation phase
  Tonic-clonic convulsions
Depression phase
  Unconsciousness
  Generalized CNS depression
  Respiratory arrest

to suppression of inhibitory neurons by the local anesthetic; the seizures result from disinhibited cortical neurons. If the concentration in the blood increases slowly enough, or if sedatives or anticonvulsants are used, there may be no excitation or seizures but instead profound sedation. In fact, administration of lidocaine in near-toxic doses shifts the dose-response curve of enflurane to the left by 0.3 MAC, indicating that the depressant effects of local anesthetics on the CNS contribute to general anesthesia. Because both local anesthetic effects and CNS toxicity are due to the effects of these drugs on neuronal sodium channels, the intrinsic anesthetic potencies of local anesthetics correlate directly with their potential to cause CNS toxicity.

Cardiovascular Toxicity

Cardiovascular toxicity occurs at greater blood concentrations of local anesthetics than does CNS toxicity and is rarely seen in clinical practice unless the local anesthetic is mistakenly injected into a blood vessel. Direct effects on the cardiovascular system depend on dose and include myocardial depression, vasodilation, and impaired cardiac conduction. Local anesthetics inhibit depolarization in cardiac muscle by preventing sodium conduction through the sodium channels. The accompanying decrease in contractility depresses cardiac output. All local anesthetics exert a dose-dependent negative inotropic action on cardiac muscle that is proportional to their abilities to suppress conduction in peripheral nerves.

As the blood concentration of local anesthetic increases, cardiovascular events follow in sequence. Concentrations of local anesthetics that cause CNS excitation result indirectly in sympathetically mediated increases in heart rate, blood pressure, and cardiac output. At nontoxic blood concentrations, a slight increase in blood pressure may occur owing to a small increase in cardiac output and heart rate due to sympathetic stimulation. Further increases in blood concentration of local anesthetics produce cardiovascular depression due to negative inotropy, peripheral vasodilation, and depressant effects on cardiac conduction and muscle contraction.

Bupivacaine exerts relatively greater cardiotoxic effects than lidocaine when the two are compared at doses equipotent for local anesthetic effects. Myocardial depression is more profound, refractory ventricular fibrillation may occur, metabolic acidosis is more severe, and resuscitation may be much more difficult with bupivacaine. The prolonged occupancy of so-dium channels by bupivacaine and depression of the rapid phase of depolarization impair contractility (by preventing complete restoration of V_{max} between beats), a problem that does not occur with lidocaine. Ropivacaine may offer a duration of effect similar to that of bupivacaine without the enhanced cardiotoxicity. The risk of cardiotoxicity has led to the abandonment of bupivacaine for intravenous regional anesthesia.

Precautions Against Systemic Toxicity

Several precautions can decrease the potential for harm due to systemic toxic reactions from local anesthetics. First, adequate drugs and equipment for treatment of reactions and resuscitation must be at hand whenever the total dose of local anesthetic being administered at one time is great enough to do harm if it were injected intravenously (1.5 mg/kg for lidocaine or the equivalent for other drugs). Included in the precautions is an intravenous catheter. Second, the patient must be monitored constantly for symptoms and signs of systemic toxicity so that the injection may be stopped and treatment begun. Third, large doses of local anesthetics are best administered in divided doses, with frequent aspiration to test for blood. Thus the dose of any drug mistakenly given intravascularly can be limited. Fourth, adding epinephrine solution not only slows the uptake of the drug but provides a sensitive marker for intravascular injection. For example, if a solution of 1.5% lidocaine with epinephrine 5 μg/ml is injected into an epidural vein, after 3 ml has been given, the 15 μg of epinephrine would produce noticeable tachycardia, but the 45 mg of lidocaine would have no systemic effects. Fifth, benzodiazepines may serve as prophylactic anticonvulsants, although the doses required may obscure the signs of CNS toxicity that warn of impending cardiovascular depression.

Treatment of Systemic Toxicity

If CNS toxicity is detected, one halts the injection of local anesthetic. Usually, oxygen and reassurance suffice because the drug is quickly redistributed and the blood concentration decreases immediately. For seizures, treatment consists of hyperventilation with 100% oxygen, since CNS toxicity is exacerbated by hypercarbia. If the seizure continues, small doses of a benzodiazepine (midazolam 1 to 3 mg) or thiopental (25 to 50 mg) may be required. The advantage of thiopental is its ready accessibility in anesthesia practice; the disadvantage is the risk of apnea with larger

Table 17-7

Algorithm for Preventing and Treating Local Anesthetic Toxicity

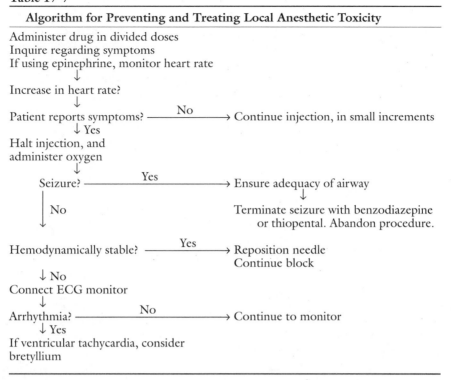

Administer drug in divided doses
Inquire regarding symptoms
If using epinephrine, monitor heart rate
↓
Increase in heart rate?
↓
Patient reports symptoms? ——— No ——→ Continue injection, in small increments
↓ Yes
Halt injection, and
administer oxygen
↓
Seizure? ——— Yes ——→ Ensure adequacy of airway
↓
| No
| Terminate seizure with benzodiazepine
| or thiopental. Abandon procedure.
↓

Hemodynamically stable? ——— Yes ——→ Reposition needle
Continue block
↓ No
Connect ECG monitor
↓
Arrhythmia? ——— No ——→ Continue to monitor
↓ Yes
If ventricular tachycardia, consider
bretyllium

doses. If ventilation is inadequate during the seizure, 20 to 40 mg of intravenous succinylcholine may allow insertion of an oral airway and success with mask ventilation. Intubation of the trachea is required if the patient has a full stomach or if mask ventilation is impossible.

Severe cardiovascular toxicity occurs in the form of ventricular tachycardia or, more commonly, electromechanical dissociation. Resuscitation includes epinephrine with atropine for electromechanical dissociation and bradycardia. Since both respiratory and metabolic acidosis can be severe and can exacerbate toxicity, blood gas analysis, adequate ventilation, and sodium bicarbonate treatments are essential. Bretylium may be required for ventricular tachycardia; direct current cardioversion is usually not helpful (Table 17-7). Protracted efforts at resuscitation are indicated, since the toxic cardiac effects of the local anesthetic will abate if the drug can be redistributed to other tissues by continued circulatory support.

Maximum Recommended Doses

The maximum recommended doses for local anesthetics are intended to prevent systemic toxic reactions. Since peak plasma drug concentrations depend greatly on the site of injection, a single maximum dose cannot be recommended for all uses of a drug. For example, injecting 300 mg of lidocaine in the intercostal region, 500 mg epidurally, 600 mg in the brachial plexus, and 1000 mg subcutaneously all result in plasma concentrations of approximately 5 µg/ml, which usually does not cause toxic reactions. However, the maximum dose of lidocaine without epinephrine that is recommended by the manufacturer is 5 mg/kg (approximately 350 mg), regardless of the site of injection. This maximum recommended amount is insufficient for brachial plexus and epidural anesthetics and does not take into account factors such as the site of injection.

The addition of epinephrine (5 µg/ml) reduces vascular absorption and peak plasma concentrations of lidocaine by 20 to 30 percent after intercostal, brachial plexus, or epidural injection and 50 percent after subcutaneous injection. The maximum recommended dose for lidocaine with epinephrine is 7 mg/kg. Some expert anesthesiologists question the logic behind these recommended dosages and may exceed them, depending on the circumstances. Although the maximum recommended doses may seem too small, they are regarded as safe and appropriate

Table 17-8

Manufacturers' Recommended Maximum Doses for Single Injections

Drug	mg/kg without Epinephrine	mg/kg with Epinephrine
Chloroprocaine	11	14
Lidocaine	4	7
Mepivacaine	4	7
Prilocaine	7	8.5
Bupivacaine	2.5	3.2
Etidocaine	6	8

Note: These doses may be exceeded depending on the block performed and the clinical situation.

limits for the neophyte. Adding epinephrine to the local anesthetic often permits increasing the dose without exceeding the manufacturer's recommendations (Table 17-8).

■ Local Tissue Toxicity

Local anesthetics may exert toxic effects on tissues at the site of injection, although they rarely produce localized nerve damage in concentrations employed clinically. However, exposing nerves in vitro to concentrations of lidocaine greater than used clinically for longer than 3 minutes produces irreversible damage. Prolonged sensorimotor deficits have occurred in patients following the subarachnoid administration of hyperbaric lidocaine through small spinal catheters. Apparently, these spinal catheters permit only the slow administration of dextrose-containing solutions of lidocaine, promoting the pooling of toxic concentrations of drug in the cauda equina.

■ Allergy

The ester-based local anesthetics are metabolized to *para*-aminobenzoic acid, which may be responsible for the allergic reactions to these drugs. The amide local anesthetics are not derivatives of *para*-aminobenzoic acid and rarely cause allergic reactions. Solutions of the amide agents may contain a preservative, methylparaben, whose chemical structure is similar to *para*-aminobenzoic acid and is often responsible for allergic reactions attributed to amide local anesthetics. Minor reactions may be manifest as erythema, urticaria, and edema; systemic reactions consist of generalized erythema, edema, bronchoconstriction, and hypotension.

Occasionally, patients indicate that they are allergic to local anesthetics. A careful history usually differentiates between true allergic responses and other more frequent reactions. The effect of added epinephrine may be remembered as a racing or irregular heartbeat, sweaty palms, or anxiety. After a systemic toxic reac-

Table 17-9

Is This Patient Truly Allergic to Local Anesthetic?

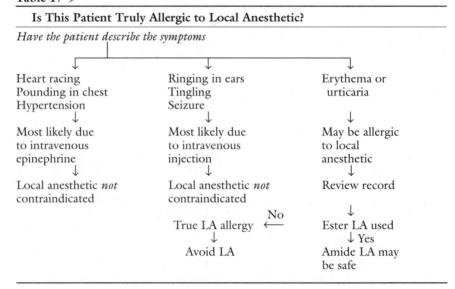

tion, the patient may describe tinnitus, visual hallucinations, anxiety, or a sense of dread. Patients who suffer vasovagal responses may recall faintness, palpitations, nausea, or sweating. Further investigation involves intradermal injection of small amounts (0.1 ml) of dilute solutions of the local anesthetic in question, the preservative methylparaben, and then progressively greater doses of local anesthetic (Table 17-9). If the patient seems to have had a genuine allergic response, it may be helpful to use preservative-free solutions or to select a local anesthetic from the class of drugs that was not implicated in the patient's previous reaction.

BIBLIOGRAPHY

Butterworth JF, Strichartz GR. Molecular mechanisms of nerve block by local anesthetics. *Anesthesiology* 1990;72:711-734.

Covino BG. Pharmacology of local anaesthetics. *Br J Anaesth* 1986;58:717-731.

Covino BG. Toxicity of local anesthetics. *Adv Anesth* 1986; 3:37-65.

Eisenach JC, Schlairet TJ, et al. Effect of prior anesthetic solution on epidural morphine analgesia. *Anesth Analg* 1991;73:119-123.

Hynson JM, Sessler DI, Glosten B. Back pain in volunteers after epidural anesthesia with chloroprocaine. *Anesth Analg* 1991;72:253-256.

Peterfreund RA, Datta S, Ostheimer GW. pH adjustment of local anesthetic solutions with sodium bicarbonate: Laboratory evaluations of alkalinization and precipitation. *Reg Anesth* 1989;14:

CHAPTER 18

Spinal, Epidural, and Caudal Anesthesia

Robert R. Gaiser

Spinal anesthesia results from the injection of local anesthetics into the cerebrospinal fluid, reached by lumbar subarachnoid puncture only. Depending on the dose, the local anesthetic may produce neurologic effects ranging from mild loss of temperature sense to complete anesthesia over an area of a few dermatomes or the entire body. The same effects result when tenfold larger doses of local anesthetic are injected into the epidural space, although the epidural space can be reached at any level below the foramen magnum. These techniques were introduced in the early twentieth century and appealed to physicians and patients alike as a means of avoiding the complications of general anesthesia. After 1950, the popularity of major conduction anesthesia waned in the United States as general anesthesia became safer and more pleasant for the patient. Beginning in 1975, it was recognized that spinal and epidural anesthesia confer benefits of their own and are not simply alternatives to general anesthesia, making these techniques essential in the care of the surgical patient.

Anatomy

■ Spine

The spinal column consists of 7 cervical, 12 thoracic, 5 lumbar, and 5 fused sacral vertebrae (Fig. 18-1). A vertebra consists of a vertebral body and an arch that comprises two pedicles anteriorly and two laminae posteriorly. At the junction of the pedicle and the lamina is the transverse process; the spinous process arises from the junction of the laminae in the posterior midline. Although the laminae and the spinous processes of successive vertebrae are joined by ligaments, the pedicles are not, forming gaps through which the spinal nerves exit the spinal canal (Fig. 18-2).

■ Spinal Cord

The spinal canal lies within the vertebral column between the foramen magnum and the sacral hiatus, bounded anteriorly by the vertebral bodies, laterally by the pedicles, and posteriorly by the laminae. The spinal cord proper extends within the canal from the brainstem to its termination at the L1-2 vertebral level in the adult. The remaining lower lumbar and sacral nerve roots continue within the spinal canal as the cauda equina.

Three membranes cover the spinal cord: the pia mater, the arachnoid mater, and the dura mater. These create three spaces. Between the pia mater, which is closely attached to the spinal cord, and the arachnoid mater, the subarachnoid space extends from the cranium caudad to the level of S2 and contains nerve roots and cerebrospinal fluid (CSF). The subdural space lies between the dura mater and the arachnoid mater; although this is a potential space only, occasionally drugs meant for the epidural or subarachnoid spaces are injected into it. The resulting subdural

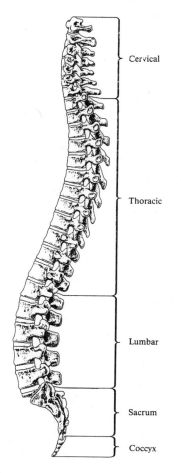

Figure 18-1

The spinal column is not straight; rather, there is a thoracic kyphosis and a lumbar lordosis.

(Reprinted by permission from the artist [Buckhöj] and Scott DB, Techniques of Regional Anaesthesia. *Norwalk, Conn: Appleton & Lange, 1989.)*

block is weak and patchy and spreads mainly in a cephalad direction. The epidural space is bounded by the dura anteriorly and the ligamentum flavum posteriorly; it extends from the base of the skull to the sacral hiatus. It contains nerves, fat, lymphatic vessels, and the veins of the epidural (Batson's) plexus.

■ Ligaments

The anterior and posterior longitudinal ligaments run between the anterior and posterior aspects of the vertebral bodies, respectively. The supraspinous ligament stretches from the seventh cervical vertebra to the sacrum, acquiring maximum thickness in the lumbar area. The interspinous ligament extends be-

tween the spinous processes. The ligamentum flavum, named for its yellow elastic fibers, runs from the anterior and inferior aspects of each vertebral lamina to the posterior and superior aspects of the lamina below and is most dense in the lumbar area. The distance between the ligamentum flavum and the dura, which defines the depth of the epidural space, is greatest in the midline at the second lumbar interspace, 5 to 6 mm. In the midthoracic region, this distance is 3 to 5 mm at the midline, and in the lower cervical region, 1.5 to 2 mm.

■ Spinal Nerves

Paired somatic spinal nerves leave the canal through the intervertebral foramina bilaterally, each supplying a region of skin known as a *dermatome* (Fig. 18-3). Visceral nervous pathways are more complex, tending to correspond to the embryonic origin of the organs rather than to their final position in the body. Frequently, the level of anesthesia required for an operation is higher than one would predict based on the overlying sensory dermatome (Table 18-1). For example, anesthesia of the viscera of the upper abdomen requires at least a T4 spinal level, even though the skin incision lies at T6 or below. Sympathetic afferents return from end-organs via prevertebral plexuses and the paravertebral chain ganglia to reach the spinal cord at multiple levels.

Preoperative Evaluation

In addition to the usual assessment of the patient, evaluation before spinal or epidural anesthesia considers the planned operation, the patient's physical condition, and any contraindications to regional techniques.

■ Surgical Considerations

Many operations on the lower extremities, pelvis, lower abdomen, and perineum can be accomplished with spinal or epidural anesthesia alone. Operations on the upper abdomen, chest, shoulder, and upper extremities can be managed with spinal or epidural anesthesia only with great difficulty. Although the operative site may be anesthetized in such cases, patients remain uncomfortable. Further, the effects of the operation or of such high levels of spinal anesthesia are likely to interfere with respiration and with

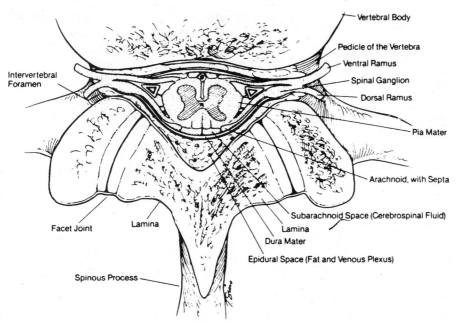

Figure 18-2

Transverse section through the spine.

(Reprinted by permission from Raj PP, Handbook of Regional Anesthesia. *New York: Churchill-Livingstone, 1985.)*

Figure 18-3

Dermatomal distribution.

(Reprinted by permission from the artist [Buckhöj] and Scott DB, Techniques of Regional Anaesthesia. *Norwalk, Conn: Appleton & Lange, 1989.)*

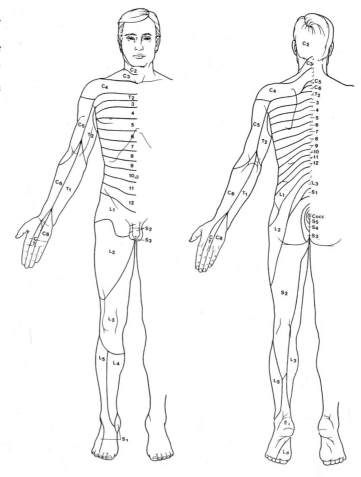

Table 18-1

Suggested Minimum Dermatome Levels for Spinal or Epidural Anesthetics	
Site of Operation	Level Required
Lower extremity	T12
Hip	T10
Prostate or bladder	T10
Testes	T6
Herniorrhaphy	T4
Intraabdominal	T4

circulation so that intubation and mechanical ventilation may be required. In these cases, epidural anesthesia may be combined with general anesthesia. In some instances, the choice of spinal or epidural anesthesia depends on the surgeon, some of whom are more accustomed than others to the gentle techniques required to make regional anesthesia practical.

■ Physical Examination

Preoperative evaluation includes examination of the thoracic and lumbar spine and the skin near the site of needle insertion. Spinal or epidural anesthesia is more difficult and more likely to fail if the patient has anatomic abnormalities such as scoliosis or limited flexion of the spine. Infection at the proposed puncture site precludes spinal or epidural anesthesia. Preexisting neurologic deficits discovered in the history or by examination must be documented to prevent misdiagnosis of postanesthetic neurologic problems.

■ Contraindications

Among the few absolute contraindications to spinal or epidural anesthesia are lack of patient consent and infection at the site of needle insertion. Spinal or epidural anesthesia is also withheld from patients with a severe coagulopathy, for fear of an epidural hematoma (Table 18-2). There is no agreement as to the safety of these techniques in patients with mild clotting disorders; epidural hematomas occur rarely in normal patients, and patients in whom epidural catheters have been inserted can safely receive heparin afterward.

Unless hypovolemia is corrected before beginning spinal or epidural anesthesia, sympathetic denervation produces catastrophic hypotension, so bleeding and

dehydration must be treated before anesthesia begins. Bacteremia is not an absolute contraindication to spinal or epidural anesthesia provided the patient receives appropriate antibiotic therapy, but many avoid either technique in these patients for fear of blood-borne bacteria seeding a small epidural hematoma and forming an abscess. Herniation of an intervertebral disk or previous back surgery does not preclude epidural or spinal anesthesia, although the associated scarring may prevent the needed spread of local anesthetic solutions or increase the susceptibility of nerve roots to injury. These problems, as well as fear of exacerbation of back pain or radiculitis, may encourage patients or anesthesiologists to choose general anesthesia. Although there is little evidence that spinal or epidural anesthesia causes or worsens neurologic diseases, many avoid these techniques when postoperative exacerbation of an existing problem is possible.

Techniques Common to Spinal and Epidural Anesthesia

As with general anesthesia, the drugs, supplies, and anesthesia machine are prepared before the patient enters the room; the standards for monitoring are the same as well. Preparations must include a vasopressor to treat hypotension and supplemental oxygen via nasal cannula or face mask to treat respiratory depression due to sedatives or the anesthetic. Administering narcotics and sedatives can make the patient more comfortable during placement of the needle, but usually the patient should remain sufficiently awake to report a paresthesia during the procedure. Persistent pain or paresthesia with needle advancement or anesthetic injection may represent trauma to a nerve root

Table 18-2

Contraindications to Major Conduction Anesthesia
Absolute
Patient refusal
Coagulopathy
Infection at site
Relative
Hypovolemia
Sepsis
Preexisting neurologic disease

and dictates that the needle or catheter be repositioned. Although epidural catheters are sometimes placed in patients under general anesthesia, some anesthesiologists are concerned that the risk of nerve damage might be increased by the absence of patient feedback.

Spinal or epidural anesthesia can be performed with the patient in the sitting, lateral decubitus, or prone position. Although it is easier for sitting patients to adopt the required flexed position with the spine in the midline, these patients may faint, so an attendant is required to assist them. A patient in the lateral or prone position requires less assistance. Throughout the procedure, the operator and assistant inform the patient of each step to be taken, providing constant reassurance. After positioning, the appropriate landmarks are identified. Precautions to avoid infection include aseptic technique, skin preparation with a bactericidal solution, a sterile drape, sterile gloves, and a careful check of the sterilization indicator included in the disposable spinal or epidural kit. To prevent administering the wrong drug or dose, identifying labels and concentrations are examined carefully.

Spinal Anesthesia

■ Technique

Positioning for lumbar puncture is determined by patient comfort, the surgical site, and the density of the local anesthetic solution. Regardless of positioning, the lumbar spine is flexed to spread the spinous processes and enlarge the interlaminar spaces. In the prone position, placing a pillow beneath the hips helps flex the lumbar spine.

At birth, the spinal cord extends to L4. After 1 year of age, the spinal cord terminates at L1-2, so performing a spinal block below L2 avoids the risk of spinal cord injury. A line connecting the iliac crests passes through the L4-5 interspace or L4 spinous process.

A midline approach is most common. The index and middle fingers of the operator's nondominant hand straddle the chosen interspace, perpendicular to the spinal column. The skin over the interspace is infiltrated with local anesthetic using a fine needle. The spinal needle is advanced in the midline sagittal plane, directed slightly cephalad (10 degrees) toward the interlaminar space. As the needle advances toward the subarachnoid space, it passes through skin, subcutaneous tissue, supraspinous ligament, interspinous ligament, and ligamentum flavum. As the needle tip advances through the ligamentum flavum, an increase in resistance is felt, followed by a "popping" sensation as the needle punctures the dura, at a typical depth of 4 to 7 cm. If the needle tip encounters bone, it must be pulled back far enough to free it from the ligaments before it is redirected in a more cephalad or caudad direction (Fig. 18-4).

After the stylet is removed, CSF flows freely from the needle. If the CSF is tinged with blood, it should clear rapidly; otherwise, the needle may lie in an epidural vein. After free flow of CSF is established, the anesthesiologist anchors the needle with the nondominant hand, which rests on the patient's back with the thumb and index finger stabilizing the hub, and attaches the syringe containing the anesthetic. Free aspiration of CSF confirms that the needle tip still lies in the CSF. Injecting rapidly through a small needle promotes mixing of the anesthetic solution with the CSF. This may promote the spread of the solution through the CSF and decreases the difference in density between the solution and the CSF. Very slow injection (a minute or more for 2 or 3 ml) avoids these effects but may promote pooling of the solution and local anesthetic toxicity (discussed later). After injection of the drug, again aspirating CSF reconfirms the position of the needle.

When the midline approach fails, as in elderly patients with calcified ligaments or in patients who are difficult to position because of limited lumbar flexion, a paramedian approach to the interlaminar space may succeed. The needle is inserted about 1 to 1.5 cm lateral to the midline and on a level with the upper border of the spinous process below the chosen interspace. The needle is advanced slightly medially and cephalad through the paraspinous muscles. If bone is encountered, it is likely to be the ipsilateral lamina, and the needle is repositioned superiorly or inferiorly into the subarachnoid space (see Fig 18–4).

An alternative to the midline or paramedian approach is the lumbosacral (Taylor) approach, which uses the largest interspace in the vertebral column, at L5-S1. The posterosuperior iliac spine is identified, and the skin is entered 1.0 cm medial and 1.0 cm inferior to this point. The needle is directed medially and cephalad to enter the spinal canal in the midline at L5-S1.

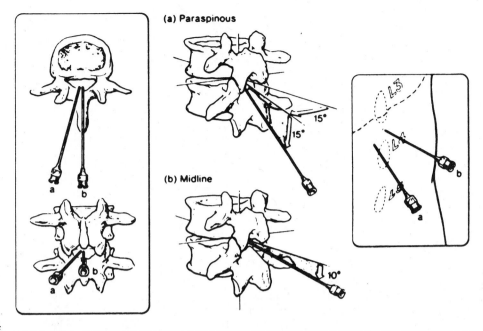

Figure 18-4

The midline and paramedian approaches for spinal or epidural anesthesia.
(*Reprinted by permission from Cousins MJ, Bridenbaugh PO, eds,* Neural Blockade, *2nd ed. Philadelphia: JB Lippincott, 1988.*)

■ Spinal Needles

The choice of spinal needle depends on the patient's age, the anesthesiologist's ability, and cost. The tips of the common Quincke needles have long bevels that incorporate a terminal orifice. They are provided in gauges 20 to 29; 22- and 25-gauge needles are used most frequently. The sharp tips of Quincke needles pass easily through tough, sometimes partially calcified ligaments, making it easy to differentiate bone from ligament. To ensure correct placement, free flow of CSF is demonstrated in all four quadrants by rotating the needle. Because it transects the fibers of the dura, this needle is more likely to produce a dural leak and subsequent headache in young patients, although using the smallest-diameter needle possible and orienting the bevel parallel to the dural fibers makes headache less likely.

Unlike the sharp beveled needle, the pencil-point needle has a tapered tip with the injection port on the side. This needle requires more force to insert, making it more difficult to differentiate bone from ligament. Examples of the pencil-point needle include the Sprotte, Whitacre, and Gertie Marx needles (Fig. 18-5). The differences among them are in the size and the location of the lateral orifices. Although more expensive than the sharp beveled needles, these needles do less damage to the dura and are less likely to result in postspinal headache.

The age of the patient largely determines the choice of needle. The more expensive pencil-point needles are most appropriate for patients at greatest risk of headache: those less than 50 years old, obstetrical patients, and same day surgery patients who would have to return to the hospital for treatment of a headache.

■ Drugs Used for Spinal Anesthesia

Satisfactory spinal anesthesia requires that the block extend to the dermatomes needed for the operation, last longer than the procedure, and be profound enough to block all sensory modalities. Limiting the extent of the anesthesia to the necessary dermatomes reduces the severity of side effects to the minimum. At present, the drugs used during spinal anesthesia include local anesthetics, opioids, and vasoconstrictors; dextrose is sometimes added to increase the specific gravity of the solution.

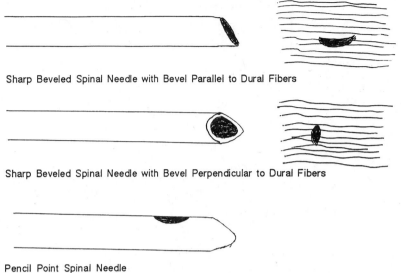

Sharp Beveled Spinal Needle with Bevel Parallel to Dural Fibers

Sharp Beveled Spinal Needle with Bevel Perpendicular to Dural Fibers

Pencil Point Spinal Needle

Figure 18-5

The pencil-point needle is designed to spread the dural fibers, resulting in less trauma to the dura and a lower incidence of headache. The sharp beveled needle cuts a hole in the dura; the least damage occurs when the bevel is oriented parallel to the dural fibers, which run cephalad-caudad. Although easier to use, it is associated with a greater incidence of headache in young patients.

Local Anesthetics

All local anesthetics are effective in producing spinal anesthesia, but in current practice the three drugs most often used are tetracaine, bupivacaine, and lidocaine. The usual criterion used to choose a drug is the duration of the operation. The first two are usually chosen for operations lasting longer than an hour and the last for briefer procedures. However, the duration of spinal anesthesia depends also on the use of vasoconstrictors and the dose and distribution of the drug. Because anesthetic effects dissipate only when the drug is washed out of neural tissue by blood flow, larger quantities of drug that are more narrowly restricted in their distribution tend to produce greater tissue concentrations and longer duration of effect. The usual doses given in Table 18-3 can be expected to produce anesthesia for the times listed.

In deciding on a dose to administer for spinal anesthesia, individual patient variables are not of great importance. In general, larger amounts of local anesthetic will produce more extensive anesthesia. When the patient's position and the density of the local anesthetic solution strongly direct the drug to one area, as in a saddle block, greater doses are inadvisable because they are confined to a limited area and may harm neural tissue.

Vasoconstrictors

The duration of blockade can be increased 1 to 2 hours by adding vasoconstrictors to the solution injected into the CSF. Both epinephrine (0.1 to 0.2 mg) and phenylephrine (1.0 to 4.0 mg) prolong the duration of spinal anesthesia. These drugs, by constricting the blood vessels supplying the dura and spinal cord, decrease vascular absorption and subsequent elimination of local anesthetic. In addition to decreasing blood flow, vasoconstrictors themselves exert a direct antinociceptive effect on the spinal cord, perhaps by means of alpha-2 sympathomimetic effects, and may contribute thereby to the quality of sensory anesthesia.

Opioids

Within the past decade, anesthesiologists have used subarachnoid opioids to improve the quality of the sensorimotor blockade and to provide postoperative analgesia. Subarachnoid narcotics act at narcotic receptors within the spinal cord. Morphine (0.1 to 0.2 mg) produces significant analgesia lasting well into the postoperative period, whereas fentanyl (25 to 37.5 µg) and sufentanil (10 µg) provide analgesia of shorter duration (Table 18-4). Side effects of sub-

Table 18-3

Local Anesthetics for Spinal Anesthesia

Drug	Concentration (%)	Dose (mg)	Duration (hours) Without Epinephrine	With Epinephrine
Lidocaine, hyperbaric	5	25–100	1	2
Lidocaine, isobaric	2	20–100	1.5	2–3
Tetracaine, hyperbaric	0.5	3–15	2	2–4
Tetracaine, isobaric	1	3–20	2–3	4–6
Tetracaine, hypobaric	0.3	3–20	2	4–6
Bupivacaine, isobaric	0.5	5–15	2–3	4–6
Bupivacaine, hyperbaric	0.75	3–15	1.5	3–4

Note: Because of irregularities in the distribution of the drug, differing definitions of the end of adequate anesthesia, and interpatient variations in anatomy, these doses and durations are only approximate.

arachnoid narcotics include pruritus, nausea, and respiratory depression.

Dextrose, Baricity, and Distribution of Anesthesia

The *density* of a local anesthetic solution is a function of its concentration and the fluid in which the drug is dissolved. The density of CSF at 37°C is 1.001 to 1.005 g/ml. The *baricity* of a local anesthetic solution is the ratio of its density to the density of CSF at the same temperature. Local anesthetic solutions with densities at 37°C greater than 1.008 g/ml are termed *hyperbaric,* those with densities between 0.998 and 1.007 g/ml are considered to be *isobaric,* and those with densities less than 0.997 g/ml are termed *hypobaric.* Local anesthetics prepared in 5% to 8% dextrose are hyperbaric; in CSF or isotonic saline, isobaric; in dilute solution with water, hypobaric (Table 18-5).

The dose of drug, the baricity of the local anesthetic solution, and the position of the patient during and just after injection largely determine the distribution of local anesthetic and the level of anesthesia.

Other factors such as age, weight, and vertebral column length are of lesser importance. In the supine position, the lumbar lordosis represents the high point of the spine at L3-4, and the thoracic kyphosis represents the low point at T5-6. Thus, if a patient is given a subarachnoid injection of a hyperbaric local anesthetic solution at L4 and placed supine, the solution moves by gravity from the high point to the two lowest regions, the sacrum and T5-6, producing a block that extends well into the thoracic dermatomes but that includes relatively sparse supplies of local anesthetic in the midlumbar roots. A saddle block provides anesthesia of the perineum, in an area that would cover a saddle if one were riding a horse. It is produced by injecting hyperbaric solutions with the patient sitting and maintaining that position for several minutes after injection.

Isobaric solutions tend to remain at the site of injection and produce more localized blocks, usually extending only to the lower thoracic dermatomes. These solutions are appropriate for lower extremity or urologic procedures.

Hypobaric solutions may be used when the patient

Table 18-4

Opioids in the Subarachnoid and Epidural Spaces

	Epidural Dose	Duration	Subarachnoid Dose	Duration
Morphine	1–5 mg	5–24h	0.1–0.2mg	8–24h
Fentanyl	25–100 μg	1–2 h	25–50 μg	1–2 h
Sufentanil	10–50 μg	2–3 h	5–10 μg	2–3 h

Table 18-5

Physical Characteristics of Commonly Used Spinal Anesthetics

Drug	Local Anesthetic Concentration (%)	Solution	Density	Baricity
Lidocaine, hyperbaric	5	Dextrose	1.0265	1.0262
Lidocaine, isobaric	2	Water	1.0007	1.0004
Tetracaine, hyperbaric	0.5	Dextrose	1.0136	1.0133
Tetracaine, isobaric	1	CSF	1.0000	0.9997
Tetracaine, hypobaric	0.33	Water	0.9980	0.9977
Bupivacaine, isobaric	0.5	Saline	0.9993	0.9990
Bupivacaine, hyperbaric	0.75	Dextrose	1.0230	1.0227

is supine, in the jack-knife position for procedures on the rectum, perineum, and anus, or in the lateral decubitus position for procedures on the side of the body opposite the one on which the patient lies. An advantage of hypobaric solutions is that tilting the table head down to reduce venous pooling in the legs also helps limit the cephalad spread of the local anesthetic.

Conduct of Spinal Anesthesia

Management after injection of the local anesthetic into CSF includes detection and treatment of side effects and evaluation of the distribution of the local anesthetic. Supplemental oxygen and pulse oximetry ensure against hypoxemia. Continuous display of the heart rate detects bradycardia, and repeated determinations of blood pressure assess hypotension.

The distribution of the block is measured by several tests. Loss of cold perception (alcohol sponge or ice to the skin) correlates with the level of sympathetic block, since these two modalities are served by nerve fibers of similar diameters and conduction velocities. Sensory levels are obtained by seeking response to a pinprick or finger scratch. Motor function is tested by asking the patient to plantar flex the toes (S1-2), dorsiflex the foot (L4-5), raise the knees (L2-3), or tense the rectus muscles by lifting the head (T6-12).

During spinal and epidural anesthesia, the level of sympathetic blockade extends higher than that of sensory blockade, which in turn extends higher than that of motor blockade. These graded degrees of block do not correspond to differential sensitivities of various kinds of nerve fibers, as was once thought, but to differences in the concentrations of local anesthetic among the various nerve roots and to concentration gradients within each root. The more peripheral sensory and sympathetic nerve fibers are more easily blocked because they are exposed to a greater concentration of local anesthetic than the deeper motor nerve fibers.

Continuous Spinal Anesthesia

Continuous spinal anesthesia entails placing a catheter into the subarachnoid space. This technique allows control of the extent and duration of spinal block by adding local anesthetic through the catheter as needed. Placing the catheter requires piercing the dura with an epidural needle; the large hole that results is so likely to produce a headache that the technique is not practical in younger patients. Microcatheters, 28 and 32 gauge, can be placed through small needles but have been removed from the market by the Food and Drug Administration (FDA) because a total of 11 neurologic injuries occurred when they were used. The small diameter of these catheters allows only the slow injection of local anesthetic, which may promote pooling and local neurotoxicity of the hyperbaric mixtures used in the reported cases.

Complications of Spinal Anesthesia

Intraoperative complications of spinal anesthesia include hypotension, high spinal anesthesia with ventilatory inadequacy, cardiac arrest, nausea, and paresthesia. Postoperative complications include headache, neurologic injury, back pain, and urinary retention.

Hypotension

Hypotension occurs often during spinal anesthesia, primarily resulting from the blockade of preganglionic vasomotor efferents of the sympathetic nervous system and loss of compensatory vasoconstriction in the lower extremities and splanchnic beds. Diminished preload (venodilation) leads to decreased cardiac output; decreased arteriolar tone contributes little to hypotension, unless peripheral vascular resistance was markedly increased (as in hypovolemia) before the spinal anesthetic. Hypovolemia, head-up postures, higher levels of anesthesia, and preanesthetic dependence on sympathetic tone all promote more severe hypotensive reactions. Block of cardioaccelerator fibers at T1 through T4 contributes to bradycardia and loss of contractility as well.

The treatment of hypotension begins with immediate measures such as correcting head-up posture, administering intravenous fluids, and giving pressors as needed. Although definitive therapy certainly includes correcting hypovolemia, therapy with excess fluid may produce bladder distension or congestive heart failure when the spinal dissipates. Further, fluids do nothing to correct bradycardia or impaired contractility. The preferable therapy for spinal hypotension is a combination of fluids to correct hypovolemia and alpha- and beta-adrenergic agonists (e.g., ephedrine) and atropine (for bradycardia) as the situation dictates.

High Spinal Anesthesia with Ventilatory Inadequacy

Patients with high sensory levels of anesthesia may complain of breathlessness. Careful differentiation of three causes allows proper treatment. Most commonly, dyspnea does not represent paralysis of the muscles of respiration but lack of proprioception that produces the sensation of dyspnea despite adequate muscle function and gas exchange. Reassurance and supplemental oxygen usually suffice. Second, respiratory embarrassment can result from hypotension and cerebral hypoperfusion; correction of the hypotension may resolve the problem. Less often, motor block to C3-5 with phrenic nerve paralysis requires treatment with assisted ventilation.

Unexpected Cardiac Arrest

Unexpected cardiac arrest has been reported in a number of healthy patients undergoing apparently satisfactory spinal anesthesia. These patients had been heavily sedated and had unremarkable hypotension until the apparently abrupt onset of cardiac arrest that proved difficult to treat. It seems likely that the combination of cardiovascular depression due to high spinal anesthesia and blunting of ventilatory and cardiovascular responses to hypercarbia and hypoxia due to the sedatives and narcotics had rendered these patients unable to respond to progressive hypoxemia, acidosis, and hypercarbia.

These cardiac arrests likely can be avoided by taking several steps. First, opioids should be used with great caution during spinal anesthesia. Satisfactory spinal anesthesia provides freedom from pain, and opioids are not good agents for producing amnesia, somnolence, or anxiolysis; these are controlled better by benzodiazepines, for example. Second, all patients undergoing spinal anesthesia require supplemental oxygen and monitoring by pulse oximetry. Third, hypotension and bradycardia require early treatment aimed at maintaining cardiac output. It is likely that atropine and agents with beta-adrenergic effects deserve earlier and more frequent use than has been customary in the past. Fourth, should a patient suffer such an abrupt episode of hypotension or a cardiac arrest, early and vigorous treatment with oxygen, hyperventilation, large doses of epinephrine (0.1 to 1 mg), and sodium bicarbonate is indicated.

Nausea

Nausea during spinal anesthesia is usually due to cerebral hypoperfusion or unopposed vagal stimulation of the gut. Often the first sign of hypotension is nausea. Also, sympathetic blockade results in unopposed excess parasympathetic tone in the gastrointestinal tract. Atropine may ameliorate refractory nausea once blood pressure and cardiac output have been restored.

Paresthesia

A paresthesia may occur during placement of the spinal needle or injection of the anesthetic. Patients may complain of pain or a shock shooting into the lower extremity, suggesting that the spinal needle may be against the nerve root. If the patient has a persistent paresthesia or a paresthesia with injection of the local anesthetic, the needle should be removed and placed at another interspace to prevent permanent damage. The presence or absence of a paresthesia is recorded on the anesthetic record.

Post-Dural Puncture Headache

Headache following dural puncture, called *spinal headache* or *post-dural puncture headache* (PDPH), was described by Bier in 1898. CSF leaking out of the subarachnoid space through the dural puncture allows the brain and its supporting structures to sag, placing traction on the pain-sensitive vascular structures. The headache is worsened by sitting or standing and is relieved by lying down. The pain may be frontal, occipital, or both and may be accompanied by symptoms such as tinnitus or diplopia. Although it may be present immediately after dural puncture, it usually occurs 24 to 72 hours later.

The incidence of PDPH is greater in younger patients and in women. As would be expected, the size of the hole in the dura affects the rate of CSF loss and thus the chance of headache and its severity. Using small needles (24 gauge or smaller) is important for patients under age 50 but less important for older patients, who are unlikely to suffer PDPH in any case. Spinal needles with blunt or rounded-point tips part the fibers of the dura, rather than transecting them, so that the hole is smaller and heals sooner. When using a conventional Quincke needle, inserting the needle with the bevel parallel to the longitudinal dural fibers offers similar benefits.

Treatment of spinal headache usually begins with conservative measures. Intravenous or oral hydration encourages CSF production and replaces lost CSF. Although patients with PDPH are more comfortable when lying down, bed rest does not prevent the headache, so there is no need to remain supine following a spinal anesthetic. Oral or intravenous caffeine may be helpful. Abdominal binders can increase pressure in the epidural space, thereby decreasing the leakage of CSF.

The definitive treatment for PDPH is an epidural blood patch. In 1960, Gormley noted that patients with bloody taps during lumbar puncture had a decreased incidence of PDPH. He postulated that clotted blood might cover the dural hole and prevent leakage of CSF. He successfully demonstrated that blood placed in the epidural space relieves the headache. To perform an epidural blood patch, 10 to 20 ml of autologous blood is obtained aseptically and slowly injected into the epidural space. The most common complication is transient back pain. Epidural blood patch is effective in greater than 95 percent of patients.

Neurologic Injury

Neurologic deficits after spinal anesthesia are rare but may result from mechanical or chemical injury. Direct trauma to a nerve root, perhaps by the needle, results in a radiculopathy with a sensory or motor deficit in a root distribution. These injuries usually resolve within 2 to 12 weeks. Epidural hematoma (unlikely unless coagulation is impaired) results in back pain, which may be masked by residual anesthe-

sia, progressive weakness, and sensory deficit. Successful treatment requires prompt recognition, confirmation with computed tomography or magnetic resonance imaging, and immediate decompressive laminectomy. Chemical injuries are more diffuse than mechanical injuries. They result from inadvertent injection of such chemicals as glutaraldehyde, contamination of local anesthetic solutions, or possibly, toxic effects of undiluted local anesthetic solutions that pool in restricted areas.

Urinary Retention

Micturition depends on intact innervation of the urethral sphincter and bladder musculature. After spinal anesthesia, lower extremity motor and sensory function recovers before bladder function, especially with the longer-acting spinal anesthetics such as tetracaine or bupivacaine. Delayed return of nerve function may lead to urinary retention and bladder distension. For longer procedures or when large amounts of intravenous fluid are required, a bladder catheter prevents this complication.

Backache

Backache is no more common following spinal anesthesia than following general anesthesia. It is probably caused by the ligamentous strain occurring with paraspinous muscle relaxation and positioning for the operation, which accompanies both regional and general anesthesia.

Epidural Anesthesia

Epidural anesthesia, which results from the injection of local anesthetic into the epidural space, resembles spinal anesthesia in many regards. The site of neural blockade is believed to be the spinal nerve roots as they emerge from the spinal cord and traverse the epidural space. Local anesthetics enter the CSF through the dura, also contributing to the anesthetic effect. Anesthesia occurs more slowly than with spinal anesthesia and develops in a segmental manner.

■ Technique

Epidural anesthesia is most readily performed in the lumbar region. In the lumbar spine, the distance between the ligamentum flavum and the dura is the greatest, about 5 to 6 mm. Spinous processes are least angled, and the interlaminar spaces are the widest.

The technique for performing epidural anesthesia and the patient's position differ little from those for spinal anesthesia. After the intradermal local anesthetic weal is raised, a thin 1.5-in needle is used to infiltrate local anesthetic in the subcutaneous tissue and to determine a suitable angle of insertion for the epidural needle.

The needles for epidural anesthesia are larger than those used for spinal anesthesia so as to permit passage of a catheter. A side-facing orifice and blunt tip reduce the chance of perforating the dura. A stylet or obturator occludes the orifice so that the needle is not occluded by skin or subcutaneous tissue.

The needle is inserted as for spinal anesthesia until it is engaged in the spinal ligaments. The stylet is then removed, and an air- or liquid-filled syringe with a freely movable plunger is attached to the needle. The dorsum of the nondominant hand is braced on the patient's back, while the thumb and index or middle finger grasp the needle shaft or hub. The nondominant hand controls the advance of the epidural needle in 2-mm increments, while the thumb intermittently depresses the plunger of the syringe. While the tip of the needle lies in the ligaments, the plunger of the syringe cannot be depressed easily and bounces back if the syringe contains air. When the needle tip enters the compliant epidural space, there is a loss of resistance (which accounts for the name of this technique), and the plunger is easily depressed and does not bounce back.

An alternative method is to place a drop of sterile fluid in the open needle hub. When the needle enters the epidural space, the fluid is drawn into the needle by the negative pressure in the epidural space. This negative pressure results from tenting of the dura and transmission of negative intrathoracic pressure. Whether a midline or paramedian approach is used, the tip of the needle enters the epidural space in the midline, where epidural veins are scarcest.

A plastic epidural catheter, with or without a stylet, is passed 2 to 4 cm into the epidural space. The epidural needle is then removed over the catheter. The catheter is never withdrawn through the needle because it may shear off and remain within the epidural space. The catheter is secured with tape, and a syringe adapter with bacterial filters is attached to the proximal end. After the operation, the catheter is removed, a dressing is placed over the entry site, and a note is entered in the patient record to document that the catheter was removed intact.

Thoracic epidural catheters provide excellent up-per abdominal and thoracic anesthesia with smaller doses of local anesthetic than are required for lumbar epidural anesthetics. Principles and procedures are similar to those for lumbar epidural anesthesia, but anatomic differences must be kept in mind. In the midthoracic region, the distance between the ligamentum flavum and the dura is only 3 to 5 mm in the midline. The greater angulation of the spinous processes requires that the needle be inserted at a steeper angle. There is a risk of producing trauma to the underlying spinal cord if dural puncture should occur. The hanging-drop method is employed frequently because of the ready transmission of negative intrathoracic pressure to the thoracic epidural space.

■ Drugs for Epidural Anesthesia

Local Anesthetics

The choice of local anesthetic for epidural anesthesia is determined by the duration of the surgical procedure and the required intensity of motor blockade. Chloroprocaine is short-acting; lidocaine and mepivacaine are intermediate in their actions; bupivacaine and etidocaine are long-acting (Table 18-6). Bupivacaine is unusual in that it produces a less intense motor blockade for any degree of sensory blockade than do other anesthetics.

Epinephrine

The addition of epinephrine (5 µg/ml) to local anesthetics injected into the epidural space not only prolongs their effect but also, by decreasing vascular absorption, reduces the blood concentration of the

Table 18-6

Local Anesthetics for Epidural Anesthesia

Drug	Concentration	Duration of Surgical Anesthesia with Epinephrine (Minutes)
Chloroprocaine	2–3%	60
Lidocaine	1.5%	60–90
Mepivacaine	1.5%	90–120
Bupivacaine	0.5%	>180
Etidocaine	1.0%	>150

Note: Lesser concentrations may be appropriate when motor block is not needed, as in analgesia for labor. More concentrated solutions, such as 2% lidocaine or 0.75% bupivacaine, produce more rapid onset of block but usually not more profound anesthesia once the block is fully developed. Studies of the duration of anesthesia with these anesthetics conflict, largely because endpoints differ and offset of block occurs gradually over time and over different dermatomes.

drug and lessens the chance of systemic toxicity. The epinephrine also serves as a marker for accidental intravascular injection (see remarks on test doses below). The small amount of epinephrine absorbed from the epidural space produces primarily beta-adrenergic effects, decreasing systemic vascular resistance and increasing heart rate.

Test Dose

Because epidural anesthesia involves the injection of large amounts of local anesthetics, the catheter must be in the proper location. Aspirating on the plunger of the syringe may draw back blood or CSF. If blood or CSF is detected, the epidural catheter is removed and placed elsewhere. Even if no blood or CSF appears in the catheter, intravascular or intrathecal placement cannot be ruled out, so a test dose is required. This consists of 3 ml of local anesthetic of a concentration appropriate for spinal anesthesia and contains 15 μg of epinephrine (1.5% lidocaine with epinephrine 1:200,000 is often used). Subarachnoid injection is recognized by the prompt onset of motor paralysis and sensory block consistent with spinal anesthesia. When the needle or catheter lies in an epidural vein, epinephrine results in an increase in heart rate of 20 beats per minute or greater within 2 minutes. In patients taking beta-adrenergic blockers, the alpha-adrenergic effects of epinephrine produce an increase of 15 mmHg or greater in systolic blood pressure, with no change or even a reflex slowing of heart rate. If the needle or catheter lies in the epidural space, there will be no anesthesia and no change in blood pressure or heart rate.

Frequently, a small amount of fluid may be aspirated prior to repeat injection of local anesthetic. This fluid may represent CSF or local anesthetic from the previous injection. A dipstick test for glucose differentiates the two, since CSF contains glucose and local anesthetic solutions do not.

Anesthetic Doses

Anesthetic drugs given in the subarachnoid space may spread through the CSF, so the extent of the anesthesia depends on the quantity of local anesthetic as well as the volume of the injectate. In contrast, the spread of the local anesthetics in the epidural space depends only on the volume injected. The concentration of the local anesthetic in the solution affects only the degree or density of the block, not its anatomic extent. The onset of anesthesia is slower with epidural anesthesia than with spinal, although the addition of

sodium bicarbonate to the local anesthetic speeds the onset dramatically. Chloroprocaine, lidocaine, and mepivacaine act more rapidly; bupivacaine and etidocaine act more slowly.

Appropriate volumes of local anesthetic solution for lumbar epidural anesthesia range from 15 to 25 ml. Studies in young volunteers indicate a mean requirement of 1.6 ml per spinal segment anesthetized. In the narrower thoracic epidural space, approximately half of this is required. Older patients, pregnant patients, and patients with increased intraabdominal pressure require lesser volumes of local anesthetic solution to achieve a given distribution.

There is little effect of posture on the distribution of epidural anesthesia. Instead, the dermatomal distribution of anesthesia tends to be centered about the tip of the needle or the catheter, although cephalad spread occurs more readily than caudad spread.

The need for additional local anesthetic is determined by the choice of anesthetic and by clinical observation. When the anesthesia has regressed by two dermatomes, the addition of one-third to one-half the original amount of local anesthetic maintains adequate anesthesia. When using epidural and general anesthesia together, additional doses are given at time intervals characteristic of the local anesthetic.

Opioids

Compared with spinal opioids, epidural opioids produce similar effects and require similar precautions, but larger amounts are administered. Opioids act synergistically with local anesthetics, enhancing the effectiveness of lesser concentrations of local anesthetic.

■ Management of Epidural Anesthesia

Management of epidural anesthesia is similar to that of spinal anesthesia, although the onset of anesthesia as well as the onset of hypotension is slower. Since position has little effect on the spread of medications in the epidural space, the patient's position is not changed to alter the distribution of anesthesia.

■ Complications

The complications of epidural anesthesia are similar to those of spinal anesthesia. There are additional risks: local anesthetic toxicity and unwanted dural puncture with a large-bore needle.

The large doses of local anesthetic used in epidural anesthesia impose risk for both immediate and delayed toxicity. Immediate toxicity results from direct intravascular administration of local anesthetic, whereas delayed toxicity follows systemic uptake of local anesthetic. In either case, the syndrome usually presents as central nervous system (CNS) toxicity, with or without cardiovascular changes. The appropriate use of test doses, in addition to aspirating prior to each local anesthetic injection, will lessen the risk of intravascular injection. The addition of epinephrine to the local anesthetic reduces the uptake of local anesthetic from the epidural space.

The risk of headache following inadvertent dura puncture is great because the diameter of the epidural needle is large. If the dura is punctured with the epidural needle, four courses of action are possible. First, a subarachnoid catheter can be passed to provide continuous spinal anesthesia. All who care for the patient must understand that this is a spinal catheter, not an epidural catheter, since much smaller volumes of local anesthetic are required. Second, a single dose of local anesthetic can be administered to produce spinal anesthesia. Third, the needle can be removed and epidural anesthesia attempted at another interspace. In this situation, less local anesthetic is required to achieve a given level because the dural puncture allows local anesthetic to enter the subarachnoid space. Fourth, the needle can be withdrawn to the epidural space and an epidural catheter passed at the same site. If an epidural catheter is placed successfully following dural puncture, a prophylactic epidural blood patch may be administered through the catheter.

Caudal Anesthesia

Caudal anesthesia is a special form of epidural anesthesia, with access through the sacral hiatus. Caudal anesthesia has decreased in popularity for adults because of a failure rate of 10 to 15 percent, related to anatomic irregularities of the sacrum. The technique is more useful in pediatric patients, in whom the landmarks are easier to identify and anesthetic spread is more consistent.

■ Anatomy

The sacrum is formed by the fusion of the five sacral vertebrae. This bone articulates with the lumbar spine superiorly, the iliac bones laterally, and the coccyx inferiorly. The caudal space is an extension of the epidural space. The sacral hiatus is formed by failure of the laminae of the fourth and fifth sacral vertebrae to fuse. The hiatus is covered by the sacrococcygeal ligament, which is formed from the supraspinous ligament, the interspinous ligament, and the ligamentum flavum. The dural sac usually ends at the lower border of S2 in the adult (Fig. 18-6).

■ Technique

Caudal anesthesia is performed with the patient in the lateral, prone, or jack-knife position. After sterile skin preparation and draping, the sacral cornua are identified, and the skin and underlying ligaments are infiltrated with local anesthetic. The needle is inserted at a 45-degree angle to the sacrum between the two cornua. After passing through the sacrococcygeal membrane, the needle tip contacts the ventral plate of the sacral canal. The needle is then withdrawn a few millimeters from the periosteum, the hub of the needle is depressed 5 to 15 degrees, and the needle is advanced 2 cm (in adults) into the canal. If the needle tip is positioned correctly within the sacral canal below the dural sac, CSF cannot be aspirated and a few milliliters of air can be injected without a sensation of crepitus over the needle tip. If desired, a catheter may be placed. The anesthetic is conducted as for lumbar epidural anesthesia; the initial volume of local anesthetic is somewhat greater.

Spinal or Epidural Anesthesia or Both?

Although spinal and epidural anesthesia are similar, there are often reasons to choose one over the other. When speed is essential, as in emergency cesarean section, spinal anesthesia is quicker in onset. When calcified ligaments or distorted anatomy presents technical difficulties, the definite endpoint provided by the flow of CSF makes spinal anesthesia appealing. By using a hyperbaric solution and performing the block with the patient sitting, spinal anesthesia can provide prompt sacral anesthesia, something difficult to do with an epidural (although a caudal anesthetic is effective). A major advantage of epidural anesthesia over spinal anesthesia is the absence of dural puncture. However, if inadvertent dural puncture occurs with the large-bore epidural needle, the risk of spinal headache is great, thus negating some of the theoreti-

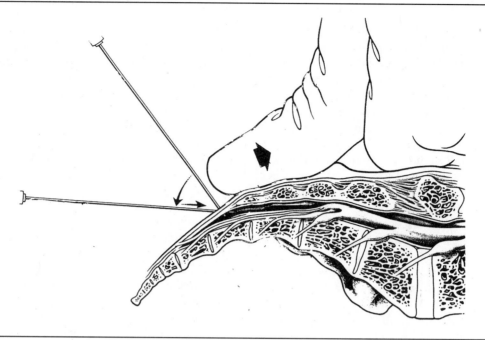

Figure 18-6

Needle placement for caudal anesthesia.
(Reprinted by permission from the artist [Buckhöj] and Scott DB, Techniques of Regional Anaesthesia. *Norwalk, Conn: Appleton & Lange, 1989.)*

cal advantages of the epidural technique. Long-term analgesia or anesthesia is commonly provided with epidural catheters and not with spinal catheters, so epidural anesthesia is usually chosen when a single injection will not suffice. After epidural anesthesia, hypotension develops more slowly than after subarachnoid block, making management easier.

Combining spinal and epidural techniques may offer some of the advantages of each but at the expense of increased complexity. The epidural space is located as described previously. However, prior to placing the epidural catheter, a long, small-diameter spinal needle is advanced through the epidural needle until CSF is obtained. The spinal anesthetic is injected through the spinal needle, the spinal needle is removed, and then an epidural catheter is passed. The onset of anesthesia is quick, but anesthesia may be maintained through the epidural catheter. The proper placing of the catheter must be ensured with test doses.

Advantages of Epidural or Spinal Anesthesia

Epidural and spinal anesthesia confer the advantages shared by all forms of regional anesthesia, in that they avoid the difficulties of general anesthesia. Although these problems have largely been overcome in modern practice, in some patients they still present hazards. With regional techniques such as spinal or epidural anesthesia, patients may remain awake, if that is important, and the patient may be more alert sooner after the operation than with general anesthesia. Endotracheal intubation or mask ventilation is rarely required. Direct depressant effects on the myocardium can be avoided, as can depression of ventilatory responses to CO_2. Complete freedom from pain can be provided, even into the early postoperative period, without the use of opioids. Regional anesthetics also provide preemptive analgesia, a concept discussed in Chapter 34.

Other benefits have been attributed to the physiologic effects of spinal and epidural anesthesia. Freedom from pain and the consequent effects on ventilation improve pulmonary function after operations that otherwise would impair movement of the diaphragm, abdomen, or thorax, such as laparotomy, herniorrhaphy, or thoracotomy. Oxygenation, the ability to cough, and vital capacity are all improved with spinal or epidural analgesia as compared with systemic narcotics.

Also attributed to major conduction anesthesia is a decreased risk of venous thromboembolism, perhaps due to improved lower limb blood flow or to blocking of the sympathetically mediated enhanced clotting and inhibited thrombolysis otherwise seen in patients undergoing operation. Blood loss during similar operations is decreased with spinal or epidural anesthesia as compared with that during general anesthesia.

Some advocate spinal or epidural anesthesia in high-risk cardiovascular patients as part of an effort to provide what has been called *stress-free management,* in the hope of reducing the incidence of cardiac complications. Yeager reported a reduction in overall cardiovascular complications in patients who received epidural anesthesia compared with general anesthesia. However, subsequent studies have not demonstrated consistent advantages in regard to postoperative cardiovascular complications when epidural or spinal anesthesia is used.

At least in part, most of these therapeutic benefits of spinal or epidural anesthesia can be achieved in other ways. Effective use of systemic narcotics intraoperatively and postoperatively, respiratory therapy, anticoagulants, induced hypotension, autologous transfusion, and techniques of intensive cardiac care often can achieve similar results. However, spinal and epidural anesthesia are now recognized as effective and inexpensive methods of obtaining these benefits.

BIBLIOGRAPHY

Bromage PR. *Epidural Analgesia*. Philadelphia: WB Saunders, 1978.

Caplan RA, Ward RJ, Posner K, Cheney FW. Unexpected cardiac arrest during spinal anesthesia: A closed claims analysis of predisposing factors. *Anesthesiology* 1988;68:5-11.

Carpenter Rl, Caplan RA, Brown DL, et al. Incidence and risk factors for side effects of spinal anesthesia. *Anesthesiology* 1992; 76:906-912.

Cousins MJ, Bridenbaugh PO, eds. *Neural Blockade*, 2nd ed. Philadelphia: JB Lippincott, 1988.

Cuschieri RJ, Morran CG, Howie JL, et al. Postoperative pain and pulmonary complications: Comparison of three analgesic regimens. *Br J Surg* 1985;72:495-498.

Greene NM. *The Physiology of Spinal Anesthesia*, 3d ed. Baltimore: Williams & Wilkins, 1983.

Hetherington R, Stevens RA, White JL, et al. Subjective experiences of anesthesiologists undergoing epidural anesthesia. *Reg Anesth* 1994;19:284-288.

Prins MH, Hirsh J. A comparison of general anesthesia and regional anesthesia as a risk factor for deep vein thrombosis following hip surgery: A critical review. *Thromb Haemost* 1990;64:497-500.

Raj PP. *Handbook of Regional Anesthesia*. New York: Churchill-Livingstone, 1985.

Tverskoy M. Postoperative pain after inguinal herniorrhaphy with different types of anesthesia. *Anesth Analg* 1990;70:29-35.

Urbano JB. Clinical observations suggesting a changing site of action during induction and recession of spinal and epidural anesthesia. *Anesthesiology* 1973;39:496-503.

Yeager MP, Glass DD, Neff RK, et al. Epidural anesthesia and analgesia in high-risk surgical patients. *Anesthesiology* 1987;66: 729-736.

CHAPTER 19

Nerve Blocks

Ray H. d'Amours

Peripheral nerve blocks are used by themselves to produce regional anesthesia for surgery, as supplements to general anesthesia, and to provide postoperative analgesia. Selected blocks are used for diagnosis and treatment of chronic pain syndromes (see Chap. 35). Although only specialists seek to master all the many nerve blocks that have been described, all anesthesiologists benefit from a basic understanding of the most commonly used nerve blocks for adult patients, as described in this chapter. (Pediatric applications are discussed in Chapter 25.)

Regional anesthesia using peripheral nerve blocks offers a number of advantages over other anesthetic techniques. Because only the involved part of the patient's body is anesthetized, the least possible physiologic disruption results from peripheral nerve blockade. As with epidural and spinal blockade, peripheral nerve blocks permit the patient to remain awake, with intact airway reflexes. It is sometimes more difficult and time consuming to provide neural blockade of peripheral nerves as compared with the relative ease and rapid onset of subarachnoid or epidural analgesia, accounting in part for the lack of popularity of peripheral nerve blocks.

Patient Preparation

Preoperative evaluation before peripheral nerve block is similar to that preceding general anesthesia, since an alternative plan for airway control and safe general anesthesia is always required. The physical examination includes examination of the site of the planned block and a search for preexisting neurologic defects. Specific tests of the coagulation system are indicated only when suggested by the patient's history.

The considerations in choosing a nerve block to replace or supplement general anesthesia are similar to those described for spinal or epidural anesthesia. Contraindications to regional anesthesia include the patient's refusal, local infection, and coagulopathy. As with spinal anesthesia, there is little reason to fear that a peripheral nerve block will worsen nerve damage already present. Nevertheless, some anesthesiologists withhold regional anesthesia from patients with neurologic disease. In many cases, one can anticipate differentiating (rare) nerve damage due to the block from damage due to operation or medical disease. For example, there can be no confusion between damage to the median nerve from axillary block and that from an operation at the wrist. In cases such as this, regional anesthesia can be performed with no fear of diagnostic confusion postoperatively.

The only absolute contraindication to nerve block anesthesia is the patient's refusal, but often this can be averted by appropriate reassurance. Patients are told that sedation will be provided during the procedure, that they need not observe the operation, and that general anesthesia will be available if needed. As described in Chapter 4, premedication often consists of intravenous sedation administered in the operating suite. Full disclosure to the patient of potential risks and benefits is documented in the preanesthetic note.

Equipment

Regional anesthesia techniques require appropriate needles, syringes, and other ancillary equipment. Sterile disposable nerve block trays or their individual components are widely available.

■ Needles

Needles for nerve blocks are small in diameter (22 gauge or smaller) and long enough to reach the intended target. Short-bevel needles, such as the 45-degree block needles or the 23-degree "B bevel" needles, are superior to the long-bevel needles used for intramuscular injections (17-degree "A bevel") because the blunter needles transmit changes in resistance as the needle passes through tissue (Fig. 19-1). Also, the shorter cutting edges do less damage to nerves. A security bead on the needle shaft prevents retraction of a distal needle segment below the skin if the shaft breaks at the hub. Needles for use with nerve stimulators include an attachment for the electrode and are usually insulated along the shaft.

■ Syringes

Syringes with finger rings allow single-handed loading and frequent aspiration during injection of local anesthetic solution, while the opposite hand stabilizes the needle. Standard syringes may require an assistant to aspirate and inject, as well as the use of flexible extension tubing to prevent needletip movement during the process.

Locating the Nerve to Be Blocked

Successful nerve blocks depend on placing the needletip near the target nerve and keeping it there throughout injection of the local anesthetic, while avoiding vital structures near the nerve, such as blood vessels. Thorough knowledge of the relevant anatomy is essential. Several methods are used to locate the nerve to be blocked. Safe blockade of nerves in close proximity to critical structures may even require radiographic guidance, an advanced technique not covered here.

■ Infiltration

Simple infiltration of local anesthetic solution around bony, vascular, or fascial landmarks can produce a successful block when the precise location of the nerve is uncertain. Only the small fraction of local anesthetic contacting the nerve produces the anesthesia, while the remainder serves to maintain the block. It is especially important to use large volumes of local anesthetic solution with this technique.

■ Paresthesias

Contact between the needletip and the nerve produces a paresthesia, often described by patients as "electricity" or "hitting the funny bone." Although a paresthesia in the distribution of the nerve sought is good evidence that the needle is in the right place, in some blocks the occurrence of paresthesias is associated with an increase in the (rare) incidence of nerve damage, which may result from trauma during localization and injection. If paresthesia persists or recurs when the injection is begun, the needle is moved slightly to avoid an intraneural injection. Since some patients do not distinguish paresthesias from other sensations and others, especially when oversedated, do not report them at all, questioning and coaching may be needed.

■ Nerve Stimulators

Using a nerve stimulator to pass weak electric currents through the needle serves to locate periph-

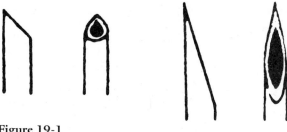

Figure 19-1

The standard sharp 17-degree angle "A bevel" needle is shown on the right, compared with the more blunt 45-degree angle block needle on the left. The block needle, or a "B bevel" needle (23-degree angle) is preferred by most for peripheral nerve blocks.

(Modified with permission from Selander D, Dhuner KG, Lundborg G: Peripheral nerve injury due to injection needles used for regional anesthesia. Acta Anaesthesiol Scand 1977; 21:186.)

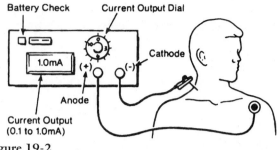

Figure 19-2

Use of a peripheral nerve stimulator.

(Used with permission from Cousins MJ, Bridenbaugh PO, eds: Neural Blockade, *2nd ed. Philadelphia: JB Lippincott, 1988.)*

eral nerves that include motor fibers. Nerve stimulators intended for monitoring of neuromuscular blockade are usable if they can provide 0.1 to 3.0 mA, with a display of the current.

The negative lead from the stimulator is attached to the insulated block needle, and the other lead is attached to the patient (Fig. 19-2). As the needletip approaches the nerve, the electric current near the tip induces depolarization of myelinated motor efferents, producing muscle contractions. The current density decreases markedly with distance from the needletip; the current required to produce a response decreases as the needletip nears the nerve. When the current required to elicit a response is 1.0 mA or less, the tip of the needle is close enough to the nerve to ensure success of the nerve block.

This technique provides an objective means of systematically guiding the needletip closer to the nerve by observing changes in electric current requirements. This technique may be used successfully in patients who are intoxicated, anesthetized, or unable to communicate effectively. Properly conducted, nerve stimulation is painless for the conscious patient, because the depolarization threshold for myelinated motor efferents is less than that for unmyelinated sensory afferents. It has been suggested that the probability of neural injury is lessened with this technique, since the needletip can be directed close to the nerve but need not touch it. Use of the nerve stimulator requires that the practitioner know which muscle contractions to expect from stimulation of the target nerve (Fig. 19-3).

Conduct of Anesthesia

Some operating suites include holding areas where nerve blocks may be performed to save operating room time and to facilitate teaching. These areas are equipped at a minimum with an electrocardiograph (ECG) and blood pressure monitors, pulse oximeters, intravenous supplies, oxygen, drugs for treating local anesthesia toxicity, and drugs and equipment for airway control and cardiopulmonary resuscitation. Otherwise, blocks may be performed in the operating room itself.

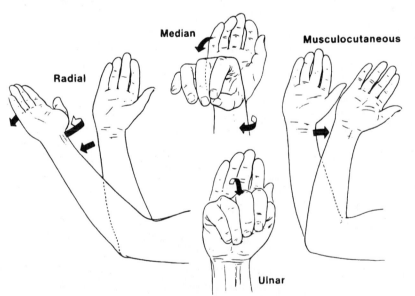

Figure 19-3

Upper extremity movements in response to stimulation of the nerves of the brachial plexus. Ulnar: Flexion at the wrist and adduction of the fingers. Radial: Extension of the elbow, wrist, and fingers, supination of the arm. Median: Flexion of the wrist, pronation of the arm. Musculocutaneous: Flexion at the elbow.

(Used with permission from Cousins MJ, Bridenbaugh PO, eds: Neural Blockade, *2nd ed. Philadelphia: JB Lippincott, 1988.)*

■ Premedication

All patients require reassurance and support during nerve blocks. In addition, some patients benefit from sedation and analgesia; midazolam and fentanyl are used commonly. Small intravenous doses given repeatedly to produce the desired effect are safest. For some blocks, patient cooperation is needed; for others, where paresthesias are not expected, profound sedation is feasible. During the block, an assistant can support the patient in the required position, as well as provide additional reassurance.

■ Needle Placement

The skin is prepared with an antiseptic solution, sterile drapes are applied, and the operator wears sterile gloves. An intradermal wheal of local anesthetic without epinephrine (with added epinephrine, these injections are more painful), placed through a 25- or 27-gauge needle, anesthetizes the skin where the block needle is to be placed. The thumb and index finger of the dominant hand hold the needle, while the wrist rests on an adjacent surface to steady the hand. Assuming a comfortable, relaxed position and advancing the needle using only the fingers, while the wrist remains fixed, provide the best control and allow fine adjustments of needle position.

When the desired endpoint is reached (paresthesia, motor response to electrical stimulation, or other landmarks), the needle position is fixed. Success now depends on maintaining the needletip near the nerve during the injection. Potential pitfalls include patient movement, failure to hold the needle firmly in place, or recoil of the needle with injection.

■ Choice of Local Anesthetic Solution

As with spinal and epidural anesthesia, the choice of local anesthetic solution depends on the expected duration of the operation and the degree of motor block needed. Chapter 17 contains information on the available local anesthetics; the section on the maximum doses is especially important in managing peripheral nerve blocks, because the use of larger volumes usually produces more certain neural blockade. For some blocks, increasing the pH of the local anesthetic solution (usually with sodium bicarbonate) speeds the onset of the block.

Because of possible direct neurotoxicity and limitations of total volume, the greatest available concentrations of local anesthetics (0.75% bupivacaine, 2.0% lidocaine) are not commonly used for peripheral neural blockade. Moderate concentrations, such as 1% to 1.5% lidocaine or 0.50% bupivacaine, are used more commonly for nerve blocks. Dilute solutions, such as 0.5% lidocaine and 0.125% bupivacaine, are used for infiltration when large volumes are required.

As in the epidural space, epinephrine (5 µg/ml) slows vascular absorption of the local anesthetic, decreasing the blood concentration and prolonging the block. The expected duration of blockade depends on vascular perfusion of the space into which the drug is injected and varies depending on the specific block. With lidocaine, peripheral nerve blocks last for 60 to 90 minutes; adding epinephrine may extend these times by 50 percent. With bupivacaine, blocks may last more than 3 hours; with epinephrine, blocks may extend for more than 12 hours. Epinephrine is not used for digital blocks or other blocks in which distal circulation may be compromised by vasoconstriction.

It is not always wise to choose the longest-acting local anesthetic mixture. First, the numb part may be at risk of injury postoperatively (e.g., from a tight cast). Second, prompt neurovascular evaluation may be important after some operations; residual neural blockade may interfere. Third, the onset of anesthesia is often delayed with such long-acting local anesthetics; this can delay the start of the operation unnecessarily.

■ Local Anesthetic Injection

For many blocks, the total dose of local anesthetic far exceeds the dose that can be given safely as an intravenous bolus. Nevertheless, appropriate precautions during the injection can prevent severe toxicity. For infiltration blocks, the use of dilute solutions of local anesthetic and moving the needle continuously about the target area ensure that only a small amount of local anesthetic will be injected if a blood vessel is entered inadvertently.

For blocks in which the needle is held in one place, one draws back on the plunger of the syringe (aspiration) before beginning the injection. If blood returns, the needle is moved slightly. Absence of blood on aspiration does not entirely rule out the possibility of intravascular injection. The local anesthetic solution is injected in increments of 5 to 10 ml, with pauses between doses so that early symptoms of intravascular injection can be detected and the injection halted.

These signs and symptoms include tinnitus, circumoral numbness, a metallic taste, tremors, agitation, or a vague sensation patients sometimes describe as "feeling funny." The ECG and blood pressure monitors are observed for signs of cardiovascular toxicity (arrhythmia, hypotension) or epinephrine effect (tachycardia, hypertension). If mild toxic symptoms appear, the block can be completed after appropriate treatment and repositioning of the needle.

■ Testing the Block

The onset of anesthesia is heralded by decreased sensitivity to cold, loss of pinprick sensation, and with concentrated local anesthetic solutions, motor block. Sufficient time is needed for local anesthetic diffusion through connective tissue barriers to the site of action. Repetitive premature testing of an unblocked area can provoke anxiety for the patient and must be avoided. Proprioception is often impossible to block, and patients must be reassured if they feel movement during the skin preparation and draping. At the time of incision, the surgeon tests the incision site (gentle probing with the scalpel or clamp) to determine the adequacy of the block. Expeditious induction of general anesthesia may be required if the block is inadequate; if general anesthesia is hazardous, the block can be repeated or supplemented with other blocks (e.g., adding a block of the ulnar nerve at the elbow if brachial plexus block leaves the little finger with sensation).

■ Intraoperative Management

Patients with adequate blocks may be sedated, and supplemental oxygen is appropriate. Monitoring during regional anesthesia is identical to that for any patient undergoing general anesthesia. It focuses on detecting delayed local anesthetic toxicity from excessive tissue absorption (usually at 15 to 60 minutes), ensuring adequate ventilation and oxygenation, and managing the consequences of surgical stress such as tourniquet pain or blood loss.

Brachial Plexus Block

■ Indications and Anatomy

Brachial plexus block is indicated for procedures involving the upper extremity from the shoulder to the hand. The plexus supplies all motor and sensory innervation to the arm. It originates from the anterior primary rami of C5-T1 and extends from the transverse processes to the apex of the axilla. The five roots of the plexus lie in the space between the anterior and middle scalene muscles and form the superior, middle, and inferior trunks as they pass over the first rib in the supraclavicular fossa. Each of these three trunks bifurcates into anterior and posterior divisions as the plexus passes under the midpoint of the clavicle. The six divisions rejoin to form the medial, lateral, and posterior cords just proximal to the axilla. In the axilla itself, the three most distal nerves of the brachial plexus (the median, radial, and ulnar nerves) encircle the axillary artery as they pass distally to the arm (Fig. 19-4).

Throughout its course, the brachial plexus is accompanied by an artery (the subclavian proximally, becoming the axillary distally), which provides an important landmark. These structures are enveloped throughout their course by a connective tissue sheath that originates from the prevertebral fascia proximally and extends to the axilla distally, known as the *neurovascular sheath*. Local anesthetic solutions injected into this space spread proximally and distally from the point of injection to anesthetize the elements of the plexus.

Three approaches to the plexus are commonly used: interscalene, supraclavicular, and axillary. Since each approach tends to produce a somewhat different distribution of anesthesia, the choice of technique depends on the surgical procedure and the desired pattern of anesthesia. In all cases, larger volumes of local anesthetic solution increase the likelihood of complete plexus blockade. The interscalene and supraclavicular blocks can be performed with the arm in any position, but the arm must be abducted for the axillary block.

■ Techniques and Complications

Interscalene Block

The interscalene approach is indicated for procedures involving the cephalad roots of the brachial plexus. This includes those about the anterior shoulder, lateral elbow, and forearm. In contrast, the inferior roots are far removed from the point of injection. As a result, C8 and T1 are frequently spared, which makes this approach less reliable for procedures on the ulnar aspect of the hand and forearm.

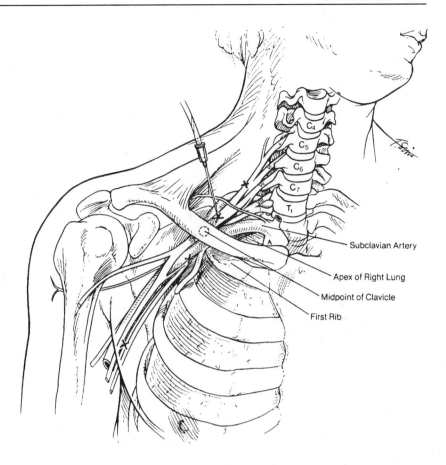

Figure 19-4

The course of the brachial plexus from its roots in the neck to the terminal nerves in the axilla. The needle is in the position for the supraclavicular block; the X above is at the site of the interscalene approach; the most distal X denotes the site of the axillary approach.

(Used with permission from Raj PP: Handbook of Regional Anesthesia. *New York: Churchill-Livingstone, 1985.)*

The patient's head is turned to the opposite side, with a roll placed between the shoulders to bring the strap muscles of the neck into relief, and the patient's ipsilateral hand is placed on the thigh to depress the clavicle. At the level of the cricoid cartilage (C6), the posterior border of the clavicular head of the sterno-cleidomastoid muscle is identified. Just posterior and deep to this, a palpating finger is rolled posteriorly over the belly of the anterior scalene muscle to sense the groove between the anterior and middle scalene muscles. This can be confirmed by asking the patient to sniff, which causes preferential contraction of the scalene muscles.

The needle is directed perpendicular to the plane of the skin, in a direction caudad, mesiad, and dorsad (Fig. 19-5). The needle contacts the cephalad roots of the plexus within the neurovascular sheath as they emerge from the neck between the anterior and middle scalene muscles. Proper position of the needle may be signaled by paresthesias extending into the arm or by responses to a nerve stimulator.

Between 30 and 40 ml of local anesthetic is injected in divided doses, with frequent aspiration. With the injection of larger volumes, the local anesthetic spreads cephalad in the interscalene groove to the nerve roots of C2, C3, and C4 to produce anesthesia of the cervical plexus as well.

Complications of the interscalene approach include Horner's syndrome and phrenic and laryngeal nerve block (hoarseness), which are common and usually well tolerated in healthy patients. The complications of epidural, subarachnoid, or intravascular injection (carotid or vertebral arteries) are rare but may require airway control and appropriate resuscitative maneuvers.

Supraclavicular Block

The roots of the brachial plexus merge to form the superior, middle, and inferior trunks as they pass over the first rib in the supraclavicular fossa. At this point the subclavian artery lies immediately anterior and inferior to the plexus within the neurovascular sheath, providing a vascular landmark. The supraclavicular

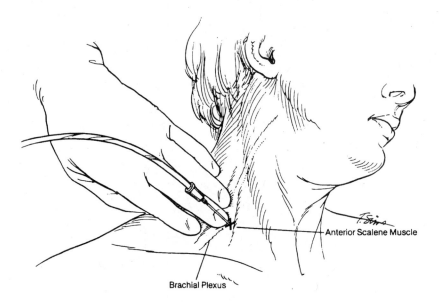

Anterior Scalene Muscle

Brachial Plexus

Figure 19-5

In the interscalene approach to the brachial plexus, the needle is directed caudad between the anterior and middle scalene muscles at the level of C6, as shown.

(Used with permission from Raj PP: Handbook of Regional Anesthesia. *New York: Churchill-Livingstone, 1985.)*

approach is appropriate for procedures involving the entire upper extremity, with the exception of the ulnar aspect of the hand (inferior trunk), which may be spared by this block (Fig. 19-6).

Patient positioning is the same as for interscalene block. The midpoint of the clavicle is identified, and the subclavian pulsation behind it palpated. Deeper palpation will reveal the shelf of the first rib, over which the subclavian artery and the brachial plexus travel as they pass laterally. The needle is introduced immediately posterior to the subclavian artery and directed caudally. The superior trunk of the plexus is most commonly encountered as it courses within the neurovascular sheath. If the first rib is encountered,

the needle is withdrawn and "walked" anteriorly along it into the plexus.

Needle position is confirmed by paresthesias or by response to a nerve stimulator. Alternatively, the subclavian artery may be punctured and the needle withdrawn a few millimeters outside the vessel (but still within the sheath). With either method, 30 to 40 ml of local anesthetic is injected after aspiration.

Complications of the supraclavicular approach are similar to those of the interscalene approach but include pneumothorax as well. Pneumothorax may be avoided by accurately identifying the first rib and advancing the needle directly toward it and not in a medial direction toward the cupola of the lung.

Figure 19-6

The supraclavicular approach to the brachial plexus. The needle is directed toward the trunks, lying just dorsal to the artery.

(Used with permission from Raj PP: Handbook of Regional Anesthesia. *New York: Churchill-Livingstone, 1985.)*

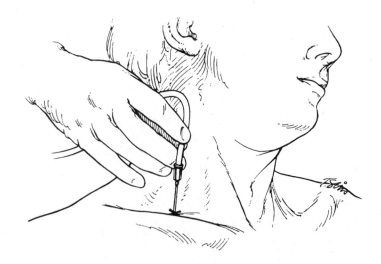

Axillary Block

In the axilla, the distal nerves of the brachial plexus (musculocutaneous, median, radial, and ulnar) are arranged circumferentially about the axillary artery. In contrast to the others, the musculocutaneous nerve lies outside the neurovascular sheath in the belly of the coracobrachialis muscle. The axillary approach is indicated for any procedure distal to the elbow, especially for hand operations (Fig. 19-7).

The arm is externally rotated and the shoulder abducted to 90 degrees or less; abduction of the arm more then 90 degrees may obliterate the axillary pulse. The axillary artery is identified lateral to the pectoralis major and carefully palpated with the index finger of the nondominant hand to determine its exact position. The needle is inserted in a cephalad direction by the dominant hand at an angle of 45 degrees in the long axis of the artery. In the transarterial approach, the artery is punctured directly and the needletip advanced just beyond the wall of the artery to lie within the neurovascular sheath. Then 20 ml of local anesthetic is injected deep to the artery, while firm pressure on the distal axillary artery promotes ceph-

alad spread of the local anesthetic. The needle is then withdrawn to a position just outside the superficial wall of the artery, and another 20 ml of local anesthetic solution is injected superficial to the artery.

If paresthesias are to be sought, or if a nerve stimulator is used, the needle is directed immediately tangential to the artery to contact nerves within the sheath. At this point, the entire dose of local anesthetic may be injected. Some advocate multiple, smaller injections into the sheath to ensure local anesthetic spread beyond septa that separate the nerves. However, the functional significance of these anatomic septa is controversial. Single-injection axillary block undoubtedly can block all the terminal nerves, indicating that the septa may not always prevent spread of local anesthetic; however, single-injection techniques sometimes result in delayed onset of block in nerves other than the one closest to the needletip.

Following local anesthetic injection, the arm is adducted and the axilla massaged to promote spread of the anesthetic flow toward the musculocutaneous nerve, which provides sensory innervation to the

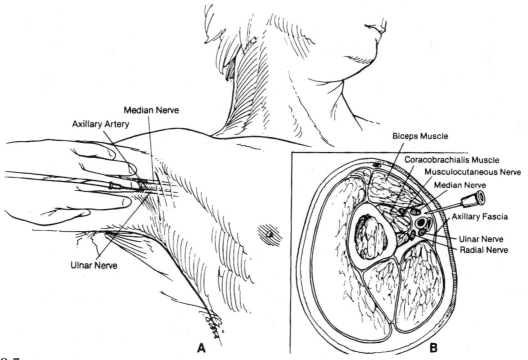

Figure 19-7

The surface anatomy of the axillary approach to the brachial plexus and a cross section of the proximal right arm, viewed from distal toward proximal. Note the position of the musculocutaneous nerve in the coracobrachialis.
(Used with permission from Raj PP: Handbook of Regional Anesthesia. *New York: Churchill-Livingstone, 1985.)*

lateral aspect of the forearm and the proximal thenar eminence. If this maneuver fails to block the musculocutaneous nerve, it may be blocked separately. Some anesthesiologists routinely include separate musculocutaneous nerve block when performing axillary block (see below).

Complications of the axillary approach include a small hematoma when the artery is punctured and intravascular injection, which can be detected by frequent aspiration and administration of small increments of local anesthetic while observing the patient.

Musculocutaneous Nerve Block

The musculocutaneous nerve supplies motor fibers to the biceps and sensory innervation to the skin of the lateral forearm. It exits the neurovascular sheath above the axilla, so proximal spread of local anesthetic from the axilla may be inadequate to reach it.

In the axilla, the nerve lies within the belly of the coracobrachialis muscle, which originates from the coracoid process of the anterior scapula and inserts onto the proximal humerus. The bulk of the muscle is palpable in the axilla immediately adjacent and cephalad to the neurovascular bundle. The nerve is blocked by wide infiltration into the belly of the coracobrachialis.

■ Intercostobrachial Nerve Block

Any of these approaches to the brachial plexus leave unanesthetized the medial aspect of the upper arm, which is served by the intercostobrachial nerve. This nerve is not part of the brachial plexus but derives from T1 and T2. Block of this nerve is important when a pneumatic tourniquet is to be used or when operations extend to the medial upper arm. The nerve passes through the axilla parallel to the neurovascular bundle but superficial to the fascia. It is often blocked inadvertently during axillary block; infiltration with 5 to 10 ml of local anesthetic solution superficial to the fascia just over the axillar artery suffices to block the nerve.

■ Distal Nerve Blocks of the Arm

Separate blocks of the median, ulnar, and radial nerves at the wrist or elbow produce anesthesia in the hand (Fig. 19-8). Accordingly, they are indicated only for procedures about the hand or to supplement an unsatisfactory brachial plexus block. Block at the elbow is technically more difficult than at the wrist,

except for the ulnar nerve, which is palpable in the ulnar groove at the elbow and is easily blocked with 5 to 10 ml of local anesthetic solution.

Median Nerve Block

The median nerve lies deep to the flexor retinaculum between the palmaris longus and flexor carpi radialis tendons. The patient flexes the wrist against counterpressure with the fingers in extension. A 5/8-in, 25-gauge needle is inserted perpendicularly between the tendons to pierce the retinaculum. Then 3 to 5 ml of local anesthetic is injected when a paresthesia is produced. If no paresthesia is produced, 5 to 8 ml is injected fanwise between the tendons.

Ulnar Nerve Block

The ulnar nerve lies between the ulnar artery and the flexor carpi ulnaris tendon, which lies medial to the artery. The needle is directed between these two structures at the wrist crease. After aspiration, 3 to 5 ml of local anesthetic is infiltrated fanwise.

Radial Nerve Block

At the wrist, the radial nerve diverges from the artery laterally and dorsally and pierces deep fascia. Three milliliters of local anesthetic is deposited lateral to the radial artery after attempted aspiration of blood. An intradermal and subcutaneous wheal is then extended laterally and dorsally over the wrist to reach those branches which have diverged near the anatomic snuff box to supply the dorsum of the hand.

Blocks of the Thoracic and Abdominal Walls

■ Intercostal Nerve Block

Indications and Anatomy

Intercostal nerve blocks are used most commonly for relief of the pain caused by rib fractures or intercostal or subcostal incisions, such as for thoracotomy or cholecystostomy. Multiple bilateral intercostal blocks, in conjunction with celiac plexus block (described in Chap. 35), give anesthesia for intraabdominal surgical procedures.

The 12 paired intercostal nerves are formed by the anterior primary rami of T1 to T12. They course circumferentially in the inferior groove of each rib, supplying skin and musculature of the chest and

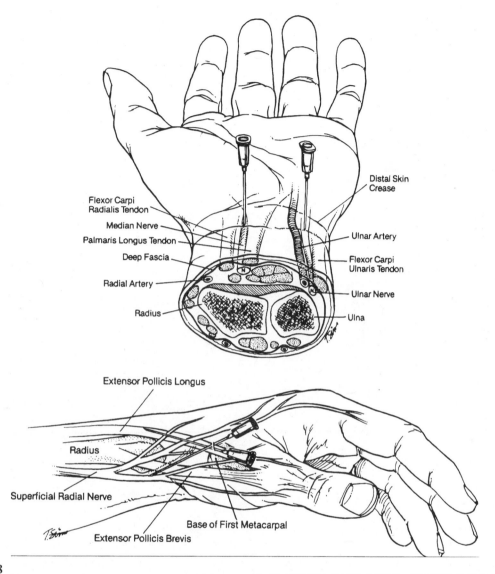

Figure 19-8

Cross section and ulnar views of the wrist showing blocks of median, ulnar, and radial nerves.
(Used with permission from Raj PP: Handbook of Regional Anesthesia. *New York: Churchill-Livingstone, 1985.)*

anterior abdominal wall (Fig. 19-9). The nerve and accompanying artery and vein are enclosed by the rib above and below and by the external and internal intercostal musculature; this constitutes a space into which local anesthetics may be injected.

Technique and Complications

Intercostal nerve block is best performed with the patient in the prone or lateral position, with the shoulder abducted to rotate the scapula superiorly and laterally. Injection is usually performed lateral to

the posterior midline at the angle of the rib. Here the intercostal space is wide, the ribs are easily palpable, and the lateral cutaneous branches have not yet left the intercostal space. Skin wheals are raised over the intercostal spaces and pulled cephalad with the nondominant hand so that they rest over the rib corresponding to the nerve to be blocked. A 1.5-in, 22-gauge needle mounted on a three-ring control syringe is inserted at a slightly cephalad angle to reach the periosteum of the rib and then is "walked" off the inferior margin to an additional depth of 3 to 5 mm.

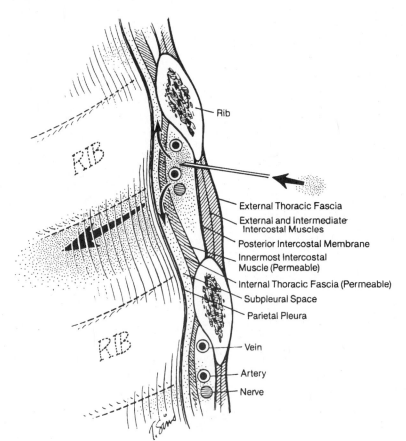

Rib

External Thoracic Fascia

External and Intermediate Intercostal Muscles

Posterior Intercostal Membrane

Innermost Intercostal Muscle (Permeable)

Internal Thoracic Fascia (Permeable)

Subpleural Space

Parietal Pleura

Vein

Artery

Nerve

Figure 19-9

Views of the tissue planes defining the space around the neurovascular bundle for the intercostal nerve block.

(Used with permission from Raj PP: Handbook of Regional Anesthesia. *New York: Churchill-Livingstone, 1985.)*

A loss of resistance may be felt as the needletip penetrates the intercostal space. Paresthesias may be elicited but are not necessary.

The syringe barrel is stabilized with the nondominant hand, and 5 ml of local anesthetic is injected after aspiration for blood. Intersegmental neural communication at the spinal cord requires that at least one nerve above and below the intended site be blocked as well.

Complications of intercostal nerve block include intravascular injection and pneumothorax owing to laceration of lung parenchyma by the needletip. Both are rare when this procedure is performed by an experienced operator and may be avoided by maintaining strict control of the needle. Local anesthetic is taken up rapidly from this site, so the resulting blood concentration of local anesthetic is great if many intercostal nerves are blocked. Epinephrine is added routinely to local anesthetic mixtures used for this block.

■Block of the Inguinal Region

Indications and Anatomy

Inguinal field block is indicated most commonly for herniorrhaphy. The technique is especially useful for outpatients or debilitated patients or as an adjunct to general anesthesia to reduce anesthetic requirements and provide postoperative pain relief.

Innervation of the inguinal region is supplied by the ventral rami of spinal nerves from T11 to L2. The peripheral nerves of interest include the subcostals (T12), ilioinguinal (T12-L1), iliohypogastric (T12-L1), genitofemoral (L1-L2), and subcutaneous ramifications of other local nerves. Autonomic fibers from the lower thoracic segments descend with and supply the spermatic cord and its contents.

Technique and Complications

The large volumes of local anesthetic solution required for the block require that dilute concentrations (1% lidocaine or 0.25% bupivacaine) be used to limit the total dose of local anesthetic.

Block of the iliohypogastric and ilioinguinal nerves is essential. As they descend and pierce the muscles of the anterior abdominal wall, they are blocked 2.5 cm medial to the anterosuperior iliac spine. A 1.5-in, 22-gauge needle is advanced through a skin wheal and directed laterally and inferiorly to touch the inside shelf of the iliac bone. Then 10 ml of local anesthetic is deposited as the needle is moved in and out in a fan to infiltrate the external oblique, internal oblique, and transversalis muscles. With experience, distinct "pops" may be felt as the needletip pierces all three layers of muscular fascia. When the depth of the muscles is sounded, the needle is directed medially through the same puncture, and 5 ml is infiltrated in a similar fashion to complete the block, bearing in mind that the peritoneal cavity becomes progressively more superficial toward the midline.

Cutaneous branches of T11 and T12, as well as stray fibers from T10, are blocked with a 3.5-in, 22-gauge needle introduced through the same point. Anesthetic solution is distributed from just lateral to the anterosuperior iliac spine to the umbilicus intradermally, subcutaneously, and intramuscularly. Thorough infiltration compensates for the variable penetration of these nerves as they descend toward the midline.

A subcutaneous wheal is then raised from the umbilicus to the pubic tubercle and from the anterosuperior iliac spine inferiorly 4 cm and then medially back to the pubic tubercle. Genitofemoral nerve block is accomplished by directing a 1.5-in, 22-gauge needle superior to the lateral pubic tubercle and infiltrating 5 ml of local anesthetic.

During the procedure, the surgeon injects the incision line, as well as the spermatic cord, to prevent visceral pain. The keys to success with this block include limiting its use to smaller reducible hernias, meticulous infiltration of the various layers of the abdominal wall, and gentle technique by the surgeon to avoid pain from peritoneal traction.

Nerve Blocks to the Lower Extremity

■ Indications and Anatomy

Virtually any surgical procedure on the lower extremity can be accomplished with a proper combination of peripheral nerve blocks. In contrast to the upper extremity, where the nerves of the brachial plexus course together, multiple blocks are required to block the lower extremity because both the lumbar and lumbosacral plexuses are involved.

The lumbar plexus and its terminal branches, the obturator, femoral, and lateral femoral cutaneous nerves, originate from the anterior primary rami of L1 to L4, form within the belly of the psoas muscle, and ramify widely to supply the anterior compartment of the thigh (Fig. 19-10). The obturator nerve originates from L2 to L4 and exits the pelvis through the obturator foramen to supply the adductors of the thigh. The femoral nerve is also derived from L2 to L4 and enters the thigh deep to the inguinal ligament, just lateral to the femoral artery. It provides motor innervation to the thigh extensors and sensory inner-

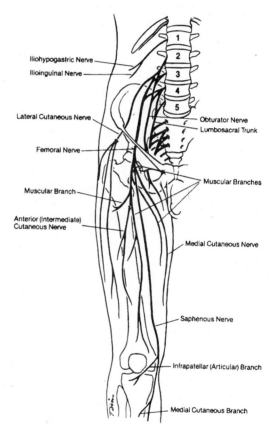

Figure 19-10

The formation of the lumbar plexus and its branches. *(Used with permission from Raj PP:* Handbook of Regional Anesthesia. *New York: Churchill-Livingstone, 1985.)*

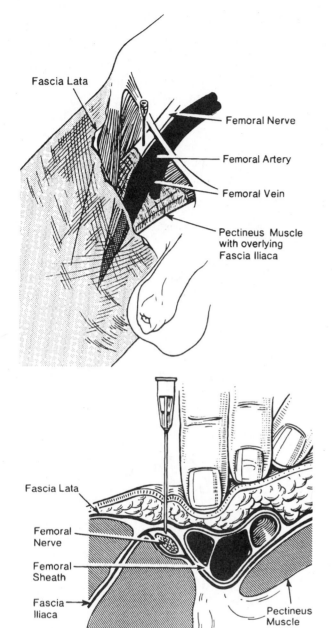

Figure 19-11

Technique of femoral nerve block. Note that the nerve is separated from the femoral sheath.

(Used with permission from Cousins MJ, Bridenbaugh PO, eds: Neural Blockade, *2nd ed. Philadelphia: JB Lippincott, 1988.)*

vation to the skin of the anterior thigh. The continuation of the femoral nerve as the saphenous nerve provides sensory innervation to the anteromedial aspect of the leg below the knee. The lateral femoral cutaneous nerve enters the thigh medial to the anterosuperior iliac spine and eventually pierces the fasciae latae to supply the skin of the lateral thigh.

The lumbosacral plexus forms from the anterior rami of L4 to S3 and lies on the anterior surface of the sacrum in a relatively inaccessible location. Its collateral branches supply the pelvis and buttocks locally, while the remaining branches give rise to the sciatic nerve. The sciatic nerve supplies the posterior thigh compartment and, through its terminal branches, the posterior tibial nerve and common peroneal nerves, the posterior and lateral compartments of the lower leg, as well as the ankle and foot.

■ Technique and Complications

Lumbar Plexus Block

All three terminal nerves of the lumbar plexus innervating the lower extremity (femoral, lateral femoral cutaneous, and obturator) may be blocked with a single injection in the psoas compartment within the belly of the psoas muscle. The patient assumes the lateral position, as for spinal or lumbar epidural anesthesia. A line connecting the iliac crests perpendicular to the spine is drawn. A second line runs parallel to the spinal column and passes through the posterosuperior iliac spine. At the intersection of these two lines, 2 to 5 cm from the midline and superior to the iliac crest, a 5- or 6-in needle is inserted perpendicular to the skin in all planes. At a depth of 5 to 8 cm, a paresthesia to the lower extremity or a thigh motor response to electrical nerve stimulation may be obtained.

Between 20 and 30 ml of local anesthetic is injected; complete anesthesia of the lumbar plexus results. If the procedure requires a sacral plexus or sciatic nerve block, this must be done separately, since local anesthetic does not spread reliably to these structures from the psoas compartment, even when given in large volumes.

Femoral Nerve Block

The femoral nerve lies immediately lateral to the femoral artery as both structures enter the leg deep to the inguinal ligament (Fig. 19-11). Infiltration, paresthesia, and nerve stimulation techniques have all been described. The femoral nerve lies in a fascial layer distinct from the artery, so a transarterial technique cannot be used. Ten milliliters of local anesthetic is injected after careful aspiration for blood. Injection of larger volumes with cephalad needle direction, which encourages proximal spread along the fascial sheath of the femoral nerve, produces anesthesia of the lateral femoral cutaneous nerve as well. It was originally thought that the obturator nerve also was blocked, but subsequent studies failed to confirm this. Apparently, the divergence of the obturator nerve from the lumbar plexus is too proximal to allow reliable blockade from an inguinal perivascular approach.

Lateral Femoral Cutaneous Nerve Block

The lateral femoral cutaneous nerve is blocked deep to the fascia lata 2 cm medial and 2 cm inferior to the anterosuperior iliac spine. A "pop" is felt as the needletip pierces the fascia, and 8 ml of local anesthetic is injected in a fan medially and laterally to cross the long axis of the nerve. Another 2 ml is injected superficial to the fascia to contact any superficial branches.

Obturator Nerve Block

The obturator nerve is blocked as it passes through the obturator foramen (Fig. 19-12). With the patient supine, the leg to be blocked is slightly abducted. A skin wheal is placed 0.5 in lateral and inferior to the pubic tubercle. The operator advances a 4-in needle medially to contact the horizontal ramus of the pubic bone inferior to the pubic tubercle. The needle is then redirected inferiorly and laterally off the bone and advanced another 1 in into the obturator foramen. After aspiration, 15 ml of local anesthetic is injected. Complications include intravascular injection and perforation of the bladder or vagina.

Sciatic Nerve Block

Combined with other nerve blocks, sciatic nerve block provides complete anesthesia of the lower extremity. During orthopedic procedures employing a thigh tourniquet, it prevents tourniquet pain. A number of anterior, posterior, and lateral approaches are possible.

The posterior approach of Labat is used most often (Fig. 19-13). The patient assumes the lateral Sims

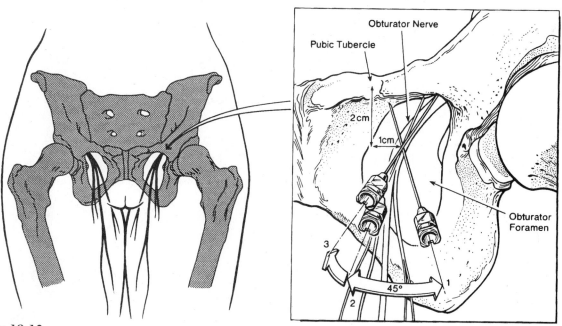

Figure 19-12

Technique of obturator nerve block (see text). The needle is directed to contact the horizontal ramus of the pubic bone near the pubic tubercle. It is then redirected laterally and inferiorly to enter the obturator foramen.
(Used with permission from Cousins MJ, Bridenbaugh PO, eds: Neural Blockade, *2nd ed. Philadelphia: JB Lippincott, 1988.)*

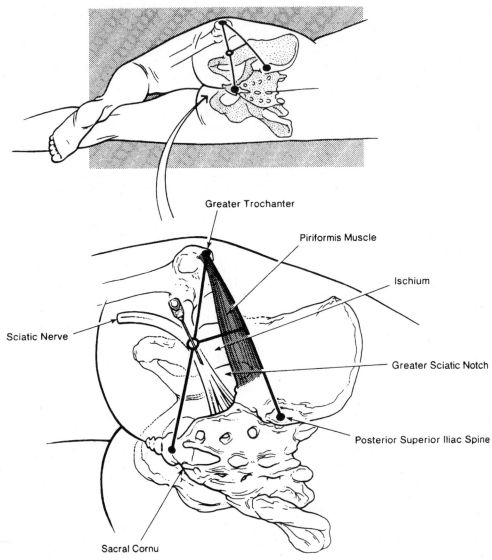

Greater Trochanter

Piriformis Muscle

Ischium

Sciatic Nerve

Greater Sciatic Notch

Posterior Superior Iliac Spine

Sacral Cornu

Figure 19-13

The classic site for the posterior approach to the sciatic nerve is found by drawing a line between the greater trochanter and the posterosuperior iliac spine. From the midpoint of that line, a line extending perpendicularly downward for 5 cm should intersect a line drawn between the greater trochanter and the distal sacrum. At this point, a needle is inserted perpendicularly in all planes to reach the sciatic nerve.

(Used with permission from Raj PP: Handbook of Regional Anesthesia. *New York: Churchill-Livingstone, 1985.)*

position, lying on the side opposite the one to be blocked with the contralateral (dependent) leg extended and the involved leg flexed at the knee and hip. A line is drawn between the greater trochanter of the femur and the posterosuperior iliac spine. From the midpoint of this line, a second line is extended perpendicularly downward for 5 cm to the point of needle insertion. Then 10 to 20 ml of local anesthetic is injected after elicitation of a lower leg paresthesia or motor response to nerve stimulation.

The sciatic nerve also can be reached via an anterior approach, with the patient supine (Fig. 19-14). A line is drawn along the inguinal ligament from the anterosuperior iliac spine to the pubic tubercle and divided into three equal parts. A perpendicular line is extended inferiorly and laterally from the junction of the

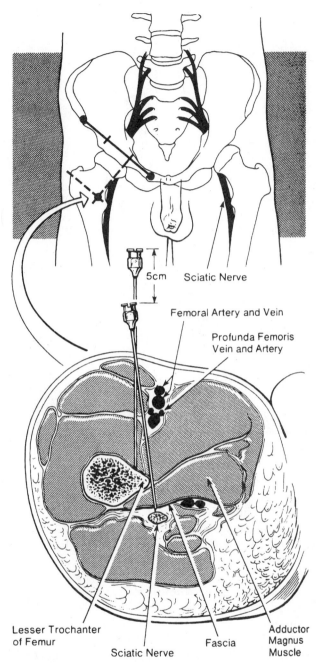

5cm Sciatic Nerve

Femoral Artery and Vein

Profunda Femoris
Vein and Artery

Lesser Trochanter
of Femur

Sciatic Nerve Fascia

Adductor
Magnus
Muscle

Figure 19-14

Anterior approach to the sciatic nerve (see text). The needle is directed to contact the lesser trochanter of the femur and then is redirected medially off the bone and toward the sciatic nerve.

(Used with permission from Cousins MJ, Bridenbaugh PO, eds: Neural Blockade, 2nd ed. Philadelphia: JB Lippincott, 1988.)

medial and middle thirds of this line. Another line originating at the greater trochanter is drawn parallel to the first line. The interaction of this line with the perpendicular line is the point of needle insertion. Beneath this point, the sciatic nerve travels medial and posterior to the femur. A 5-in needle is inserted perpendicular to the skin and advanced until bone is contacted. The needle is then redirected medially past the bone and advanced another 2 in, using parasthesias or nerve stimulation to signal proximity to the sciatic nerve. After aspiration, 20 to 30 ml of local anesthetic is injected.

Ankle Block

Infiltration block at the ankle is indicated for procedures distal to the malleoli. The terminal branch of the femoral nerve, the saphenous nerve, and the four terminal branches of the sciatic nerve (the posterior tibial, deep and superficial peroneal, and sural nerves) are readily accessible in the subcutaneous tissue as they cross the ankle joint (Fig. 19-15).

The patient lies prone or supine with the ankle to be blocked elevated. Omitting epinephrine in the local anesthetic mixture avoids arterial vasoconstriction and possible ischemia. The posterior tibial nerve is infiltrated behind the medial malleolus as it passes posterior to the pulsation of the posterior tibial artery. The sural nerve is blocked superficially by infiltration from the lateral malleolus to the Achilles tendon. The deep peroneal nerve is blocked where it lies deep to the extensor retinaculum between the tendons of the extensor hallicus longus and tibialis anterior muscles. Superficial infiltration from this point to the medial and lateral malleoli blocks the saphenous and superficial peroneal nerves, respectively.

Intravenous Regional Anesthesia

■ Indications and Anatomy

Intravenous regional anesthesia (Bier block) entails intravenous injection of large volumes of dilute local anesthetic while the circulation to the extremity is isolated by a tourniquet. The apparent mechanism of action is diffusion of local anesthetic from blood vessels to local nerves. The technique is indicated for brief procedures, especially about the forearm or hand, such as ganglion cyst excision. The duration of anesthesia is limited not by the duration of the effect of the local anesthetic but by the patient's tolerance of

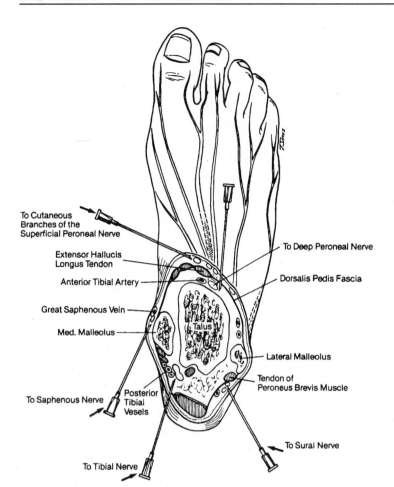

To Cutaneous Branches of the Superficial Peroneal Nerve

Extensor Hallucis Longus Tendon

Anterior Tibial Artery

Great Saphenous Vein

Med. Malleolus

To Saphenous Nerve

Posterior Tibial Vesels

To Tibial Nerve

To Deep Peroneal Nerve

Dorsalis Pedis Fascia

Talus

Lateral Malleolus

Tendon of Peroneus Brevis Muscle

To Sural Nerve

Figure 19-15

A transverse section of the ankle showing the approaches to blocking the five nerves at the ankle.

(Used with permission from Raj PP: Handbook of Regional Anesthesia. *New York: Churchill-Livingstone, 1985.)*

the tourniquet, usually 40 to 60 minutes. Lidocaine 0.5% is used most commonly. Chloroprocaine may produce thrombophlebitis, and bupivacaine is avoided because of cardiovascular toxicity.

■ Technique and Complications

The operator places an intravenous cannula distally in the limb to be anesthetized and attaches it via extension tubing to a syringe containing local anesthetic. A double pneumatic tourniquet is placed proximally, and the limb is elevated to drain venous blood. If possible, an elastic Esmarch bandage wrapped tightly around the limb beginning distally completes the venous exsanguination. The distal tourniquet is inflated, followed by the proximal tourniquet, both to 300 mmHg. The distal tourniquet is then released. At this point, the extremity has a mottled, cadaveric appearance.

Lidocaine 0.5% without epinephrine, 3 mg/kg (approximately 40 ml in a 70-kg patient), is then injected slowly from the reservoir syringe. Anesthesia begins virtually immediately. Usually, tourniquet pain develops after 40 minutes. Additional time may be gained by inflating the distal tourniquet and then deflating the proximal tourniquet. This extends the duration of anesthesia to approximately 60 minutes.

At the conclusion of the procedure, the tourniquet is deflated. Circulation returns to the limb, washing the local anesthetic into the systemic circulation and allowing sensation to return within minutes. Deflation of the tourniquet must be delayed a minimum of 30 minutes after injection to allow fixation of the local anesthetic to tissues; premature deflation of the tourniquet results in toxic blood concentrations of local anesthetic. Peak blood concentrations also can be reduced by releasing the local anesthetic from the limb in small aliquots, deflating the tourniquet intermittently for no more than 10 seconds at a time.

Toxic reactions are rare but do occur. They usually take the form of transient cardiovascular changes, such as bradycardia. The most feared complication is premature accidental tourniquet release leading to fulminant local anesthetic toxicity. For this reason, a separate intravenous cannula in another extremity and the immediate availability of resuscitation equipment are required.

BIBLIOGRAPHY

Cousins MJ, Bridenbaugh PO, eds. *Neural Blockade*, 2nd ed. Philadelphia: JB Lippincott, 1988.

Katz J. *Atlas of Regional Anesthesia*, 2nd ed. Norwalk, Conn: Appleton and Lange, 1985.

Raj PP. *Handbook of Regional Anesthesia*. New York: Churchill-Livingstone, 1985.

Winnie A. *Plexus Anesthesia*, Vol I: *Perivascular Techniques of Brachial Plexus Block*. Philadelphia: WB Saunders, 1984.

Patients with Special Requirements

20

Cardiopulmonary Resuscitation

Frederick W. Campbell

Cardiopulmonary resuscitation (CPR) employs temporary measures to deliver oxygen to the heart and brain while specific therapies are administered to restore the native circulation and ventilation. Cardiopulmonary resuscitation is an essential skill for everyone who administers anesthetics or other sedative or analgesic medications that depress consciousness, ventilation, or circulation.

Cardiopulmonary Resuscitation: Restoration of Oxygen Delivery

Deficiency of oxygen delivery is fundamental to all cardiopulmonary arrests, regardless of the initial cause. Basic life support (BLS) consists of temporarily providing oxygen delivery to the lungs with airway opening and rescue breathing and providing oxygen transport from the lungs to the body tissues with cardiac compression. Advanced cardiac life support (ACLS) adds specific treatments that restore natural cardiopulmonary function so that the patient's ventilation and circulation maintain oxygen delivery to the body. In the final phase of resuscitation, postresuscitation life support, the primary cause of the arrest is defined, and treatment is provided to achieve long-term recovery (Table 20-1).

Basic life support with manual airway opening, mouth-to-mouth exhaled air ventilation, and closed chest compression has been taught to the public and medical personnel alike as a first step in the treatment of cardiopulmonary arrest (Fig. 20-1 and Table 20-2). However, BLS produces arterial oxygenation and cardiac output that are far less than physiologic, which do not permit successful resuscitation unless ACLS therapy follows rapidly (Table 20-3). The most effective therapeutic approach to cardiopulmonary arrest is immediate application of definitive treatment that restores the patient's native cardiac output and ventilation. Basic life-support measures must not delay the start of specific therapy when it is immediately available.

Cardiopulmonary resuscitation outside the hospital may be limited by lack of trained personnel or support equipment to enhance temporary oxygen delivery during BLS and delayed arrival of ACLS-capable providers. In the hospital, CPR administered by anesthesiologists or other trained personnel avoids these limitations. Specifically, the anesthesiologist's definition of BLS includes securing the airway by intubation, use of ventilating devices that deliver 100% oxygen, and use of adjuncts to increase perfusion during chest compression. Further, ACLS treatment specific to the cause of the arrest can be administered promptly. Once ACLS begins, BLS continues until restoration of natural ventilation and circulation occurs or resuscitation is stopped.

Respiratory Resuscitation

Respiratory insufficiency and arrest lead to carbon dioxide retention and hypoxemia. Although extreme

Table 20-1

Component Parts of CPR	
BLS: Temporary oxygen delivery	Vascular access
Airway opening	Peripheral/central venous
Manual maneuvers	Endotracheal
Pharyngeal airways	Intraosseous
Tracheal intubation	Pharmacologic therapy
Cricothyrotomy	Chronotropes
Artificial ventilation	Antiarrhythmics
Oxygen	Inotropes
Mouth-to-mouth	Vasopressors
Mouth-to-mask	Volume expanders/blood
Cricoid pressure	Narcotic, benzodiazepine antagonists
Manually powered ventilators	Thrombolytic therapy
Oxygen-powered ventilators	Invasive procedures
Automatic transport ventilators	Pericardiocentesis
Transtracheal jet ventilation	Needle thoracostomy
Artificial circulation	Chest tube insertion
Closed chest compression	Aortic clamping
Cardiac back board	PRLS: Definition of the primary cause of arrest and treatment of the consequences of cardiopulmonary arrest
Epinephrine	Continuous monitoring
Open chest cardiac massage	Diagnostic evaluation
Cardiopulmonary bypass	General intensive care
ACLS: Restoration of native oxygen delivery	Definitive treatment of the cause of arrest
Electrical therapy	
Cardioversion	
Cardiac pacing	
Precordial thump	

Abbreviations: BLS, basic life support; ACLS, advanced cardiac life support; PRLS, postresuscitation life support.

Figure 20-1

Decision tree illustrating the American Heart Association (AHA) one-rescuer basic life support (BLS) sequence for adult CPR. Patient assessment, activation of emergency medical system (EMS), and airway opening are the initial steps (section A in diagram). For unconscious, apneic subjects, artificial ventilation is begun (section B). If unable to ventilate the lungs after repositioning the airway and a second effort to ventilate, lay rescuers are taught to apply therapy for airway foreign bodies (in unconscious adults, a repeated series of five Heimlich maneuvers, a finger sweep of the hypopharynx, and repeated attempts to ventilate). Trained rescuers may use airway opening and ventilating adjuncts, including laryngoscopy, to open the airway or visualize and remove a foreign body, if present. Artificial circulation of the pulseless subject is provided by closed chest compression (section C). A single rescuer performs a repeating series of 15 chest compressions and 2 rescue breaths for adult victims. The pulse is reassessed for return of native circulation after the first minute of CPR and every few minutes thereafter. The BLS sequence for infant and child victims is the same as that applied to adults. The performance of specific ventilation, foreign-body treatment, and chest compression steps differs from those described for adults and varies according to age (see Table 20-2). When two or more lay rescuers are present, they alternate the performance of one-rescuer CPR. Rescuers monitor correct technique and the pulse generated by each other's CPR. Two or more trained professionals may administer two-rescuer CPR. The ratio of compressions to ventilations during two-rescuer CPR is 5:1; one rescuer performs chest compression, pausing briefly after every fifth compression to permit the second rescuer to provide artificial ventilation with a 1.5- to 2-second inspiratory time. Once tracheal intubation has been accomplished and gastric inflation prevented, chest compression is performed without pauses, and ventilations are delivered simultaneously with chest compression or quickly interjected between compressions. Advanced cardiac life support modalities are administered by trained professionals as soon as equipment is available.

(Reproduced with permission from Chandra NC, Hazinski MF, eds: Textbook of Basic Life Support for Healthcare Providers. Dallas: American Heart Association, 1994.)

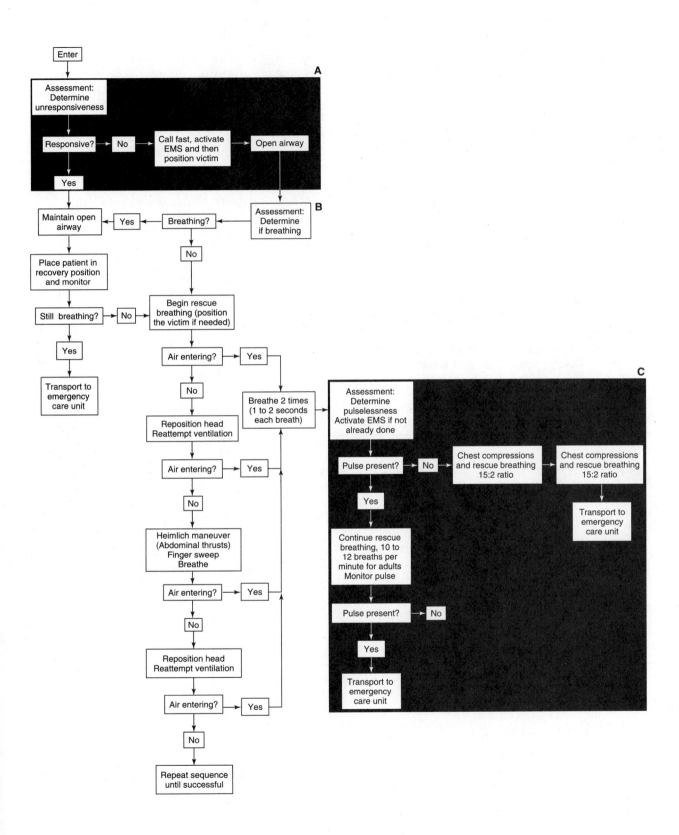

hypercarbia exerts arrhythmogenic and negative inotropic actions, hypoxemia is the disorder primarily responsible for the morbidity and mortality of respiratory arrest. Patient outcome from respiratory arrest depends on the duration of cerebral hypoxia and whether secondary cardiac arrest has occurred. Recovery is swift and complete if gas exchange is restored within 3 to 4 minutes of unconsciousness and prior to cardiac arrest. Outcome after secondary cardiac arrest is extremely poor in both children and adults.

Several nonspecific steps apply universally to patients with respiratory insufficiency:

1. Permit the conscious patient with respiratory difficulty to assume whatever body position is most comfortable. This will likely be a forward-leaning sitting position.
2. Administer 100% oxygen. If apnea then occurs in a subject dependent on hypoxic ventilatory drive (a rare occurrence), provide artificial ventilation until the FIO_2 is adjusted.
3. Monitor vital signs, electrocardiogram (ECG), and oxygen saturation, and establish intravenous access.

Prompt restoration of normal breathing is desired and can be achieved when the cause of the respiratory difficulty is identified and specific therapy (e.g., bronchodilators, thoracentesis, narcotic antagonist) is given. Airway opening and artificial ventilation with oxygen are provided as needed until native respiration returns.

■ Opening the Airway in Obtunded and Unconscious Patients

Airway obstruction occurs with loss of consciousness because of relaxation of the muscles supporting the mandible, tongue, and epiglottis. The base of the tongue and epiglottis fall posteriorly into the airway, impeding gas flow into the trachea (Fig. 20-2). Placing the unconscious patient in a lateral or prone position does not ensure an open airway.

Manual Airway Opening

The fundamental maneuver to open the airway is anterior displacement of the mandible to lift the epiglottis and base of the tongue from the airway. This is accomplished by the chin lift (see Fig. 20-2) or jaw thrust maneuver (Fig. 20-3).

Pharyngeal Airways

When airway obstruction persists despite maximal mandibular displacement, an oropharyngeal or nasopharyngeal airway is indicated. These augment the elevation of the epiglottis and base of the tongue from the posterior pharyngeal wall. The oropharyngeal airway is more effective but may induce vomiting in responsive patients. Improper insertion or use of an undersized oral airway can exacerbate airway obstruction by pushing the tongue back into the posterior pharynx. Mandibular displacement must be maintained during use of pharyngeal airways.

Tracheal Intubation

When a patient's altered consciousness is not quickly reversible, measures are taken to prevent gastric inflation during artificial ventilation and protect the airway from aspiration of regurgitated gastric contents. Tracheal intubation accomplishes these goals and provides an alternative drug delivery route during resuscitation.

Attempts at tracheal intubation must not delay oxygenation of the patient; ventilation by bag and mask with manual airway opening or insertion of a pharyngeal airway precedes attempts at tracheal intubation. Tracheal intubation is described in Chapter 13.

Alternative artificial airways that may be inserted without visualization of the glottis have been used by rescuers unskilled in the technique of tracheal intubation. Use of the esophageal obturator airway (EOA) (Fig. 20-4) or esophageal gastric tube airway (EGTA) often results in inadequate ventilation. The efficacy of the esophageal-tracheal Combitube, the pharyngotracheal lumen airway, and the laryngeal mask airway (LMA) during CPR is not established. Tracheal intubation is the preferred means to achieve airway protection and ventilation during CPR.

■ Artificial Ventilation

With the airway open, ventilation and oxygenation must begin immediately. Without special equipment, mouth-to-mouth ventilation provides the quickest means of delivering adequate tidal volumes. Fear of infection has lead to the use of face shields and mouth-to-mask ventilating devices. The mask devices include a filter and nonrebreathing valve to protect rescuer and patient from direct contact and exhaled droplets.

While transmission of hepatitis B and human immunodeficiency virus (HIV) between health care

Table 20-2

Performance of Basic Life Support Maneuvers for Adults, Children, and Infants

Maneuver	Adult (>8 years)	Child (1–8 years)	Infant (<1 year)
Airway opening	Head tilt-chin lift, jaw thrust	Head tilt-chin lift, jaw thrust	Head tilt-chin lift, jaw thrust
Breathing Initial breaths	Mouth-to-mouth 2 breaths, 1.5–2 seconds inspiratory time.	Mouth-to-mouth 2 breaths, 1–1.5 seconds inspiratory time	Mouth-to-mouth and nose 2 breaths, 1–1.5 seconds inspiratory time
Tidal volume	10–15 ml/kg, or produce chest expansion	10–15 ml/kg, or produce chest expansion	10–15 ml/kg, or produce chest expansion
Rate (approximate)	10–12/min	20/min	20/min
Foreign-body airway obstruction Conscious victim	Heimlich maneuver, repeat until effective or patient unconscious	Heimlich maneuver, repeat until effective or patient unconscious	Back and chest blows, alternate 5 of each maneuver until effective or patient unconscious
Unconscious victim	Attempt to ventilate, Heimlich maneuver (5 times), finger sweep, repeat sequence	Attempt to ventilate, Heimlich maneuver (5 times), finger sweep only if object visualized in mouth, repeat sequence	Attempt to ventilate, back blows (5), chest thrusts (5), finger sweep only if object visualized in mouth, repeat sequence
Circulation Pulse check	Carotid or femoral artery	Carotid or femoral artery	Brachial or femoral artery
Compression area	Lower half of sternum	Lower half of sternum	Lower half of sternum
Compression source	Two hands	Heel of one hand	2–3 fingers
Depth	1.5–2 inches or more if needed to produce a pulse	1–1.5 in, or one-third to one-half of the depth of the chest if needed to produce a pulse	0.5–1 in, or one-third to one-half of the depth of the chest if needed to produce a pulse
Rate	80–100/min	100/min	At least 100/min
Compression-ventilation ratio	15:2 for one rescuer or two lay rescuers; 5:1 for ventilation for two professional rescuers	5:1 (pause for ventilation)	5:1 (pause for ventilation)

Adapted from Chandra NC, Hazinski MF, eds: *Textbook of Basic Life Support for Healthcare Providers.* Dallas: American Heart Association, 1994.

providers and patients has occurred as a result of blood exchange or penetrating injury by blood-contaminated instruments, transmission of these infections during mouth-to-mouth resuscitation has not been documented. There is a greater theoretical risk of transmission of herpes simplex, tuberculosis, and other respiratory infections. Barrier devices, including mouth-to-mask or bag-valve-mask ventilating devices, latex gloves, and eye protection are recommended for use by health care workers who perform CPR.

Exhaled air ventilation techniques provide an FIO_2 of 0.16 to 0.17, limiting alveolar oxygen tension to less than 80 mmHg. Decreased cardiac output and increased intrapulmonary shunting during CPR further impair arterial oxygenation. These patients require ventilation with 100% oxygen as soon as possible.

Manually Powered Ventilators

Self-inflating resuscitators or portable anesthesia ventilating circuits administer oxygen and effective ventilation via mask or endotracheal tube. The FIO_2 delivered by a simple self-inflating resuscitation bag (Fig. 20-5) is limited to 0.4 to 0.6 (oxygen inflow 10 to 15 liters/min) because the self-inflating bag

Table 20-3

Relation of Survival from Cardiac Arrest (Witnessed Out-of-Hospital Ventricular Fibrillation) to Promptness of Basic Life Support (BLS) and Advanced Cardiac Life Support (ACLS)

Time to BLS (min)	Time to ACLS (min)	Survival Rate (%)
0–4	0–8	43
0–4	>16	10
8–12	8–16	6
8–12	>16	0
>12	>12	0

Data reproduced from Eisenberg MS, Bergner L, Mallstrom A: Cardiac resuscitation in the community: Importance of rapid provision and implications for program planning. *JAMA* 1979;241:1905–1907.

refills itself at a rate exceeding the oxygen inflow, thereby entraining room air. Oxygen reservoirs that can be attached to these permit inspired oxygen concentrations near 0.9 to 1.0 (oxygen inflow 10 to 15 liters/min).

Portable anesthesia ventilating systems administer an FIO_2 of 1.0 when supplied by an oxygen source, but oxygen inflow rates must be properly set to minimize rebreathing of exhaled gas and over- or underinflation of the breathing bag.

Gastric inflation occurs during mouth-to-mouth, mouth-to-mask, and bag-to-mask ventilation when inflation pressure exceeds esophageal opening pressure (approximately 20 cmH_2O). Distension of the stomach is minimized by using slow inspiratory flow rates (administering each breath over a 1.5- to 2-second inspiratory time), limiting tidal volume to that needed to raise the chest, and correcting airway obstruction in order to avoid unnecessary inflation pressure. When the number of rescuers permits, cricoid pressure (Sellick's maneuver) is applied during artificial ventilation prior to tracheal intubation in order to reduce gastric inflation and prevent regurgitation. As soon as tracheal intubation is accomplished, cricoid pressure is released, and ventilation may be provided using more rapid inspiratory times and greater airway pressures. The stomach may be decompressed by a gastric tube.

Oxygen-Powered Ventilators

Manually triggered oxygen-powered ventilators deliver 100% oxygen and prevent rebreathing. These

devices administer oxygen at inspiratory flow rates up to 100 liters/min for as long as the control lever or button is depressed or until the inspiratory pressure relief valve opens at 60 to 80 cmH_2O airway pressure. Chest excursion is observed during inflation to avoid overinflation. Inspiratory flow rates greater than 40 liters/min produced by many of these devices cause gastric distension when used with a mask during artificial ventilation.

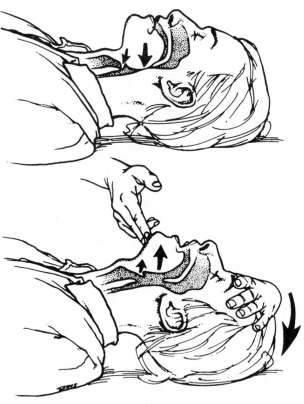

Figure 20-2

Airway obstruction and the chin lift airway opening maneuver. The fingers of one hand, grasping the mentum or ramus of the mandible, lift the jaw anteriorly. This elevates the epiglottis and lifts the base of the tongue from the posterior pharyngeal wall. Care must be taken not to compress the soft tissue under the chin, thereby obstructing the airway. The rescuer's other hand is used to extend the victim's head or operate manually powered ventilating devices. If the patient has dentures, they are left in place to help maintain a normal facial contour, facilitating adequate lip or mask seal for ventilation.

(Reproduced with permission from Chandra NC, Hazinski MF, eds: Textbook of Basic Life Support for Healthcare Providers. Dallas: American Heart Association, 1994.)

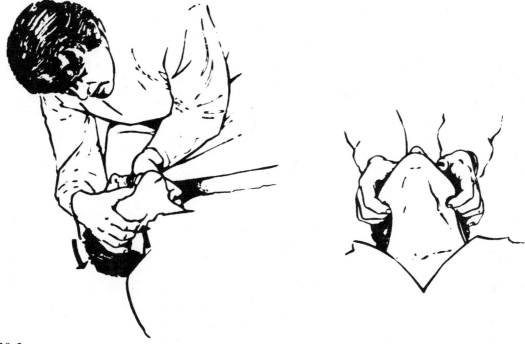

Figure 20-3

Two-handed jaw thrust maneuver. The mandible is pulled forward by the fingers of both hands behind the angles of the jaw. This maneuver is often effective when the one-handed chin lift has not opened the airway. Simultaneous extension of the head augments airway opening. A second person is needed to operate manual ventilating devices. The jaw thrust without cervical extension generally provides a patent airway in patients with suspected cervical spine injury.

(Reproduced with permission from Safar P, Bircher JG: Cardiopulmonary Cerebral Resuscitation, *3rd ed. London: WB Saunders, 1988.)*

Automatic Transport Ventilators

Automatic transport ventilators (ATVs) are portable, compact ventilators designed for prehospital use. ATVs generate a constant inspiratory flow to provide a tidal volume and respiratory rate set by the operator. When used with a mask, the devices permit rescuers to use both hands for airway and mask control. In intubated patients, use of ATVs frees the rescuer for other tasks. An oxygen source is required.

Monitoring Artificial Ventilation

The efficacy of ventilation and arterial oxygenation is assessed throughout resuscitation using observation (e.g., chest excursion, breath sounds) or quantitative measures. In the presence of effective native circulation, pulse oximetry and capnometry measure blood oxygen saturation and carbon dioxide tension, respectively. During artificial circulation, arterial blood gas analysis is required to quantitate oxygenation and ventilation.

■ Treatment of Airway Obstruction Caused by a Foreign Body

The management of airway obstruction after foreign-body aspiration depends on the magnitude of obstruction and adequacy of gas exchange. Partial airway obstruction with adequate gas exchange is recognized when the conscious choking victim can speak and generate an effective cough despite some respiratory distress. A rescuer does not interfere with the subject's efforts to expel the foreign object as long as adequate oxygenation continues. Artificial cough techniques produce less expulsive pressure and flow than natural coughs and may move the object to a more critical position in the airway, converting a partial obstruction to a more severe obstruction.

Partial obstruction with ineffective air exchange and complete airway obstruction are characterized by inability to speak and a weak or absent cough. In the unwitnessed arrest, foreign-body airway obstruction

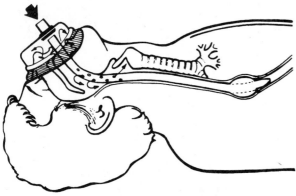

Figure 20-4

Structure and function of the esophageal obturator airway (EOA). The EOA is a 9.5-mm inside diameter tube with multiple air outlets along its proximal portion and a 30-cc inflatable cuff just proximal to its occluded distal tip. The proximal end of the tube snaps into a face mask and is inserted blindly into the esophagus of the unconscious subject with the mask in place on the obturator. The EOA is inserted maximally so that the mask seats properly on the face and ensures a sealed external airway. The cuff rests in the distal esophagus below the level of the carina in the adult patient. After inflation of the esophageal cuff, ventilation is provided by attaching any ventilating device to the proximal end of the obturator. Since the esophagus is occluded, inspiratory gas flow passes through the multiple openings of the EOA in the hypopharynx into the trachea. If it is properly positioned, the esophageal balloon precludes air entry into the stomach, and the mask prevents air leak from the mouth and nose. Adequate ventilation is often not achieved because of a retrograde air leak from the mouth and nose owing to difficulty obtaining a good mask fit and obstruction of the air ports by the base of the tongue when the mandible is not held in a displaced position. The anesthesiologist is most likely to encounter the EOA in place in a patient transported to a medical facility. It is replaced with a tracheal airway to ensure effective ventilation. After preoxygenation and ventilation using the EOA, the mask is detached from the obturator, which remains in place at the left side of the mouth during tracheal intubation to prevent regurgitation. Once the trachea is intubated, the esophageal cuff may be deflated and the EOA removed. *(Reproduced with permission from Safar P, Bircher NG: Cardiopulmonary Cerebral Resuscitation, 3rd ed. London: WB Saunders, 1988.)*

is suspected if the rescuer cannot ventilate the lungs despite several attempts to open the airway. Treatment must begin immediately.

Artificial Cough Techniques

Heimlich's abdominal thrust is the manual artificial cough technique administered for the treatment of foreign-body airway obstruction in adults and children over 1 year of age (Fig. 20-6). A variation of this technique, the chest thrust, is used for treatment of choking victims who are pregnant near term or less than 1 year of age.

Series of chest thrusts and back blows in combination are recommended for infants less than 1 year of age with foreign-body obstruction. When back blows are administered to an infant whose head and torso are supported by the opposite hand or thigh of the rescuer, intrathoracic pressure rises as a result of both the direct blow and compression of the thorax in a manner analogous to the chest thrust.

As the conscious choking victim becomes asphyxiated and unconscious, glottic muscles relax, and maneuvers that were previously ineffective may dislodge the object. With relaxation it also may become possible to ventilate around the obstruction and to remove the obstructing object with a finger sweep of the posterior pharynx administered in conjunction with a tongue-jaw lift maneuver (Fig. 20-7).

Direct Laryngoscopy

Direct laryngoscopy and removal of the obstructing body may be used by rescuers skilled in these

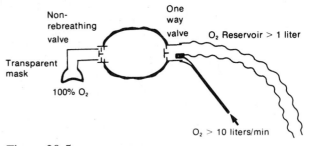

Figure 20-5

Manually powered self-inflating resuscitator (bag-valve device). Bag-valve devices consist of a hand-powered, self-inflating bag with inflow and nonrebreathing valves. On bag compression, the inflow valve closes, stopping oxygen and air inflow, and the nonrebreathing valve opens, delivering the bag's gas mixture to the patient. During exhalation, the recoil of the bag draws in oxygen and air via the opened inflow valve. The nonrebreathing valve directs the patient's exhaled gases to the atmosphere, preventing reentry into the bag. An attached oxygen reservoir at the inflow valve accumulates oxygen during inspiration. When bag reinflation occurs, oxygen enters the bag from the oxygen source and the reservoir, thereby minimizing the volume of room air entrained and increasing the oxygen concentration in the ventilating bag. *(Reproduced with permission from Safar P, Bircher NG: Cardiopulmonary Cerebral Resuscitation, 3rd ed. London: WB Saunders, 1988.)*

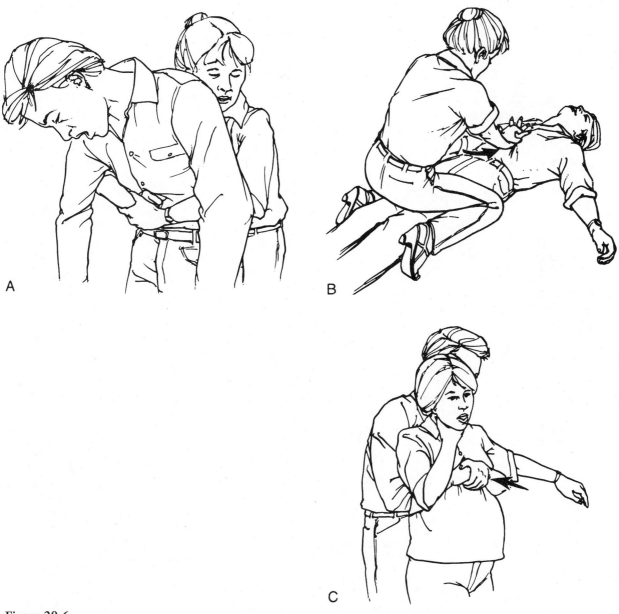

Figure 20-6

Manual artificial cough techniques. (A, B) Abdominal thrust (Heimlich maneuver) applied to a standing or supine subject. The rescuer places the fist or heel of one hand against the abdomen, in the midline slightly above the navel and well below the xiphoid process. After grasping the first hand with the second, the rescuer uses both arms to provide a quick inward and upward thrust. With rapid compression of the epigastrium, the diaphragm is forced cephalad, compressing the air volume trapped in the lungs. The airway pressure and airflow generated move the foreign body from its position in the airway. (C) Chest thrusts, manual thrusts applied to the middle or lower chest, compress the intrathoracic gas volume directly and produce airway pressures and flows comparable with those achieved with abdominal thrusts. In infants and pregnant women, chest thrusts may be more effective and cause fewer complications than abdominal thrusts.

(Reproduced with permission from Chandra NC, Hazinski MF eds: Textbook of Basic Life Support for Healthcare Providers. *Dallas: American Heart Association, 1994.)*

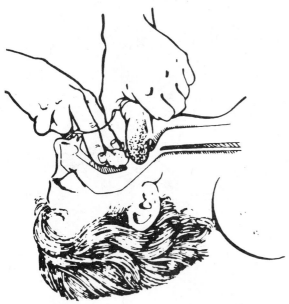

Figure 20-7

Tongue-jaw lift maneuver and finger sweep of the hypopharynx. Firmly grasping the victim's mandible and tongue between the thumb and fingers of one hand, the rescuer pulls this block of tissue anteriorly, thereby dislodging supraglottic foreign bodies or, at least, providing more space in the hypopharynx for the finger sweep. Caution must be exerted during blind probing of the pharynx to avoid impaction of an object deeper into the airway. Because this risk is greatest in the small mouths of infants and children, finger sweeps of the posterior pharynx are not recommended in these groups unless the foreign object is visualized.

(Reproduced with permission from Safar P, Bircher NG: Cardiopulmonary Cerebral Resuscitation, 3rd ed. London: WB Saunders, 1988.)

techniques (e.g., anesthesiologists). Once the subject is unconscious, direct visualization can be accomplished with a laryngoscope and the object grasped with a long forceps or clamp. Blind grasping attempts in the posterior pharynx using forceps or clamps are avoided.

Cricothyrotomy and Transtracheal Ventilation

Percutaneous cricothyrotomy may permit ventilation when the obstruction is at or above the glottis, but this is tried only after simpler measures are unsuccessful. Transtracheal catheter ventilation (TCV, or jet ventilation) requires an oxygen source, a specialized ventilation system, and a large-bore intravenous cannula inserted into the airway through the cricothyroid membrane. The cannula is connected by a length of intravenous extension tubing to a hand-operated release valve that is connected to a source that delivers 100% oxygen at 50 lb/in². The source may be a wall oxygen outlet, an oxygen tank with a pressure-reducing valve, or an anesthetic machine. Transtracheal catheter ventilation also may be accomplished with simplified equipment, using an ordinary wall oxygen flowmeter set at the maximum flush position (approximately 30 liters/min) and a piece of standard oxygen tubing with a sidehole cut near its distal end. This end is connected via a stopcock or other connector to the transtracheal cannula. Lung inflation occurs when the sidehole in the tubing is occluded by the rescuer's thumb, and exhalation occurs passively when the thumb is removed.

If effective ventilation and oxygenation are to be achieved, insertion of a transtracheal cannula of adequate size and use of an appropriate ventilating device are mandatory. A 12-, 14-, or 16-gauge intravenous catheter can be used in adults and children in conjunction with jet ventilation systems. Transtracheal ventilation with bag-valve devices or anesthesia ventilating systems require a 3.0-mm inside diameter or larger cannula.

Once cricothyrotomy is performed and the catheter is connected to the ventilating device, a jet of oxygen introduced into the trachea produces lung inflation despite a retrograde air leak. Because exhalation during TCV occurs passively through the upper airway, complete obstruction at or above the glottis prevents exhalation and may produce dangerous airway pressures. In this situation, the transtracheal cannula permits apneic oxygenation by insufflation of oxygen to meet basal metabolic requirements. Although marked hypercarbia develops, arterial oxygenation is maintained while an adequate airway is established. Subsequent tracheostomy, controlled orotracheal intubation, or endoscopic examination may be performed while ventilation continues. (See Chapter 13 for details of jet ventilation, endotracheal intubation, and tracheostomy.)

Artificial Circulation

■ Closed Chest Compression

Absence of a central (i.e., carotid or femoral) arterial pulse is the indication to immediately begin artificial circulation and provide ACLS measures to restore native circulation. Closed chest compression (Fig. 20-8) accompanied by ventilation and oxygenation is indicated throughout the period of resuscitation. Closed chest compression is not indicated for patients with palpable central pulses and systolic blood pressures greater than 50 mmHg, even though peripheral pulses may be undetectable due to peripheral vasoconstriction. These patients are best treated with specific measures that augment circulation, such as fluids and drugs.

External chest compression can produce systolic blood pressure of 100mmHg and greater, but diastolic pressures range from 10 to 40 mmHg. As a result of the decreased aortic diastolic pressures, myocardial perfusion during closed chest compression seldom exceeds 5 to 10 percent of normal levels. Carotid artery blood flow is generally less than one-third normal. Although these blood flows temporarily sustain cerebral viability, prompt restoration of native circulation and coronary perfusion is critical for survival.

Efforts to develop more effective external chest compression techniques have led to the understanding that two mechanisms are responsible for blood flow during CPR: compression of the heart between the sternum and spine (cardiac pump) and phasic increases in arterial perfusion pressure produced by compression of the thorax (thoracic pump). Blood flow produced by direct cardiac compression is directly related to compression rate, and thoracic pump blood flow is directly related to the magnitude and duration of intrathoracic pressure produced by sternal depression.

Rapid compression rates improve perfusion during closed chest CPR as a result of rate-dependent effects on cardiac output (cardiac pump) and increases in the systolic-to-diastolic duration ratio (thoracic pump). Compression rates of 80 to 100 per minute are recommended for adults and children (see Table 20-2). Adequate depth of sternal displacement is essential to achieve complete cardiac compression (cardiac pump) and produce a substantial increase in intrathoracic pressure (thoracic pump).

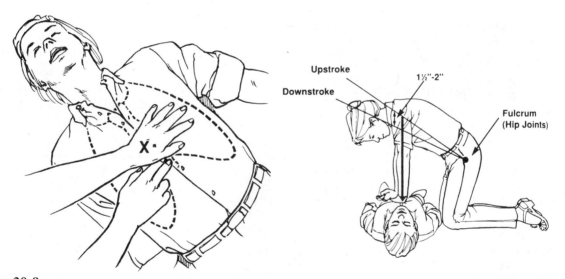

Figure 20-8

Chest compression. Proper hand position is achieved by placing the heel of one hand on the lower one-half of the victim's sternum in the midline and above the xiphoid process. The weight of the rescuer's torso is used to apply downward pressure to the sternum, thereby permitting effective compression and minimizing arm and shoulder fatigue. The rescuer's arms and elbows are locked, and the shoulders are positioned directly over the hands. The fingers may be interlaced or extended but should not apply pressure to the rib cage. In the adult patient, the sternum is depressed 1.5 to 2 in during each compression. Optimal depth of sternal compression is gauged by the generation of a palpable carotid or femoral pulse, intraarterial pressure monitoring, or capnometry. During upstroke, sternal compression is completely released to permit venous return to the chest; however, correct hand position may be lost if the hands are lifted off the chest.

(Reproduced with permission from Chandra NC, Hasinski MF, eds: Textbook of Basic Life Support for Healthcare Providers. *Dallas: American Heart Association, 1994.)*

Alternative chest compression techniques that augment the intrathoracic pressure increase (simultaneous compression-ventilation CPR, pneumatic vest CPR) or increase compression rate (up to 120 per minute) produce superior perfusion compared with conventional CPR. Improved survival after CPR using these methods has not been documented. Interposition of abdominal compressions between chest compressions, interposed abdominal compression CPR, increases diastolic perfusion of the heart and brain in a manner analogous to intraaortic balloon counterpulsation. This technique has not consistently improved survival from CPR. In active compression-decompression CPR (ACD-CPR), a device consisting of a rubber suction cup with a compression handle is applied to the chest and used to provide manual chest compression during artificial systole and active chest expansion during diastole. In preliminary trials, ACD-CPR is more effective than standard CPR. More experience is needed with this CPR technique before its clinical effectiveness can be determined.

Artificial circulation is enhanced when intravenous epinephrine and the supportive equipment described below are employed to increase the cardiac output and perfusion pressure produced by closed chest compression.

■ Supportive Equipment and Epinephrine

The patient undergoing external chest compression must lie on a firm surface. A cardiac back board, operating table, floor, or food tray may be used.

Mechanical chest compressors reduce fatigue resulting from manual chest compression and permit longer periods of CPR. However, they provide no hemodynamic advantage over manual CPR.

Epinephrine and norepinephrine improve cerebral and coronary blood flow during artificial circulation as a result of alpha-adrenergic-mediated vasoconstriction, which limits blood flow to peripheral tissues and increases aortic blood pressure. The enhanced myocardial oxygen delivery may result in spontaneous cardiac contraction or increased response to electrical defibrillation.

Epinephrine remains the vasopressor of choice during CPR; the recommended dose is 1 mg for the adult patient given every 3 to 5 minutes during artificial circulation. Improvements in perfusion pressure and myocardial blood flow are directly related to

epinephrine dose. Despite the hemodynamic benefits of increasing epinephrine dose (to as great as 200 µg/kg), clinical trials show no improvement in survival of adults from CPR using larger epinephrine doses.

■ Open Chest Cardiac Massage

Although closed chest compression has replaced direct cardiac massage during CPR, direct compression of the heart generates superior cardiac output and coronary perfusion. Coronary perfusion and survival from arrest in animals are improved when open cardiac massage is instituted in place of closed chest compression within 15 minutes of cardiac arrest. There are indications for open chest cardiac massage in a hospital setting when trained rescuers are present (Table 20-4).

■ Monitoring Artificial Circulation

An index of cardiac output produced during CPR would be a useful guide to chest compression rate and depth, epinephrine dose, or need for alternative artificial circulation techniques. Palpation of a central pulse during chest compressions has served this purpose, but it provides little information about blood flow and oxygen delivery.

Exhaled end-tidal carbon dioxide tension is an index of cardiac output and may predict outcome from resuscitation. When cardiac output is depressed

Table 20-4

Indications for Thoracotomy and Direct Cardiac Compression

Operating room
  Thorax or upper abdomen already open
Conditions prohibit effective artificial circulation by closed chest compression
  Severe anatomic thoracic cage abnormalities
  Flail chest
  Cardiac tamponade
  Tension pneumothorax
  Major mediastinal shift, e.g., postpneumonectomy, massive pleural effusion
Cause of arrest is defined and treated by thoracotomy or pericardiotomy
  Cardiac tamponade
  Tension pneumothorax
  Penetrating chest injury
  Infradiaphragmatic exsanguination
  Hypothermia
  Thromboembolic and air embolism

and ventilation is constant, end-tidal CO_2 tension reflects the rate of CO_2 delivery to the lungs and is directly related to cardiac output. In humans undergoing closed chest compression, greater exhaled end-tidal CO_2 values are observed in eventual survivors than in those who do not survive. End-tidal CO_2 tensions of less than 10 to 15 mmHg obtained after tracheal intubation during closed chest compression imply a poor prognosis for survival.

■ Emergent Cardiopulmonary Bypass

The institution of cardiopulmonary bypass (e.g., percutaneous femoral-femoral bypass) in place of conventional artificial circulation techniques can improve resuscitation and survival when begun immediately upon cardiac arrest. This can be used when the necessary equipment and expert personnel are immediately available, as with hospitalized patients known to be at risk for cardiac arrest. It is also useful for the rewarming and resuscitation of victims of cardiac arrest due to accidental hypothermia.

Restoration of Native Oxygen Delivery

Rescue of the unresponsive patient entails rapid assessment, temporary oxygen delivery, and specific treatment of the cause of collapse (Fig. 20-9). Prompt recognition of ventricular fibrillation (VF) and pulseless ventricular tachycardia (VT) permits early defibrillation, which is vital to the resuscitation of patients in cardiac arrest due to these rhythm disorders. When cardiac arrest occurs without established electrocardiographic (ECG) monitoring, the heart rate and rhythm can be determined most rapidly using defibrillator chest paddles that incorporate ECG electrodes so that definitive therapy can be administered immediately.

■ Specific Therapy of Cardiac Arrest from Tachydysrhythmias

Ventricular tachycardia (VT) and ventricular fibrillation (VF) are the most common cardiac dysrhythmias causing cardiopulmonary arrest. Ventricular tachycardia is a life-threatening rhythm disturbance that results in hypotension and shock. It is an electrically unstable rhythm and may degenerate to VF. Ventricular fibrillation is a lethal dysrhythmia; cardiac output is absent. Hypotension and shock also may be caused by very rapid supraventricular tachycardia (SVT). Electrical cardioversion is the most rapidly effective therapy for these rhythm disturbances and is the mainstay of advanced cardiac life support.

Synchronized and Unsynchronized Cardioversion

Electrical cardioversion, rather than pharmacologic therapy, is indicated for the treatment of tachydysrhythmias when the pulse is absent or when there is stupor or unconsciousness, severe arterial hypotension, pulmonary edema, or angina pectoris.

Cardioversion delivers an electric current that depolarizes a critical mass of myocardium and permits a more stable pacemaker, such as the atrioventricular or sinus node, to assume control. The amount of current passing through the heart and depolarized myocardial mass depends directly on the energy delivered from the paddles and inversely on the transthoracic resistance to current flow (Table 20-5).

The energy dose selected for cardioversion during cardiac arrest is based on the need for rapid resolution of the rhythm disturbance. Unnecessarily large doses, however, produce myocardial injury, often manifested as transient conduction blocks following cardioversion. Thus cardioversion starts with the least energy dose that is expected to be effective for the patient's hemodynamic condition and cardiac rhythm (Table 20-6). If this dose is ineffective, the energy level is increased for each succeeding shock.

For treatment of VF or pulseless VT, as soon as a defibrillator is available, a series of rapidly repeated shocks is delivered until cardioversion is achieved or three to four shocks and maximum defibrillator output, 360 J, have been administered (Figure 20-10). The pulse or ECG is reevaluated immediately after each shock. When the rhythm disturbance persists after the first series of three to four shocks, efforts are directed at oxygenating the myocardium and enhancing its susceptibility to cardioversion. These steps include increased ventilation, chest compression and epinephrine administration, correction of metabolic abnormalities, and antiarrhythmic drug therapy specific to the dysrhythmia. Subsequent cardioversion attempts using maximum energy are delivered as two successive shocks, because diminished transthoracic resistance is observed on repeated shocks.

Defibrillation can be synchronized to the ECG in the presence of a rhythm with a QRS complex, such as VT or SVT (the QRS deflection can be sensed and discharge of the paddles timed accordingly)

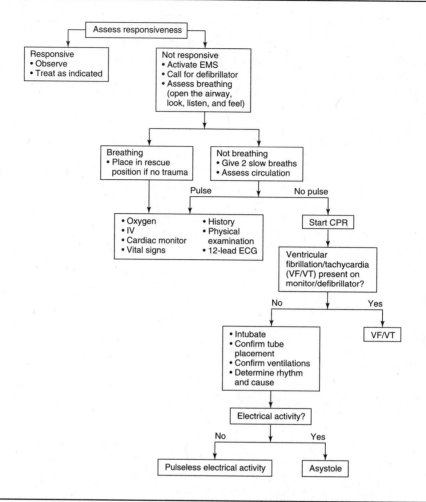

Figure 20-9

American Heart Association universal algorithm of initial assessment and management of the unresponsive victim suspected to be in cardiac arrest. This AHA algorithm, as well as the others reproduced in this chapter, were developed to teach a generic and fundamental treatment plan for a broad range of patients. Some patients may require care not specified herein. The algorithm must not be construed as prohibiting such flexibility. Suspected causes of unresponsiveness in the presence of native circulation include drug overdose, metabolic disturbances (e.g., hypo-hyperglycemia, hyponatremia), hypoxemia and hypercarbia (respiratory failure), neurologic conditions (e.g., seizure, head injury, stroke), hypothermia, and hypovolemic, septic, or cardiogenic shock. Cardiogenic shock may result from tachydysrhythmias, bradydysrhythmias, myocardial infarction, advanced cardiomyopathy, acute valvular insufficiency, cardiac tamponade, and pulmonary embolism. Oxygen, airway and ventilatory support, vascular access and continuous monitoring are provided for these patients while evaluation and therapy is begun. These steps may prevent deterioration of the patient's condition and permit prompt recognition and therapy of cardiac arrest, should it occur.

(Reproduced with permission from the American Medical Association, Emergency Cardiac Care Committee and Subcommittees, American Heart Association: Guidelines for cardiopulmonary resuscitation and emergency cardiac care: III. Adult advanced life support. JAMA 1992; 268: 2199-2241.)

(Fig. 20-11). Synchronized defibrillation requires smaller electrical doses and avoids delivering a shock during the period of vulnerability immediately prior to the T wave, which can provoke VF. Unsynchronized cardioversion is used for the treatment of VF, whereas synchronized cardioversion may be used for termination of all other tachydysrhythmias. The syn- chronization mechanism is deactivated for defibrillation of VF because no QRS deflection exists and the paddles would not be discharged.

Precordial Thump

Precordial thump is a mechanical form of unsynchronized cardioversion that generates a small electric

Table 20-5

Factors That Increase Current Flow During Electrical Cardioversion

1. Paddles of large surface area that permit complete electrode contact with chest surface
2. Conductive gel, paste, or pads. Saline-soaked gauze sponges are an acceptable alternative; alcohol swabs are not.
3. Correct paddle position: The heart must lie between the paddles. In the standard paddle position, one paddle is placed on the upper right thorax below the clavicle, and the other is lateral to the apex of the heart on the lower left chest at the midaxillary line.
4. Firm pressure on paddles
5. Exhalation of air from lungs
6. Repetitive shocks

current in the heart and occasionally converts acute tachydysrhythmias. A single thump is delivered to the sternum by the rescuer's fist. It may be administered to a monitored patient at the onset of VF or pulseless VT or to an unmonitored patient without a pulse. If a single blow fails to restore a pulse or organized rhythm, BLS measures are instituted until a defibrillator becomes available. The precordial thump is used only in the absence of the more effective defibrillator and only for pulseless patients, since induction of VF is possible.

Drug Therapy

In addition to epinephrine, antiarrhythmic drugs are administered for tachyarrhythmias during cardiac arrest to promote sustained cardioversion. Lidocaine and bretylium tosylate are equally effective during resuscitation from VF and pulseless VT. Lidocaine is the drug of choice because of its rapid effect. Phar-macologic cardioversion of stable VT not requiring rapid electrical cardioversion is achieved with lidocaine or procainamide (Fig. 20-12).

Adenosine is the drug of choice for pharmacologic cardioversion of paroxysmal supraventricular tachycardia (PSVT) involving atrioventricular (AV) node reentry when vagal maneuvers are not effective (Fig. 20-12). Verapamil and diltiazem are as effective as adenosine but may decrease blood pressure. These calcium channel blockers are indicated when PSVT continues after adenosine therapy. Adenosine will not terminate rhythms caused by mechanisms other than nodal reentry (e.g., atrial flutter, atrial fibrillation, or ventricular tachycardia). Calcium channel blockers and procainamide are used for heart rate control and rhythm conversion, respectively, in cases of atrial fibrillation or flutter. Beta-adrenergic antagonists slow ventricular response rate during atrial fibrillation and flutter but are less effective in the termination of PSVT. The long onset time of digoxin limits the drug's use. Table 20-7 is a summary of drug therapy during CPR.

■ Specific Therapy of Cardiac Arrest from Bradydysrhythmias

Asystole is a lethal dysrhythmia, and severe bradycardias are life-threatening when the resulting heart rate is insufficient to generate effective cardiac output (usually less than 30 beats per minute). Extreme bradycardias, including heart blocks, also may be the progenitors of VF or asystole.

Emergent Cardiac Pacing

In instances of ventricular standstill due to acute complete heart block, activating an artificial pace-

Table 20-6

Recommended Initial Energy Dose for Emergent Cardioversion*		
Dysrhythmia	Energy Dose (J)	Synchronized or Unsynchronized†
Ventricular fibrillation	200	Unsynchronized
Ventricular tachycardia	100	Synchronized
Paroxysmal supraventricular tachycardia	50	Synchronized
Atrial fibrillation	100	Synchronized
Atrial flutter	50	Synchronized

*Any dysrhythmia is treated as if it were ventricular fibrillation if there is no pulse.
†Unsynchronized cardioversion is used for hemodynamically unstable patients if synchronization process will cause delay in therapy.

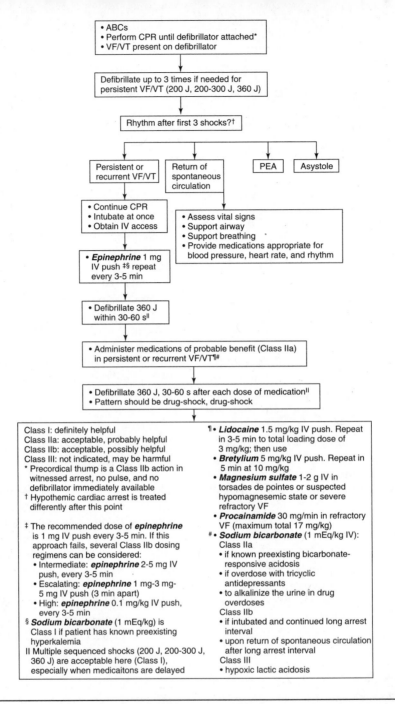

Figure 20-10

American Heart Association treatment algorithm for cardiac arrest due to ventricular fibrillation (and pulseless ventricular tachycardia). Flow of algorithm presumes that VF (or VT) is continuing. Check pulse and rhythm after each shock. If VF (or VT) recurs after transiently converting (rather than persisting without ever converting), use the energy level which has previously been successful for subsequent defibrillation. Use of epinephrine as the first drug administered for VF refractory to defibrillation is empiric. Alternatively, lidocaine may be administered prior to epinephrine. This AHA algorithm, as well as others reproduced in this chapter, incorporates the following system of classifying interventions based on the strength of the supporting scientific evidence:

Class I. A therapeutic option that is usually indicated, always acceptable, and considered useful and effective;

Class II. A therapeutic option that is acceptable, is of uncertain efficacy and may be controversial;

Class IIa. A therapeutic option for which the weight of evidence is in favor of its usefulness and efficacy;

Class IIb. A therapeutic option that is not well established by evidence, but may be helpful and probably not harmful;

Class III. A therapeutic option that is inappropriate, is without scientific supporting data, and may be harmful.

(Reproduced with permission from the American Medical Association, Emergency Cardiac Care Committee and Subcommittees, American Heart Association: Guidelines for cardiopulmonary resuscitation and emergency cardiac care: III. Adult advanced life support. JAMA 1992; 268: 2199-2241.)

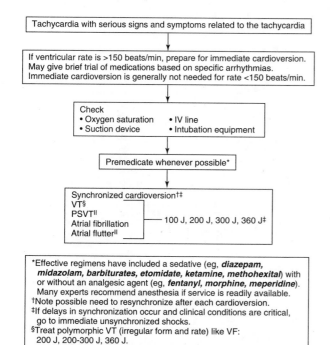

Tachycardia with serious signs and symptoms related to the tachycardia

↓

If ventricular rate is >150 beats/min, prepare for immediate cardioversion. May give brief trial of medications based on specific arrhythmias. Immediate cardioversion is generally not needed for rate <150 beats/min.

↓

Check
• Oxygen saturation   • IV line
• Suction device   • Intubation equipment

↓

Premedicate whenever possible*

↓

Synchronized cardioversion†‡
VT§
PSVT‖
Atrial fibrillation ── 100 J, 200 J, 300 J, 360 J‡
Atrial flutter‖

*Effective regimens have included a sedative (eg, *diazepam, midazolam, barbiturates, etomidate, ketamine, methohexital*) with or without an analgesic agent (eg, *fentanyl, morphine, meperidine*). Many experts recommend anesthesia if service is readily available.
†Note possible need to resynchronize after each cardioversion.
‡If delays in synchronization occur and clinical conditions are critical, go to immediate unsynchronized shocks.
§Treat polymorphic VT (irregular form and rate) like VF:
  200 J, 200-300 J, 360 J.
‖PSVT and atrial flutter often respond to lower energy levels (start with 50 J).

Figure 20-11

American Heart Association algorithm of electrical cardioversion for tachydysrhythmias. Use of sedative premedication is associated with risks of regurgitation and aspiration, hypotension, and hypoventilation; it is not indicated in the presence of coma, pulmonary edema, or severe hypotension.

(Reproduced with permission from the American Medical Association Emergency Cardiac Care Committee and Subcommittees, American Heart Association. Guidelines for cardiopulmonary resuscitation and emergency cardiac care: III. Adult advanced life support. JAMA 1992; 268: 2199-2241.)

maker already in place is the best treatment. This is possible when a hospitalized patient is known to be at risk for the development of complete heart block (e.g., new conduction defect during anterior wall myocardial infarction, pulmonary artery catheterization in the presence of preexisting left bundle branch block, or emergency operations for a patient with syncope and trifascicular block on ECG). Pacemaker therapy becomes ineffective if delayed even minutes following cardiac standstill.

If a pacing wire is not already in place, external transcutaneous pacing electrodes are as effective as transthoracic pacing wires and offer fewer complications. Alternatively, repeated precordial thumps ("fist

pacing") may be used for monitored acute ventricular asystole, provided each thump produces ventricular depolarization.

Drug Therapy

Epinephrine is the drug of choice for restoration of cardiac impulse formation and contraction in cardiac arrest due to asystole (Fig. 20-13). Drugs withpredominantly beta-adrenergic actions, such as isoproterenol and dobutamine, are not used because coronary perfusion during CPR is diminished by beta-adrenergic-mediated peripheral vasodilation.

Atropine is used when bradycardia or heart block in the sinus or atrioventricular node produces hypotension (Fig. 20-14). Atropine-refractory bradycardia and second- or third-degree heart block occurring below the atrioventricular node are indications for dopamine or epinephrine until a cardiac pacer is placed.

■ Specific Therapy for Cardiac Arrest from Pulseless Electrical Activity

A patient with an organized ECG pattern but no pulse or blood pressure has pulseless electrical activity (PEA). This disorder may be a terminal phenomenon, the result of extensive myocardial damage, or may be due to conditions that interfere with venous return to the heart or ventricular output, such as cardiac tamponade, tension pneumothorax, severe hypovolemia, or inhalational anesthetic overdose. Prompt treatment (pericardiocentesis, needle decompression of the pleural space, volume and vasopressor therapy, and discontinuation of the anesthetic) restores cardiac output. Massive pulmonary embolism with air or thrombus also may produce PEA.

When PEA cannot be reversed immediately, epinephrine enhances myocardial oxygen delivery during CPR and augments cardiac inotropy (Fig. 20-15). Calcium chloride increases contractility in patients with hypocalcemia and is useful in cases of cardiac arrest due to hyperkalemia, hypermagnesemia, and calcium channel blocker toxicity.

Table 20-8 lists the features and treatment of specific CPR situations.

■ Vascular Access

Peripheral arm veins are the first sites of vascular access during resuscitation because they are easily cannulated with few complications. Effective closed

Text continued on page 274

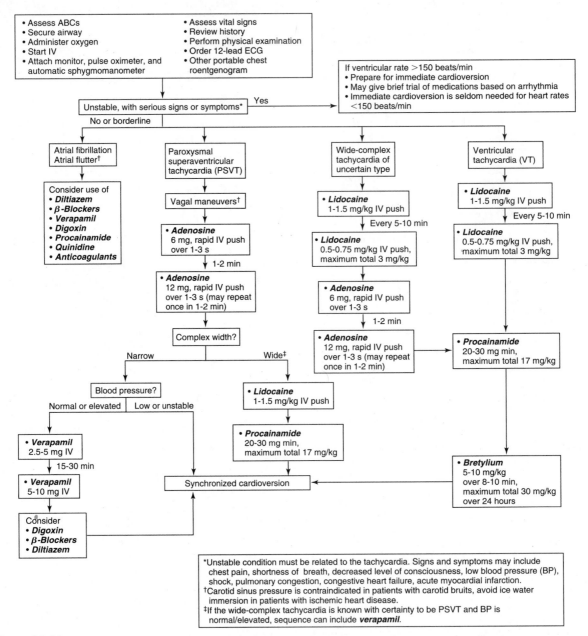

Figure 20-12

American Heart Association treatment algorithm for tachydysrhythmias other than ventricular fibrillation and pulseless ventricular tachycardia. The algorithm emphasizes the need to avoid use of calcium channel antagonists in patients with wide-complex tachycardia that may be ventricular in origin. A wide-complex tachycardia is most likely to be ventricular tachycardia. Other wide-complex tachycardias are supraventricular tachycardia (SVT) with aberrant atrioventricular (AV) conduction (e.g., due to preexisting bundle branch block) and SVT with ventricular activation via an accessory pathway [e.g., Wolff Parkinson-White (WPW) syndrome]. Unstable tachycardias are treated with cardioversion regardless of origin. Stable SVT with aberrancy is treated according to the supraventricular rhythm disturbance (atrial or nodal reentry, atrial fibrillation/flutter) present. Lidocaine and procainamide are the drugs of choice for stable VT and wide-complex tachycardia in patients with WPW syndrome. Adenosine may be used as a diagnostic or therapeutic agent in wide- complex tachycardias of uncertain type. This drug will terminate wide-complex SVT with aberrancy resulting from AV nodal reentry. In the presence of tachycardias caused by mechanisms other than nodal reentry, adenosine may produce transient AV block that exposes the underlying atrial activity and clarifies the rhythm diagnosis. The drug is not likely to produce hemodynamic collapse in the presence of VT because of its lack of hypotensive effects and its short duration of action.

(Reproduced with permission from the American Medical Association Emergency Cardiac Care Committee and Subcommittees, American Heart Association: Guidelines for cardiopulmonary resuscitation and emergency cardiac care: III. Adult advanced life support. JAMA 1992; 268: 2199-2241.)

Table 20-7

CPR Pharmacology

Drug	Indication	Bolus Dose*	Infusion Rate	Remarks
Oxygen	All cardiac arrests All patients in near arrest		$F_iO_2 = 1.0$	Never withheld; support ventilation as required
Chronotropes Atropine sulfate	Asystole	1.0 mg IV		Total dose 3 mg (children 1.0 mg)
	Bradycardia, heart block	0.4–1.0 mg IV (children 0.02 mg/kg)		Dose selected by degree of hemodynamic compromise; beware of tachydysrhythmia, myocardial ischemia
Antidysrhythmics Lidocaine	Cardiac arrest ventricular fibrillation, tachycardia	1.0–1.5 mg/kg IV; repeat 0.5 mg/kg every 5 minutes to total dose 3 mg/kg		
	Ventricular ectopy, stable ventricular tachycardia	1.0–1.5 mg/kg IV; repeat 0.5 mg/kg every 5 minutes to total dose 3.0 mg/kg *or* use loading infusion	Loading infusion: 15 mg/min to total dose 3 mg/kg; maintenance infusion: 2–4 mg/min (children 30–50 µg/kg/min)	Titrate to effect; central nervous system toxicity at plasma levels > 9 µg/ml; reduce dose in patients with congestive heart failure, hepatic disease, advanced age
Procainamide	Ventricular ectopy; stable ventricular tachycardia; atrial fibrillation, flutter		Loading infusion: 20–50 mg/min to total dose 17 mg/kg or toxicity; maintenance infusion 1–4 mg/min	Titrate to effect; toxicity: hypotension, atrioventricular block, QRS widening (> 50%); reduce dose in patients with congestive heart failure, renal failure; check blood levels
Bretylium tosylate	Cardiac arrest, ventricular fibrillation, tachycardia	5 mg/kg IV; repeat 10 mg/kg every 5–15 minutes to total dose 35 mg/kg		
	Stable ventricular tachycardia	5–10 mg/kg IV over 10 minutes; repeat in 30 min if necessary, then infusion	Maintenance infusion: 1–2 mg/min	Side effects: postural hypotension, nausea/vomiting; use with caution in digitalis toxicity

Table continued on following page

Table 20-7

CPR Pharmacology *Continued*

Drug	Indication	Bolus Dose*	Infusion Rate	Remarks
Adenosine	Reentrant atrio-ventricular node tachycardia	6 mg IV; repeat 12 mg every 2 minutes twice (children, 50–100–200 µg/kg)		Inject rapidly; metabolized in < 1 minute; beware of transient heart block
Verapamil	Reentrant atrio-ventricular node tachycardia; atrial fibrillation, flutter; MAT	0.05–0.15 mg/kg IV (max 10 mg) (children 0.1–0.3 mg/kg); repeat in 15 minutes as necessary		Beware of hypotension; use with caution in congestive heart failure, atrioventricular block, hypotension, presence of beta blockade; not recommended for WPW with preexcitation
Diltiazem	Reentrant atrio-ventricular node tachycardia; atrial fibrillation, flutter; MAT	0.25 mg/kg IV; repeat 0.35 mg/kg in 15 min as necessary	5–15 mg/h; titrate to effect	See Verapamil
Esmolol	Reentrant atrio-ventricular node tachycardia; atrial fibrillation, flutter; MAT; sinus tachycardia; ventricular ectopy	0.1–0.5 mg/kg IV	25–200 µg/kg/min; titrate to effect	Beware of heart failure, bronchospasm; not recommended for WPW with pre-excitation
Propranolol	Reentrant atrio-ventricular node tachycardia; atrial fibrillation, flutter; MAT; sinus tachycardia; ventricular ectopy	0.01–1.0 mg IV; titrate cautiously to total dose 0.1 mg/kg		See Esmolol
Magnesium	Refractory ventricular fibrillation, tachycardia; torsades de pointes	1–2 g IV		
Digoxin	Atrial fibrillation, flutter, supraventricular tachycardias (except MAT)	0.25–0.5 mg IV; repeat every 4 h as necessary to total loading dose 10–15 µg/kg		Reduce dose in elderly and in patients on digoxin therapy
Inotropes				
Epinephrine	All cardiac arrests	1.0 mg IV (children 10 µg/kg); repeat every 3–5 minutes; consider larger doses in refractory arrest, up to 100–200 µg/kg		Prefilled syringes 1:10,000 = 100 µg/ml (10 ml = 1 mg); beneficial effect results from alpha-adrenergic action, increases perfusion pressure during CPR

Table 20-7

CPR Pharmacology *Continued*

Drug	Indication	Bolus Dose*	Infusion Rate	Remarks
	Hypotension, low cardiac output, atropine-refractory bradycardia		Initial rate 2–4 μg/min (children 0.1 μg/kg/min); titrate to effect	Beta-adrenergic 1–2 μg/kg; alpha-adrenergic effect predominates > 12 μg/min; beware of tachydysrhythmias, myocardial ischemia
Dopamine	Hypotension, low cardiac output, atropine-refractory bradycardia		Initial rate 2–5 μg/kg/min; titrate to effect	Dopaminergic 2–5 μg/kg/min; beta-adrenergic 5–10 μg/kg/min; alpha-adrenergic effect predominates > 20 μg/kg/min; beware of tachydysrhythmias, myocardial ischemia
Dobutamine	Low cardiac output, atropine-refractory bradycardia		Initial rate 2–5 μg/kg/min; titrate to effect	Beware of tachydysrhythmias, myocardial ischemia; do not use during CPR, reduces perfusion pressure
Isoproterenol	Low cardiac output, atropine-refractory bradycardia		2–20 μg/min (children 0.1–0.5 μg/kg/min); titrate to effect	See Dobutamine
Calcium chloride, CaCl₂	Hypotension, low cardiac output	5–10 mg/kg IV; repeat every 10 minutes as necessary		Useful in hypocalcemia, hyperkalemia; CaCl₂ preferred to calcium gluconate because it produces greater, more predictable concentrations of ionized calcium
Amrinone	Low cardiac output	Loading dose 0.75 μg/kg IV over 10 minutes	5–10 μg/kg/min; titrate to effect	Beware of hypotension due to vasodilation
Milrinone	Low cardiac output	Loading dose 50 μg/kg IV over 10 minutes	0.25–0.75 μg/kg/min; titrate to effect	See Amrinone
Vasopressors				
Norepinephrine	Hypotension		Initial rate 0.1–0.5 μg/kg/min; titrate to effect	
Phenylephrine	Hypotension	50–200 μg IV	Initial rate 100–200 μg/min; titrate to effect	

Table continued on following page

Table 20-7

CPR Pharmacology *Continued*

Drug	Indication	Bolus Dose*	Infusion Rate	Remarks
Methoxamine	Hypotension	1–5 mg IV		
Vasodilators				
Sodium nitro-prusside	Low cardiac output, pulmonary edema		Initial rate 0.25–0.5 µg/kg/min; titrate to effect	Beware of cyanide toxicity at infusion rates > 8–10 µg/kg/min; beware of hypotension
Trimethaphan	Low cardiac output, pulmonary edema	1–2 mg IV	Initial rate 1–2 mg/min; titrate to effect	Beware of hypotension
Nitroglycerin	Myocardial ischemia, pulmonary edema	50–100 µg IV	Initial rate 0.25–0.5 µg/kg/min; titrate to effect	Beware of hypotension
Morphine sulfate	Myocardial ischemia, pulmonary edema	2–5 mg IV		Beware of hypotension, respiratory depression
Miscellaneous				
Sodium bicarbonate	Hyperkalemia, preexisting metabolic acidosis; after resuscitation to buffer washout acidosis	1 mEq/kg IV, or one-half the dose calculated to neutralize the base deficit from arterial blood gas analysis		Avoid alkalosis, hyperosmolality; carbon dioxide is generated by bicarbonate neutralization of acid, increase ventilation
Naloxone	Opioid-induced respiratory depression	0.1–2.0 mg IV (children 0.005–0.1 mg/kg); repeat every 3 min as necessary	Initial rate 2 µg/kg/h; titrate to effect	Beware of recurrence of respiratory depression after bolus therapy
Flumazenil	Benzodiazepine-induced respiratory depression	0.2 mg IV; repeat 0.2–0.5 mg every 3 min as necessary to total dose 5 mg		See Naloxone

*Drugs are administered only by bolus dose to patients with cardiac arrest. Epinephrine, atropine, lidocaine, and naloxone boluses may be given via the endotracheal tube. The endotracheal dose of these drugs is 2 to 3 times the IV bolus dose.

Abbreviations: MAT = multifocal atrial tachycardia, WPW = Wolff-Parkinson-White syndrome.

chest compression circulates drugs from peripheral venous sites, although circulation time is prolonged. Drug delivery from peripheral vascular sites is accelerated by a flush of intravenous fluid after drug injection. It is inappropriate to withhold medications for subsequent administration through a yet unestablished central venous catheter when peripheral access is present.

Central venous drug administration reduces the time to onset of drug effect and is the ideal route when cardiac output is reduced. Central venous cannulation, most commonly via the internal jugular or subclavian vein, is performed if circulation is not restored following initial therapy and peripheral drug administration. Although femoral vein cannulation does not interfere with defibrillation, airway management, or chest compression, drug delivery by catheters lying below the diaphragm is unreliable because of poor flow in the inferior vena cava during closed chest compression.

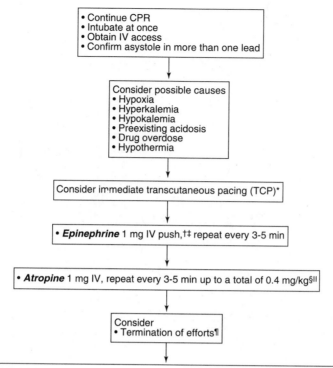

Figure 20-13

American Heart Association treatment algorithm for cardiac arrest owing to asystole. Asystole is confirmed by checking two ECG leads, paddle or ECG lead contact and cable connections, and oscilloscope gain adjustment to avoid improper therapy of VF or other cardiac rhythm. For witnessed ventricular asystole in the presence of a rapidly applied external pacemaker, cardiac pacing is provided as initial therapy.

(Reproduced with permission from the American Medical Association Emergency Cardiac Care Committee and Subcommittees, American Heart Association: Guidelines for cardiopulmonary resuscitation and emergency cardiac care, III: Adult advanced cardiac life support. JAMA 1992; 268:2199–2241.)

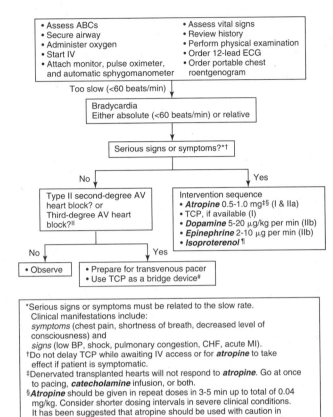

- Assess ABCs
- Secure airway
- Administer oxygen
- Start IV
- Attach monitor, pulse oximeter, and automatic sphygomanometer

- Assess vital signs
- Review history
- Perform physical examination
- Order 12-lead ECG
- Order portable chest roentgenogram

Too slow (<60 beats/min)

Bradycardia
Either absolute (<60 beats/min) or relative

Serious signs or symptoms?*†

No / Yes

Type II second-degree AV heart block? or
Third-degree AV heart block?‖

Intervention sequence
- *Atropine* 0.5-1.0 mg‡§ (I & IIa)
- TCP, if available (I)
- *Dopamine* 5-20 μg/kg per min (IIb)
- *Epinephrine* 2-10 μg per min (IIb)
- *Isoproterenol* ¶

No / Yes

- Observe

- Prepare for transvenous pacer
- Use TCP as a bridge device#

*Serious signs or symptoms must be related to the slow rate.
Clinical manifestations include:
symptoms (chest pain, shortness of breath, decreased level of consciousness) and
signs (low BP, shock, pulmonary congestion, CHF, acute MI).
†Do not delay TCP while awaiting IV access or for *atropine* to take effect if patient is symptomatic.
‡Denervated transplanted hearts will not respond to *atropine*. Go at once to pacing, *catecholamine* infusion, or both.
§*Atropine* should be given in repeat doses in 3-5 min up to total of 0.04 mg/kg. Consider shorter dosing intervals in severe clinical conditions. It has been suggested that atropine should be used with caution in atrioventricular (AV) block at the His-Purkinje level (type II AV block and new third-degree block with wide QRS complexes) (Class IIb).
‖Never treat third-degree heart block plus ventricular escape beats with *lidocaine*.
¶*Isoproterenol* should be used, if at all, with extreme caution. At low doses it is Class IIb (possibly helpful); at higher doses it is Class III (harmful).
#Verify patient tolerance and mechanical capture. Use analgesia and sedation as needed.

Figure 20-14

American Heart Association treatment algorithm for brady-cardias. Need for treatment is based on the site of conduction block and the patient's degree of hemodynamic compromise. Bradycardia is treated when heart rate slowing produces signs or symptoms of hypotension or permits ventricular escape complexes. Many patients tolerate sinus bradycardia with heart rates of 45 beats per minute or less without hemodynamic compromise. Mobitz type II second-degree atrioventricular (AV) heart block and third-degree AV (complete) heart block occurring below the AV node in the His-Purkinje system (the infranodal site of conduction block is manifested by the widened QRS complexes of the escape ventricular beats) are generally atropine refractory. These heart blocks are electrically unstable rhythms that may degenerate to asystole; external transcutaneous or transvenous cardiac pacing is indicated. TCP = transcutaneous pacing.

(Reproduced with permission from the American Medical Association, Emergency Cardiac Care Committee and Subcommittees, American Heart Association: Guidelines for cardiopulmonary resuscitation and emergency cardiac care: III. Adult advanced life support. JAMA 1992; 268: 2199-2241.)

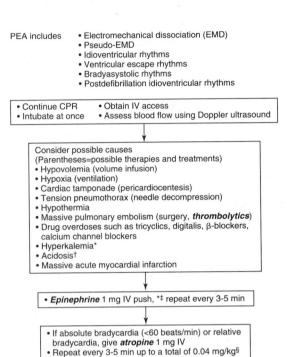

PEA includes
- Electromechanical dissociation (EMD)
- Pseudo-EMD
- Idioventricular rhythms
- Ventricular escape rhythms
- Bradyasystolic rhythms
- Postdefibrillation idioventricular rhythms

- Continue CPR
- Intubate at once
- Obtain IV access
- Assess blood flow using Doppler ultrasound

Consider possible causes
(Parentheses=possible therapies and treatments)
- Hypovolemia (volume infusion)
- Hypoxia (ventilation)
- Cardiac tamponade (pericardiocentesis)
- Tension pneumothorax (needle decompression)
- Hypothermia
- Massive pulmonary embolism (surgery, *thrombolytics*)
- Drug overdoses such as tricyclics, digitalis, β-blockers, calcium channel blockers
- Hyperkalemia*
- Acidosis†
- Massive acute myocardial infarction

- *Epinephrine* 1 mg IV push, *‡ repeat every 3-5 min

- If absolute bradycardia (<60 beats/min) or relative bradycardia, give *atropine* 1 mg IV
- Repeat every 3-5 min up to a total of 0.04 mg/kg§

Class I: definitely helpful
Class IIa: acceptable, probably helpful
Class IIb: acceptable, possibly helpful
Class III: not indicated, may be harmful
Sodium bicarbonate 1 mEq/kg is Class I if patient has known preexisting hyperkalemia.
†*Sodium bicarbonate* 1 mEq/kg:
  Class IIa
- if known preexisting bicarbonate-responsive acidosis
- if overdose with tricyclic antidepressants
- to alkalinize the urine in drug overdoses
  Class IIb
- if intubated and long arrest interval
- upon return of spontaneous circulation after long arrest interval
  Class III
- hypoxic lactic acidosis
‡The recommended dose of *epinephrine* is 1 mg IV push every 3-5 min. If this approach fails, several Class IIb dosing regimens can be considered.
- Intermediate: *epinephrine* 2-5 mg IV push, every 3-5 min
- Escalating: *epinephrine* 1 mg-3 mg-5 mg IV push (3 min apart)
- High *epinephrine* 0.1 mg/kg IV push, every 3-5 min
§Shorter *atropine* dosing intervals are possibly helpful in cardiac arrest (Class IIb).

Figure 20-15

American Heart Association treatment algorithm for cardiac arrest from pulseless electrical activity (PEA). Reversible causes of PEA are considered immediately upon recognition of the condition, and specific therapy is provided before or simultaneously with drug administration and intubation.

(Reproduced with permission from the American Medical Association, Emergency Cardiac Care Committee and Subcommittees, American Heart Association: Guidelines for cardiopulmonary resuscitation and emergency cardiac care: III. Adult advanced life support. JAMA 1992; 268: 2199-2241.)

Table 20-8

Special CPR Situations

Cause of Arrest	Pathophysiology	Treatment
Trauma	Arrest due to massive blunt head and visceral injury, uncorrectable Reversible arrest caused by exsanguination, tension pneumothorax, cardiac tamponade, airway obstruction (due to loss of consciousness or airway injury) Associated cervical injuries, hypothermia	BLS with cervical spine precautions for airway opening Transport to advanced trauma center without delay Rapid primary survey for reversible causes of arrest and specific treatment See Exsanguination below Consider thoracotomy for direct cardiac massage, treatment of pneumothorax and tamponade, clamping of aorta or pulmonary hilum
Exsanguination	Respiratory and cardiac arrest due to loss of cerebral and myocardial perfusion Chest compression ineffective in absence of venous return	Control hemorrhage Restore blood volume via ≥ 2 large IVs with crystalloid solutions and O negative or type-specific blood BLS and ACLS as indicated; ACLS not effective until artificial circulation achieved
Electrocution	Primary apnea followed by secondary cardiac arrest due to hypoxemia, *or* Primary VF or asystolic cardiac arrest Associated burns, muscle destruction, myoglobinuria, bone fractures	Do not become a second victim! Artificial ventilation as soon as possible Chest compression and ACLS as indicated Better prognosis for asystole than in other conditions
Near drowning	Submersion-induced asphyxiation followed by secondary cardiac arrest due to hypoxemia Full stomach due to swallowed water Pulmonary edema Hypothermia, cervical spine injury possible	Do not become a second victim! Artificial ventilation as soon as possible; start mouth-to-mouth ventilation in water. Do not attempt to expel gastric water Chest compression and ACLS as indicated
Hypothermia	Bradycardia, dysrhythmias, myocardial depression, coma, when $T < 28°C$ Cardiac arrest due to VF or asystole Refractory to drugs, defibrillation, pacing until warmed Metabolic acidosis Diuresis	ECG monitoring Dry patient Core warming: IV fluids; heated inspired gas; warm lavage of pericardium, body cavities, and viscera: esophageal warming tubes; cardiopulmonay bypass BLS and ACLS as indicated; ACLS not effective until central warming achieved
Carbon monoxide poisoning	Displacement of O_2 from hemoglobin, myoglobin, cytochrome binding sites by CO Airway obstruction due to unconsciousness, ventilatory depression Seizures Myocardial depression, dysrhythmias	BLS and ACLS as indicated Ventilation with 100% oxygen Hyperbaric oxygen: CO elimination half-life 1.5 h in 100% O_2 at 1 atm; 0.5 h in 100% O_2 at 3 atm
Cocaine intoxication	Central nervous system, sympathetic stimulation Ectopy, SVT, VT, VF Hypertension, myocardial ischemia and infarction Seizures	BLS and ACLS as indicated Benzodiazepines decrease CNS and sympathetic activity Beta-adrenergic antagonists for dysrhythmias refractory to usual therapy Limit epinephrine in ACLS for VF
Narcotic intoxication	Hypoventilation, airway obstruction associated with CNS depression Pulmonary edema due to drug contaminants, CNS anoxia Victims may be hepatitis B- or HIV-positive	BLS and ACLS as indicated Naloxone

Transthoracic intracardiac injection is the least desirable route of drug administration because of complications and the availability of safer alternatives for drug delivery.

Endotrachael Drug Administration

If intravenous access is delayed, most drugs can be instilled directly into the endotracheal tube diluted to 10 ml in sterile saline. Onset is comparable with that of peripheral intravenous injection, but plasma concentrations are somewhat less and persist longer. Endotracheal drugs are given at two to three times the recommended intravenous dose in order to achieve an equivalent effect. Hyperventilation after endotracheal injection promotes dispersion of the drug.

Intraosseous Administration

Intraosseous administration of fluids and drugs can be used in pediatric patients when intravenous access cannot be achieved. The anterior surface of the tibia below the tibial tuberosity is pierced with a needle that is 18 gauge or larger. Volume expanders, blood, and drugs are flushed into the marrow cavity by gravity-fed or pressurized infusions. Intraosseous drug doses greater than the intravenous dose may be needed to produce an equivalent effect.

■ Acid-Base Therapy

Diminished tissue perfusion during cardiopulmonary arrest results in the accumulation of carbon dioxide and lactic acid in body tissues. Effects of the resulting acidosis in the heart and vascular system include depression of myocardial contractility, reduced myocardial and vasomotor responsiveness to catecholamines, a diminished threshold for the induction of VF, and increased energy dose requirements for cardioversion.

Tissue acidosis and outcome from resuscitation are not improved by administration of sodium bicarbonate to neutralize lactate in the blood, despite correction of arterial pH. The carbon dioxide and lactate generated in tissues, as well as the carbon dioxide liberated by the neutralization of acid by bicarbonate, are not cleared from tissues because of the low blood flow produced by CPR. Other buffers that do not liberate CO_2 also fail to correct intracellular acidosis, probably because of inadequate tissue perfusion.

No pharmacologic therapy is now available that corrects tissue metabolic acidosis during CPR; only improved tissue perfusion and pulmonary blood flow, coupled with effective ventilation, appears efficacious. Acidosis is best avoided by prompt therapy that restores native circulation and ventilation.

Bicarbonate therapy during CPR may be helpful in specific conditions (e.g., hyperkalemia, preexisting metabolic acidemia, certain drug overdoses). After restoration of native circulation and ventilation, bicarbonate can be administered to buffer the lactic acid washed out of tissues after prolonged arrest.

■ Postresuscitation Life Support

After resuscitation, the patient is evaluated to determine the extent of cerebral, cardiovascular, pulmonary, and renal function salvaged during BLS and ACLS, as well as the primary underlying cause of the cardiopulmonary arrest. If a primary condition can be identified, prompt definitive treatment may prevent recurrence of arrest.

The patient who is awake and breathing spontaneously after successful resuscitation is monitored in an intensive care unit for recurrence of cardiac arrest. A continuous prophylactic antiarrhythmic infusion, most commonly lidocaine, is indicated for 24 hours following resuscitation from VF and VT. Other supportive measures are needed for the patient who remains apneic or who has cardiovascular instability; these may include mechanical ventilation, pressors, inotropes, and other treatment for cardiogenic shock.

Support of cerebral function after global ischemic injury caused by cardiopulmonary arrest entails general measures that maintain cerebral oxygen delivery (e.g., avoiding hypotension, correcting hypoxemia) and control cerebral metabolic rate (e.g., preventing hyperthermia, treating seizures). Specific therapies such as hyperventilation, neuromuscular blockade, and barbiturates have not been shown to improve neurologic outcome from global cerebral ischemic injury. Corticosteroids, calcium channel blocking agents, and iron chelators remain controversial.

BIBLIOGRAPHY

Brown CG, Martin DR, Pepe PE, et al. Multicenter High-Dose Epinephrine Study Group: A comparison of standard-dose and high-dose epinephrine in cardiac arrest outside the hospital. *N Engl J Med* 1992;327:1051-1055.

Chandra NC, Hazinski MF, eds. *Textbook of Basic Life Support for Healthcare Providers.* Dallas: The American Heart Association, 1994.

Cummins RO, ed. *Textbook of Advanced Cardiac Life Support.* Dallas: The American Heart Association, 1994.

Emergency Cardiac Care Committee and Subcommittees, American Heart Association. Guidelines for cardiopulmonary resuscitation and emergency cardiac care. *JAMA* 1992;268:2171-2302.

Jaffe AS. New and old paradoxes: Acidosis and cardiopulmonary resuscitation. *Circulation* 1989;80:1079-1083.

Kette F, Weil MH, von Planta M, et al. Buffer agents do not reverse intramyocardial acidosis during cardiac resuscitation. *Circulation* 1990;81:1660-1666.

Lurie KG, Shultz JJ, Callaham ML, et al. Evaluation of active compression-decompression CPR in victims of out-of-hospital cardiac arrest. *JAMA* 1994;271:1405-1411.

Ornato JP. Should bystanders perform mouth-to-mouth ventilation during resuscitation? *Chest* 1994;106:1641-1642.

Paradis NA, Koscove EM. Epinephrine in cardiac arrest: A critical review. *Ann Emerg Med* 1990;19:1288-1301.

CHAPTER 21

Cardiovascular Disease

Stuart J. Weiss and Constance F. Neely

Cardiovascular Disease

Cardiovascular complications are the leading causes of postoperative morbidity and mortality, and meticulous perioperative management of cardiovascular disease can improve outcomes significantly. This chapter addresses the basic pathophysiology, evaluation, and perioperative management of ischemic heart disease, valvular dysfunction, hypertension, tamponade, vascular disease, and congestive heart failure. The first section describes the preoperative evaluation, cardiac testing, and perioperative care of patients with cardiovascular disease. The second part focuses on specific cardiac pathology and the hemodynamic management of these conditions.

Preoperative Evaluation

Routine preoperative evaluation is described in Chapter 2. The relationship between preexisting cardiovascular disease and adverse perioperative outcome is illustrated by risk classification schemes such as those from Goldman, Eagle, Parsonette, and Detsky. The multivariate analysis of preoperative risk factors relates clinical indicators to postoperative morbidity. Preoperative screening to detect these risk factors is most helpful in high-risk patients or those undergoing major vascular procedures. About 40 percent of patients who require vascular operations have coronary artery disease, and the incidence of postoperative cardiac morbidity and mortality is significantly increased in this subset of patients. Combined medical and invasive management of ischemic heart disease (e.g., drug therapy plus coronary bypass surgery or percutaneous angioplasty if indicated) decreases the incidence of infarction after major vascular surgery as compared with medical therapy alone. However, the value of such extensive therapy before procedures associated with a low incidence of adverse outcomes, such as ophthalmic surgery, has not been established.

The history, physical examination, and laboratory testing of the patient with cardiovascular disease are directed at the cardiac, vascular, neurologic, and renal systems. A history of angina, palpitations, syncope, dysrhythmia, recent myocardial infarction, congestive heart failure, transient ischemic attack, or cerebral vascular accidents suggests that a detailed preoperative evaluation is required. In the absence of such history, a functional assessment that documents exercise capacity may be the only evaluation required. The necessity of further testing also depends in part on the planned operation. Limited evaluation may be adequate before minor operations performed under local anesthesia, whereas extensive evaluation is required before major vascular abdominal or thoracic operations. A patient who can easily climb one or two flights of stairs without chest pain or dyspnea is likely to have adequate myocardial reserve for the demands of anesthesia and minor operation. More formal classification of functional status and anginal symptoms is offered by the New York Heart Association (Table 21-1).

When activity is limited by other diseases, or when the history and physical examination suggest significant cardiovascular dysfunction, specific testing may be required to evaluate cardiopulmonary reserve. Noninvasive testing, using either radioactive multiple gated acquisition (MUGA) scans or echocardiogra-

Table 21-1

Symptom Classification of the New York Heart Association

	Limitation of Physical Activity	Symptoms
Class I	None	Asymptomatic with normal level of physical activity
Class II	Slight	Fatigue, dyspnea with ordinary activity, but comfortable at rest
Class III	Marked	Symptomatic with less than ordinary activity, but comfortable at rest
Class IV	Symptomatic at rest	Symptomatic at rest and exacerbation with activity

phy, is often suitable for assessing general left ventricular performance. MUGA scans provide an accurate measure of left ventricular ejection fraction but not of regional myocardial wall motion abnormalities caused by ischemic heart disease. Echocardiography is less invasive and less expensive, and it provides visual assessment of valvular function, global ventricular function, and regional wall motion abnormalities. However, neither MUGA scans nor echocardiography is a good screening technique for coronary artery disease, since patients with severe coronary disease may have normal left ventricular function at rest.

Three noninvasive tests assess coronary artery disease: analysis of ST segments, assessment of regional wall motion abnormalities (Fig. 21-1), and distribution of a radioactive nucleotide marker, thallium-201 (Table 21-2). The accuracy of ST-segment analysis is limited by abnormalities in the baseline electrocardiogram (ECG) due to left ventricular hypertrophy, electrolyte imbalance, bundle branch block, or digoxin. The use of echocardiography to detect abnormalities of ventricular wall motion may be limited by electrical conduction abnormalities, loading conditions, and technical problems of quantitating the data. Myocardial perfusion scanning by thallium scintigraphy is used to detect areas of flow maldistribution under conditions of increased demand (i.e., exercise) and at rest (i.e., redistribution). Whereas a persistent defect is suggestive of infarcted myocardium, a perfusion defect that later disappears suggests ischemic but viable myocardium. Increased

lung uptake of thallium is indicative of poor global ventricular function or increased left atrial pressures.

Most testing for ischemic heart disease involves the use of provocative stresses produced by either exercise or drugs. The value of exercise stress testing is often limited by the patient's inability to reach the target heart rate, due either to poor conditioning or to other physical limitations. Alternative strategies test coronary flow reserve by employing the coronary vasodilator dipyridamole to produce a relative flow reduction in diseased arteries or dobutamine to mimic the cardiovascular effects of exercise. The advantages and disadvantages of these tests are presented in Table 21-2. No current diagnostic test is 100 percent sensitive or specific, and test results may be of limited value in select populations of patients. Nevertheless, the results of testing plus history and physical findings give an overall impression of risks and possible perioperative complications.

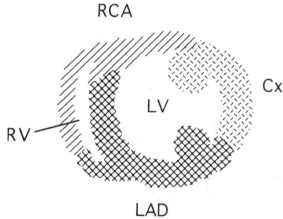

Figure 21-1

A schematic cross-sectional view of the heart at the level of the papillary muscles. The portions of the walls of the right ventricle (RV) and left ventricle (LV) perfused by the coronary arteries are shown as *(striped)* right coronary artery (RCA), *(light stippled)* circumflex artery (CX), and *(cross-hatched)* left anterior descending (LAD). The distribution of the coronary arteries, the ECG leads showing ischemia in the corresponding myocardium, and areas of wall motion are related as shown:

ECG	Coronary Artery	Distribution
II, III, AVF	RCA	Posterior, inferior walls
V_2-V_5	LAD	Septum, anterior wall
I, AVL, V_4-V_6	CX	Lateral wall

Table 21-2

Myocardial Ischemia: The Strategies for Challenging Coronary Reserve and Techniques for Detecting Ischemia

		Advantages	Disadvantages
Techniques of Ischemia Detection			
ECG	Quantitative ST-segment changes	Simple, available, standard for ischemia detection	Limited by an abnormal ECG bundle branch block, strain pattern, pacer, digoxin (effect)
Echocardiography	Image of LV, for wall motion abnormalities	Image of wall motion abnormalities and ischemic MR	Poor assessment of right ventricle, technical limitations
Thallium-201	Localization of perfusion defects	Visualize distribution of myocardium at risk	Exposure to radioactivity
Modes of Challenge			
Exercise stress	Use exercise bicycle or treadmill	Previous standard, inexpensive, can be performed in outpatients	Limited by poor conditioning, musculoskeletal problems
Atrial pacing	Increase heart rate to increase demand	Independent of patient conditioning	Limited availability
Dobutamine	Inotrope to mimic the increased demand of exercise	Independent of patient conditioning, very sensitive and specific	Arrhythmias
Dipyridamole	Vasodilator to test reserve of coronary arteries	Independent of patient conditioning	Contraindicated with COPD, asthma, recent MI or unstable angina; may fail to detect severe CAD in vascular patients

Perioperative Management of Patients with Cardiovascular Disease

■ Anesthetic Technique

Most studies suggest that morbidity and mortality correlate with patient and surgical risk factors and not the specific anesthetic technique or drug. A possible exception occurs with vascular surgery on the lower extremity; regional anesthesia improves graft patency. However, the successful conduct of anesthesia in patients with cardiovascular disease requires meticulous attention to hemodynamic variables such as heart rate, blood pressure, and vascular resistance, which can have a profound effect on cardiac function and which are altered by specific anesthetics.

A skillfully conducted regional anesthetic limited to an extremity produces minimal physiologic alterations and blocks the pain that causes tachycardia and hypertension. Given adequate sedation, ventilation, and oxygenation, this is a satisfactory form of anesthesia for many patients at risk for myocardial infarction, myocardial pump failure, or arrhythmias. The modest sympathectomy associated with limited regional anesthesia may reduce left ventricular afterload and even improve cardiac performance. Continuing regional anesthesia into the postoperative period provides analgesia and reduces the hemodynamic stresses (e.g., tachycardia) associated with pain. Regional anesthesia also may be used during or after major procedures. For example, thoracic epidural anesthesia may confer an additional benefit in patients with coronary artery disease by treating angina and decreasing the incidence of ischemic ECG changes and regional wall motion abnormalities.

The potent inhaled anesthetics are used widely in the management of patients with cardiovascular disease because they provide for rapid changes in depth of anesthesia to manage alterations in heart rate and blood pressure during operations. A well-planned general anesthetic incorporates the best aspects of several different agents in hopes of providing anesthesia while minimizing the risk of poor outcomes. Of the inhalational anesthetics, halothane is noted for myocardial depression and isoflurane for decreased systemic vascular resistance; all reduce blood pressure when administered in clinical concentrations. Under very specific laboratory conditions, isoflurane may produce "coronary steal" in animals by promoting blood flow to areas of the myocardium perfused by normal vessels and away from areas supplied by diseased coronary arteries, but this is an extremely rare event in humans, and the drug is used widely in patients with coronary artery disease. The combination of a potent anesthetic vapor and nitrous oxide allows control of arterial pressure without excessive myocardial depression. The addition of nitrous oxide increases systemic vascular resistance slightly, but arterial pressure is usually not changed because cardiac output decreases.

Of the intravenous anesthetics, thiopental and propofol produce dose-dependent depression of myocardial contractility. Etomidate produces minimal hemodynamic changes or alterations in myocardial function and is useful in situations such as pericardial tamponade or congestive heart failure. Opiates have gained a special place in managing patients with cardiovascular disease; they are given in moderate doses to supplement general anesthesia and in much larger doses to provide nearly complete general anesthesia (see Chap. 10). They have little effect on myocardial performance, cardiac output, or arterial pressure in the supine patient, and they decrease requirements for the more potent inhaled anesthetics.

■ Intraoperative Monitoring

The choice of invasive cardiovascular monitoring depends on the preoperative cardiac status, type of operation, anticipated hemodynamic alterations, and requirements for vascular access (see Chap. 6). Enhanced monitoring in high-risk patients allows closer control of the patient's cardiovascular system, with the hope of improving outcome. Intensive monitoring and aggressive medical management during the operative and postoperative periods have been shown to decrease the incidence of reinfarction in high-risk patients. However, even when blood pressure and heart rate are carefully maintained near preoperative values, patients may still suffer unanticipated ischemia.

Electrocardiography is the most commonly used monitor for the intraoperative detection of rhythm disturbances or ischemia. Lead II is the most sensitive

for detecting the P waves of atrial depolarization, important for the diagnosis of tachycardia, bradycardia, and conduction rhythm disturbances. Myocardial ischemia by ECG is defined as 0.1 mV or more of ST-segment depression or greater than 0.2 mV of ST-segment elevation 60 to 80 ms beyond the J-point. Electrocardiographic changes consistent with ischemia occur in 18 to 74 percent of patients with coronary artery disease undergoing noncardiac surgical procedures. Most of the changes are ST-segment depression, and 90 percent of these occur in leads V_4 and V_5. The combination of leads II, V_4, and V_5 detects ischemia with 96 percent sensitivity.

Intraarterial blood pressure monitoring is used commonly for patients with cardiovascular disease, especially those with hypertension or associated pulmonary diseases and in those undergoing operations that result in major hemodynamic alterations. Advantages include continuous recording of the blood pressure and access for sampling of arterial blood for such measurements as arterial blood gases, electrolytes, and hemoglobin concentration.

Monitoring the patient at risk for myocardial failure, whether from myocardial dysfunction or from valve disease, includes the invasive measurement of arterial pressure, cardiac filling pressures, and cardiac output. Strategies for managing cardiac failure using these data are given in Chapter 29. In patients with poor left ventricular function (ejection fraction less than 0.40 or with significant wall motion abnormalities), changes in central venous pressure (CVP) do not predict changes in pulmonary artery occlusion pressure (see Chap. 6). Although useful in managing pump failure, the pulmonary artery catheter is not a sensitive or specific monitor for cardiac ischemia. An increased pulmonary artery occlusion pressure (more than 25 mmHg) has been associated with a greatly increased risk of perioperative reinfarction, however.

Transesophageal echocardiography (TEE) can be used to assess regional ventricular wall motion, wall thickening, ejection fraction, valvular function, and intracardiac pathology. The first detectable alterations of myocardial ischemia are segmental wall motion and wall thickening abnormalities, which are followed by ECG changes. However, the application of TEE for ischemia monitoring during routine operations is limited because of expense, availability, and the training required. TEE may have a use during the perioperative period for assessing dynamic diastolic and systolic cardiac function in high-risk patients having major vascular, cardiac, or thoracic operations.

■Hemodynamic Management

A major goal in the anesthetic management of patients with cardiovascular disease is maintenance of hemodynamic stability by anticipating episodes of potential hypotension, hypertension, or tachycardia. The target range for intraoperative blood pressure is determined by the blood pressure in the days before surgery, the presence of associated disease, and the type of operation. Usually the goal is to maintain blood pressure within ±20 percent of baseline, but closer control may be needed for patients with vascular disease. For example, blood pressure during carotid endarterectomy is maintained within a narrow predetermined range, often at or above the preoperative value, in an effort to avoid cerebral ischemia during carotid occlusion.

Hypotension in the presence of severe coronary artery stenosis decreases coronary perfusion pressure and may produce myocardial ischemia. The combination of hypotension and tachycardia increases the risk of myocardial ischemia more than does hypotension alone. Strategies for managing hypotension are directed toward increasing peripheral vascular resistance or improving cardiac output (Table 21-3). When hypotension is the result of decreased peripheral resistance, vasopressors such as those listed in

Table 21-4 are appropriate. In the case of decreased cardiac output, rational therapy is directed at one or more of the following: increasing preload, decreasing afterload, improving contractility, or treating dysrhythmias. In patients with severe left ventricular dysfunction, medical therapy may be insufficient to support systemic perfusion so that a mechanical device, such as an intraaortic balloon pump, may be required. Specific strategies to treat hypotension in patients with cardiac valvular disease are discussed in the later sections and are presented in Table 21-5.

Acute episodes of hypertension are common during the perioperative period. Increased blood pressure does not imply increased blood flow, since blood pressure is the product of cardiac output and systemic vascular resistance. Hypertension may reflect an increased vascular resistance and reduced blood flow to vital organs. In addition, hypertension impairs the balance between cardiac oxygen utilization and delivery by increasing ventricular wall stress and decreasing coronary perfusion. Intraoperative hypertension is often a sign of an underlying anesthetic problem, not a primary condition requiring antihypertensive therapy.

Intraoperative hypertension often follows acute noxious stimuli, such as laryngoscopy, intubation, skin incision, sternotomy, manipulation of the aorta,

Table 21-3

Strategies for Treating Hypotension (BP = CO × SVR)*

Cardiac Output	Systemic Vascular Resistance
Increase preload	Discontinue vasodilators
Head-down position	Administer vasoconstrictor
Infusion of fluids	
Restore sinus rhythm	
Decrease mean intrathoracic pressure by adjusting ventilator settings	
Decrease afterload	
Vasodilator	
Intraaortic balloon pump	
Improve contractility	
Discontinue myocardial depressants	
Administer inotropic agent	
Treat ischemia	
Alter heart rate	
Increase heart rate if bradycardia limits output	
Decrease heart rate if tachycardia limits left ventricular filling, as in mitral stenosis	
Restore normal sinus rhythm	

*Arterial blood pressure is actually the product of cardiac output and the difference between mean arterial pressure and mean central venous pressure. Central venous pressure is so small as to be negligible in this calculation.

Table 21-4

Common Vasopressors Used During the Perioperative Period

	Adrenergic Receptor Activity	Single Dose Adults	Continuous Dose, µg/kg/min
Phenylephrine (Neosynephrine)	Alpha	50–200 µg	0.2–3
Methoxamine (Vasoxyl)	Alpha	2–10 mg	
Ephedrine	Alpha, beta	5–15 mg	
Epinephrine (Adrenaline)	Alpha, beta	8–100 µg	0.02–0.2
Norepinephrine (Levophed)	Alpha > beta		0.02–0.2
Dopamine (Intropin)	Alpha, beta, dopaminergic		2–15
Dobutamine (Dobutrex)	Alpha < beta		2–20

Note: Dosage and choice of drug are based on the severity of hypotension, underlying cardiac pathology, and response of the patient during treatment.

pain on emergence, or light anesthesia, especially in patients with histories of preexisting hypertension. Increased sympathetic nervous system activity produces both hypertension and tachycardia, which are best prevented by increasing the depth of inhalation anesthesia or giving opioids. Administration of short-acting beta-adrenergic antagonists, such as esmolol, attenuates the tachycardia and hypertension produced by stimuli such as laryngoscopy and tracheal intubation. Preoperative administration of clonidine or beta-adrenergic blockers also reduces the incidence of intraoperative hypertension and tachycardia.

Hypertension also may result from disorders such as hypervolemia, hypercarbia, hypoxia, or intracranial hypertension. Once these causes have been ruled out, intravenous administration of vasodilators can be considered. A list of the most commonly used vasodilators is presented in Table 21-6. Because of the prevalence of coronary artery disease in patients having major vascular operations, nitroglycerin is often used prophylactically for its coronary, pulmonary, and systemic vasodilating effects.

■Postoperative Care

The immediate postoperative period is associated with significant hemodynamic stress. The risk of postoperative respiratory and cardiac complications is increased in patients with cardiac disease, especially following upper abdominal or thoracic surgery or when large amounts of fluids are administered. Postoperative care begins as the patient is transferred to a recovery room or intensive care unit. Patients such as those having open-heart operations, craniotomies, major vascular operations, or surgical procedures associated with large volume replacement are transported with continuous hemodynamic monitoring. Also, patients receiving infusions of vasoactive drugs or those at risk for major blood pressure fluctuations are monitored during transport because hyperten-

Table 21-5

Strategies for Treating Hypotension in the Patient with Cardiac Disease*

	Afterload	Preload	Heart Rate	Myocardial Contractility
Aortic stenosis	↑	↑	↓	
Mitral stenosis		↑	↓	
Aortic insufficiency	↓		↑	↑
Mitral regurgitation	↓		↑	↑
Tamponade		↑	↑	↑
Congestive heart failure	↓			↑

*These are suggestions for initial therapy that must be modified to suit circumstances. For example, although it is helpful to avoid tachycardia in aortic stenosis so as to avoid limitations on diastolic coronary flow, extreme bradycardia would limit cardiac output.

Table 21-6

Common Vasodilators Used During the Perioperative Period

	Mechanism of Action	Single Dose Adults	Initial Dose for Continuous Infusion, µg/kg/min
Sodium nitroprusside	Activation of nitric oxide		0.5
Hydralazine	Activation of nitric oxide	5–20 mg	
Trimethaphan	Ganglionic blocker	0.5–2 mg	0.5
Phentolamine	Alpha antagonist	5 mg	
Nitroglycerine	Activation of nitric oxide		0.5
Nicardipine	Calcium channel blocker		0.1

Note: Dosage must be individualized depending on the severity of hypertension and response of the patient during treatment.

sion, hypotension, or tachycardia occur commonly during this interval.

Hypertension and tachycardia are frequent in the immediate postoperative period. Postoperative hypertension is usually brief in duration; 80 percent of postoperative hypertensive episodes begin within 30 minutes of admission to the recovery room and end within 3 hours. Factors that increase postoperative blood pressure include preexisting hypertension, pain, emergence delirium, anxiety, hypoxia, hypercarbia, hypothermia, and hypervolemia. The most common contributing factor to the development of postoperative hypertension is a history of hypertension preoperatively. Physiologic responses to hypothermia include vasoconstriction, which increases afterload, and shivering, which markedly increases oxygen consumption. Hypothermia is treated aggressively because it is associated with an increased incidence of ischemia and hypoxemia. In some cases, prevention of the stress response to hypothermia may require postoperative paralysis, sedation, and mechanical ventilation. Hypoxemia in the immediate postoperative period also increases the risk of cardiac complications and must be prevented as described elsewhere (see Chaps. 22 and 25).

Effective postoperative pain management, including epidural analgesia, may decrease stress and the risk of cardiac morbidity by alleviating pain and consequent hypertension and tachycardia. Aggressive pain management is part of the anesthetic care for patients at risk of myocardial ischemia. High-risk surgical patients who receive epidural anesthesia for intraoperative and postoperative analgesia have lower inci-

dences of morbidity and mortality as compared with those who receive conventional postoperative care only.

Postoperative hypertension also is related to the type of operation. Cardiac, aortic, and carotid artery operations produce the greatest incidence of postoperative hypertension. With carotid operations, postoperative hypertension may compensate for cerebral vascular ischemia or result from abnormal baroreceptor function.

After the other treatable causes of hypertension and tachycardia have been addressed, specific pharmacologic therapy is considered. Medical therapy of hypertension is usually limited to parenteral administration of drugs having rapid onsets, such as labetalol or hydralazine. Potent short-acting vasodilators such as sodium nitroprusside, trimethaphan, or nicardipine are used to treat refractory or profound hypertension and may require use of an arterial catheter for appropriate monitoring.

Management of Patients with Specific Cardiovascular Diseases

Many patients who require operation have either clinically symptomatic or occult cardiovascular disease. To improve the care of this increasing portion of the patient population, the anesthesiologist must understand the effects of anesthetics and surgical stresses on individual pathologic conditions. The following subsections focus on specific cardiovascular diseases.

■ Hypertension

Hypertension is defined as a systolic blood pressure greater than 140 mmHg or a diastolic blood pressure greater than 90 mmHg. It is the most common cardiovascular disease and the leading cause of coronary artery, cerebrovascular, and renal diseases. The pathophysiology of chronic hypertension involves vascular remodeling that decreases arterial lumen diameter and the number of small arterioles and capillaries. Such structural changes render the tissues at increased risk for cellular hypoxia, especially during conditions of decreased blood flow.

Multiple organs systems are affected by chronic hypertension, including the kidney, brain, and heart. Structural changes in the walls of blood vessels, combined with alterations in circulating hormones and vasoactive substances such as angiotensin, result in increased renal vascular resistance and impaired renal blood flow and function. Chronic exposure to systemic hypertension causes a shift in end-organ pressure requirements so that the autoregulatory curve for blood flow is shifted to the right (i.e., greater arterial pressure is required to maintain perfusion). In patients with chronic systemic hypertension, increased cerebral perfusion pressure is required to avoid ischemia; a rapid decrease in blood pressure to "normotensive values" may result in cerebral ischemia.

The direct pathophysiologic effect of hypertension on the heart is left ventricular hypertrophy. Systemic hypertension increases left ventricular systolic wall stress, which in turn is compensated by hypertrophy of the left ventricle. Even in the absence of coronary artery occlusion, myocardial ischemia may occur. Hypertrophy of the left ventricle increases oxygen consumption without a proportional increase in coronary blood flow. In addition, coronary artery blood flow to the subendocardium may be compromised by the increase in wall thickness and decrease in coronary perfusion pressure.

The importance of systemic hypertension as a risk factor for predicting perioperative complications is controversial. Most studies do not account for the presence of subclinical organ dysfunction or the response to chronic medical management. Some chronic antihypertensive therapy is associated with regression of left ventricular hypertrophy, improvement of diastolic function, and decrease in the prevalence of ventricular arrhythmias and central neurologic events. Although mild to moderate hypertension with diastolic blood pressure less than 100 mmHg may not be associated with adverse cardiac outcome, it predisposes to increased intraoperative blood pressure lability and heart rate variability. Although this too is controversial, some investigators have found that intraoperative hemodynamic lability in hypertensive patients correlates with postoperative renal and cardiac complications.

Perioperative management is guided by the severity of end-organ dysfunction, current antihypertensive medications, and preoperative baseline blood pressure. Some antihypertensive medications (beta-adrenergic blockers, clonidine, and calcium channel blockers) permit rebound increases in sympathetic outflow when they are discontinued abruptly; thus they are continued on the day of surgery. Diuretics are often discontinued because they decrease intravascular volume, making the hypertensive patient more susceptible to hypotension with blood loss, fluid restriction, and the vasodilating effects of general or spinal anesthesia. The usual goal is to maintain the blood pressure and heart rate within a range of about 20 percent of baseline so as to prevent ischemia to vital organs. In general, these patients have exaggerated reductions in blood pressure in response to inhalational anesthetics, to antihypertensive therapy, or to the sympathectomy associated with spinal or epidural anesthesia. In addition, these patients often require intravenous fluids or vasopressors to prevent hypotension with anesthesia because of contracted plasma volumes due to the disease process, diuretic therapy, or associated dehydrating factors such as administration of radiocontrast media or laxatives for bowel preparation.

■ Coronary Artery Disease

The risk of perioperative myocardial infarction in the general population of noncardiac surgical patients is less than 1 percent, as compared with about 5 percent for patients who have had a previous infarction. Since coronary artery disease is often silent, the absence of symptoms and good exercise tolerance do not guarantee freedom from cardiac disease. To better diagnose heart disease and improve outcome, studies have sought to identify risk factors predictive of coronary artery disease and perioperative myocardial infarction. The accepted risk factors for coronary artery disease are listed in Table 21-7. Patients with peripheral vascular disease or histories of hyperten-

Table 21-7

Risk Factors for Coronary Artery Disease

Age
Hypertension
Obesity
Family history
Diabetes mellitus
Smoking
Hyperlipidemia
Peripheral vascular disease

---

sion, diabetes, or cigarette smoking have a increased incidence of coronary artery disease. The presence of Q waves on the ECG, evidence of congestive heart failure, and a previous myocardial infarction are also associated with an increased perioperative risk.

The risk of reinfarction is a function of the type of surgical procedure and the duration since the previous infarction. The risk of postoperative reinfarction associated with major abdominal operation performed more than 6 months after previous infarction is 5 percent; between 3 and 6 months, the infarction rate increases to 10 to 15 percent; within 3 months, there is a 30 percent risk of reinfarction. However, these data are from older studies and may be overestimates for patients managed by current methods. The combination of aggressive preoperative therapy, careful intraoperative hemodynamic management, and postoperative intensive care may improve outcome. In contrast to major abdominal or thoracic operations, minor procedures such as ophthalmic surgery are not associated with markedly increased risk of reinfarction.

The assumption that intraoperative ischemic events signal an increased incidence of postoperative cardiac morbidity has been challenged. Most recommendations for managing patients with coronary artery disease during operations focus on detecting, preventing, and treating episodes of myocardial ischemia (including the guidelines that follow in this chapter). However, silent transient ischemic episodes occur often in these patients, before, during, and after operation, and are not usually followed by infarction. Whatever measures are taken to detect and manage ischemia during anesthesia must extend into the postoperative period, when pain, vasoconstriction, tachycardia, and hypoxemia can all provoke ischemia.

Preventing myocardial ischemia may begin for some patients with such aggressive management as coronary artery bypass grafting or angioplasty. These patients include those with severe but correctable coronary occlusion who are to undergo major aortic operations. Other management requires attention to factors that affect the balance of myocardial oxygen supply and demand. The supply of oxygen to the heart is a function of coronary blood flow, hemoglobin concentration, and the arterial partial pressure of oxygen. Determinants of myocardial oxygen demand (MVO_2) include systolic wall tension, which is a function of aortic systolic pressure and end-diastolic pressure and volume; the contractile state of the myocardium; and the heart rate (Table 21-8). Under normal conditions, the coronary vascular bed autoregulates blood flow over coronary perfusion pressures (difference between the systemic diastolic pressure and the left ventricular end-diastolic pressure) in the range of 60 to 130 mmHg. When MVO_2 exceeds the supply, ischemia occurs. During such periods, coronary vasodilator reserve is exhausted, and coronary flow becomes a direct function of perfusion pressure. In these circumstances, physiologic conditions that increase left ventricular end-diastolic pressure, such as left ventricular hypertrophy, aortic stenosis, or aortic insufficiency, decrease coronary perfusion pressure.

Other determinants of coronary ischemia include heart rate, collateral circulation, coronary vasomotor tone, and intramyocardial compression forces, which vary during systole and diastole. Increases in heart rate not only increase myocardial oxygen consumption but also decrease the time for diastolic perfusion of the coronary arteries and for diastolic ventricular filling. About 75 percent of left coronary artery flow occurs during diastole because of the extravascular compression that occurs with systolic contraction. A greater fraction of right coronary flow (30 to 50 percent) occurs during systole in the thin-walled right ventricle because intramyocardial compressive forces are less.

Table 21-8

Determinants of Myocardial Oxygen Supply and Demand

Increase Oxygen Supply	Increase Oxygen Demand
↑ Coronary blood flow	↑ Systolic wall stress
↑ Oxygen transport	↑ Aortic systolic pressure
↑ O_2 saturation	↑ LVEDP*
↑ Hemoglobin	↑ Heart rate
	↑ Contractile states

*Left ventricular end-diastolic pressure.

Table 21-9

Diagnostic Features of Valvular Disease

	Auscultatory Features	Other Clinical Features
Aortic stenosis	S_4, systolic murmur at right second intercostal space transmitted to the carotid arteries	LVH by ECG, powerful PMI, delayed carotid upstroke
Aortic regurgitation	S_3, decrescendo diastolic murmur at sternal border	Widened pulse pressure, rapid upstroke and collapse
Mitral stenosis	Middiastolic rumble, loud S_1	Atrial fibrillation, ECG finding of LA enlargement, RVH, right axis deviation
Mitral regurgitation	Holosystolic murmur at the apex which radiates to the axilla	V wave on PA catheter occlusion pressure trace

Note: RVH, right ventricular hypertrophy; LA, left atrium; PMI, point of maximal impulse.

The goals of perioperative management include increasing blood flow while reducing myocardial demand by maintaining a normal heart rate and coronary perfusion pressure. Both increased heart rate and hypotension are associated with myocardial ischemia. Treatment of myocardial ischemia may involve not only coronary vasodilators but also reduction of heart rate and myocardial contractility with beta blockers. Another strategy is to decrease oxygen consumption through decreasing systolic wall stress by reducing afterload using nitroglycerin, sodium nitroprusside, or nicardipine.

■ Cardiac Valvular Diseases

Valvular abnormalities affect not only valve function but also the pulmonary vasculature, cardiac contractility, and diastolic function. Patients with valvular disease generally have reduced margins of safety for fluid management and require close attention to control intravascular volume, heart rate, and systemic vascular resistance. Patients with valvular disease have an increased risk of perioperative morbidity and may require additional preoperative testing, including echocardiography and cardiac catheterization, to determine the extent of myocardial and valvular impairment.

Aortic Stenosis

Aortic stenosis is the most common cardiac valvular disease. The severity of symptoms correlates with progression of the disease and the extent of cardiac decompensation. Life expectancy is 5 years after the onset of angina, 3 years after the onset of syncope, and 2 years after congestive heart failure. The characteristic physical finding is a harsh systolic ejection murmur that radiates to the carotid arteries and is associated with a delayed carotid upstroke (Table 21-9). The severity of aortic stenosis can be evaluated with echocardiography or cardiac catheterization, by measuring the aortic to left ventricular pressure gradient, and by calculating the effective value area. The transvalvular pressure gradient varies as the square of the cardiac output. Therefore, a minimum pressure gradient may reflect either the absence of significant obstruction or diminished cardiac output with poor cardiac function.

Anatomic obstruction to ventricular ejection leads to chronic pressure overload of the left ventricle. The increased left ventricular systolic pressure increases ventricular wall stress, which in turn produces hypertrophy. Hypertrophy is associated with a decrease in diastolic compliance, increasing the importance of the atrial contribution to diastolic filling. In addition, left ventricular hypertrophy and increased left ventricular end-diastolic pressure increase susceptibility to endocardial ischemia.

The goals of perioperative management are to avoid increases in heart rate and decreases in preload, afterload, or coronary perfusion pressure. Appropriate sedation is important to prevent excitement and anxiety that increase heart rate. Both regional and general anesthetic techniques can be performed safely. However, the sympathectomy associated with epidural and spinal anesthesia may result in an acute decrease in preload and afterload, resulting in hypotension and myocardial ischemia. Spinal and epidural anesthesia are rarely used for patients with aortic stenosis. The choice of monitoring depends on the severity of the disease and the magnitude of the operation. Invasive cardiovascular monitoring, including a pulmonary artery catheter, is required for major vascular, thoracic, or cardiac operations.

Perioperative hypotension must be treated aggressively with vasopressors and volume resuscitation (see Table 21-5). Atrial arrhythmias, such as junctional rhythms, atrial tachycardia, or atrial fibrillation, can result in hypotension and ischemia. As the disease progresses and ventricular compliance decreases, maintenance of normal sinus rhythm becomes more important. Depending on the severity of hypotension, management of these arrhythmias may include antiarrhythmics such as verapamil, vasopressors such as phenylephrine, or electrical cardioversion to reestablish sinus rhythm.

Mitral Stenosis

Mitral stenosis is a common cardiac disease often associated with a history of rheumatic heart disease. An asymptomatic patient may manifest symptoms of stenosis unexpectedly during conditions of stress such as pregnancy, sepsis, or operations. The impediment to blood flow from the left atrium into the left ventricle results in not only inadequate left ventricular filling but also increased left atrial, pulmonary arterial, and right ventricular pressures. Early in the disease, increased pulmonary pressures are associated with an increased incidence of pulmonary edema. Later in the disease, increased pulmonary artery pressures are associated with right ventricular failure. Physical findings in patients with mitral stenosis include a low-pitched diastolic murmur, jugular venous distension, right ventricular heave, and often the irregular rhythm of atrial fibrillation (see Table 21-9). As with aortic stenosis, patients with severe mitral stenosis may benefit from valvuloplasty prior to elective operations. The resulting increased valve area and decreased pressure gradient can be expected to decrease perioperative morbidity.

Patients can be managed with either general or regional anesthesia. The goals of anesthetic management include maintaining adequate preload to overcome the obstruction of flow and a slow heart rate to allow time for diastolic filling of the left ventricle. Mitral stenosis limits increases in cardiac output that ordinarily compensate for decreases in peripheral resistance. Careful administration of intravenous fluids or vasopressors provides for increased preload to overcome mitral stenosis (see Table 21-5), but pulmonary edema, fluid overload, and beta-adrenergic effects that produce tachycardia must be avoided.

Aortic Regurgitation

In contrast to aortic stenosis, in which concentric hypertrophy compensates for excessive pressure load, aortic insufficiency causes progressive ventricular dilation due to excessive volume load. The retrograde flow of blood during diastole decreases the effective cardiac output and systemic diastolic blood pressure, which decreases the coronary perfusion pressure. Preoperative assessment of the severity of regurgitation and left ventricular dysfunction is important. Physical examination reveals a blowing decrescendo diastolic murmur along the left sternal border and widened pulse pressures (see Table 21-9).

The goals of operative management include decreasing afterload to improve forward flow and maintaining normal to slightly increased heart rate to limit the time for retrograde flow during diastole. Both regional and general anesthetic techniques are compatible with the hemodynamic goals of maintaining heart rate and vasodilation while avoiding myocardial depression. However, intravascular volume must be augmented to compensate for the arterial vasodilation and decreased preload of anesthesia. The vasodilation associated with isoflurane and desflurane promotes forward flow and may improve cardiac performance. Intraoperative hypotension is treated with intravenous fluids and positive inotropic agents (see Table 21-5). Vasopressors such as phenylephrine or methoxamine increase afterload, promoting retrograde flow and exacerbating left ventricular dysfunction.

Mitral Regurgitation

The incompetent mitral valve decreases the effective stroke volume of the left ventricle by permitting regurgitant flow into the left atrium. The resulting increase in left atrial volume increases left atrial and pulmonary artery pressures. The physical examination includes a systolic murmur at the apex that radiates to the axilla and pulmonary rales (see Table 21-9). Right-sided heart catheterization reveals increased pulmonary artery pressures and a pathologic V wave in the pulmonary artery occlusion pressure tracing. Left ventricular ejection fraction is overestimated because it reflects the sum of both antegrade and retrograde flow out of the left ventricle.

As in aortic insufficiency, the goals of management

are to promote forward flow by decreasing afterload and to maintain a normal to slightly increased heart rate. Both regional and general anesthesia techniques are consistent with these goals. Use of the pulmonary artery catheter is especially important for those patients having severely depressed left ventricular function or significant pulmonary hypertension. Hypertension related to increased systemic vascular resistance is treated with arterial vasodilators, but not beta blockers, to avoid depression of myocardial function. Problems most often encountered during the postoperative management of these patients are pulmonary congestion and right ventricular failure, including hepatic insufficiency.

■ Cardiac Tamponade

Cardiac tamponade is due to pericardial effusion or bleeding sufficient to impede right atrial and ventricular filling, thereby decreasing left ventricular preload, which results in hypotension. As tamponade worsens, the stroke volume gradually declines and eventually becomes fixed. Small effusions that occur rapidly, as with trauma or aortic dissection, can alter cardiac output profoundly. Chronic processes, such as a malignancy or uremia, lead to the slow accumulation of large effusions with modest clinical effects, except under conditions of hypovolemia or controlled ventilation. The physical examination reveals a decreased systolic pressure, a narrow pulse pressure, and pulses paradoxus (a decrease in systemic

pressure with inspiration). In addition, jugular venous distension, tachycardia, and distant or faint cardiac sounds are common. The ECG may demonstrate low voltage, ST-segment elevation, or electrical alternans (beat-to-beat variation in the R wave amplitude). Echocardiography demonstrates the presence of pericardial fluid and invagination (or collapse) of the right atrium and ventricle (Fig. 21-2). With tamponade, right-sided heart catheterization demonstrates equalization of the right atrial, ventricular, and pulmonary artery pressures.

The goals of management are to maintain a rapid heart rate and increased intravascular volume. Induction of anesthesia can result in profound hypotension from the effects of peripheral vasodilation, myocardial depression, or controlled ventilation. Ketamine is a rational choice for intravenous induction of anesthesia. Percutaneous pericardiocentesis performed under local anesthesia may improve the patient's condition and permit safer induction. Hypotension is treated with vasopressors and fluid administration (see Table 21-5).

■ Congestive Heart Failure

Congestive heart failure (CHF) results when adaptive mechanisms fail to compensate for dysfunction of the right side of the heart, left side of the heart, or both. Right ventricular failure produces hepatic engorgement, ascites, and peripheral edema. Left ventricular failure produces pulmonary edema

Figure 21-2

Transesophageal echocardiogram showing a pericardial effusion, pericardium (PC), right ventricle (RV), left ventricle (LV), right atrium (RA), tricuspid valve (TV), and intraatrial septum (IAS).

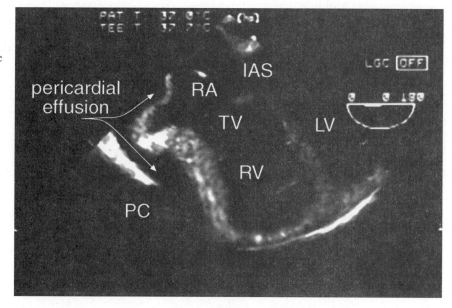

and right-sided heart failure. Patients with active heart failure are at greatly increased risk for serious postoperative cardiovascular complications. Those with well-controlled CHF are less liable for such sequelae. Patients having clinical evidence of CHF, manifested by third heart sounds or jugular venous distension, had a 16 percent incidence of postoperative complications after noncardiac operations, as compared to 6 percent for patients having only the prior history of heart failure.

Anesthetic techniques and drugs are chosen to minimize cardiac depression and decrease systemic vascular resistance. Invasive monitoring during the operative and postoperative periods is often required. Perioperative CHF is treated with diuretics, nitroglycerin, inotropes, and afterload reduction to decrease ventricular wall stress and myocardial oxygen consumption. Hypotension resulting from poor cardiac performance may require the use of inotropic infusions such as dopamine, epinephrine, or dobutamine (see Tables 21-4 and 21-5).

■ Vascular Disease of the Aorta

The most common etiologies of aortic disease include atherosclerosis, fibromuscular dysplasia, hypertension, inflammatory arteriopathies, and trauma. Coronary artery disease is especially prevalent in vascular surgical patients. The risk of perioperative cardiac complications is decreased by coronary artery revascularization or coronary angioplasty prior to elective aortic surgery.

Intraoperative management during these operations emphasizes avoiding major hemodynamic perturbations. For example, placement of the aortic cross-clamp results in proximal hypertension with an acute increase in left ventricular wall stress. These effects are more dramatic with more proximal placement of the aortic cross-clamp. Vasodilators such as nitroglycerine or nitroprusside blunt the acute increase in cardiac afterload and decrease the risk of cardiac dysfunction. Later, release of the aortic cross-clamp results in a marked decrease in systemic blood pressure that is related to blood loss, decreased vascular resistance, increased venous capacitance, and decreased ventricular preload. If not anticipated and prevented, the subsequent hypotension results in decreased coronary perfusion and ischemia. Prophylactic administration of fluids to increase cardiac preload and sodium bicarbonate to treat the impending acidosis attenuate the decrease in blood pressure

following the release of the aortic cross-clamp. Postoperatively, continued hemodynamic monitoring and effective management of analgesia are required.

Conclusion

Despite recent progress in managing patients at risk through careful hemodynamic control and the other measures described here, a significant number of patients suffer cardiac complications during the perioperative period. Further improvements in care will require better understanding of the mechanisms of thrombosis, vessel spasm, and hypertension and reliable means of ensuring oxygen delivery to vital organs during the perioperative period.

BIBLIOGRAPHY

Frank SM, Beattie C, Christopherson R, et al. Unintentional hypothermia is associated with postoperative myocardial ischemia: The Perioperative Ischemia Randomized Anesthesia Trial Study Group. *Anesthesiology* 1993;78:468-476.

Fleisher LA, Skolnick ED, Holroyd KJ, Lehmann HP. Coronary artery revascularization before abdominal aortic aneurysm surgery: A decision analytic approach. *Anesth Analg* 1994;79: 661-669.

Mangano DT. Perioperative cardiac morbidity. *Anesthesiology* 1990;72:153-184.

Mangano DT, Browner WS, Hollenberg M, et al. Association of perioperative myocardial ischemia with cardiac morbidity and mortality in men undergoing noncardiac surgery. *N Engl J Med* 1990;323:1781-1788.

Mantha S, Roizen MF, Barnard J, et al. Relative effectiveness of four preoperative tests for predicting adverse cardiac outcomes after vascular surgery: A meta-analysis. *Anesth Analg* 1994; 79: 422-433.

Prys-Roberts C. Anesthesia and hypertension. *Br J Anaesth* 1984; 56:711-724.

Rao TK, Jacobs KH, El-Etr AA. Reinfarction following anesthesia in patients with myocardial infarction. *Anesthesiology* 1983;59: 499-505.

Saada M, Catoire P, Bonnet F, et al. Effect of thoracic epidural anesthesia combined with general anesthesia on segmental wall motion assessed by transesophageal echocardiography. *Anesth Analg* 1992;75:329-335.

Shah KB, Kleinman BS, Rao TLK, et al. Angina and other risk factors in patients with cardiac diseases undergoing noncardiac operations. *Anesth Analg* 1990;70:240-247.

Slogoff S, Keats AS. Randomized trial of primary anesthetic agents on outcome of coronary bypass operations. *Anesthesiology* 1989; 70:179-188.

van Rugge FP, van der Wall EE, Bruschke AV. New developments in pharmacologic stress imaging. *Am Heart J* 1992;124: 468-485.

Wong T, Detsky AS. Preoperative cardiac risk assessment for patients having peripheral vascular surgery. *Ann Intern Med* 1992;116:743-753.

CHAPTER 22

Anesthesia and Respiratory Disease

C. William Hanson, III, and Gordon R. Neufeld

Although the idea that a patient might be too sick for anesthesia seems incongruous today, in the past, patients were sometimes denied operations because of pulmonary disease. Advances in care now permit operations on patients despite crippling respiratory disease. This remarkable record of success is due in part to the development of short-acting muscle relaxants, narcotics, and narcotic antagonists; increasing use of laparoscopic surgical procedures; improvements in postoperative nursing, acute pain management, and intensive care medicine; early recognition of the patient at risk; and meticulous intraoperative anesthetic management. This chapter reviews the salient features of normal pulmonary gas exchange, the impact of pulmonary disease on respiratory gas exchange, and the principles of clinical management of patients with pulmonary disease based on an understanding of gas exchange.

Anatomy and Physiology of the Lung

■ Anatomy of the Lung

The human lung consists of conducting airways and alveolated airways that are tightly coupled to the vascular supply. The conducting airways include the air passages of the nose, nasopharynx, and tracheobronchial tree down to the level of the terminal bronchioles. The airways of the lung consist of a series of branchings or bifurcations beginning at the tra-

cheal carina; the number of airways doubles with each generation of branching. Alveoli first appear at the level of the respiratory bronchioles (generation 17). Each successive generation incorporates more alveoli, leading to the alveolar ducts (generations 20 to 22) and terminating as alveolar sacs at generation 23. This organization and classification are summarized in Figure 22-1.

The pulmonary arterial blood supply to the lung is organized similarly. The pulmonary artery bifurcates within the mediastinum and divides successively as the vessels follow the course of the bronchial airways, eventually reaching the alveolated airways. The capillaries of the alveoli form a dense network between the layers of the alveolar membrane, creating a rich, thin interface between the capillary blood and the alveolar gas. Returning pulmonary venous blood is collected by successive orders of converging vessels that culminate in the pulmonary vein and left atrium.

■ Pulmonary Ventilation

Pulmonary ventilation is the bulk flow (convection) of gas in and out of the lung. The conducting airways distribute inspired gas down to the respiratory zone where gas exchange takes place in the alveolated airways. In quantitative terms, the process of ventilation and gas exchange is shown in Figure 22-2. The expansion in total cross-sectional area of the lung with each successive generation causes gas velocity to decrease through each lung generation. For a typical

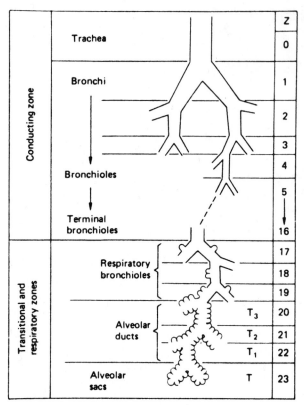

Figure 22-1

The airways of the human lung are organized into conducting and respiratory zones in a dichotomous branching system. The respiratory zone begins with the first alveolated airways at generation 17 (the respiratory bronchioles).

(Reproduced with permission from Weibel ER: Morphometry of the Human Lung. *Berlin: Springer-Verlag, 1963.)*

inspiratory flow rate at rest of 200 ml/s (12 liters/min), the velocity of gas within the trachea is approximately 100 cm/s (see Fig. 22-2). As airway cross section increases, convective velocity decreases until at generation 13 it is about 5 cm/s, approximately equal to the diffusive velocity of O_2 at 37°C. Within the alveolated airways beginning in generation 17, the convective velocity of gas transport is much less than the diffusive velocity of O_2 or CO_2 (see Fig. 22-2). Within the terminal acinus (generation 23), the convective velocity is two orders of magnitude less than the diffusive velocity. This means that within the alveolated airways, diffusion largely accounts for the exchange of gas between the freshly inspired tidal volume and the residual alveolar gas. Even when ventilation increases tenfold during exercise (see Fig.

22-2), diffusion predominates in the airways below generation 17.

For the purpose of understanding the gas transport process, the lung is divided into a number of volumes and capacities (Fig. 22-3). The *total lung capacity* (TLC) is the volume of gas contained within the lungs during a maximal inspiration. The *residual volume* (RV) is the lung volume at maximal exhalation. The functional ability of the lung to move gas by convection is incorporated in the *vital capacity* (VC), which is the difference between TLC and RV. Within the VC, normal breathing takes place by the exchange of the *tidal volume* (VT), which increases or decreases to accommodate the metabolic needs for O_2 uptake and CO_2 elimination. The volume of gas within the lung at the end of normal exhalation is the *functional residual capacity* (FRC). *Expired minute ventilation* ($\dot{V}_E$) is the total convective exchange per unit time (a function of VT and respiratory frequency f).

Compliance

During spontaneous ventilation, the convection of gas in and out of the lung results from expansion of the chest cavity by the diaphragm and muscles of the chest wall. With mechanical ventilation, convection is achieved by applying positive pressure to the airway, inflating the lungs and expanding the chest. The volume of gas moved in and out of the lung during mechanical ventilation at a given applied airway pressure is determined by the compliance of the lung and chest wall, as well as by the resistance to flow in the airways and the viscous resistance of the tissues of the lung and chest wall.

Compliance is the change in lung volume per unit of applied pressure. The nonlinear relationship between pressure and volume (compliance curve), along with the greater volume excursion of the lower chest and diaphragm as compared with that of the upper chest and apex of the lung, causes the base of the lung to receive a larger specific ventilation (ventilation volume per unit lung volume) than does the apex (Fig. 22-4). Compared with the apex, the base of the lung receives an excess of ventilation relative to its actual volume. Changes in static compliance of the lung and chest wall are reflected in the end-inspiratory airway pressure required for a given inspired volume.

Resistance

The pressure decrease that occurs along the airways during the process of ventilation is determined by the instantaneous flow rate multiplied by the

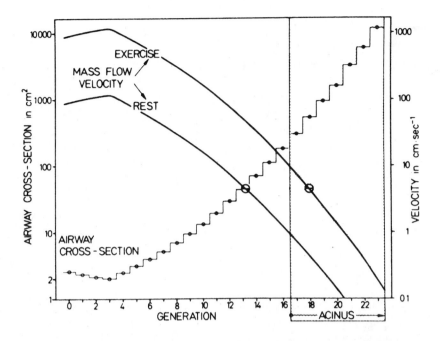

Figure 22-2

As total airway cross section increases with airway branching, the convective velocity of inspired air decreases rapidly such that by generation 17 (striped area) as fresh gas enters the acinus, the diffusive velocity of equilibration exceeds the convective velocity. By the time the fresh gas reaches generations 20 to 23, the speed of diffusion exceeds convection by one or two orders of magnitude.

(Reprinted by permission of the publisher from The pathway for oxygen *by ER Weibel, Cambridge, Mass: Harvard University Press, copyright © 1984 by the President and Fellows of Harvard College.)*

airflow resistance of the airways. Any process that increases airways resistance increases the pressure difference required for a given flow rate. In the case of spontaneous ventilation, an increase in airways resistance results in a more negative intrathoracic pressure during inspiration and an increased positive intratho-

racic pressure on exhalation. This is evidenced by characteristic physical findings on inspiration and expiration and by large respiratory excursions on the central venous pressure trace (if present). In mechani-

Figure 22-3

The total lung capacity (TLC) is subdivided into the residual volume (RV) and vital capacity (VC). Breathing takes place within the limits of the VC by increasing or decreasing the tidal volume (VT).

(Reproduced with permission from Biological Handbooks: Respiration and Circulation. *Federation of American Societies for Experimental Biology, 1971, chap 3.)*

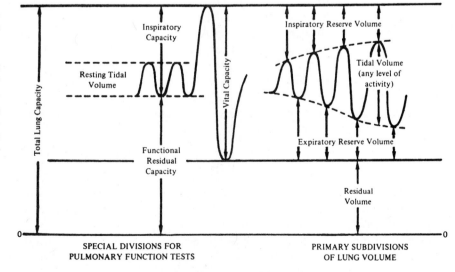

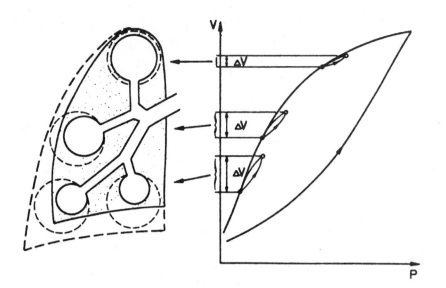

Figure 22-4

During quiet ventilation, the base of the lung receives a larger specific ventilation than the apex, owing to the greater expansion of the lower chest cavity and nonlinear pressure-volume curve of the lung and chest wall.

(Reprinted by permission of the publisher from The Pathway for Oxygen *by E.R. Weibel, Cambridge, Mass: Harvard University Press, Copyright © 1984 by the President and Fellows of Harvard College.)*

cal ventilation, during inspiration, a larger positive intraairway pressure is required for a given flow rate when airways resistance is increased; during exhalation, greater airways resistance is reflected by a decreased flow rate for a given intrathoracic pressure.

Disease processes that decrease chest wall or lung compliance or that increase airways resistance impair convective gas exchange. In these cases, gas is distributed to the alveolated airways according to the distribution of the local airways resistances and compliances. For example, when a patient lies in the left lateral decubitus position for a right thoracotomy, a larger fraction of VT enters the more compliant right lung than the dependent left lung because of the large discrepancy in compliance between the two sides of the chest. Uneven ventilation in the lateral position is exacerbated as well in patients with chronic bronchitis, since airway resistance in the dependent lung is increased by the accumulation of secretions in the dependent lung. Similarly, increases in local airways resistance at any level of the bronchial tree impair the distribution of gas to all airways subtended by that branch. For example, in chronic obstructive pulmonary disease (COPD), radionuclide scans show quite uneven distribution of ventilation.

■ Pulmonary Perfusion

Gas exchange between the capillary blood and alveolar gas occurs across the alveolar membrane. The quantity of gas exchanged between the blood and gas phase is determined by the difference between alveolar gas tension and mixed venous gas tension, the solubility of the gas in blood, and the blood flow. Just as ventilation is not uniform throughout the lung, neither is blood flow, which generally decreases from base to apex. This gradient has been ascribed to the difference between the hydrostatic pressure in the lung (determined by gravity) and the driving pressure in the pulmonary artery (Fig. 22-5). More recent evidence indicates that gravity may be a minor determinant of the pattern. Regardless of the mechanism, the distribution of blood flow complements the distribution of ventilation, and as a result, blood flow and ventilation are fairly well matched (Fig. 22-6).

This proportional distribution of ventilation and blood flow ($\dot{V}/\dot{Q}$ distribution) is maintained not only by the passive mechanisms described above but also by reflex pulmonary vasoconstriction responding to regional hypoxia, called *hypoxic pulmonary vasoconstriction* (HPV). Many mechanisms combine to account for the disordered distribution of $\dot{V}/\dot{Q}$ commonly seen among anesthetized patients, including abnormal posture, elevation of the diaphragm, decreased cardiac output, and inhibition of HPV by anesthetic agents. Studies of HPV in isolated lungs, intact animals, and humans do not all agree. However, it appears that the potent inhaled anesthetics and some direct-acting vasodilators (especially sodium nitroprusside) directly inhibit HPV in a dose-related fashion. Other concomitant changes, such as a decrease in cardiac output that potentiates HPV, will ameliorate this effect in patients. Thus it is possible that substituting an increased dose of a potent inhaled agent for nitrous oxide might fail to improve arterial oxygenation in a patient with atelectasis who requires active HPV to maintain a normal $\dot{V}/\dot{Q}$ distribution. Intravenous anesthetic agents do not seem to inhibit HPV.

Figure 22-5

The vertical distribution of blood flow in erect humans is determined by the driving pressure in the pulmonary artery and the vertical hydrostatic pressure gradient within the vascular space of the lung. The apex is less well perfused than the base under resting conditions.

(Reproduced with permission from West JB: Ventilation/Blood Flow and Gas Exchange, 3rd ed. Oxford: Blackwell Scientific Publications, 1977.)

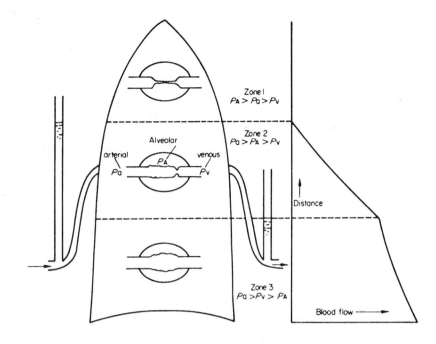

■ Gas Transport Through the Alveolar Membrane

Gas exchange across the alveolar membrane is governed by ventilation and perfusion of the alveoli and by diffusion through the alveolar membrane. The transport process for a given gas is described by the mass balance between gas transported in blood and gas entering and leaving the lung.

Ventilation and Perfusion

Many calculations in pulmonary physiology are derived from mass balance equations that are rooted in the law of conservation of mass. The most funda-

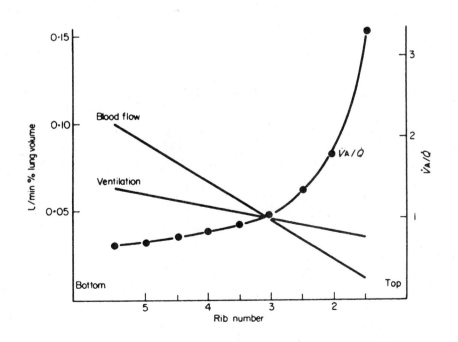

Figure 22-6

The distribution of ventilation-perfusion ratio ($\dot{V}/\dot{Q}$) in erect humans is the consequence of the independent distribution of ventilation and perfusion. The $\dot{V}/\dot{Q}$ is less than 1 in the base of the lung and increases vertically, becoming much greater than 1 at the apex.

(Reproduced with permission from West JB: Ventilation/Blood Flow and Gas Exchange, 5th ed. Oxford: Blackwell Scientific Publications, 1990.)

mental of these relate the net quantity of gas exchanged by ventilation to the quantities transported in blood (Fick's equation):

Amount of gas transported by arterial blood = amount of gas delivered in the mixed venous blood + amount of gas uptake (or elimination) by pulmonary ventilation

$$Ca_g \times \dot{Q}_T = C\bar{V}_g \times \dot{Q}_T + (CI_g - C\bar{E}) \times \dot{V}_E \qquad (22.1)$$

where Ca_g = arterial blood gas concentration (milliliter of gas per milliliter of blood)

$\dot{Q}_T$ = total pulmonary flow

$C\bar{V}_g$ = mixed venous blood gas concentration (content)

CI_g = inspired gas concentration

$C\bar{E}_g$ = concentration of gas in mixed expired air

$\dot{V}_E$ = expired minute volume

The amount of gas transported by arterial blood is equal to the arterial blood gas concentration (content) multiplied by the total blood flow ($\dot{Q}_T$ or cardiac output). Similarly, the amount of gas transported by mixed venous blood is equal to the mixed venous content multiplied by $\dot{Q}_T$. To increase the systemic arterial O_2 supply or reduce arterial CO_2 content, O_2 must be supplied and CO_2 eliminated by the lung. This uptake and elimination can only occur through blood vessels that come in contact with alveolar gas (blood flow through a ventilated acinus), which is designated as *capillary blood flow* ($\dot{Q}_C$). Mixed venous blood that does not participate in gas exchange is called *shunt blood flow* ($\dot{Q}_S$). $\dot{Q}_T$ is the sum of $\dot{Q}_C$ and $\dot{Q}_S$ and thus can be incorporated into the mass balance equation to yield

$$Ca_g \times \dot{Q}_T = C\bar{V}_g \times (\dot{Q}_C + \dot{Q}_S) + (CI_g - C\bar{E}_g) \times \dot{V}_E \quad (22.2)$$

These underlying concepts and equations are fundamental to pulmonary pathophysiology and provide the information necessary to calculate or derive virtually all the relationships among ventilation, perfusion, and gas exchange.

Any process that interferes with the ventilation of perfused alveoli increases the apparent shunt and decreases the capacity of the lung to exchange gas. Similarly, redistribution of blood flow from well-ventilated acini to poorly ventilated acini also impairs gas exchange. Anesthesia and pulmonary pathology exert both these effects; anesthesia has a significant impact on gas exchange, particularly in patients with pulmonary disease.

Diffusion

Gas transport between pulmonary capillary blood and the gas in the alveoli occurs by diffusion across alveolar membranes. Fick's law of diffusion relates the quantity of gas transported per minute ($\dot{V}_g$) to the partial pressure decrease across the membrane (ΔP_g), the membrane thickness (ΔX), the membrane area (A), and the diffusivity of the gas in the membrane (D_g):

$$\dot{V}_g = D_g \times A \times \frac{\Delta P_g}{\Delta X} \qquad (22.3)$$

The quantity of gas transported by diffusion ($\dot{V}_g$) is equal to the diffusivity of the gas multiplied by the area and the partial pressure difference and divided by the membrane thickness. The measure of carbon monoxide diffusion capacity in the pulmonary function laboratory combines D, A, and X into a single term (DL_{CO}) such that the diffusing capacity becomes

$$DL_{CO} = \frac{\dot{V}_{CO}}{\Delta P} \qquad (22.4)$$

Diffusing capacity is the ratio of gas uptake to the partial pressure difference for carbon monoxide.

Diseases that result in increases in functional alveolar membrane thickness (e.g., alveolar proteinosis, pulmonary edema) or reduce alveolar cross section (e.g., pneumonia, pulmonary embolus, pneumonectomy) reduce diffusing capacity. A reduction in diffusing capacity is clinically important when it becomes the limiting factor in the exchange between alveolar gas and pulmonary capillary blood.

■ Gas Transport Between Alveolar Gas and Tidal Volume

Combining the physical processes of convection and diffusion (see Fig. 22-2) with the lung volumes and capacities of tidal breathing (see Fig. 22-3) yields a picture of the gas exchange process in the airways that is consistent with the anatomy of the lung and the physics of gas transport. At end-exhalation, the lung contains only FRC gas. During inspiration, the FRC retreats into the lung, pulling fresh gas (VT) into the airways. This process effectively creates a moving boundary or interface between VT and the FRC with a sharp concentration gradient across it; the interface rapidly propagates down the conducting airways during inspiration. As the airway cross section of the VT/FRC interface expands and the convective velocity decreases, the concentration differences across the interface cause diffusive exchange to take place. CO_2 moves into the VT from the FRC gas and alveolar capillary blood as O_2 moves from the VT into the FRC and alveolar capillary blood. The large cross-sectional area available in the alveolated airways enhances this diffusive exchange so that equilibration is virtually complete over the course of each breath cycle in a healthy person.

Thus convection, or bulk flow, brings fresh inhaled gas from the upper airway into the respiratory zone. The rapid expansion in total airway cross-sectional area slows the velocity of convective gas transport once the tidal volume enters the alveolated airways. Gas exchange between the inhaled tidal volume and the residual FRC gas occurs by the diffusive equilibration of these two gas volumes within the respiratory airways. This air-phase diffusive equilibration is very rapid in healthy lungs but can be impaired by processes that reduce either the number or the caliber of alveolated airways. Infant respiratory distress syndrome, bronchopulmonary dysplasia (BPD), adult respiratory distress syndrome (ARDS), and emphysema are examples of lung diseases in which reduced airway cross-sectional area may limit gas transport.

This increase in diffusive resistance can be overcome to a limited extent by increasing the concentration gradient for the gases between the tidal volume and the FRC. Increasing inspired O_2 tension or tolerating higher CO_2 tension in the arterial and mixed venous blood compensates for an increased diffusive resistance at a given minute ventilation.

Evaluating Patients before Anesthesia and Operation

Recognition and management of patients who are susceptible to perioperative respiratory difficulties require identifying respiratory risk factors. These problems may be latent, chronic, or acute. Latent respiratory problems, such as hiatal hernia, gastroesophageal reflux, or obstructive sleep apnea, may not cause the patient respiratory distress during the nor-

mal activities of daily life yet may present significant difficulties in the perioperative period. Chronic active respiratory diseases are more apparent. The derangements of gas exchange they produce interfere with the patient's daily activities and produce abnormalities in the physical examination and respiratory pattern.

Improvements in anesthetic management and the accomplishments of modern intensive care have created a third population of operative patients: patients with acute lung diseases requiring mechanical ventilation or intensive respiratory therapy. Congestive heart failure (CHF) and adult respiratory distress syndrome (ARDS) are increasingly common among critically ill patients who require operation.

■ History of Cardiopulmonary Disease

The best indicator of potential perioperative respiratory difficulties is lack of exercise tolerance. Patients with dyspnea at rest or during mild exercise such as walking are at great risk of perioperative ventilatory failure. Those who can climb a flight of stairs without dyspnea usually have adequate reserve pulmonary function. Despite the absence of symptoms, latent pulmonary diseases such as asthma may become apparent during the course of anesthesia. Any history of wheezing warns of the possibility of bronchospasm with anesthesia. Patients who smoke experience increased pulmonary complications, but the risks decrease several months after they stop smoking provided that permanent damage, such as COPD, has not occurred (Table 22–1).

Table 22-1

Smoking Cessation and Pulmonary Complication Rate after Cardiac Operation

Smoking	Rate of Pulmonary Complications
Never stopped	50%
Stopped < 2 weeks	> 50%
Stopped 2–4 weeks	> 50%
Stopped 4–8 weeks	50%
Stopped > 8 weeks	< 20%
Nonsmokers	< 20%

Note: The risk of pulmonary complication for patients undergoing cardiac operations increases at first when patients stop smoking. After 8 weeks, the rate of complication is similar to that for comparable patients who have never smoked.

From Warner MA, Divertie MB, Tinker JH: Preoperative cessation of smoking and pulmonary complications in coronary artery bypass patients. *Anesthesiology* 1984;60:380–383.

Table 22-2

Risk Factors for Postoperative Pulmonary Complications

Advanced age (> 60 years)
Major abdominal operation (particularly upper abdominal)
Emergency operation
History of COPD
Operation > 3 hours
ASA > 2
Obesity
Prolonged preoperative stay

Advanced age and excess body weight correlate directly with perioperative pulmonary complications, as does the site of incision: Upper abdominal and thoracic incisions result more often in atelectasis and pneumonia than do more peripheral incisions (Table 22-2). These conditions all reduce functional residual capacity below the closing volume of the lung. Intraabdominal or intrathoracic processes that compress the lung (e.g., tumor, ascites, gravid uterus, pleural effusion) also reduce FRC to the point of airway closure and thereby promote atelectasis.

■ Physical Examination

Dyspnea is the unifying symptom of patients with respiratory diseases. The physical examination often reveals the underlying etiology. Inspection, percussion, and auscultation distinguish COPD from restrictive disease and give substantial information about the severity of the disease. For example, in a patient with COPD, a spontaneous inspiratory-to-expiratory ratio of less than 1:3 suggests that a similar ratio will be necessary during positive-pressure ventilation to prevent air trapping and decreased venous return to the right side of the heart.

Patients with chronic obstructive lung disease may have emphysema, with destruction of the architecture of the lung, or bronchitis, with excessive secretions in the airways and bronchial smooth muscle proliferation. Usually, the pathophysiology lies between these extremes, which serve as useful reference points. Patients with emphysematous disease have a high proportion of lung units with ventilation in excess of perfusion (physiologic dead space), whereas patients with bronchitis have a high proportion of units with perfusion in excess of ventilation (physiologic shunt).

Patients with emphysema are asthenic with promi-

nent sternocleidomastoid musculature, barrel chests, and scaphoid abdomens. Exhalation is prolonged, and pursed-lip breathing is common. Patients with bronchitis appear plethoric (from chronic hypoxemia and erythrocytosis) and may show signs of right ventricular failure. Exhalations are prolonged, with wheezing. Many patients with COPD have a combination of hypoxemia and hypercarbia due to ventilation-perfusion mismatch and increased dead space.

Patients with restrictive lung diseases such as sarcoidosis have small lung volumes with airways of normal calibers; cyanosis, tachypnea, and audible crackles on auscultation are common. Severe ventilation-perfusion mismatch causes hypoxemia, treated with supplemental oxygen therapy.

In each case, the patient adopts a respiratory pattern that is most efficient given the limits imposed by the disease. COPD results in normal to increased compliance and increased resistance, especially on exhalation when the airways collapse. These patients breathe slowly with a prolonged expiratory phase, which allows the alveoli to empty fully and avoids air trapping. Patients with restrictive lung disease have decreased compliances and normal resistances. The energy cost for expanding the lung is large, but there are no constraints on expiratory flow. These patients breathe rapidly with small tidal volumes, the most efficient pattern in restrictive diseases.

■ Laboratory and Special Studies

Although often the history and physical examination suffice, in some cases laboratory studies are required to determine the severity or mechanisms of the disorders. Such studies may include arterial blood gas determinations, pulmonary function tests (including measurement of volumes, flows, and the flow-volume loop), radiographic studies, and in cases of chronic cyanosis, the hematocrit or hemoglobin.

Blood Gas Determinations

An analysis of the arterial blood obtained while the patient breathes room air may be required in patients with severe pulmonary disease, as indicated by limited exercise tolerance, recent hospitalization for respiratory care, a requirement for chronic medication, or a recent history of CHF. Hypoxemia (corrected for age) is common, whereas hypercarbia is less common and more ominous. Four problems account for hypercarbia at rest: increased inspired CO_2, increased

CO_2 production (as in sepsis), hypoventilation, or increased dead space. Although hypoventilation, respiratory obstruction, and restrictive processes are occasional causes of preoperative hypercapnia, the most common cause for increased $PaCO_2$ is the combination of increased alveolar dead space and decreased ventilatory capacity seen in patients with COPD or severe asthmatic episodes just prior to respiratory collapse.

Pulmonary Function Testing

Pulmonary function tests (PFTs) are used to establish diagnoses, to estimate the severity of the disorder, and to assess the effectiveness of therapy. The decision to obtain PFTs before anesthesia and operation is not a simple one. PFTs are not ordered as a matter of routine but are best used to make management decisions. A patient with severe pulmonary disease nevertheless requires no testing when it is anticipated that a peripheral operation will cause no impairment of ventilatory function. Likewise, little testing is required when it is clear that a major procedure will necessitate postoperative ventilatory support. The flow-volume loop sometimes is used to diagnose airway obstruction and to distinguish between fixed and variable intra- and extrathoracic obstruction (Fig. 22-7).

The most commonly employed PFTs are the forced vital capacity (FVC) and the forced expired volume in 1 second (FEV_1), which are sensitive to restrictive and obstructive disease, respectively. The FVC is an index of the reserve available to increase the tidal volume. An FVC of 1.0 liter or less indicates no reserve and severe disease. The FEV_1 is a measure of expiratory flow, so a reduced FEV_1 indicates obstructive disease. An FEV_1 of less than 1.0 liter represents severe disease. The use of PFTs in preoperative evaluation has not been standardized. They are of particular use in designing a perioperative plan in patients scheduled for upper abdominal, cardiac, and thoracic operations, all of which impair pulmonary function.

Radiographic Studies

Radiographic studies are obtained selectively, not as a routine (see Chap. 2). The chest radiograph is useful in the diagnosis of hiatal hernia, acute and chronic lung disease, tracheal obstruction, or intrapleural processes. Lateral views of the neck reveal extrinsic compression of the trachea and epiglottis. More esoteric studies such as computed tomography (CT) and magnetic resonance imaging (MRI) are used to evaluate lesions of the lung parenchyma, mediastinum, and airway. Nuclear medicine scans are used to determine regional ventilation-perfusion relationships prior to lung resection.

Hypercarbia on a preoperative room air blood gas determination, a forced vital capacity of less than 15 ml/kg, or significant airway obstruction detected by PFTs or radiographic studies identifies a patient who is at substantially increased risk for perioperative respiratory complications.

Figure 22-7

Maximum flow-volume loops for a healthy subject *(outer loops)*, a patient with moderate obstruction to the intrapulmonary airways *(inner right-hand loop)*, and a patient with obstruction to extrathoracic airways *(inner left-hand loop)*. PEFR is the peak expiratory flow rate (the maximum that can be sustained for 10 ms). FEF_{50} and FIF_{50} are the forced expiratory and inspiratory flow rates at the midpoint of the vital capacity.

(Reproduced with permission form Cotes JE: Lung Function: Assessment and Application in Medicine, 3rd ed. Oxford: Blackwell Scientific Publications, 1979.)

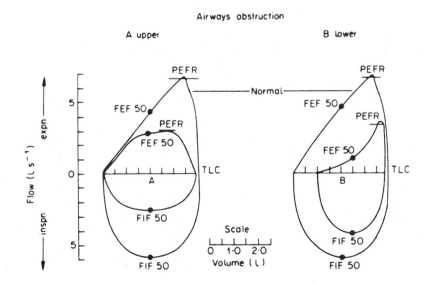

■ Preoperation Management

Medical management before the operation can reduce risks for patients susceptible to respiratory complications, if time and the patient permit.

Abstinence from smoking reduces postoperative pulmonary complications and is recommended to patients at least 8 weeks prior to elective operation (see Table 22-2). Refraining from smoking for at least 24 hours may increase oxygen-carrying capacity somewhat by eliminating exposure to carbon monoxide. Patients with reversible bronchoconstriction require treatment preoperatively. Appropriate agents include inhaled beta-adrenergic agonists (preferably selective beta-2 agents), membrane-stabilizing drugs such as cromolyn sodium, anticholinergics, and inhaled corticosteroids. Antibiotics reduce secretions and airway inflammation in patients with chronic bronchitis.

Obesity predisposes patients to postoperative atelectasis and pneumonia. When an elective procedure is planned and the patient is obese, it is best to defer surgery until the patient has lost weight if this is possible.

The preoperative period is often the ideal time to train patients in the proper technique for incentive spirometry, which reduces the incidence of atelectasis after operations.

The risk of pulmonary complications after anesthesia of any kind is minimal in a healthy young patient undergoing a peripheral operation. Risk clearly increases beyond this baseline in patients who suffer from any form of respiratory disease, from CHF, or who undergo thoracic or upper abdominal operations. In addition, risks may be increased in the elderly, in patients who fall in ASA physical status classes III, IV, or V, and in those having lengthy or emergency operations. An anesthetic plan that takes into account the pathophysiology of these problems reduces risk to a minimum. Specific advice for managing a number of common conditions follows.

Acute Respiratory Tract Infections

It is clear that patients with pneumonia or severe bronchitis benefit from postponing elective operations for 4 to 6 weeks to allow recovery and reduce the rate of pulmonary complications. Adults with viral infections limited to the upper respiratory tract do not seem to suffer an increased rate of respiratory complications. This makes it acceptable to proceed with their planned elective operations, especially if the operative site does not involve the chest or abdomen.

For patients recovering from mild bronchitis or other infections involving the larynx or structures below it, it is debatable whether to proceed with anesthesia. Effects on the tracheobronchial mucosa persist for 5 to 6 weeks after infection, and the patients may experience coughing, wheezing, and postoperative bronchitis and atelectasis. However, in adults, these complications may not be severe and do not occur at a greatly increased rate.

CHF and ARDS

Congestive heart failure (CHF) is a primary cardiac disease with secondary effects on the lung. It is the primary cardiac disease that guides anesthetic management. Preload and afterload reduction, fluid limitation, and if necessary, inotropic support are treatments that improve the performance of the failing ventricle and limit pulmonary congestion.

Acute lung injury (ALI), known in its more severe form as *adult respiratory distress syndrome* (ARDS), was first described in the 1960s. Despite 30 years of research, its mortality remains at about 50 percent. It is defined by the following criteria: acute onset, bilateral infiltrates on frontal chest radiograph, and $PaO_2/FIO_2 < 300$ mmHg (ALI) or $PaO_2/FIO_2 < 200$ mmHg (ARDS). It is distinguished from CHF by pulmonary artery occlusion pressures less than 18 mmHg. These patients require respiratory therapy to sustain life and in many cases are supported by highly sophisticated controlled mechanical ventilation.

The pathophysiology of ARDS places significant constraints on the anesthesia plan: Because these patients require mechanical ventilation, general anesthesia is a virtual necessity. The required increased oxygen concentrations limit the use of nitrous oxide, so potent inhaled or intravenous agents are used. During transportation of patients with CHF and ARDS to and from the operating room, the settings on the mechanical ventilator are reproduced as nearly as possible, including I/E ratio, flows, PEEP, and FIO_2.

Asthma

Regional anesthesia is preferred for peripheral procedures in patients with asthma. For abdominal operations, as for patients in respiratory distress from asthma, tracheal intubation and positive-pressure ventilation may be required to ensure adequate ventilation. Intravenous corticosteroids are often administered to patients with asthma perioperatively or during the procedure when bronchospasm occurs but has not been anticipated. Intravenous steroids require 4 to 6 hours before effect.

Thiopental may provoke or at least permit bronchoconstriction when given in small doses. Bronchodilation occurs at greater doses (> 5 mg/kg), which seem to be safe for patients with asthma. Potent inhaled agents are used for induction and maintenance of anesthesia in asthmatic patients because of their direct bronchodilating effects. Ketamine produces bronchodilation, whereas morphine and some neuromuscular blocking agents (e.g., atracurium, curare) release histamine when given rapidly, which might provoke or aggravate bronchospasm. Topical or intravenous lidocaine obtunds airway reflexes and is a useful adjunct to other induction agents.

Induction of general anesthesia and intubation of the trachea in patients with active or chronic asthma can produce the abrupt onset of severe bronchospasm. Successful endotracheal intubation can be mistaken for esophageal intubation if there is no exhaled carbon dioxide, the pulse oximeter indicates desaturation, and no breath sounds can be heard. When this occurs, correct endotracheal tube placement must be verified immediately by direct vision with a laryngoscope or fiberoptic bronchoscope. Effective treatments include potent inhaled anesthetics, epinephrine, inhaled bronchodilators, and isoproterenol or aminophylline.

Regional versus General Anesthesia

The potential advantages of regional anesthesia for patients with respiratory disease are considerable, but the decision to use regional anesthesia alone or in combination with a general anesthetic is complex and requires careful consideration of the individual patient and operation. Often, the apparent advantages of regional anesthesia cannot be realized in practice or are too slight to affect outcome very much.

In the past, the reason most often cited for preferring regional anesthesia was to avoid the ill effects of general anesthesia on the respiratory system. These include inhibition of the tracheobronchial mucociliary function, the risk of infection after tracheal intubation, atelectasis and small airways closure, intraoperative hypoxemia, respiratory depression, deconditioning of respiratory muscles, and weakness in the

immediate postoperative period due to the residual effects of muscle relaxants. Modern management has reduced these risks so much that studies comparing the outcomes of general and regional anesthesia for peripheral procedures (e.g., repair of fractured hips) show no significant differences in outcome. Nevertheless, regional anesthesia offers clear benefits in certain circumstances.

Operations on the periphery (extremities, head and neck, lower abdomen) are unlikely to interfere directly with ventilatory function either during the procedure or postoperatively. For these patients, regional anesthesia provides a simple means of avoiding respiratory difficulties without taking complicated precautions. However, sedation to the point of near unconsciousness or the unwise use of opioids amounts to poorly managed general anesthesia with all of its expected respiratory complications. When such heavy sedation may be needed for anxious patients, or when a regional anesthetic fails to make the patient comfortable, general anesthesia may be preferable.

Operations on the upper abdomen and thorax interfere directly with breathing and oxygenation during the operation. Although some of these operations (e.g., open cholecystectomy) can be managed with regional anesthesia alone, this plan is workable only in healthy patients. Otherwise, general anesthesia is required to gain the beneficial effects of tracheal intubation, positive-pressure ventilation, PEEP, or maximal FIO_2. The role of regional anesthesia in these cases is to alleviate postoperative pain that otherwise would impair movement of the diaphragm, thorax, and abdomen. This impaired ventilation produces respiratory complications by several mechanisms.

First, vital capacity is markedly decreased, to as little as 30 percent of preoperative values after thoracotomies and upper abdominal operations. For patients without other risk factors, such as obesity or smoking, who have normal preoperative vital capacities, this reduction in vital capacity is not enough to precipitate ventilatory failure. For those with severe respiratory disease who come to operation on the verge of respiratory failure, postoperative mechanical ventilation will be required regardless of anesthesia management. Postoperative respiratory failure may be inevitable even if the patient is comfortable, so supple-mental epidural anesthesia cannot be expected to eliminate the need for mechanical ventilation. For those with moderately severe disease (VC in the range of 15 to 30 ml/kg), providing fully effective postoperative pain relief with an epidural catheter or intercostal nerve blocks can be the deciding factor that allows removal of the endotracheal tube.

Second, impaired respiratory motion reduces the FRC to less than the closing capacity (CC) so that small airways closure occurs during each breath. Age, obesity, and COPD all produce the same effect, perhaps explaining the relationship between these risk factors and perioperative respiratory problems. This closure of small airways produces maldistribution of the ventilation-perfusion ratio and hypoxemia. Usually, this effect is treatable with oxygen. Other effects include increased atelectasis, ventilatory failure, pneumonia, prolonged stay in the ICU and in the hospital, and death.

Postoperative supplemental epidural analgesia has been adopted widely to prevent these complications and to provide other benefits (see Chap. 34). Only a few studies have been done to demonstrate the overall effects of this practice. Beneficial effects are likely to be strongest for borderline patients with moderately severe respiratory disease; an example would be a 72-year-old man with COPD who has a PO_2 while breathing room air of 70 mmHg, who is able to walk two blocks, and who requires a colectomy. The respiratory benefits of regional anesthesia are less apparent in a healthy younger patient (e.g., an otherwise healthy 30-year-old who requires laparoscopic cholecystectomy) or in a desperately ill patient (the first patient when admitted for ventilatory failure, who then requires an emergency laparotomy for a perforated ulcer while he still requires mechanical ventilation for his COPD). Offering these patients epidural analgesia may not reduce the expected rate of perioperative respiratory complications but may allow more rapid weaning from mechanical ventilation.

Intraoperative Management

■ General Considerations

Several interventions during anesthesia improve lung function in patients at risk for pulmonary complications. Endotracheal secretions require frequent removal by suction to prevent the development of atelectasis. Periodic large tidal volume breaths (sighs) reexpand atelectatic lung and limit shunting. Intrave-

nous fluids must be administered conservatively; excessive volume replacement results in decreased lung compliance, increased work of breathing, and eventually, pulmonary edema. Despite two decades of investigation, it is not clear that colloid solutions are superior, making it reasonable to use crystalloids for their lower cost.

Bronchospasm is treated by deepening the level of anesthesia, adding a volatile agent with bronchodilatory properties, administering beta-2-adrenergic agonist aerosols, or giving aminophylline. Beta agonists and aminophylline must be used cautiously during general anesthesia to avoid arrhythmias. Bronchospasm may worsen as the concentration of a potent inhaled anesthetic agent decreases at the conclusion of an anesthetic.

The patient must not be allowed to become hypothermic, in order to avoid shivering and excessive oxygen consumption during recovery from anesthesia. Similarly, complete reversal of neuromuscular blockade at the end of the procedure is essential. Adequate analgesia on emergence prevents splinting from a painful incision, but one must avoid respiratory depression from opioids or residual anesthetics.

■ Positive-Pressure Ventilation

Positive-pressure ventilation during anesthesia in patients with respiratory disorders should mimic the respiratory pattern employed by the patient during spontaneous breathing (Table 22-3). The use of usual tidal volumes and respiratory rates in the patient with COPD may result in unrecognized air trapping, decreased venous return, and hypotension. Adequate expiratory time is essential to allow time for alveolar emptying. Evidence of bronchospasm or expiratory obstruction is reflected in the time required for complete exhalation and by the presence of expiratory wheezing. The time required for complete exhalation is estimated by examining the filling of the bellows of the ventilator. If exhalation is incomplete or complete just prior to the next inhalation, then the expiratory time should be lengthened by increasing the expiratory pause, reducing respiratory frequency, decreasing the inspiratory-expiratory (I/E) ratio, or increasing inspiratory flow rate. Conversely, patients with restrictive disease and reduced compliance develop increased peak and plateau inspiratory pressures when ventilated with usual tidal volumes and rates.

Intrinsic or extrinsic airway compression with fixed

Table 22-3

Strategies for Mechanical Ventilation in Patients with Pulmonary Disease						
Lung disease	Pathology	Rate	Tital Volume	Inspiratory Flow	PEEP	I:E
Obstructive disease						
Emphysema	↑ compliance	↓	–↑	–	–	↓
Bronchitis	↑ resistance	↓	–	–↓	–	↓
Restrictive disease	↓ compliance	↑	↓	–	–	–↑
Fixed airway lesion	↑ resistance	↓	–↓	↓	–	–↑
ALI/ARDS*	↓↓ compliance	↑	↓	↑	↑	–↑
Atelectasis	Alveolar collapse	–	–↑	–	↑	↑

*May require ICU ventilator in the operating room.

or variable airway obstructing lesions requires different ventilation strategies. Fixed lesions of the airway (such as extrinsic compression of the trachea) impede both inspiratory and expiratory flow and must be managed with slower respiratory rates, minimal inspiratory flows, and prolonged expiratory times. Variable extrathoracic lesions (such as vocal cord paralysis) cause dynamic restrictions to inspiratory flow and usually can be alleviated by positive-pressure ventilation (especially with endotracheal intubation). Variable intrathoracic lesions (such as mass lesions of the trachea) result in dynamic restriction to expiratory flow, which may be relieved by applying constant positive airway pressure (CPAP) to hold the airway open during exhalation.

The heterogeneous nature of ARDS and CHF causes ventilation to be preferentially distributed to regions of normal lung because of compliance mismatch. This creates the potential for overdistension and damage of normal alveoli. Lung-sparing modes of ventilation have been developed for these patients and include the use of minimal tidal volumes or pressure-controlled ventilation. Anesthesia ventilators are often inadequate, so intensive care ventilators are often used for intraoperative care of these selected patients.

■ Monitoring Gas Transport Intraoperatively

Modern anesthetic and respiratory equipment provides a wealth of information about gas exchange (see Chaps. 5 and 6). It is important to chart initial data following induction of anesthesia so that changes that develop intraoperatively or postoperatively can be documented. This careful record provides early warning of deterioration and saves time in arriving at the diagnosis (Table 22-4).

Monitoring Pulmonary Ventilation

Once anesthesia begins and the airway is secured, tidal volume, breathing frequency, minute ventilation, end-tidal CO_2, and airway pressure are recorded at regular intervals. Airway pressure includes peak

Table 22-4

Monitoring During Anesthesia for Patients with Lung Disease

All patients
  Breath sounds
  Movement of chest wall and abdomen
  Airway pressure: peak and plateau
  Ventilatory volumes: tidal volume, expired minute volume
  Expired CO_2: end-tidal CO_2 and waveform
  Pulse oximeter reading
Moderate disease (choices depend on disease process)
  Arterial blood gases
  $(A\text{-}a)DO_2$ at F_1O_2 1.0
  $a\text{-}ETCO_2$
  Apparent dead space: expired minute ventilation to maintain physiologic $PaCO_2$
Severe pulmonary disease or cardiopulmonary disease
  Pulmonary artery catheter: CVP, PCWP, cardiac output
  Pulmonary vascular resistance
  Shunt fraction
  Mixed venous gases or O_2 saturation

airway pressure and plateau pressure. Plateau pressure is the airway pressure sustained during the inspiratory pause (i.e., at zero flow) and is an index of total lung and chest wall compliance. Increases in plateau pressure indicate a decrease in compliance that may be extrathoracic (abdominal retractors or compression of the chest wall), intrathoracic (hemothorax, pneumothorax), or intrapulmonary (edema). Increases in peak airway pressure may indicate increased airway resistance owing to endotracheal tube obstruction, accumulation of secretions, blood, or edema fluid in the airways, or a change in bronchial smooth muscle tone.

Monitoring Pulmonary Perfusion

Pulmonary perfusion is normally monitored using a thermal dilution pulmonary artery (PA) catheter. Cardiac output (CO or $\dot{Q}_T$) measurements are very useful in patients with preexisting cardiac disease or pulmonary hypertension or during procedures requiring large volumes of blood or electrolyte solutions. Pulmonary artery systolic, diastolic, mean, and occlusion pressures may be recorded at intervals along with calculated pulmonary vascular resistance (PVR):

$$PVR = \frac{(\overline{PAP} - PAOP) \times 80}{CO} \qquad (22.5)$$

where PVR = pulmonary vascular resistance
$\qquad$ (dyn–cm s^{-5})
$\quad \overline{PAP}$ = mean pulmonary arterial pressure (mmHg)
$\quad$ PAOP = pulmonary artery occulusion pressure (mmHg)
$\qquad$ CO = cardiac output (liters/min) $\qquad$ (22.5)

An increase in PVR with an increasing arterial to end-tidal CO_2 difference is pathognomonic of pulmonary embolus.

Monitoring CO_2 Transport

Once a stable anesthetic depth has been attained, the minute ventilation and $P_{ET}CO_2$ are recorded regularly. The difference between arterial and end-tidal CO_2 ($PaCO_2 - P_{ET}CO_2$) is an index of pulmonary function in general and of alveolar dead space in particular. Alveolar dead space increases with pulmonary embolization (air, amniotic fluid, fat, or blood clots). The relation between dead space (VD) and tidal volume (VT) is generally

$$\frac{VD}{VT} = 1 - \frac{P\overline{E}CO_2}{PaCO_2} \qquad (22.6)$$

(The Bohr dead space fraction substitutes $P_{ET}CO_2$ for $PaCO_2$ in the preceding equation. Bohr dead space fraction does not include alveolar dead space and thus is insensitive to pulmonary embolic processes or decreases in pulmonary perfusion.)

Unfortunately, mixed expired CO_2 ($P\overline{ET}CO_2$) is not generally available from clinical CO_2 monitors despite the fact that the technology to monitor it is available on modern anesthetic machines. To overcome this problem, dead space fraction can be monitored indirectly by recording $\dot{V}_E$ with the associated $PaCO_2$ or $P_{ET}CO_2$. Assuming that CO_2 production remains unchanged, as is usual in anesthetized patients, if $\dot{V}_E$ must be increased to maintain a fixed $PaCO_2$ (or conversely if $PaCO_2$ increases while $P_{ET}CO_2$ decreases with a fixed $\dot{V}_E$), then CO_2 elimination is impaired. Thus analysis of $\dot{V}_E$ and arterial or end-tidal CO_2 measurements detects intraoperative changes in dead space fraction.

Dead space fraction increases if pulmonary perfusion is compromised, as when cardiac output decreases. When cardiac output decreases, less lung is perfused, and the unperfused lung becomes alveolar dead space. This routinely accompanies general anesthesia and mechanical ventilation, when the dead space fraction increases from 30 to 40 percent and even greater in patients with respiratory or cardiac disease.

Monitoring Oxygen Transport

Monitors that measure end-tidal CO_2 and peripheral oxygen saturation have not completely eliminated the need for measuring blood gases intraoperatively in patients with lung diseases. Changes in PaO_2 and arterial-alveolar tension differences precede peripheral hemoglobin desaturation or obvious reductions in end-tidal CO_2. The measurement of arterial oxygen tension as related to the alveolar oxygen tension or (more easily) to the inspired oxygen concentration is a useful index of alveolar function in patients under anesthesia. Normally, $P(A-a)DO_2$ while breathing 100% O_2 is less than 50 to 100 mmHg. Any increase in this difference is a clear warning of an increased shunt fraction ($\dot{Q}_S/\dot{Q}_T$).

In patients with pulmonary or cardiac disease, pulmonary artery catheters are useful for monitoring central pressures, cardiac output, and systemic and pulmonary vascular resistance. The catheters also allow the calculation of $\dot{Q}_S/\dot{Q}_T$ (using the mass balance shunt relationship of Eq. 22.2), which is reflected in the $P(A-a)DO_2$. Despite the widespread use of pulmonary artery catheters in monitored patients and the frequency of blood gas determinations, the calculation of shunt fraction remains neglected. The interrelationship of mixed venous, arterial, and expired gas tensions provides a clear picture of cardiopulmonary function in critically ill patients. For example, a decrease in PaO_2 under conditions of unchanged ventilation or FIO_2 may reflect deterioration in lung function, a pulmonary embolus, a change in cardiac output, or the development of sepsis. Monitoring cardiac output and pulmonary arterial pressures is of help, but measuring mixed venous PO_2 and PCO_2 in conjunction with the other variables may define the problem exactly.

Any of the foregoing monitoring techniques are valuable in caring for critically ill patients. Of the measurements described, those which receive less emphasis than they deserve in current practice are $P(a-A)DCO_2$, $P(A-a)DO_2$, and $\dot{Q}_S/\dot{Q}_T$, which are sensitive to changes in pulmonary or cardiovascular status. A systematic approach to monitoring provides early warning of developing problems, making diagnosis more certain.

■ Evaluating Patients for Extubation

The decision to remove the endotracheal tube at the conclusion of routine surgical procedures in healthy patients usually can be made using objective criteria that depend on level of consciousness and strength (described in Chap. 13). Some patients (such as those with bronchospasm) are appropriate candidates for deep extubation. While the patient is still in the third stage of anesthesia, the endotracheal tube is removed with the patient breathing spontaneously, and mask ventilation is used until consciousness is regained and the airway is secure.

Patients with respiratory disease who meet the usual criteria for extubation must be monitored carefully in the immediate postoperative period. These patients have limited respiratory reserve and are prone to acute respiratory failure. Precipitating causes include the administration of narcotic analgesics, somnolence, residual neuromuscular blockade, partial airway obstruction, or difficulty in clearing accumulated airway secretions. These issues are particularly important in patients who have undergone procedures on the upper abdomen, chest, oropharynx, tongue, or upper airway. Supplemental oxygen is administered to avoid hypoxemia, but serial blood gas determinations are required to reveal the trend in $PaCO_2$. Progressive hypercarbia is an indication for reintubation and mechanical ventilation.

Patients with severe respiratory disease may not meet the usual criteria for extubation of the trachea. Each patient requires careful evaluation prior to extubation. If the patient is alert and cooperative but dyspneic, a trial of spontaneous ventilation can be used prior to extubation. Conversely, if the patient is alert but restless and complaining of the presence of the endotracheal tube, then a trial of extubation is warranted. In these cases, reintubation is required if dyspnea increases and the $PaCO_2$ increases over time. An increased $PaCO_2$ may not be an indication for reintubation of the trachea; the direction of the change in $PaCO_2$ is most significant.

Postoperative Management

For more than 50 years, it has been known that measures such as early mobilization, incentive spirometry, chest physiotherapy, and appropriate analgesia to prevent splinting can reduce the incidence of postoperative complications such as atelectasis and pneumonia. Along with mechanical ventilation when needed, these measures remain the bases of the postoperative care of the surgical patient with respiratory disease.

BIBLIOGRAPHY

American College of Physicians. Preoperative pulmonary function testing. *Ann Intern Med* 1990;112:793-794.

Hall JC, Tarala RA, Hall JL, Mander J. A multivariate analysis of the risk of pulmonary complications after laparotomy. *Chest* 1991; 99:923-927.

Pedersen T, Viby-Mogensen J, Ringsted C. Anaesthetic practice and postoperative pulmonary complications. *Acta Anaesthesiol Scand* 1992;36:812-818.

Warner MA, Divertie MB, Tinker JH. Preoperative cessation of smoking and pulmonary complications in coronary artery bypass patients. *Anesthesiology* 1984;60:380-383.

West JB. *Respiratory Pathophysiology,* 5th ed. Oxford: Blackwell Scientific Publications, 1990.

Yeager MP, Glass DD, Neff RK, Brinck-Johnsen T. Epidural anesthesia and analgesia in high-risk surgical patients. *Anesthesiology* 1987;66:729-736.

23

Patients with Hepatic and Renal Disease

Mitchell D. Tobias

The management of anesthesia for patients with hepatic and renal diseases requires an understanding of the type and extent of organ dysfunction. A healthy, asymptomatic patient requires no specific testing for kidney or liver disease, and a patient with mild, stable disease may require limited evaluation and little special perioperative management. At the other extreme, very careful management is required in patients with severe liver or kidney disease in order to preserve remaining organ function and to avoid the complications of the disorder. Medical judgment is critical in prescribing the right level of care for these patients; it is an error to insist on extensive laboratory testing, invasive cardiovascular monitoring, and the administration of albumin and clotting factors for a patient with mild disease and little physiologic disturbance, just as it is an error to neglect these measures for a patient with severe disease.

This chapter reviews the pathophysiology of hepatic and renal disease from the point of view of determining proper anesthesia care for patients suffering from these problems.

Patients with Liver Disease

■ Hepatic Blood Flow

Management of patients with liver disease depends on an understanding of the physiology of liver blood flow, since success often depends on preserving re-

maining hepatocytes. The liver receives approximately 25 percent of the total cardiac output; two-thirds of liver blood flow derives from the portal vein and one-third from the hepatic artery, which together provide the total hepatic blood flow (THBF). Because portal blood is desaturated, the hepatic artery provides about half the total oxygen requirement. Although flow through the hepatic artery increases in response to diminished portal flow, portal vein circulation does not increase with decreases in hepatic arterial blood flow. This limited compensatory mechanism is impaired in liver disease or by halothane anesthesia, increasing the risk of liver hypoxia.

Hepatic blood flow is affected by factors related to both operation and anesthesia. The stress response to laparotomy can greatly diminish splanchnic and therefore portal blood flow. Other causes of diminished THBF may be mechanical, related to traction, dissection, or patient position; THBF decreases in response to increased $PaCO_2$ and sympathetic tone also. Positive-pressure ventilation and positive end-expiratory pressure (PEEP) may increase hepatic venous pressure and decrease both cardiac output and hepatic blood flow; abdominal operations are associated with greater decreases in hepatic blood flow than are operations at other sites.

Both general and spinal or epidural anesthetics may decrease total hepatic blood flow or worsen the ratio between hepatic oxygen supply and demand. Mechanisms include decreased cardiac output, decreased splanchnic arterial blood flow, arterial hypotension, and increased hepatic venous pressure. Splanchnic arterial flow (and thus portal venous flow) is decreased by inhalation anesthetics, although the effect is most prominent with halothane and less with isoflurane or desflurane. Hepatic arterial flow is decreased most by halothane, which produces hepatic artery vasoconstriction. Fentanyl increases oxygen consumption by the liver but also increases THBF, thus maintaining the supply-demand ratio. Barbiturates, benzodiazepines, relaxants, and spinal and epidural anesthesia all reduce hepatic blood flow in proportion to decreases in blood pressure. Nitrous oxide limits FIO_2 and promotes bowel distension, which may decrease splanchnic flow.

The conduct of anesthesia is as important as the choice of anesthetic in preserving hepatic perfusion. Decreases in arterial blood pressure and cardiac output, due to positive-pressure ventilation or PEEP, decrease hepatic blood flow. Hypocarbia diminishes hepatic blood flow, and respiratory alkalosis favors conversion of ammonium ion to ammonia, which more readily crosses the blood-brain barrier. Conversely, hypercarbia causes increases in sympathetic tone and decreases in hepatic blood flow; normocarbia is the best compromise for these patients.

Surgical site and position alter splanchnic hemodynamics. The portal circulation, even in end-stage liver disease (ESLD), is a low-pressure system. Gravity affects drainage, and positions that markedly increase abdominal or chest pressures can adversely affect hepatic blood flow.

■ Hepatitis

Hepatitis is of special concern in anesthesia practice both because the patient may carry the virus and because anesthesia management may be associated with postoperative hepatitis. Although precautions against transmission of viral illness are always appropriate, particular care is indicated in managing patients with liver disease. These patients can be presumed to carry hepatitis virus, either because their primary disease is hepatitis or because of repeated blood transfusions.

When a specific cause for postoperative jaundice cannot be found, the disease is sometimes attributed to the inhaled anesthetic, especially halothane. Although there may be no distinctive chemical, immunologic, or microscopic signs of anesthesia-induced liver injury, estimates of the incidence of severe hepatic dysfunction are given as 1 in 6000 to 1 in 20,000

halothane anesthetics. Those at greatest risk appear to be middle-aged obese women, especially those who receive repeated halothane anesthesia at intervals of a few weeks. There is no evidence that preexisting liver disease increases the risk of anesthesia-induced hepatitis, but it may be prudent to avoid halothane in a patient who has had halothane in the previous few months or who reports a history of unexplained hepatitis after anesthesia. The available data do not implicate sevoflurane, desflurane, or isoflurane. Hepatitis is attributed to enflurane less often than to halothane, and the incidence after halothane is especially small in children. Proposed mechanisms of "halothane hepatitis" include hepatic hypoxia, toxic effects of reductive metabolites, and an autoimmune response to liver proteins bound to metabolites of halothane, particularly trifluoroacetate.

Because the incidence of "halothane hepatitis" is much less than the incidence of hepatitis from other causes, and because good animal models are lacking, the existence of the syndrome has been the subject of debate. A survey of 7600 healthy patients scheduled for elective operations uncovered 11 with preoperative liver disease by laboratory test. The operations were canceled for these 11 patients, and 3 went on to become jaundiced. Thus, in this population, between 1 in 2000 and 1 in 700 healthy surgical patients developed liver disease without anesthesia or operation.

In evaluating a patient with jaundice or hepatic dysfunction after anesthesia, other causes are sought, including obstructive jaundice, hemolysis, hematoma resorption, and viral hepatitis. The diagnosis of anesthesia-related hepatitis remains one of exclusion. Postmortem examination can only exonerate a volatile anesthetic as the cause of hepatitis when an unsuspected infectious agent is discovered.

■ Pathophysiology of Liver Disease

Hepatic diseases fall into three categories: obstructive disease and acute or chronic hepatocellular disorders. In obstructive disease, due to tumors or to gallstones, hepatic function is usually preserved. Operations are directed at restoring biliary tract patency; mortality and morbidity usually result from renal failure, sepsis, or hemorrhage. Acute hepatocellular disease is usually viral, toxic, or thrombotic in origin. These patients come to operation only for emergency treatment of life-threatening illnesses or for orthotopic liver transplantation. Chronic hepatocellular disease results from repeated bouts of acute hepatitis (e.g., alcohol) or deranged immune mechanisms (e.g., primary biliary cirrhosis or chronic active hepatitis). Less commonly, inborn errors of metabolism (Wilson's disease, hemochromatosis) impair hepatic function.

Cirrhosis is a final common pathway for all forms of chronic liver disease. Its pathologic hallmarks, necrosis, fibrosis, and disordered architecture, represent the extremes of the disturbances of the flow of blood, lymph, and bile and of metabolic function that characterize liver diseases in general. These produce significant effects on other organ systems, which must be taken into account in planning anesthesia care (Table 23-1).

The Cardiovascular System

Patients with severe liver disease typically have markedly increased cardiac outputs and diminished systemic vascular resistances, owing in part to arteriovenous anastomoses resulting from altered concentrations and action of estrogens. Despite a cardiac output as great as 20 liters/min, functional intravascular volume and perfusion of organs such as the liver and kidney may be inadequate. A dilated cardiomyopathy is likely if ethanol is the etiologic agent of cirrhosis. The combination of impaired myocardial performance with a diminished, fixed peripheral vascular resistance compromises the patient's ability to cope with hypovolemia or medications that depress cardiovascular function.

Renal System

With cirrhosis and, to a lesser degree, in acute liver disease, the main renal defect is impaired excretion of salt and water, probably due to decreased effective circulating volume and renal blood flow. Regardless of salt intake, the urine in advanced liver disease may be almost free of sodium. There is a marked increase in extracellular fluid, evident as ascites and edema.

Hepatorenal syndrome (HRS) is a progressive form of oliguric renal failure that is almost always fatal and is found in patients with cirrhosis, hepatoma, or acute hepatitis. HRS resembles prerenal azotemia, which must be ruled out before making this diagnosis.

Pulmonary System

Chronic hypoxemia in liver disease results from several causes. Intrapulmonary arteriovenous shunting increases the shunt fraction. Increases in interstitial lung water from hypoalbuminemia and hy-

ponatremia contribute to defects in O_2 diffusion. Ascites and pleural effusions produce a restrictive pulmonary disorder. Many patients with alcoholic cirrhosis also smoke heavily. Hypoxic pulmonary vasoconstriction is blunted by circulating vasodilator substances. The oxyhemoglobin dissociation curve is shifted rightward due to increased 2,3-DPG concentrations, an effect that is offset by the respiratory alkalosis of chronic hyperventilation. Consequently, maintaining arterial oxygenation is a major challenge during anesthesia in these patients.

Nervous System

Hepatic encephalopathy is thought to result from accumulation of circulating toxic wastes normally cleared in the liver. Asterixis, somnolence, obtundation, and eventually coma are common neurologic signs. Ammonia has long been considered the cause, but there is no clear correlation between serum concentrations and symptoms. Other candidate molecules include mercaptans, octopamine, phenol, and short-chain fatty acids. The blood-brain barrier is thought to be more permeable in liver failure, and intracranial pressure is often increased. Anesthetic plans for such patients must reduce to a minimum the chances of postoperative somnolence and increased intracranial pressure.

Gastrointestinal System

Malabsorption and inanition are common accompaniments of liver dysfunction. Cirrhosis increases portal resistance, engorging the portal circulation and promoting bleeding, especially from esophageal varices. Bacterial overgrowth predisposes the patient to encephalopathy from bacterial metabolic wastes. Peptic ulceration is a common, potentially fatal problem in cirrhotic patients.

■ Other Physiologic Consequences of Hepatic Disease

Albumin Synthesis

The healthy liver produces 10 g of albumin each day, with a half-life of about 20 days. There may be no albumin deficiency in the first few days of acute liver failure, but hypoalbuminemia is a feature of severe chronic liver disease, especially in malnourished patients. Edema and ascites result, affecting the pharmacokinetics of water-soluble and protein-bound drugs.

Table 23-1

Physiologic Disorders Due to Liver Disease that Affect Management of Anesthesia

Disorder	Consequence
Cardiovascular	
Arteriovenous shunting	Limited ability to increase cardiac output further
Fixed, decreased peripheral resistance	Intolerant of hypovolemia
Increased cardiac output at rest, diverted to shunts	Marginal or inadequate perfusion of kidney, liver
Cardiomyopathy (alcohol use)	Unable to tolerate myocardia depressants
Renal	
Decreased effective renal blood flow	Impaired excretion of salt and water
Increased ADH secretion	Dilutional hyponatremia
Ascites and edema	Decreased effective circulating blood volume; mechanical effects of ascites
Hepatorenal syndrome	Progressive renal and hepatic failure, death
Pulmonary	
Intrapulmonary A-V shunts	Hypoxemia due to increased shunt fraction
Increased interstitial water	Hypoxemia due to diffusion defects
Ascites elevates restricts diaphragm	Restrictive lung disease, reduced FRC
Pleural effusions	Restrictive lung disease, reduced FRC
History of smoking is common	Associated COPD and bronchitis
Circulating vasodilators	Impaired hypoxic pulmonary vasoconstriction
Nervous system	
Accumulation of circulating toxins	
Impaired blood-brain barrier	Asterixis, somnolence, obtundation, coma; hepatic encephalopathy
Intracranial hypertension	
Gastrointestinal	
Malabsorption	Malnutrition
Portal hypertension	GI bleeding, bowel edema
Peptic ulcers	
Impaired albumin synthesis	
Hypoalbuminemia	Ascites
	Decreased binding of drugs, bilirubin
Ascites	
Increased ECF volume	Volume of distribution increased for hydrophilic drugs
Diaphragm displaced upward	Decreased FRC, restrictive lung disease
Decreased splanchnic venous capacity	Reduced circulating blood volume; abrupt hypotension when ascites is drained
Impaired bilirubin metabolism	Direct toxic effects of bilirubin on mitochondria
	Encephalopathy, kernicterus
Hematologic	
Deficient factors II, VII, IX, X	Coagulopathy due to deficiency of soluble factors
Failure to clear activated coagulation factors	Consumption coagulopathy
Hypersplenism	Thrombocytopenia
Impaired storage or synthesis of B_{12}, haptoglobin, transferrin, ceruloplasmin	Anemia
Pharmacokinetics	
Impaired phase I and II biotransformation	Delayed drug metabolism
Portosystemic shunts	Enhanced action of oral medications otherwise subject to first-pass metabolism by the liver
Hypoalbuminemia	Enhanced action of drugs bound to albumin
Ascites and edema = increased ECF volume	Decreased effect, due to increased volume of distribution, of water soluble drugs
Hypogammaglobulinemia	Blunted effects of drugs bound to gamma globulin
Glucose	
Impaired glycogen storage	Rarely, hypoglycemia (in severe hepatocellular disease)
Hormone metabolism	
Increased estrogens, ADH, thyroid-stimulating hormone	Hyperdynamic circulation, stigmata of cirrhosis

Ascites

Three factors contribute to the ascites seen in patients with liver failure. Oncotic pressure decreases with chronic hypoalbuminemia, cirrhosis causes hepatic lymphatic obstruction, and there is dilutional hyponatremia. Ascitic fluid accumulating under pressure in the abdomen has predictable pathophysiologic effects: The volume of distribution of hydrophilic compounds increases, splanchnic capacitance decreases, venous return and cardiac output diminish, and the diaphragm is displaced cephalad.

When ascitic fluid is drained during an operation, intraabdominal pressure decreases abruptly, allowing splanchnic vasodilation, which may precipitate cardiovascular collapse. Aggressive fluid replacement is required to allow patients to tolerate this abrupt decrease in portal pressure.

Bilirubin Secretion

Bilirubin is culled by the reticuloendothelial system from hemoglobin and other hemoproteins. It is normally bound to albumin, conjugated by the liver, and excreted in the bile. Even small additional amounts of bilirubin can overwhelm a patient with hypoalbuminemia and diminished conjugating capacity. Unconjugated bilirubin unbound to albumin is toxic to mitochondria; it causes encephalopathy and, in neonates, kernicterus. Treatment consists of intravenous albumin or hemodialysis.

Coagulation and Hematologic Effects

Most soluble coagulation factors derive from the liver. Disorders of coagulation rapidly follow severe hepatic damage because the half-lives of some factors are brief (e.g., factor VII, 6 hours). Deficiency of the vitamin K-dependent factors II, VII, IX, and X is linked to impaired bile secretion, as occurs in obstructive jaundice.

The liver is responsible for clearing activated coagulation products. Failure to extract these complexes leads to factor consumption and primary fibrinolysis. Important anticoagulant and fibrinolytic factors are essential hepatic hemostatic products also.

Platelet quantity and quality may suffer in liver disease. Normally, 30 percent of circulating platelets may be found within the spleen, but up to 90 percent are sequestered in hypersplenism accompanying portal hypertension. Intravascular coagulation consumes platelets, and uncleared dialyzable toxins disable them. Perioperative management includes blood component therapy with platelets, fresh frozen plasma, cryoprecipitate, or vitamin K as dictated by laboratory studies (see Chap. 15).

Anemia in patients with hepatic disease is due to many factors. Bleeding is exacerbated by derangements of hemostasis. Effective erythropoiesis depends on a normal liver for iron and heme transport with serum proteins such as haptoglobin, transferrin, and ceruloplasmin. Vitamin B_{12} is stored in the liver.

Drug Metabolism and Pharmacokinetics

Most drug metabolism occurs in the liver. In patients with severe liver disease, diminished phase I and II biotransformation may increase the serum half-lives of drugs. Other effects of liver disease may increase the relative potency of some drugs. Portosystemic shunts permit orally administered drugs to bypass the liver, thus reducing first-pass metabolism, and hypoalbuminemia allows an increase in free plasma drug concentration. In contrast, other effects of liver disease may require that drug doses be increased. Ascites and other increases in extracellular volume produce increased volumes of distribution for water-soluble drugs, and gamma-globulins are increased in most hepatic diseases so that drugs bound to these proteins have a larger volume of distribution.

Glucose and Glycogen Metabolism

Despite the role of the liver in glycogen storage, fasting hypoglycemia is rare in liver disease; as little as 20 percent of the hepatic parenchyma suffices for this function. Measurements of serum glucose ensure that hypoglycemia does not go unrecognized during anesthesia.

Hormone Metabolism

The hormonal abnormalities associated with hepatic dysfunction are multiple and complex. Estrogens, antidiuretic hormone, and thyroid-stimulating hormone are all increased.

■ Anesthesia Management of Patients with Liver Disease

Preoperative Preparation

Preoperative assessment begins with establishing the presence of liver disease and its effects on organ systems (see Table 23-1). For patients with disorders of mild severity, there may be no pathophysiologic consequences of the disease, since the liver possesses remarkable reserve; function can be normal in animals even after resection of up to 90 percent of the liver. For patients with severe liver disorders, the following measures are used to improve the patient's condition:

1. Correct hypovolemia and electrolyte disorders.
2. Treat coagulopathy with vitamin K, soluble coagulation factors, and platelets.
3. Drain ascites as appropriate to relieve the effects of increased intraabdominal pressure; correct resulting hypotension with crystalloid solutions (usually) or colloid solutions (if the volume of ascitic fluid exceeds 4 liters).
4. Control infection.
5. Sterilize the bowel with neomycin or inhibit bacterial urease with lactulose to treat encephalopathy.
6. Treat anemia with packed red cell transfusions.
7. Monitor intracranial pressure and control cerebral edema.

Premedication

Sedative-hypnotic premedication is not contraindicated in these patients. Doses must be reduced and prolonged effects anticipated because of alterations in the blood-brain barrier, pharmacodynamics, and pharmacokinetics.

Monitoring

The choice of invasive cardiovascular monitoring depends on the severity of the patient's disease and the magnitude of the planned surgical procedure. For patients with severe liver disease, direct determinations of urine output, arterial pressure, central venous pressure, pulmonary artery pressures, and cardiac output are required for all but the least invasive of operations. The coagulopathy due to the liver disease is treated before placing internal jugular vein or subclavian vein catheters because of the risk of hematoma. Frequent determinations of glucose, electrolytes, blood gases, acid-base status, coagulation state, and hematocrit are required as well (Table 23-2).

Choice of Anesthesia: Regional versus General Anesthesia

For minor or peripheral procedures, regional anesthesia produces the least physiologic disturbance and is preferred, with some caveats. Severe coagulopathy may limit the choice of block, although for all but spinal or epidural anesthesia this risk does not usually constitute an absolute contraindication. Spinal or epidural anesthesia may result in hypotension and reduced hepatic blood flow, especially if high levels of anesthesia are required. Reduced hepatic metabolism of local anesthetics may lead to unexpected toxicity as the drug accumulates with repeated administrations.

General anesthesia offers significant advantages that make it advisable for management of major operations or for patients with severe liver disease. Intubation of the trachea assures the tidal volume and FIO_2, and reduces the risk of aspiration pneumonitis, an especially important problem in patients with severe ascites and impaired pulmonary function. Rapid-sequence intubation or awake intubation may even be needed. Avoiding nitrous oxide helps maintain oxygenation and avoid bowel distension. Hypocarbia should be avoided, as should halothane, which decreases hepatic arterial flow. The combination of isoflurane or desflurane in oxygen, with small doses of narcotics, seems to be a rational choice for maintaining hepatic oxygen delivery.

Intravenous Anesthetics

Although chronic abuse of alcohol produces tolerance to some anesthetics, cardiomyopathy and altered pharmacokinetics may accentuate the effects of intravenous anesthetics in patients with cirrhosis. For patients with liver disease, it is best to give the initial dose of drug in small increments until the desired effect is achieved. If a rapid-sequence induction and intubation are required, choosing an agent such as ketamine may reduce the risk of hypotension that can occur when an excessive dose of thiopental is chosen. Successive small doses are given only when indicated, since drug metabolism is likely to be impaired.

Muscle Relaxants

The choice of muscle relaxant depends on the duration of the planned procedure. Although pseudocholinesterase production is decreased, the duration of effect of succinylcholine is not markedly prolonged. Most nondepolarizing muscle relaxants are acceptable for use. The duration of effect of atracurium is unaffected by liver disease, making it a good choice when rapid recovery of neuromuscular function is required after anesthesia. The increased volume of distribution requires greater initial doses of most muscle relaxants, but many patients with ESLD suffer inanition and reduced skeletal muscle mass, reducing the total amount of neuromuscular blocking agents necessary.

Table 23-2

Anesthesia Management of Patients with Liver Disease

Consideration	Management
Hepatitis	Avoid halothane in preexisting liver disease, after recent exposure, or with history of reaction to previous exposure.
	Use special care with universal precautions.
	Desflurane, isoflurane, sevoflurane seem to be entirely safe.
Maintaining hepatic blood flow	Avoid excess catecholamine secretion: "stress free" management may be of value.
	Avoid hypercarbia or hypocarbia.
	Avoid PEEP, which reduces HBF.
	Avoid systemic hypotension.
Hypovolemia and electrolyte disorders	Frequent determinations of electrolytes.
	Generous fluid administration, guided by CVP or PA pressures, with crystalloid or albumin as dictated by measurements.
Coagulopathy	Correct preoperatively after measurements.
	Monitor intraoperatively; the patient will need soluble factors and platelets.
Ascites	Paracentesis if respiratory and circulatory compromise demand.
	Expect hypotension when ascites is drained with abdominal incision; treat with pressors and volume.
Anemia	Transfuse as needed; minimum Hct is higher than usual, due to compromised blood flows.
Encephalopathy and pulmonary edema	Monitor ICP as indicated, treat increases in the usual way.
	Sterilize bowel with neomycin or inhibit urease with lactulose.
Premedication	Reduce doses.
Monitoring	Monitor ABGs, glucose, electrolytes, urine output.
	Invasive cardiovascular monitoring for severe cases; use care to avoid hematomas.
Regional anesthesia	Prefer peripheral blocks where possible.
	Expect cumulation with successive doses of local anesthetic.
	Profound hypotension with spinal or epidural anesthesia, if ascites or portal hypertension present.
General anesthesia	Consider need for rapid sequence induction.
	Reduced doses of intravenous agents.
	Choose agents that do not compromise hepatic blood flow or that are implicated as causes of hepatitis.
Muscle relaxants	Expect larger volume of distribution, slower metabolism for drugs such as pancuronium, vecuronium.
	Atracurium is a good choice if predictable offset of effect is needed.
	Though pseudocholinesterase production is decreased, succinylcholine effect is nearly normal.
Fluids	Maintain urine output, cardiac output, CVP or PA pressures.
	Saline acceptable unless albumin is required to treat hypoalbuminemia.

Fluid Management

Many patients with liver failure have decreased intravascular volumes and A-V shunting, both of which can cause hyperaldosteronemia; despite markedly increased total-body water, restoration of effective circulation is often necessary prior to the induction of anesthesia. Colloid-containing solutions (5% albumin) may be better suited for those patients with hypoalbuminemia, decreased plasma oncotic pressure, and anasarca. Crystalloid solutions effectively restore intravascular volume and maintain urine output in most situations, although colloid solutions (e.g., albumin) may be required if the volume of ascitic fluid removed exceeds approximately 4 liters or if major hepatic resection is performed. If diuretics are required, mannitol is preferred over furosemide, which exacerbates hypokalemic alkalosis. Either diuretic may further diminish intravascular volume.

Patients with Renal Disease

Mild kidney disease affects perioperative risk and anesthesia management only slightly. Signs and symptoms of renal failure occur only after loss of 60 percent of the 2 million nephrons. Conservative medical therapy suffices to treat renal insufficiency until only 10 percent of the nephrons remain, at which time renal failure requires dialysis. The management of the patient with impaired renal function focuses on preserving remaining function and altering therapeutic approaches to compensate for renal dysfunction.

■ Pathophysiology of Renal Failure

Renal failure affects acid-base regulation, water and fluid volume maintenance, electrolyte balance, elaboration of some hormones, and waste excretion (Table 23-3).

Loss of Renal Function

The kidneys normally receive about 25 percent of the adult's cardiac output (renal blood flow is 1250 ml/min), of which 10 percent is filtered (glomerular filtration rate is 125 ml/min). Although autoregulation normally keeps renal blood flow within narrow limits for a wide variety of mean arterial pressures, the functioning of the nephron is subject to neurohumoral regulation by antidiuretic hormone, aldosterone, renin, and catecholamines, all of which are secreted in response to the stress of operation.

In renal failure, the 50 mEq of hydrogen ions produced daily are not fully excreted, and metabolic acidosis results. Phosphate and sulfate ions accumulate, producing an anion gap. There is a subsequent pH-dependent shift of the oxyhemoglobin dissociation curve to the right that partially offsets the severe anemia occurring in end-stage renal disease (ESRD). Acidemia exacerbates the hyperkalemia that usually coexists.

Patients with some forms of renal insufficiency are unable to produce concentrated urine. Salt and water wastage with resulting hypovolemia occurs, especially when patients fast. More commonly, the ability to excrete water fails, and the patient with oliguria or anuria must depend on dialysis to eliminate exogenous and endogenous water. The patient easily develops volume overload. Pulmonary edema and hypoxia may occur with modest infusions of intravenous fluids.

Disturbances of electrolyte balance occur, with predominant hyponatremia, hypocalcemia, and increased serum concentrations of chloride, potassium, phosphate, and magnesium ions. Patients with renal insufficiency who have not received dialysis may have potassium concentrations of 6 to 7 mEq/liter; the chief electrocardiographic (ECG) findings are tall, peaked T waves. Acute exacerbation of hyperkalemia may be precipitated by respiratory acidosis, potassium-sparing diuretics, or intravenous succinylcholine. When the serum potassium reaches 8 mEq/liter, the PR interval becomes prolonged, and the QRS complex widens. At concentrations greater than 9 mEq/liter, the P wave disappears, and the QRS complex widens to a sine-wave form. Immediate treatment of hyperkalemia includes hyperventilation and the administration of insulin with glucose. In life-threatening hyperkalemia, calcium is administered to reverse the effects of potassium on excitable membranes.

Hematologic System

In renal failure, anemia results from gastrointestinal bleeding, decreased erythropoietin secretion, and decreased red cell life span. Preoperative treatment to correct anemia is with recombinant human erythropoietin or with transfusion with packed red blood cells, taking care to avoiding fluid overload. Because patients adapt to chronic anemia, correction must be based on physiologic function and not an arbitrary value for hemoglobin or hematocrit.

There is a qualitative defect in platelet adhesiveness and aggregation in renal failure related to dialyzable toxin(s). Transfusion of platelets is ineffective unless dialysis is performed also. In the absence of dialysis, platelet function can be restored with administration of 1-deamino-(8-D-arginine)-vasopressin (DDAVP), cryoprecipitate, or conjugated estrogens.

Cardiovascular System

Hypertension, often due to increased renin excretion, is an almost universal finding in renal insufficiency and renal failure. Left ventricular hypertrophy results from hypertension and from increased cardiac output due to anemia. High-output cardiac failure occurs in some patients due to arteriovenous shunts created for hemodialysis. Uremic pericarditis may cause tamponade.

Table 23-3

Physiologic Disorders of Renal Failure that Affect Management of Anesthesia

Disorder	Consequences
Cardiovascular	
Increased renin secretion	Hypertension
Increased cardiac output, due to anemia	High-output failure
Left ventricular hypertrophy	Myocardial ischemia
AV shunt for dialysis	High-output renal failure
Volume overload or deficiencies following dialysis	CHF or hypovolemic hypotension
Associated diabetes > accelerated atherosclerosis	Myocardial infarction, stroke
Renal: Failure to excrete potassium	Progressive hyperkalemia
	7 mEq/L: tall peaked T waves
	8 mEq/L: prolonged PR interval, QRS widening
	9 mEq/L: P wave disappears, QRS widens further
Renal: Failure to excrete fixed acid	Progressive acidemia
Renal: Water excretion	
Failure to excrete water (oliguria or anuria)	Volume overload, pulmonary edema
Failure to concentrate urine	Fasting dehydration, hypotension, salt wasting
Pulmonary	
Pulmonary calcification	Decreased diffusing capacity
Diaphragmatic elevation with peritoneal dialysis	Decreased FRC, restriction
Nervous system	
Uremic toxemia	Mental slowing, fatigue, seizures, myoclonus, coma
Sensory peripheral neuropathy	Lower extremity numbness
Dysautonomia	Orthostatic hypotension, gastroparesis
Gastrointestinal	
Increased volume and acidity of gastric contents	Increased risk of aspiration pneumonitis
Ulcers	GI bleeding
Anorexia, nausea, vomiting	
Hematologic	
Erythropoietin secretion decreases	Anemia
Decreased red cell life span	Anemia
Dialyzable toxins impair platelet aggregation	Platelet dysfunction
Immune system	
Uremia impairs leukocyte chemotaxis	Infection, sepsis
Steroid treatment	
Loss of immunoglobulins	
Pharmacokinetics	
Diminished excretion of water soluble drugs and metabolites	Accumulation of active metabolites of morphine, demerol, benzodiazepines
Hypoalbuminemia	Increased free fraction of drugs bound to albumin
Acidosis	Drugs with acid pKa are less ionized, have greater volumes of distribution and longer half lives
Impaired function of blood brain barrier	Accentuated effects of drugs with CNS effects

Intravascular volume overload may occur between dialysis treatments, whereas acute volume depletion may result from vigorous hemodialysis. Accelerated atherosclerosis and coronary artery disease associated with diabetes mellitus and hypertension commonly accompany severe renal disease.

Pulmonary System

Pulmonary edema in kidney disease results from volume overload and from the decreased oncotic pressure caused by hypoproteinemia. Calcification occurs in pulmonary tissues, contributing to a diminution in diffusion capacity. Peritoneal dialysis restricts diaphragmatic motion, decreasing functional residual capacity.

Gastrointestinal System

Anorexia, hiccup, nausea, and vomiting are common in uremia. Gastrointestinal ulceration occurs in up to 25 percent of patients with renal failure. Patients have increased gastric acidity and volumes, suggesting the use of appropriate precautions against aspiration of gastric contents, including preoperative cimetidine and metoclopramide, and rapid-sequence induction or awake intubation of the trachea.

Immune System

Uremia impairs leukocyte chemotaxis. Immunity is further embarrassed by loss of humeral globulins in proteinuria and steroid treatments for some causes of renal failure. Sepsis is the major cause of death in patients with renal failure.

Nervous System

Uremic toxemia presents as mental slowing, fatigue, and malaise; it progresses to seizures, myoclonus, and coma if left untreated. Many patients receiving chronic hemodialysis suffer from depression or experience personality changes. Peripheral sensory neuropathies usually affect the lower extremities; motor deficits occur less often. Dysautonomia occurs with severe disease and produces orthostatic hypotension, gastroparesis, or vomiting.

■ The Effects of Anesthesia on Renal Function

Inhalational anesthetics themselves produce a dose-dependent reversible depression of renal function as a result of reduced renal blood flow and glomerular filtration rate, although fluid administration produces diuresis in anesthetized subjects. The risk of permanent renal damage from inhalational anesthetics has been studied extensively since it was recognized that metabolism of methoxyflurane releases quantities of fluoride ion that are toxic to the distal convoluted tubule and collecting ducts. After prolonged exposure to large doses of methoxyflurane, patients suffer polyuria and are unable to concentrate urine in response to antidiuretic hormone.

Subclinical nephrotoxicity has been demonstrated in healthy volunteers following enflurane exposure for 9.6 MAC-hours (i.e., dose, in multiples of MAC, times hours of administration). Obesity and isoniazid therapy increase free fluoride release from enflurane. Patients with renal disease and some remaining renal function are not good candidates for enflurane anesthesia. Isoflurane, sevoflurane, and desflurane are not extensively metabolized and produce no ill effects on the kidneys after prolonged administration, support-

ing the choice of these inhalational agents for anesthesia of patients with impaired renal function.

■ Perioperative Renal Failure

Distinct from the reversible decrement in renal function due to anesthesia itself, acute renal failure sometimes follows operation and anesthesia. Perioperative acute renal failure usually involves acute tubular necrosis, with a precipitating event such as cross-clamping of the aorta, a severe bout of hypotension or reduced cardiac output, sepsis, prolonged use of large doses of vasopressors, cardiopulmonary bypass, or relative overdoses of nephrotoxic drugs such as gentamicin. In healthy patients undergoing limited operations, when these circumstances are not present, oliguria under anesthesia is almost always due to reduced GFR and requires no treatment. In the presence of these risk factors, simultaneous treatment and diagnosis of oliguria can be accomplished by administering fluids and ensuring that the CVP, blood volume, and cardiac output are adequate. If these measures do not produce diuresis, then the onset of acute tubular necrosis (ATN) is likely. In such cases, diuretics (both loop diuretics and osmotic agents) may be of use, but the prognosis is poor.

■ Dialysis-Related Conditions

Dialysis controls many of the ill effects of renal failure described in Table 23-3: volume overload, volume-dependent hypertension, electrolyte imbalances, platelet defects, and acidosis. Encephalopathy can be prevented and largely reversed. Red cell transfusion may be accomplished without volume change during hemodialysis. Dialysis does not improve renin-dependent hypertension, impaired immunity, anemia, hypoproteinemia, increased cardiac output, accelerated atherosclerosis, or gastrointestinal ulceration.

Dialysis can provoke specific problems that affect anesthesia care. High-output cardiac failure can result from the A-V shunt created to support hemodialysis. Although therapy ameliorates the hemostatic defect of uremia, bleeding tendencies occur in up to 75 percent of patients undergoing dialysis. Rebound heparinization has been recognized following hemodialysis, owing to the differences in the rates of clearance of heparin and protamine after dialysis. In general, rebound heparinization is preferable to thrombosis of the hemodialysis shunt in patients who do not require operation.

After vigorous dialysis, some patients suffer hypovolemia. This can be detected by questioning the patient about body weight and by testing for orthostatic hypotension. Lastly, hepatitis is endemic in patients with end-stage renal disease.

■ Anesthesia Management in Patients with Renal Failure

Mild disorders of renal function that have not produced the ill effects described above require little special management. For patients with more severe disease, thorough evaluation involves assessment of intravascular volume, electrolyte balance, hypertension, remaining renal function, and the effects of renal failure on other organ systems. The results of this evaluation dictate management (Table 23-4).

Preoperative Preparation

Specific therapy for hypertension, anemia, coagulopathy, fluid overload, or hyperkalemia may be needed. Often, dialysis will prove effective treatment for all these disorders and is required within a day preceding elective operations for patients with renal failure.

Premedication

Sedative premedication is administered only in reduced doses. Premedication includes an H_2 receptor antagonist and metoclopramide to reduce gastric acidity and volume.

Monitoring

Monitoring depends on the patient's condition and the operation proposed. The site of vascular access for dialysis is protected from blood pressure cuffs or intravenous access to reduce the chance of thrombosis or infection. If possible, arterial catheters are not used so as to preserve future access sites. A bladder catheter is a source of urinary tract infection; it is used only if absolutely necessary, as in a long operation. In many patients, oliguria or anuria is well established, and there is no value to monitoring urine output. A central venous pressure cannula or a pulmonary artery catheter is useful if the patient has significant heart failure or fluid overload or the patient's blood volume is expected to change rapidly, as from severe bleeding. A nerve stimulator is essential if neuromuscular blockers are to be used.

Positioning

Careful positioning of the patient is required because these patients may have little subcutaneous tissue as well as peripheral neuropathies and are subject to skin necrosis. Renal osteodystrophy makes fractures more likely. The hemodialysis access sites should be available for monitoring (by palpation or Doppler flowmeter) during the operation, and mechanical obstruction by the blood pressure cuff or positioning is avoided to prevent stasis and thrombosis.

Choice of Anesthesia: Regional versus General

Regional anesthetic techniques confer significant advantages for patients with ESRD since the potential ill effects of general anesthesia on the cardiovascular system can be avoided, and blood flow may be better maintained at the site of an arteriovenous shunt.

However, the presence of renal failure imposes limitations on the use of regional anesthesia techniques. Coagulopathy may contraindicate regional techniques such as spinal and epidural anesthesia. If fluid administration is used to maintain arterial blood pressure following the sympathectomy of spinal or epidural anesthesia, patients who cannot excrete sodium or free water will suffer hypervolemia, with possible pulmonary edema, when the effects of the block dissipate and vasoconstriction returns. Acidemia predisposes to greater serum concentrations of local anesthetics, with increased risk of toxicity.

General anesthesia is often required. Rapid intravenous induction, combined with cricoid pressure and immediate intubation of the trachea, may be appropriate for uremic patients with evidence of dysautonomia or nausea and vomiting. However, these patients often have associated coronary artery disease, labile hypertension, or volume depletion, making the rapid induction of anesthesia risky.

Inhalational agents have an advantage over intravenous agents because they are eliminated primarily via the lungs and not the kidneys. The effects of small doses of intravenous drugs dissipate predictably, due to redistribution. With large or repeated doses, effects may be prolonged, since renal elimination of the drugs and their metabolites is impaired.

Muscle Relaxants

Since succinylcholine increases serum potassium concentrations transiently by less than 1 mEq/liter, it may be used for rapid-sequence induction of anesthe-

Table 23-4

Anesthesia Management of Patients with Renal Failure

Consideration	Management
Preoperative preparation	Dialysis is the first and most important measure to correct most preoperative defects
Hypervolemia, hypovolemia	Diuresis (if possible) or fluids as appropriate; invasive cardiovasc. monitoring if CHF is a risk
Hyperkalemia	Glucose, insulin, bicarbonate
Hypertension	Vasodilators, ACE inhibitors, and other antihypertensive drugs
Platelet dysfunction	DDAVP (not platelet transfusions)
Anemia	Transfuse only for physiologically significant anemia; these patients often tolerate chronic anemia well
Premedication	
Impaired excretion	Administer small doses of sedative and narcotics, IV, to effect
Increased volume and acid in stomach	Premedicate with H_2 blockers, antacids, metoclopramide
Monitoring	
Impaired left ventricular function	Consider invasive cardiovascular monitoring
Anticipated major blood losses, fluid shifts	Consider invasive cardiovascular monitoring
Need to monitor remaining urine output	Weigh infection risk from Foley catheter vs. need for accurate measurement of urine output
Positioning	
Skin breakdown	Padding for skin
Osteodystrophy	Careful positioning to avoid fractures
Hemodialysis shunts	No bp or IV on side of A-V shunt; monitor pulse and flow in shunt intraoperatively
Regional anesthesia	
Coagulopathy	Correct coagulopathy or select blocks that do not risk hematoma
Spinal hypotension	Use only moderate doses of fluids for spinal hypotension; use vasopressors
Vascular access procedures	Prefer regional anesthesia for vascular access procedure, to enhance blood flow
General anesthesia	
Full stomach	Full stomach precautions, including rapid sequence induction
Associated coronary artery disease	Evaluate for coronary artery disease; appropriate precautions
Impaired excretion of IV anesthetics	Limit IV anesthetics to induction or choose those not excreted in urine
Muscle relaxants	
Hyperkalemia with succinylcholine	Withhold succinylcholine if potassium exceeds 5 mEq/L
Impaired excretion of drugs	Avoid pancuronium, d-tubocurarine and doxacurium; prefer atracurium, except for long procedures
Fluid management	
Hyperkalemia	No exogenous potassium; monitoring serum potassium; glucose, insulin, bicarbonate if needed
Polyuric renal failure	Administer fluids and electrolytes to match obligate renal losses as well as operative losses
Anuria	Restrict water, sodium to amounts needed to maintain blood volume; monitor CVP, PA, electrolytes

sia in these patients, provided that the serum potassium is not excessive before the succinylcholine is given. Rapidly acting nondepolarizing neuromuscular blocking agents can be used in place of succinylcholine. Rocuronium or vecuronium produces rapid paralysis for intubation of the trachea without further increases in serum potassium.

Impaired drug excretion in renal failure makes the effects of pancuronium, D-tubocurarine, or doxacurium prolonged and unpredictable. Mivacurium, vecuronium, and atracurium are more suitable choices. Despite the theoretical advantages enjoyed by these drugs, careful monitoring and limited doses are still required to avoid unwanted paralysis at the end of anesthesia. Reversal of neuromuscular blockade with anticholinesterase and anticholinergic drugs is effective in patients with renal failure. These drugs have even longer durations of action in the presence of renal failure than do the nondepolarizing neuromuscular blocking drugs. Reports of late unopposed muscarinic effects (bradycardia, bronchospasm, and hypersecretion) have appeared, but these are not common problems.

Fluid Management

For patients with polyuria and renal failure, fluid management consists of matching blood loss and urine output with a suitable mixture of red cells, electrolytes, and water, as determined by measurements of urine and blood, and careful assessment to detect hypovolemia. For anuric patients undergoing operations, replacement blood and fluids are limited to those required to replace blood loss and third space losses. Determining these requirements when they are large, as during major operations, often requires invasive cardiovascular monitoring to measure CVP or pulmonary arterial pressures. In severely ill patients or victims of trauma, who require large amounts of blood or who suffer tissue hypoperfusion, accumulation of fixed acid and potassium may require aggressive treatment with glucose, insulin, and bicarbonate or even immediate dialysis.

BIBLIOGRAPHY

Brown BR Jr. *Anesthesia in Hepatic and Biliary Tract Disease.* Philadelphia: FA Davis, 1988.

Gelman S, Dillard E, Bradley EL Jr. Hepatic circulation during surgical stress and anesthesia with halothane, isoflurane, or fentanyl. *Anesth Analg* 1987;66:936-943.

Mazze RI, Calverley RK, Smith NT. Inorganic fluoride nephrotoxicity: Prolonged enflurane and halothane anesthesia in volunteers. *Anesthesiology* 1977;46:265-271.

Moore K, Wendon J, Frazer M, et al. Plasma endothelin immunoreactivity in liver disease and the hepatorenal syndrome. *N Engl J Med* 1992;327:1774-1778.

Murray JM, Rowlands BJ, Trinick TR. Indocyanine green clearance and hepatic function during and after prolonged anaesthesia. *Br J Anaesth* 1992;68:168-171.

Priebe HJ, ed. The kidney in anesthesia. In *International Anesthesiology Clinics,* vol 22. Boston: Little, Brown, 1984.

Schemel WH. Unexpected hepatic dysfunction found by multiple laboratory screening. *Anesth Analg* 1976;55:810-812.

CHAPTER 24

Metabolic and Endocrine Disorders

Clifford S. Deutschman

Operations result in a profound alteration in systemic metabolism and physiology that is frequently referred to as the *stress response*. This adaptive response represents an attempt to minimize tissue damage and effect recovery. All aspects of the perioperative care of surgical patients, especially those with metabolic disorders or endocrinopathies, are most easily understood when viewed within the framework of these physiologic, hormonal, and metabolic responses to tissue damage. Some responses, especially those that are poorly understood, seem essential; others, such as pain, can be circumvented without apparent harm. Perioperative medical management supports the adaptive portions of the stress response and modifies those that are harmful. This chapter reviews the nature of the hypermetabolic response and the implications of preexisting metabolic and hormonal disorders.

Physiologic Responses: Shock and Hypermetabolism

■ Initial or Shock Response

The time course of the stress response is depicted in Figure 24-1. Following either traumatic injury or an elective operation, there is an initial phase of several hours in which energy expenditure decreases below baseline levels. This period corresponds to *circulatory shock,* an initial phase that allows for the preservation of vital organs and ultimately survival. Basal metabolism decreases and blood flow to organs other than heart or brain diminishes as cardiac output decreases. The duration of this shock phase is reduced by fluid administration and attenuated by both regional and general anesthesia, as it is initiated and driven primarily by sympathetic neural mechanisms, including pain responses. With anesthesia and appropriate fluid management, shock may be transient and barely detectable. Failure of the ebb phase to resolve is incompatible with survival.

■ The Period of Hypermetabolism

After shock resolves, there follows a period of obligatory hypermetabolism. To limit further damage and initiate tissue repair, white cells are activated, hepatic protein synthesis is directed toward the manufacture of acute-phase reactants, and somatic muscle is mobilized into constituent amino acids both for synthesis of structural and enzymatic protein and as a source of energy. Fat is mobilized as an energy source, glucose production by the liver increases, and blood flow is directed toward injured tissue and those organs involved in the provision of energy and material for repair. The overall metabolic rate increases, in part to meet the needs of leukocytes (which use the bulk of the glucose) and hepatocytes (which burn fat) and in part reflecting the protein synthetic requirements of the wound. In the initial subphase of this response, substrate does not reach damaged tissue, which is

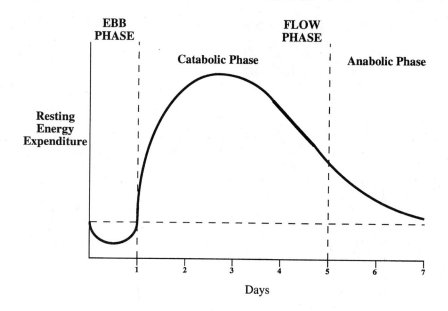

Figure 24-1

Schematic diagram of the time course of the stress response. See text for details.

essentially avascular. Thus the signal stimulating the increase in metabolism, which appears to originate in the substrate-deprived wound tissue, intensifies. This period, which Moore termed the *catabolic phase* because of the dramatic consumption of endogenous tissue, is accompanied by decreased vascular tone, increased cardiac output, capillary recruitment, and leaking of fluid out of the vascular space and into the tissue matrix. The result is anasarca and an increased need for fluid, which also leads to renal salt and water retention and movement of water out of cells and into the extracellular space.

By about the fourth postinjury day, angiogenesis is complete, and neovascularization of damaged tissue has occurred. Substrate needed by damaged tissue is delivered, and demand decreases. The capillary leak seals, the vasculature constricts, fluid is mobilized to be excreted or to move back into cells, metabolic rate and cardiac output decrease, and metabolism is geared toward repletion of the body cell mass. This second subphase is termed *anabolism*. Actual repletion can take months, but in the absence of complications, the increased metabolism usually recedes to baseline levels by day 6 or 7. In general, the time course of the hypermetabolic phase is consistent and difficult to modify using current therapy. High epidural anesthesia blocks the response, but once the epidural is discontinued, anabolism follows the predicted time course. This implies that the response is obligatory and essential. The magnitude of the response is a function of the magnitude of the injury. It

may be difficult to detect any change in the metabolism of an elderly patient undergoing an elective herniorrhaphy, while the victim of severe trauma may develop a resting energy expenditure of up to three times normal.

The mediators of the hypermetabolic phase include at least local tissue products (histamine, bradykinin, serotonin, nitric oxide, endothelins), white blood cell mediators (cytokines, nitric oxide, and growth factors), eicosanoids (prostaglandins, leukotrienes and thromboxanes), the sympathetic nervous system, and other hormonal mediators. Serum epinephrine concentrations increase during the course of operation and then return to baseline in most elective operations but remain increased after trauma and sepsis. In contrast, norepinephrine concentrations are increased for as long as 5 days after elective surgery; the source of this increase appears to be sympathetic nerve terminals and not the adrenal medulla. Cortisol secretion is increased, and the response of the adrenal cortex to ACTH is doubled. Arginine vasopressin may increase as much as 50-fold for up to 5 days, while changes in the renin-angiotensin system are inconsistent. However, aldosterone secretion is uniformly increased after elective operation, and activation of renin-angiotensin is more predictable in more profoundly ill patients. Serum glucose concentrations tend to increase due to increased secretion of catechols, glucagon, and cortisol. Finally, there are transient increases in total and free T_4, free T_3, and thyroid-stimulating hormone (TSH) secretion, followed by reductions in T_3 and T_4 that persist for about a week. There is often a significant increase in reverse T_3, a pattern of altered deiodination similar to the euthyroid sick syndrome (see below).

These profound changes in metabolic and endocrine function make it evident that preexisting endocrine and metabolic disorders exert profound impacts on the responses to surgical and traumatic stress, both in the operating room and postoperatively.

Preexisting Metabolic States

▪ Malnutrition

Malnutrition is by definition the inappropriate loss of body cell mass. When this loss is due to the inadequate intake of macronutrients (protein, carbohydrate, and fat), the process is referred to as *protein-energy malnutrition* (PEM). PEM represents a broad continuum of abnormalities, but two are common among patients presenting for operation. PEM can result from starvation without an increase in metabolic rate. Metabolic rate decreases, and there is a uniform loss of fat and muscle and a proportionate loss of total-body water. In contrast, PEM can be brought about by hypermetabolism due to the stress response described above or cancer, thyrotoxicosis, hyperadrenergic states, or inflammatory diseases. In hypermetabolism, protein in skeletal muscle is spared relative to visceral protein and fat stores, and water is retained in the extracellular compartment despite depletion of intracellular water.

Starvation and hypermetabolism have important but different implications for perioperative management. Malnutrition is the most common metabolic or endocrinologic abnormality among surgical patients. The patient suffering from starvation presents the classic cachectic appearance. Although total quantities of such serum transport proteins as albumin decrease because of decreased hepatic protein synthesis, concentrations in circulation may not decrease until malnutrition is severe, because water loss parallels protein loss. Conversely, the anasarca associated with hypermetabolism may mask significant loss of body cell mass, since the retention of water may maintain or increase body weight. At the same time, the alterations in hepatic protein synthesis and expansion of the vascular compartment brought about by stress may lead to a decrease in serum protein concentrations before significant depletion of body cell mass.

Treatments of the two forms of malnutrition differ. Simple starvation responds to provision of substrate in any form, but the neurohormonal milieu of hypermetabolism impairs glucose utilization, so glucose administration may lead to hyperglycemia, hyperinsulinemia, osmotic diuresis, dehydration, lactic acidosis, and increased risks for cerebrovascular abnormalities and intrahepatic fat deposition. Outcomes are poor because of the specific abnormalities associated with severe malnutrition in cardiac, pulmonary, renal, gastrointestinal (GI), hepatic, central nervous system (CNS), and immunologic function.

Appropriate perioperative management of the malnourished patient first requires repletion if the operation can be delayed. When this is not possible, the management plan must deal with the pathophysiologic consequences of malnutrition. Since cardiac muscle atrophies in proportion to other muscle, the patient may have inadequate cardiac reserve. Electrocardiographic (ECG) abnormalities consistent with ischemia have been noted, as have escape beats and ventricular tachycardia. Anesthetics with potential for myocardial depression must be used judiciously, and inotropic or antiarrhythmic agents may be needed. There is wasting of respiratory muscle, a decrease in surfactant production, and loss of functional residual capacity. Parenchymal lung mass is also reduced; severe malnutrition may produce emphysema. Prolonged ventilatory support may be necessary. Renal clearance of creatinine, free water, and most solutes diminish as does the ability to concentrate the urine. Thus salt and water loads may be poorly tolerated, and renal metabolism and excretion of drugs and toxins may be limited. Impaired GI motility may increase the risk of pulmonary aspiration, and altered absorption may make oral medications ineffective. Unpredictable hepatic metabolism and lower amounts of transport proteins may alter pharmacokinetics and drug action. Impaired immune function mandates strict adherence to sterile technique for invasive procedures. Peripheral neuropathy that often accompanies malnutrition may influence the use of regional and major conduction anesthesia.

▪ Obesity

Although obesity is defined as a body weight of 20 percent greater than ideal, marked alterations in perioperative risk occur only in patients who are morbidly obese. Those who are either twice their ideal weight or who weigh 100 lbs more than the ideal suffer excess perioperative mortality. Morbidly obese men between the ages of 25 and 35 experience a mortality rate 11 times that of the population as a whole.

Obesity has significant effects on pulmonary, cardiovascular, GI, and renal function. Overall metabolic demand in these patients is increased in direct proportion to body mass; oxygen consumption, carbon dioxide production, and minute ventilation increase to compensate. Respiratory muscles appear to be less efficient in obese patients, primarily reflecting the loss of compliance associated with increased chest wall mass. Functional residual capacity (FRC), expiratory reserve volume, vital capacity, and total lung volume are markedly reduced. This contributes not only to baseline hypoxemia but also to hypoxemia occurring with apnea, hypoventilation, or the supine position. Obesity has been demonstrated to be a significant predictor of cardiovascular disease, especially coronary artery atherosclerosis, hypertension, stroke, congestive heart failure, arrhythmias, myocardial infarction, and sudden death. Gastrointestinal function is altered; increased gastric volume and acidity place obese patients at risk for aspiration pneumonitis. In addition, hepatic drug metabolism may be affected because fatty infiltration, inflammation, focal necrosis, and cirrhosis occur in the livers of obese individuals. Enhanced biotransformation of volatile agents has been reported, and this, in combination with the large adipose compartment and altered volume of distribution, makes the pharmacokinetics not only of inhaled anesthetics but of all drugs less predictable. Renal changes in obesity include proteinuria, changes consistent with diabetic nephropathy (even in patients without glucose intolerance) and an increased glomerular filtration rate (GFR), but there is no report documenting consistent appearance of renal dysfunction in the obese patient.

A subset of morbidly obese patients of particular concern in the perioperative period are those with the obesity-hypoventilation, or Pickwickian, syndrome. These are patients who retain carbon dioxide as the result of alveolar hypoventilation. Chronic hypercarbia increases pulmonary artery pressure, impedes right ventricular outflow, limits left-sided venous return, and causes passive congestion of the liver. The risk of operation is great for these patients.

The physiologic abnormalities of obesity carry implications for perioperative management. It is essential to reduce pulmonary risk, for example, by cessation of smoking, and to evaluate the patient for cardiac disease. In the morbidly obese, blood gas analysis may identify those who retain CO_2. Premedication is best avoided in individuals with respiratory compromise. Prophylaxis against aspiration is unproven but seems to be prudent. Technical considerations may preclude regional anesthetic techniques, but issues of airway management and loss of FRC may restrict the use of general anesthesia. Continuous positive airway pressure (CPAP) may help overcome the loss of FRC and may also improve pulmonary compliance, but it may impair ventricular filling. Postoperative hypoxemia and hypoventilation are major concerns. In addition, the obese may be at increased risk for deep venous thrombosis and pulmonary embolism. Finally, the increased risk of myocardial ischemia calls for careful management and early intervention for this potentially avoidable complication.

Preexisting Endocrine Disorders

■ Diabetes Mellitus

Diabetes is a complex disease that affects perioperative management. In type I, or juvenile-onset diabetes, pancreatic insulin production is deficient; in type II, or adult-onset diabetes, responses to insulin are abnormal. Insulin not only alters glucose homeostasis but also affects cellular handling of fat and amino acids and has significant effects on cell growth and differentiation. This global disorder of metabolism produces complications due to hyperglycemia or hypoglycemia, and the associated organ dysfunction predisposes to morbidity and mortality.

The hormonal milieu associated with the stress response promotes hyperglycemia. In the type I diabetic patient, the lack of insulin exacerbates this response because of loss of the inhibitory effects exerted by insulin. Insulin blocks fat release from adipocytes, inhibits liberation of amino acids from skeletal (but not smooth) muscle, opposes the gluconeogenic effects of the counterregulatory hormones, promotes glycogenesis, and prevents ketone formation. This last explains why ketoacidosis is prominent in type I but not in type II patients who produce insulin.

The surgical patient with diabetes is at risk for hyperglycemia, but no study has documented the benefits of close control of blood glucose in the perioperative period. In fact, one could argue that

Table 24-1

Diseases and Disorders Associated with Diabetes

System	Diseases and Disorders
Cardiovascular	Coronary artery disease
	Myocardial infarction
	Congestive heart failure
	Hypertension
	Peripheral vascular disease, including aortic aneurysms
	Cerebrovascular disease and stroke
Urologic	Urosepsis, voiding abnormalities due to diabetic neuropathy
Renal	Renal insufficiency
Neurologic	Stroke
	Peripheral diabetic neuropathy
	Autonomic neuropathy
	Loss of heart rate variability
	Resting tachycardia
	Palpitations
	Loss of exercise tolerance
	Orthostatic hypotension
	Syncope
Gastrointestinal	Decreased esophageal and gastric motility
Airway	Stiff joints in cervical and thoracic spine and jaw
	Increased incidence of "difficult intubation"

overtreatment, leading to hypoglycemia and cerebral high-energy phosphate depletion, is potentially as harmful as undertreatment. However, it is important to manage blood glucose appropriately. Hyperglycemia and the accompanying osmotic diuresis may produce dehydration, especially because the renal threshold for spilling sugar appears to be decreased by inflammation. Hyperglycemia has been associated with poor neurologic outcome following cerebral ischemic events; this has been shown convincingly in animals, and may apply in humans.

Overall, it seems best to maintain blood glucose in the range of 150 to 250 mg/dl, prevent dehydration, and treat osmotic diuresis with aggressive fluid administration. This may be accomplished by withholding or reducing morning doses of intermediate-acting insulin, measuring glucose concentrations frequently, and administering glucose or short-acting insulin as necessary. In the "brittle" diabetic patient, the best strategy may be early use of continuous intravenous insulin.

Good care also allows for the effects of diabetes-induced organ system dysfunction on the stress re-sponse. Diabetic patients are at increased risk for a number of diseases that affect perioperative management (Table 24-1).

■ Disorders of the Adrenal Cortex

Adrenal cortical steroids produce three effects: glucocorticoid effects, which involve substrate metabolism (Table 24-2); mineralocorticoid effects on sodium, potassium, and acid-base homeostasis (Table 24-3); and androgenic or estrogenic effects. A listing of common exogenous glucocorticoids and their relative glucocorticoid and mineralocorticoid potencies is noted in Table 24-4.

Glucocorticoids

The primary glucocorticoid in humans is cortisol. Glucocorticoid action is primarily permissive, that is, glucocorticoids typically potentiate the effects of other hormones, most notably catecholamines. Secretion of cortisol is controlled by a complex series of negative feedback loops involving all the components of the hypothalamic-pituitary-adrenal axis. States that alter cortisol-binding globulin concentrations, noted in Table 24-5, are important in determining cortisol effects. Similarly, cortisol is inactivated via hepatic transformation; disorders that affect the liver may alter the metabolism of cortisol.

Causes of glucocorticoid deficiency are noted in Table 24-6, but the most common are idiopathic (presumably autoimmune) and the withdrawal of chronic steroid therapy. Glucocorticoid deficiency leads to hypoglycemia and impaired responses to catechols and glucagon. Of primary concern in the perioperative period are the cardiovascular changes:

Table 24-2

Biologic Activity of Glucocorticoids

Carbohydrate metabolism
1. Increased hepatic gluconeogenesis
2. Inhibition of glucose uptake by adipocytes, fibroblasts, lymphoid cells and perhaps skeletal muscle
3. Increased hepatic glycogen deposition
4. Peripheral glycogenolysis

Lipid metabolism
1. Increased peripheral lipolysis
2. Diminished reesterification, especially hepatic

Protein metabolism
1. Stimulation of hepatic protein synthesis
2. Decreased peripheral protein synthesis
3. Stimulation of peripheral protein catabolism

Table 24-3

Biologic Activity of Mineralocorticoids
Sodium conservation
Potassium secretion
Hydrogen ion secretion

Table 24-5

Conditions Associated with Altered Concentrations of Corticosteroid-Binding Globulin

Increased	Decreased
Pregnancy	Liver disease
Oral contraceptive use	Multiple myeloma
Hyperthyroidism	Hypothyroidism
Diabetes	Obesity
Hematologic disorders	Nephrosis

hypotension and decreased cardiac output despite adequate fluid therapy. Altered renal function leads to retention of potassium, acid, and water and to hypercalcemia. Severe glucocorticoid deficiency may require treatment in the perioperative period with inotropes or vasoconstrictors, and it may be prudent to avoid agents with vasodilator or myocardial depressant properties if such a diagnosis is suspected.

Cortisol excess results in increases in basal energy expenditure, oxygen consumption and carbon dioxide production, as well as hyperglycemia. Generalized muscle wasting affects the heart and the diaphragm as well. Free fatty acids are mobilized, but reesterification is impaired; this may account for the deposition of fat in the truncal region characteristic of Cushingoid patients. Blood pressure is increased, perhaps as a result of enhanced sensitivity to catecholamines. Glomerular filtration rate (GFR) is increased, renal acid and potassium wasting may occur, and calcium and phosphate may be lost as well. There may be impaired inflammatory responses, increased rates of infection, and perhaps inhibition of wound healing. Adrenocorticoid excess may be due to exogenous steroid administration or to endocrine-active tumors such as adrenal or pituitary adenomas, oat cell carcinoma of the lung, thymoma, islet cell tumors, carcinoid tumors, medullary cancer of the thyroid, or

pheochromocytoma. Acute treatment consists of control of heart rate, blood pressure, alkalosis and deficiencies of potassium and phosphate.

Mineralocorticoids

The major mineralocorticoid is aldosterone, but both cortisol and 11-hydroxycorticosterone also act on renal, GI, salivary, vascular, and neural tissues to conserve sodium. Secretion is largely controlled by the renin-angiotensin system; angiotensin II is the most potent stimulator of aldosterone. Unlike cortisol, aldosterone circulates essentially unbound, but excretion depends on hepatic conversion and thus on hepatic blood flow.

Mineralocorticoid deficiency causes hypovolemia, hyperkalemia, hyponatremia, hypochloremic acidosis, and hemoconcentration. In the absence of stress, this is well tolerated, but in stress states or with reduced sodium intake, hypotension, vascular collapse, dysrhythmias, and cardiac arrest can occur. The most common cause of this disorder is the exogenous administration of glucocorticoids with little mineralo-

Table 24-4

Relative Potency of Exogenous Steroid Preparations

Compound	Relative Glucocorticoid Potency	Relative Mineralocorticoid Potency
Cortisone (as acetate)	1	1
Hydrocortisone (Cortisol)	0.8	0.8
Prednisone	3.5–4.5	
Prednisolone	4	0.8
Methylprednisolone	5	0.5
Triamcinolone	5	0
Dexamethasone	30	0
Fluorocortisone	10	125

Table 24-6

Conditions Associated with Glucocorticoid Deficiency

Withdrawal of glucocorticoid drugs
Idiopathic (autoimmune)
Tuberculosis
AIDS
Lymphoma
Enzyme inhibitors
Inborn errors of metabolism
Fungal infections
Metastatic cancer
Pituitary disease
Cytotoxic agents

corticoid activity (Table 24-4); heparin and nonsteroidal anti-inflammatory drugs also may be associated with mineralocorticoid deficiency. Therapy involves simply administering appropriate amounts of salt and water.

Primary hyperaldosteronism (Conn's syndrome), most often the result of adrenal tumors or hyperplasia, is characterized by hypokalemia, sodium retention, and hypertension. Alkalosis may occur, but only in severe cases do polyuria, polydipsia, nocturia, weakness, paraesthesias, and tetany become manifest. Secondary hyperaldosteronism reflects underlying conditions such as congestive heart failure (CHF), nephrosis, cirrhosis, dehydration (as with chronic diuretic use), pregnancy (especially in the preeclamptic patient), oral contraceptive use, and other states in which the effective blood volume may be reduced. Therapy is most often directed toward the underlying condition.

Glucocorticoids, the Stress Response, and Replacement Therapy

The stress response to surgery or trauma and anesthesia includes increases in secretions of glucocorticoids. Because it is feared that they will be unable to achieve the usual response, patients likely to suffer a deficiency of endogenous glucocorticoid secretion are often given replacement therapy with large doses of glucocorticoids. The controversy about this practice involves four issues: identifying patients incapable of responding to surgical stress; the effects of relative glucocorticoid deficiency; the risks of overreplacement; and choosing rational recommendations for potentially steroid-dependent patients.

The patients most often thought to be at risk are those treated with corticosteroids who are expected to suffer adrenal suppression. The potential for adrenal suppression is well founded; even a single dose of steroids may be sufficient to reduce the adrenal response to stimulation. However, it is not clear what ill effects can be expected from attenuation of the adrenal response. A series of anecdotal reports, beginning in the 1950s, implicated glucocorticoid deficiency as the cause of unexplained perioperative hypotension. Prior to operation, most of these patients had received steroids for a variety of conditions, and these medications were discontinued on hospitalization. In animals, it is clear that glucocorticoid deficiency impairs normal recovery from operation. On the other hand, many patients have had steroids withdrawn before operation and suffered no ill effects. Thus, although Addisonian crisis is possible with surgical stress and some basal glucocorticoid level appears necessary, it is difficult to predict who is truly in need of supplementation.

Current practice frequently involves the administration of large doses (i.e., 300 mg of cortisol per day) to patients undergoing surgical procedures. Where and why this practice originated is unclear. Blood concentrations that extrapolate to this dose have been measured in patients undergoing cardiopulmonary resuscitation (CPR). However, the use of such doses may be associated with an increase in complications, including death, sepsis, infection, wound dehiscence, immune suppression, salt and water wasting, and exacerbations of hypertension, diabetes, and CHF.

In light of these data, Salem has presented a rational scheme for replacement of steroids in the perioperative period based on the dose of steroids taken preoperatively, the duration of this therapy, and the type of procedure (Table 24-7). As an alternative, it is reasonable to administer the normal daily dose of steroids prior to operation and to supplement with small doses (25 mg cortisol equivalent) if otherwise unexplained hypotension develops.

Anesthetics and Corticosteroids

The only directly demonstrated interactions between anesthetic agents and corticosteroids are the suppressive effects of etomidate and the potentiation by exogenous steroids of the duration of action of steroid-based muscle relaxants. This last has been reported to result in muscle degeneration and a need for prolonged ventilatory support.

Table 24-7

Recommendations for Perioperative Glucocorticoid Supplements in Patients Believed to Have Adrenocorticoid Deficiency

Level of Stress	Recommendation (Hydrocortisone Equivalent/day)
Minor surgical stress (e.g., inguinal herniorrhaphy)	25 mg × 1 day
Moderate surgical stress (e.g., open cholecystectomy, lower extremity revascularization, subtotal colectomy, total joint replacement, abdominal hysterectomy)	50–75 mg × 2 days
Major surgical stress (e.g., Whipple's procedure, esophagogastrectomy, total proctocolectomy, cardiopulmonary bypass)	100–150 mg × 2–3 days

Adapted from Salem M, Tainsh RE, Bromberg J et al: Perioperative glucocorticoid coverage; A reassessment 42 years after emergence of a problem. *Ann Surg* 1994;219:416.

■ Disorders of Thyroid Function

Thyroid Physiology and Pharmacology

Physiologically active thyroid hormone circulates as either T_4 (levothyroxine) or the more potent T_3 (triiodothyronine). Most T_4 or T_3 is bound to T_4-binding globulin (TBG); only the free form of the hormone is metabolically active. This distinction is important when binding-protein concentrations or affinities are altered in states such as sepsis, in which TBG as well as albumin may be depleted, or pregnancy, in which TGB levels are increased. Thyroid hormone stimulates metabolism by increasing metabolic rate, accelerating protein turnover, and facilitating lipolysis. The role actually played by thyroid hormones in the stress response is undetermined. In the early perioperative period T_4 generally increases, while T_3 decreases, but both decrease as the response progresses for several days.

Hyperthyroidism

The clinical manifestations of hyperthyroidism range from asymptomatic abnormalities of laboratory values to the severe metabolic derangements seen in thyroid storm. The two most characteristic symptoms are heat intolerance and weight loss. Other signs and symptoms are noted in Table 24-8. It is not appropriate for routine preoperative screening to include laboratory testing for thyroid disease; detection depends on a carefully taken history and the physical examination. Most commonly, thyrotoxicosis is a consequence of Graves' disease, an autoimmune disorder otherwise known as *diffuse toxic goiter*. Goiter is commonly associated with all forms of hyperthyroidism, with the exception of exogenous thyroid hormone intake. Airway abnormalities may accompany goiter, including recurrent laryngeal nerve compression, tracheal deviation, and airway narrowing. The lack of hyperkinesis in the elderly may obscure the diagnosis.

Hyperthyroidism produces dysfunction in a number of different organ systems that must be taken into account when planning anesthesia (Table 24-9). Although thyrotoxicosis resembles sympathetic excess, plasma catecholamine concentrations are normal. It is possible that plasma concentrations do not correlate with biologic effect or that thyroid hormone increases the sensitivity of adrenergic receptors to stimulation. The most extreme form of hyperthyroidism is thyroid storm, characterized by arrhythmias, increased cardiac output, pulmonary edema, nausea and vomiting, sweating, dehydration, and increased core temperature; these symptoms mimic malignant hyperthermia. Most often, thyroid storm is found in either undiagnosed or incompletely treated patients or patients in whom a stress response has been provoked by concomitant illness. Left untreated, thyroid storm is often fatal.

Definitive treatment of hyperthyroidism consists of suppression of thyroid hormone synthesis or release

Table 24-8

Signs and Symptoms of Thyroid Excess
Nervousness
Diaphoresis
Heat intolerance
Palpitations
Dyspnea
Weakness and fatigability
Fluctuations in weight
Increased appetite
Diarrhea and increased colonic motility
Goiter
Tachycardia
Atrial fibrillation
Hyperkinesis
Proptosis

Table 24-9

Changes in Organ System Function Associated with Hyperthyroidism

Organ System	Functional Alteration
Cardiovascular	Resting tachycardia
	Increased stroke volume
	Increased cardiac output
	Widened pulse pressure
	Arrhythmias
	Premature contractions
	Atrial fibrillation
	Congestive heart failure
	Valvular dysfunction
	Mitral valve prolapse, insufficiency
Pulmonary	Ventilatory failure
	Respiratory muscle myopathy
	Increased carbon dioxide production
	Decreased vital capacity
	Hypoxemia
	Increased oxygen consumption
	Altered Hb affinity for oxygen
Renal/electrolyte	Polyuria
	Hypomagnesemia
	Hypercalcemia and hypercalcuria
GI	Hypermotility
Hepatic	Increased transaminases
	Intrahepatic cholestasis
Musculoskeletal	Myopathies
	Protein wasting
CNS	Nervousness, emotional lability
Metabolic	Increased resting energy expenditure

using methimazole, propylthiouracil (PTU), or iodide. Symptomatic relief can be obtained with beta blockers, which are the mainstays of therapy for hyperthyroid patients requiring immediate operation. Definitive therapy requires 2 to 3 weeks to be effective. The best course of action is to render the patient euthyroid prior to operation. Regional techniques are advantageous, but vasopressors or inotropes used to treat hypotension must be given in reduced doses because of hypersensitivity.

Hypothyroidism

The most common causes of hypothyroidism are hyposecretion of the hormone due to idiopathic atrophy, medical treatment of hyperthyroidism, or surgical removal of the gland. Among those of particular interest in the perioperative period are lithium therapy and the administration of sodium nitroprusside. The effects of hypothyroidism on organ function are listed in Table 24-10.

The pathophysiologic changes associated with mild to moderate hypothyroidism alter perioperative management, but they do not appear to warrant the cancellation of elective surgery, since replacement can begin intraoperatively and management can be tailored to minimize risk. Titration of myocardial and respiratory depressants and careful use of opioids often suffice. There are exceptions, including patients with severe hypothyroidism, myxedema coma, or

Table 24-10

Changes in Organ System Function Associated with Hypothyroidism

Organ System	Functional Alteration
Cardiovascular	Bradycardia at rest
	Decreased stroke volume
	Decreased cardiac output
	Decreased cerebral, renal, and skin blood flow
	Pericardial effusions
	Orthostatic hypotension
	Arrhythmias
	Reentrant tachyarrhythmias
	Prolonged QRS
Pulmonary	Ventilatory failure
	Decreased maximal breathing capacity
	Loss of hypercapnic and hypoxic drives
	Pleural effusions
	Decreased alveolar ventilation
Renal/electrolyte	Decreased plasma volume
	Decreased GFR
	Decreased creatinine clearance
	Peripheral edema
	Hyponatremia
GI	Delayed gastric emptying
	GI bleeding
	Constipation
Hematologic	Anemia
	Platelet hyperaggregability
	Factor VIII and IX deficiency
Musculoskeletal	Myopathies
	Increase of creatinine kinase can produce renal failure
Metabolic	Decreased resting energy expenditure

severe respiratory and cardiovascular instability. These patients require treatment prior to any surgical intervention and do not undergo elective operations until rendered euthyroid. In the event of an emergency in a severely depleted patient, replacement should be started, but cardiovascular and respiratory support may be needed and only minimal doses of anesthetics will be tolerated. Owing to the long half-lives (7 to 10 days) of most thyroid preparations, discontinuing them temporarily is of little consequence.

The Euthyroid Sick Syndrome

The euthyroid sick syndrome is most often noted in debilitated elderly patients or individuals with severe illnesses or prolonged hospital courses, particularly in the intensive care unit. Free T_4 concentrations are often normal, but circulating T_3 is decreased; in addition, reverse T_3 (rT_3) is increased, indicating either increased breakdown of T_4 or failure to metabolize rT_3. Thyroid-stimulating hormone is often normal and the signs and symptoms of hypothyroidism may be absent, but patients are functionally hypothyroid and have poor perioperative outcomes. The role of thyroid replacement in the treatment of euthyroid sick syndrome has not been determined. Management of the syndrome includes preparation for cardiorespiratory collapse.

■ Disorders of the Parathyroids

Calcium homeostasis is under the regulation of three hormones. Parathyroid hormone (PTH) comes from the parathyroid glands. Calcitonin comes from the thyroid and acts to decrease serum calcium levels via bone formation and renal excretion. Vitamin D, which is hydroxylated by the liver and kidney, acts in conjunction with PTH to increase serum calcium levels via bone resorption, GI absorption and renal retention of calcium and loss of phosphate. Calcitonin is of little physiologic consequence in humans, but PTH and Vitamin D are highly important. PTH excretion is stimulated by hypocalcemia and adrenocorticosteroids. Similarly, vitamin D and hypermagnesemia inhibit PTH release.

Hyperparathyroidism

Primary hyperparathyroidism, implying excessive, uncontrolled secretion by the parathyroid glands, is almost entirely the result of benign adenomas; rarely, it is caused by carcinoma or hyperplasia. On occasion,

parathyroid adenomas appear along with medullary carcinoma of the thyroid and pheochromocytoma as part of the multiple endocrine neoplasia type II syndrome. The physiologic effects of PTH excess are those of hypercalcemia, hypomagnesemia, and hypophosphatemia (Table 24-11). Diagnosis is made by measuring serum ionized calcium and PTH concentrations. Treatment is most often accomplished with saline diuresis; mithramycin, a highly cytotoxic antibiotic, is reserved for extreme cases. Calcium abnormalities also can be corrected with dialysis.

The primary perioperative hazard is cardiac arrhythmia. In addition, the hypophosphatemia can predispose to both cardiac and respiratory depression. Neuromuscular blocking agents must be used with care because both increased and decreased sensitivity have been reported. Treatment of hyperparathyroidism most often involves resection of the offending gland.

Hypoparathyroidism

Hypocalcemia resulting from hypoparathyroidism most commonly occurs following intentional resection of the parathyroid glands. Secondary hypoparathyroidism may result from peripheral resistance to PTH, which accompanies congenital defects, hypomagnesemia, renal insufficiency, malabsorption, or

Table 24-11

Changes in Organ System Function Associated with Hyperparathyroidism

Organ System	Functional Alteration
Cardiovascular	Hypertension
	Peripheral vasoconstriction
	Renin excess
	Elevated levels of vasoactive amines
	Arrhythmias
	Short QT
	Prolonged PR
	Respiratory and cardiac failure
Renal/electrolyte	Decreased GFR
	Nephrolithiasis
	Nephrocalcinosis
	Hypercalcemia
	Hypomagnesemia
	Hypophosphatemia
GI	Peptic ulcers
Musculoskeletal	Osteopenia
	Weakness and fatigue
CNS	Depression
	Lethargy and coma

Table 24-12

Changes in Organ System Function Associated with Hypoparathyroidism (Hypocalcemia)

Organ System	Functional Alteration
Cardiovascular	Arrhythmias
	Increased QT interval
	Increased ST interval
	2:1 heart block
	Ventricular dysrhythmias
	Atrial arrhythmias
	Congestive heart failure
	Cardiac standstill
CNS	Irritability
	Seizures
	Coma
	Hyperreflexia
	Tetany
	Laryngospasm

anticonvulsants. The cardinal sign of this hypocalcemia is tetany, the manifestations of which include Chvostek's (facial nerve hyperreactivity) and Trousseau's (carpopedal spasm) signs; other manifestations of hypocalcemia are noted in Table 24-12. Particularly worrisome is a predisposition to laryngospasm. Altered responses to neuromuscular blocking agents may be present just as in hypercalcemia. In the patient whose PTH decreases following surgical resection,

the onset of hypocalcemia may be abrupt. This is less well tolerated than a slow decrease. Treatment is by administration of calcium gluconate or calcium chloride. Avoiding rapid overcorrection is important; magnesium can be administered acutely to treat tetany and allow for a slow repletion of calcium.

BIBLIOGRAPHY

Bessey PQ, Watters JM, Aoki TT, Wilmore D. Combined hormonal infusion simulates the metabolic response to injury. *Ann Surg* 1984;200:264.

Bistrian BR, Blackburn GL, Hallowell E. Protein status of general surgical patients. *JAMA* 1974;230:858.

Breslow MJ. Neuroendocrine responses to surgery. In Breslow MJ, Miller CF, Rogers MC, eds: *Perioperative Management.* St Louis: Mosby–Year Book, 1990, p 180.

Cerra FB. Hypermetabolism, organ failure and metabolic support. *Surgery* 1987;101:1.

Cork RC, Vaughan RW, Bentley JB. General anesthesia for morbidly obese patients: An examination of postoperative outcomes. *Anesthesiology* 1981;54: 310.

Cuthbertson D, Tilstone W. Metabolism in the post-injury period. *Adv Clin Chem* 1977;12:1.

Moore FD, Olesen KH, McMurrey JC, et al. *The Body Cell Mass and Its Supporting Environment.* Philadelphia: WB Saunders, 1978.

Salem M, Tainsh RE, Bromberg J, et al. Perioperative glucocorticoid coverage: A reassessment 42 years after emergence of a problem. *Ann Surg* 1994;219: 416.

Udelsman R, Ramp J, Gallucchi WT, et al. Adaptation during surgical stress: A reevaluation of the role of glucocorticoids. *J Clin Invest* 1986;77:1377.

25

Pediatric Anesthesia

Eugene K. Betts and John J. Downes

Infants and children requiring anesthesia present unique challenges to the anesthesiologist. This chapter presents an approach to the management of these challenges.

Pediatric Physiology

The essential features of physiologic function that form the basis of rational anesthesia management of children are presented here to serve as a basis for the subsequent discussions of pharmacology and clinical care.

■ Pulmonary and Cardiovascular Systems

Fetal Cardiopulmonary Development

At 16 weeks of gestation, the tracheobronchial tree has achieved 16 branching generations ending in the terminal bronchiole, the distal growth center for development of the essential functional pulmonary unit, the acinus. If through disease, genetic defect, or the pressure of a space-occupying lesion (e.g., diaphragmatic hernia) the lungs fail to develop all 16 branches by this stage, pulmonary hypoplasia results.

At 24 weeks the pulmonary capillaries come into closer approximation with the primitive alveolar saccules, and the type II alveolar epithelial cells begin to secrete an immature form of alveolar phospholipid lining that can function as a surfactant at a gas-liquid interface. The potential for alveolar gas exchange with pulmonary capillary blood thus begins. The diffusion barrier for oxygen, the matching of capillary flow with the alveolar epithelial membrane and alveolar gas, the stability of the alveoli, and the central control of breathing remain inadequate for effective spontaneous and unsupported ventilation in most infants until at least 28 weeks gestation.

At birth, the total lung volume, crying vital capacity, and functional residual capacity (FRC) are all significantly less per unit body mass than they are at over age 7 years, but especially less when compared with the infant's metabolic needs and alveolar ventilation. In the normal newborn, the average FRC of 30 ml/kg is only somewhat less than the mean adult value of 34 ml/kg, but the ratios of FRC to alveolar minute ventilation differ greatly (newborn 0.23, adult 0.56), indicating a much greater reserve volume of gas in the lung of the adult in relation to alveolar ventilation (Table 25-1).

Cardiopulmonary Adaptation to Extrauterine Life

The fetal cardiovascular system, well established by the eighth week of gestation, performs admirably with the placenta as the organ of fetal external gas exchange. The flow pattern depicted in Figure 25-1, a parallel circuit, must adapt to increased pulmonary blood flow at birth, accompanied by closure of the ductus arteriosus and foramen ovale, resulting in a series circuit. The central feature in this adaptation consists of an abrupt and substantial reduction in the pulmonary vascular resistance of the fetal circuit, which in utero allows only 10 percent of the right ventricular output to flow through the lungs (see Fig. 25-1).

Table 25-1

Pulmonary Function (Mean Values)	Newborn	Adult
Body weight (kg)	3	70
Cal/kg/h [large calories (kcal)]	2	1
Oxygen consumption ($\dot{V}O_2$) (ml/kg/min)	7.0	3.5
CO_2 production ($\dot{V}CO_2$) (ml/kg/min)	5.5	3.0
Expired minute volume $\dot{V}CO_2$ ($\dot{V}E$) (ml/kg/min)	200–210	90–100
Tidal volume (V_T)(ml/kg)	6	6
Respiratory rate (*f*) (breaths/min)	35–60	15–20
Anatomic dead space (V_D) (ml/kg)	2.5	2.0
Physiologic dead space–tidal volume ratio (V_D/V_T)	0.3	0.3
Alveolar ventilation ($\dot{V}A$) (ml/kg/min)	130	60
Total lung capacity (TLC) (ml/kg)	63	82
Vital capacity (VC) (ml/kg)	35	70
Functional residual capacity (FRC) (ml/kg)	30	34
FRC/$\dot{V}A$	0.23	0.56
Tracheal internal diameter (mm)	4	16
Tracheal length (mm)	57	120

Adapted with permission from Fisher BJ, Carlo WA, Doershak CF: Pulmonary function from infancy through adolescence. In Scarpelli EM, ed: *Pulmonary Physiology: Fetus, Newborn, Child, Adolescent,* 2nd ed. Philadelphia: Lea and Febiger, 1990, p 429.

The cardiac output of the newborn meets changing metabolic demands primarily by adjustments in heart rate because the stiff ventricular walls limit the ability to vary stroke volume. A reduction in heart rate greater than 20 to 30 percent below normal values in a newborn or young infant (i.e., a rate less than 100 beats per minute) invariably causes a reduction in cardiac output.

The principal differences in the blood of the fetus compared with that of the older infant are the presence of fetal hemoglobin and relatively small concentrations of 2,3-diphosphoglyceraldehyde (2,3-DPG) in the red cells. Fetal hemoglobin binds oxygen more readily than does adult hemoglobin; this is characterized by a left-shifted oxyhemoglobin dissociation curve (Fig. 25-2). Combined with lesser 2,3-DPG concentrations, this favors uptake of oxygen in the placenta (or lung) but results in lesser volumes of oxygen unloaded in the peripheral tissues at physiologic capillary oxygen tensions (Table 25-2).

Failure of the newborn to establish or maintain adequate alveolar ventilation or pulmonary blood flow causes persistent acidemia and hypoxemia, which in turn causes opening of the ductus, pulmonary vasoconstriction, increased pulmonary vascular resistance, diminished pulmonary blood flow, and a decrease in the left atrial pressure below that in the right atrium, opening the foramen ovale. Fatal asphyxia ensues unless this cycle is interrupted quickly by controlled alveolar ventilation with oxygen.

The integrated control of breathing is not well developed even in the full-term newborn (37 to 42 weeks gestation). Over 70 percent of preterm newborns experience periodic breathing, with nearly half of these suffering prolonged apneic episodes accompanied by bradycardia and arterial hemoglobin desaturation well below 90 percent. The development of ventilatory control parallels the gestational (or postconceptual) age from 25 weeks, when protracted apnea with severe hypoxemia nearly always occurs if the fetus is born, through 40 weeks, when apnea causing serious hypoxemia rarely occurs (see Table 25-2).

Cardiopulmonary Development in the Neonate and Infant

The neonate (age 1 to 28 days) and infant (age 1 to 12 months) undergo cardiopulmonary development that strengthens considerably their abilities not only to meet basic metabolic needs but also to withstand infection or trauma (such as that incurred in surgical operations). These include the following:

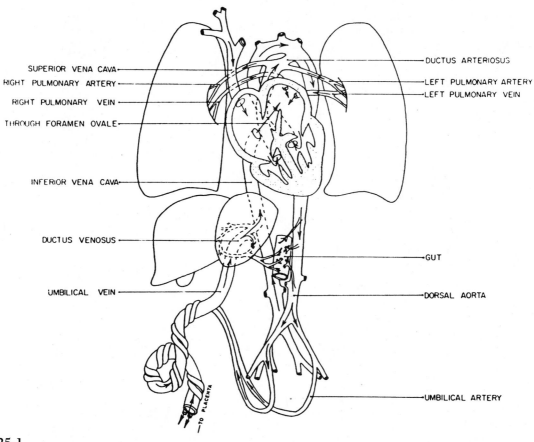

Figure 25-1

Schematic representation of the fetal circulation (not to scale).
(Reproduced with permission from Avery ME: The Lung and Its Disorders. *Philadelphia: WB Saunders, 1964.)*

1. Integrated central control of ventilation matures.
2. Expansion of total lung volume continues.
3. Stiffening of the thoracic wall provides tethering forces that help maintain small airways.
4. Maturation of the diaphragm and chest wall muscles increase the power available for breathing and coughing.
6. Pulmonary vascular resistance is reduced further.
7. The left ventricular wall thickens relative to the right ventricle.
8. Stroke volume increases and heart rate decreases (Fig. 25-3).
9. Physiologic anemia reaches its nadir at 12 weeks, but by age 6 months, fetal hemoglobin is replaced and total hemoglobin concentration is well above 10 g/dl.

Thus, by the end of infancy at 12 months of age, the cardiopulmonary system approaches that of the adult (see Table 25-2 and Figs. 25-3 and 25-4). Maturation continues throughout childhood and adolescence until functional adulthood at age 15 (Table 25-3).

■ Central and Autonomic Nervous Systems

A detailed review of nervous system development lies beyond the scope and purpose of this chapter; the features significant to anesthesia management include the following:

1. The newborn brain constitutes 12 percent of the body weight and receives approximately 34 percent of the cardiac output compared

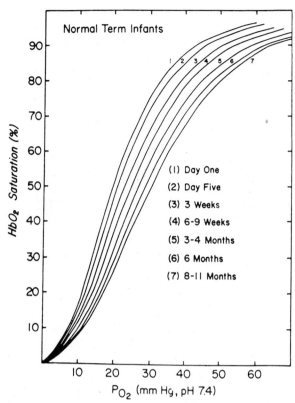

Figure 25-2

The P_{50} of 19 mmHg on day 1 shifts to 30 mmHg at 11 months of age.

(Reproduced with permission from Smith CA, Nelson NM: Physiology of the Newborn Infant, *4th ed. Springfield, Ill: Charles C Thomas, 1976.)*

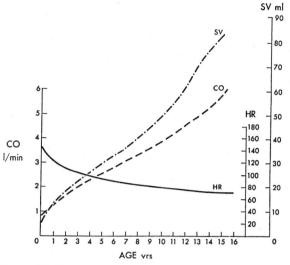

Figure 25-3

Postnatal changes in cardiac output (CO), heart rate (HR), and stroke volume (SV) from birth to 16 years.

(Reproduced with permission from Rudolph AM: Congenital Heart Disease. *Chicago: Year Book Medical Publishers, 1974.)*

with the adult, whose brain represents 2 percent of body weight and receives about 14 percent of the cardiac output.

2. The newborn's blood-brain barrier is far more permeable than that of the older child or adult to molecules that are lipid-soluble (e.g., bilirubin and barbiturates).

3. The fetus, by the time of viability (24 to 25 weeks gestation), responds to noxious stimuli with facial grimaces as well as significant

Table 25-2

Normal Arterial pH, Blood Gas Tensions, Hematocrit (Mean ± SD)

	Age				
	1 h	**24 h**	**1–24 mos**	**Child**	**Adult**
pHa	7.33	7.37 (.03)	7.40 (.03)	7.39 (.02)	7.40 (.03)
$PaCO_2$ (mmHg)	36 (4)	33 (3)	34 (4)	37 (3)	39 (5)
Base excess (mEq/liter)	−6.0 (1)	−5.0 (1)	−3.0 (3)	−2.0 (2)	0.0 (2)
PaO_2 (21% O_2) (mmHg)	63 (11)	73 (10)	—	95 (4)	95 (4)
Hematocrit (vol%)	53 (5)	55 (7)	35 (2.5)	38 (2)	45 (4)

Adapted with permission from Koch G, Wendel H: Adjustment of arterial blood gases and acid base balance in the normal newborn infant during the first week of life. *Biol Neonate* 1968;12;136–161; Levison H, Featherby EA, et al: Arterial blood gases, alveolararterial oxygen difference, and physiologic dead space in children and young adults. *Am Rev Respir Dis* 1970;101;972; Albert MS, Winters R: Acid-base equilibrium of blood in normal infants. *Pediatrics* 1966;37;728–732.

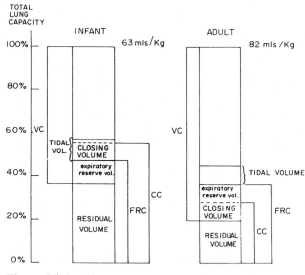

Figure 25-4

Lung volumes in the infant and adult.

(Reproduced with permission from Smith CA, Nelson NM: The Physiology of the Newborn Infant, 4th ed. Springfield, Ill: Charles C Thomas, 1976.)

cardiovascular and metabolic changes, indicating probable perception of pain.

4. At term, the parasympathetic nervous system appears to be well developed, but sympathetic functions do not seem to fully mature until 4 to 6 months of age. The bradycardic response to hypoxemia characteristic of the newborn, and its attenuation by atropine, illustrates the parasympathetic predominance of reactions to this as well as other major autonomic stimuli, such as laryngoscopy.

Whether the infant's responses imply the perception of pain remains conjectural. The issue seems moot because if only nitrous oxide analgesia is used, the ensuing hyperglycemia and systemic arterial hypertension may place the infant at an increased risk of intracranial hemorrhage. Thus the anesthesiologist ordinarily seeks to prevent these manifestations of the stress response as well as the possible perception of pain by providing sufficient anesthesia.

■ Renal System and Fluid Balance

Despite apparent structural maturity, the kidney of the preterm or term newborn is not functionally mature. Glomerular filtration rate, renal blood flow, the tubular maximum for *p*-aminohippuric acid, and maximal concentrating ability increase with advancing postconceptual age (Table 25-4).

The preterm newborn exhibits renal function that is far less effective than that of the term newborn, but with striking improvement by age 6 months; renal function approaches that of an adult by 12 months. The preterm infant is ill equipped to conserve or excrete sodium in response to sodium deprivation or excess. Also, the concentrating ability of the preterm newborn kidney during water deprivation or excess loss reaches only 35 percent and that of the term newborn only 50 percent of adult capacity. However, the term newborn's capacity to dilute urine following an excessive water load approaches the adult's by age 6 weeks but remains reduced in the preterm infant for many weeks or months.

The newborn's total-body water contributes 70 to 75 percent of its body mass compared with 50 to 60 percent in the child and adult. Extracellular water

Table 25-3

Normal Cardiovascular Function (Mean and Range)

	Age				
	1–30 days (term infant)	1–24 mos	2–6 years	7–13 years	14–18 years
Heart rate (beats/min)	125 (100–190)	120 (80–160)	100 (80–120)	90 (70–110)	80 (55–95)
Systemic arterial pressure (mmHg)	55–90 / 40–60	80–120 / 45–65	75–115 / 50–75	95–125 / 60–80	105–140 / 65–85
Cardiac output (ml/kg/min)	200–250	170–200	150–170	100–140	90–115

Adapted with permission from Behrman RE, Kliegman RM, Nelson WE, et al: *Nelson's Textbook of Pediatrics,* 14th ed. Philadelphia: WB Saunders, 1992, pp 1127–1130 and Smith CA, Nelson NM: *The Physiology of the Newborn Infant,* 4th ed. Springfield, Ill: Charles C. Thomas, 1976.

Data from Blumenthal S, Epps RP, Heavenrich R, et al. Report of the task force on blood pressure control in children. *Pediatrics* 1977;797–820.

Table 25-4

Normal Basal Fluid Volumes and Characteristics (Range or Mean ± SD)

	Age		
	1–30 days	1–24 mos	2 yrs–Adult
Urine volume (ml/kg/h)	1–4	1–4	1–4
Urine osmolality (mOsmol/liter)	100–600	50–1400	50–1600
Extracellular volume (% body wt)	42 (6)	34 (4)	25
Blood volume (ml/kg)	80–90	70–75	65–70

Data from Friis-Hansen B: Changes in body water compartments during growth. *Acta Paediatr Scand* 1957;110(suppl):36–42; Mollison PL: *Blood Transfusion in Clinical Medicine.* Philadelphia: FA Davis, 1967, p 145.

comprises over half the total-body water or roughly 40 to 45 percent of body mass in the newborn, decreasing rapidly over the first few postnatal days to approximately 30 to 33 percent of body mass. The extracellular fluid compartment appears to remain proportionately similar throughout infancy, thereafter declining gradually to approximately 20 percent of body mass in the older child and adult. Blood volume, a component of the extracellular fluid compartment, varies with age in relation to body mass from approximately 90 ml/kg in the preterm and 80 ml/kg in the term newborn to 70 to 75 ml/kg in the infant and child and 65 to 70 ml/kg in the adult (see Table 25-4).

Water requirements and their variability in preterm neonates differ considerably from those in term neonates, infants, and older children or adults. The preterm infant, especially if less than 1500 g birth weight, has immature skin and an exceptionally great ratio of surface area to body mass, resulting in unusually large evaporative water losses in relation to metabolic rate; these losses are further increased by exposure to ambient warmers and phototherapy units. These concerns prevail in larger preterm and full-term newborns also, but to a lesser extent, since their evaporative losses are more predictable.

■ Metabolism and Thermal Homeostasis

Oxygen consumption in the newborn averages 5 ml/kg per minute on day 1, increasing to 7 to 8 ml/kg per minute by day 7. This increased oxygen consumption persists throughout infancy, declining gradually in later childhood and thereafter to adult values of 3 to 4 ml/kg per minute.

Metabolism drives minute ventilation and cardiac output, which in infants are double the values observed in older children. Both increased ventilation and increased cardiac output are achieved by increased rates of activity (breaths or beats per minute) (see Tables 25-1 and 25-3). Thus minute volume in the infant is approximately 200 ml/kg per minute with a frequency of 35 to 60 breaths per minute, compared with 90 ml/kg per minute with a frequency of 15 to 20 breaths per minute in the adult. Cardiac output averages 200 ml/kg per minute at heart rates of 100 to 190 beats per minute in the newborn and 100 ml/kg per minute with heart rates of 55 to 95 beats per minute in the adult. Similarly, basic resting caloric requirements of the newborn are more than double those of the older child and young adult (120 versus 35 to 50 kcal/kg per day). Responses to cold environments increase metabolic activity even further. A 10-degree difference between skin temperature and room air temperature (e.g., 34 and 24°C, respectively) will double a neonate's oxygen consumption.

Pediatric Pharmacology

The commonly used anesthetics, muscle relaxants, narcotics, and other adjuvant drugs differ in their pharmacokinetics and pharmacodynamics in the newborn and infant as compared with the older child and adult. Major variations that concern the anesthesiologist include the following:

1. The greater relative volumes of total-body water and of the extracellular fluid compartment in the newborn and infant result in substantially greater volumes of distribution for drugs.

2. The brain, heart, liver, and kidneys constitute

18 percent of the body weight in the newborn but only 5 percent in the adult, so a relatively larger fraction of a dose of an inhaled or injected drug is distributed to these organs rather than to muscle or fat.

3. Neonates, especially if born preterm, have significantly less plasma protein concentrations, with predictable pharmacokinetic results.

4. Lipid-soluble drugs diffuse more readily into the neonatal brain because of the permeability of the neonatal blood-brain barrier.

5. Most hepatic enzyme systems involved in microsomal drug metabolism are either inactive or immature unless induced by exposure to a drug such as phenobarbital.

6. The lesser glomerular filtration rate causes slower elimination of most drugs and their metabolites.

Pediatric Anesthesia Equipment

Anesthetic and airway equipment, as well as vascular cannulas, infusion sets, and monitoring devices, must be appropriate for the size of the infant or child requiring anesthesia.

The two popular breathing systems for infants and small children (under 25 kg) are the various modifications of the Mapelson-D system and the circle absorber system (see Chap. 5). The Mapelson modification most widely used over the past decade has been the Bain system, in which the fresh gas flows through a tube that lies inside the expiratory tube, through which warm expired gas flows. These pediatric partial rebreathing systems waste large volumes of gases and vapors because they depend on large total flows to clear CO_2. The cost of the newer volatile anesthetics made circle absorber systems popular again, with modifications including small-bore delivery system tubing, a 0.5- to 1.0-liter rebreathing bag, and pediatric bellows for the mechanical ventilator.

For the infant under 6 months to 1 year of age, unless anesthesia is brief and the operation superficial, tracheal intubation ensures airway patency and adequate ventilation. Pediatric laryngoscope blade configurations vary, but the most widely employed in the United States is the Miller series. The Miller-0 and Miller-1 blades are available with a cannula paralleling the light tube along the side of the blade and a proximal nipple attachment for continuous oxygen flow (2 liters/min) during laryngoscopy. This simple device reduces the likelihood of hypoxemia in infants undergoing awake tracheal intubation.

Uncuffed Magill and Murphy polyvinylchloride tubes in conventional shape and in angled configurations for procedures involving the head and neck are most commonly employed in the United States today. Cuffed tubes have not proven necessary for most patients under age 8 years. By that age, the funnel shape of the laryngeal and cricoid structures found in younger children no longer persists, and the internal diameter of the trachea approximates the largest internal diameter of the glottis, requiring a cuffed tracheal tube.

Management Before the Induction of Anesthesia

■ Preanesthetic Evaluation

A number of age-related considerations affect the preanesthetic evaluation of the pediatric patient. The spectrum of common pediatric diseases and abnormal conditions differs considerably from that in the adult. Younger patients cannot give their own medical history, so this must be obtained from parents. Some toddlers cooperate reluctantly or cry during a physical examination.

Children over 6 months of age vary in their emotional responses to a proposed anesthetic and operation. Despite the brevity of the preanesthetic visit, the anesthesiologist can attempt to gain the confidence of the infant or child and establish rapport with the parents prior to any physical examination of the patient.

The pediatric preanesthetic physical examination emphasizes the upper airway, lungs, and heart. Small nares, purulent rhinitis, adenoid and tonsillar hypertrophy, or a small mandible with a protruding maxilla frequently herald the development of upper airway obstruction after premedication or anesthetic induction. Children older than 6 years may have loose deciduous teeth that could be dislodged by an oropharyngeal airway or laryngoscope.

Many syndromes peculiar to pediatric-age patients have anesthetic implications. When confronted with a child with such abnormalities, one can consult a textbook on pediatric anesthesia for a table listing these syndromes and their anesthetic problems (see Bibliography).

Prematurity (birth at less than 37 weeks after conception) predisposes the patient to anemia, as well as postoperative apnea and bradycardia. A hemoglobin nadir of 11 ± 2 g/dl occurs at 2 to 3 months of age in the infant born at full term. In prematurely born infants weighing less than 1.2 kg at birth, the expected minimum hemoglobin is 7.7 g/dl. As with adults, this anemia is no threat to life during ordinary operations.

An upper respiratory infection (URI) occurs an average of five times per year in pediatric patients and persists up to 10 days. In adults, mucus clearance remains impaired for up to a week and pulmonary mechanics abnormal for up to 5 weeks after symptoms have cleared. Healthy children demonstrate no detrimental effects from anesthesia administered during a URI. However, preoperative wheezing and rales indicate lower airway disease, which contraindicates elective anesthesia.

Patients who could be infectious from exposure to an exanthem have their operations postponed to prevent them from infecting other patients. If their operation cannot be postponed, they must be isolated from others in the hospital.

Many children manifest functional heart murmurs that have no physiologic significance. Functional murmurs sound soft and do not radiate; they can be difficult to differentiate from organic murmurs at a single examination. When an anesthesiologist detects such a murmur, confirmation of the diagnosis with the parent (tact is required; the parent may not be aware of the murmur) or directly with the pediatrician is advisable. If the implications of a murmur seem uncertain, consultation with a pediatric cardiologist should be obtained.

Healthy children need few laboratory studies. Hemoglobin and hematocrit determinations are done in those at risk for physiologic anemia (less than age 1 year) and those scheduled for surgical procedures associated with significant blood loss. In order to avoid administering anesthesia to pregnant patients, human chorionic gonadotropin determinations are done in postmenarche girls.

■ Preanesthetic Preparation

Preoperative Reassurance

Many children, including some adolescents, psychologically regress under the stress of anesthesia, operation, and separation from parents. Some children develop disturbing psychological changes manifested by nightmares, enuresis, and temper tantrums. Various approaches have served to ameliorate the unpleasant aspects of hospitalization, including (1) eliminating intramuscular injections, (2) preoperative puppet shows and a visit with an anesthesiologist, and (3) minimizing the length of time the child is separated from parents by having the parents present during anesthesia induction and by performing the operation on the day of admission. One of the most effective measures, yet sometimes one of the most difficult to achieve, is for the parents to demonstrate confidence and cheerfulness. Many parents have difficulty hiding their fears and tensions and transmit them to the child. During the preanesthetic visit with the parents, away from children who are old enough to understand, the parents are counseled about this as well as about the risks of anesthesia for their child.

Preanesthetic Medication

The numerous regimens and drugs advocated for preanesthetic sedation of the pediatric patient testify to the lack of an overall solution. In young patients, tachycardia often is desirable; atropine is employed most commonly in pediatric patients. Doses are twice those used in adults, but the drug is as effective given by mouth as intramuscularly (Table 25-5). Scopolamine can substitute for the atropine (in the same dose), providing additional preoperative sedation, but it significantly increases the incidence of emergence delirium. Glycopyrrolate does not produce tachycardia and induces such an intense antisialagogue effect that children complain of pharyngeal soreness for up to 7 hours.

Sedation and analgesia can be achieved with barbiturates or benzodiazepines combined with narcotics in flavored oral preparations that infants and children find acceptable. We favor an oral premedication consisting of atropine and midazolam (see Table 25-5).

Preoperative Fasting

We recommend that children abstain from solid food and milk for 12 hours prior to induction of anesthesia. This fasting interval is based on the frequency of recovery of milk from the stomachs of infants after tracheal intubation. In contrast, the rapid turnover of body water in young infants predisposes them to dehydration. Recent studies demonstrate that children drinking up to 240 ml of clear liquids (depending on body size) 2 hours prior to anesthetic

Table 25-5

Drugs for Preanesthetic Sedation		
Age (mos)	Inpatient	Outpatient
0–6	Atropine IM or PO	Atropine PO
6–12	Atropine + pentobarbital IM or PO	Atropine PO
Over 12	Atropine + pentobarbital + narcotic IM or PO	Atropine + midazolam PO

	Doses	
	Atropine	≤ 4 kg: 0.04 mg/kg IM or PO > 4 kg: 0.02 mg/kg, minimum 0.16 mg, maximum 0.6 mg IM or PO
	Diazopam	0.2 mg/kg PO
	Meperidine	1 mg/kg IM: 1.5 mg/kg PO in outpatients: 3 mg/kg PO in inpatients
	Midazolam	0.5 mg/kg PO
	Morphine	0.1 mg/kg IM, maximum 10 mg IM
	Pentobarbital	4 mg/kg IM or PO maximum 100 mg IM (one injection)
	Scopolamine	0.02 mg/kg IM or PO
	The narcotic and belladonna drugs can be mixed and given with one injection	

induction have gastric residual volumes and acidity no different from those fasting for 4 to 12 hours. We therefore offer clear liquids until 2 hours prior to induction of anesthesia.

Intraoperative Anesthetic Management

■ Selection of Anesthetic Agents and Adjuvant Drugs

Pediatric anesthesiologists use most of the common anesthetic agents and techniques. Halothane, isoflurane, and desflurane have replaced narcotics as the basal anesthetic agent in the healthy infant. Fentanyl is the agent of choice in sick infants with cardiopulmonary instability. Nitrous oxide remains the most common carrier gas. Pancuronium, vecuronium, rocuronium, and mivacurium have replaced

curare. The tachycardia of pancuronium particularly benefits neonates whose cardiac output depends predominantly on heart rate. Preparing a written list of the appropriate weight-adjusted doses of the drugs to be used during the anesthetic (Table 25-6), including the common emergency drugs, helps avoid errors in administration. Those most likely to be used are prepared in appropriate syringes before induction of anesthesia.

■ Induction

A rapid, unthreatening anesthetic induction reduces psychological trauma to the pediatric patient. We allow the child some control of the situation, including the choice of sitting in the anesthesiologist's lap, being held by the circulating nurse, or sitting or lying on the operating room table. A soft, caring, and reassuring voice combined with firm, honest direction of events despite the child's hesitation improves the child's confidence in most instances. Distracting the child with a story that involves the sensations the child may experience during the induction helps allay anxiety. In the healthy child, we often delay applying monitoring devices and cannulating a vein until the patient is unconscious.

■ Inhalation Induction

Halothane enjoys a clear superiority as an inhalation induction agent. Disguising the odor of the mask and initial gas flow with a drop of a common liquid food flavoring, such as those found in grocery stores, makes the mask more acceptable to most children. Doubling the halothane concentration ev-

ery two to four breaths while the patient breathes spontaneously without assistance reduces the duration of the induction.

Other inhalational agents present difficulties in inhalation induction. Enflurane, isoflurane, and desflurane are more pungent and disagreeable than halothane. Laryngospasm occurs in 5 percent of isoflurane inductions, and seizures occur in 7 percent of children anesthetized with enflurane. Excitement (100 percent), breath holding (50 percent), coughing (36 percent), and laryngospasm (30 percent) are common during inductions in infants and children with desflurane. Sevoflurane holds promise of being nonirritating.

Table 25-6

Intravenous Drug Dosages in Infants During Anesthesia

Adjuvant Drug	Newborns	Infant
Atracurium	0.4 mg/kg initial dose	0.4 mg/kg initial dose
Maintenance	25% initial dose	25% initial dose
Atropine	0.04 mg/kg (≤ 4 kg)	0.02 mg/kg (> 4 kg), minimum 0.16 mg IV
Fentanyl	1–2 µg/kg	1–2 µg/kg
Ketamine	2 mg/kg	2 mg/kg
Mivacurium	Not established	0.2 mg/kg
Morphine	0.1–0.2 mg/kg	0.1–0.2 mg/kg
Neostigmine	0.07 mg/kg	0.07 mg/kg
Pancuronium		
Initial	0.05 mg + 0.05 mg increments to effect	0.1 mg/kg
Maintenance	20% initial dose	20% initial dose
Rocuronium	Not established	0.6 mg/kg
Succinylcholine	2 mg/kg	1 mg/kg
Thiopental (2.5%)	4 mg/kg	4 mg/kg
Vecuronium	0.1 mg/kg initial dose	0.1 mg/kg initial dose
Maintenance	15% initial dose	15% initial dose

Cardiovascular Drugs	Dosage
Calcium chloride (10%)	10–12 mg/kg
Calcium gluconate (10%)	15–60 mg/kg
Dobutamine	2.5–10 µg/kg/min
Dopamine‡	1–20 µg/kg/min
Epinephrine†	
Initial*	1–10 µg/kg/min
Maintenance	0.1–2.0 µg/kg/min
Furosemide	0.5–1.0 mg/kg
Isoproterenol†	0.1–2.0 µg/kg/min
Lidocaine (1%)	1.0 mg/kg
Sodium bicarbonate	1–3 mEq/kg (depending on pHa and base deficit)

*Start with a small dose; double the dose periodically until desired effect is achieved or maximum dose is reached.
†Dilute in syringe to 1 or 10 µg/kg/ml; give with calibrated syringe pump.
‡Dilute in syringe to 10 or 100 µg/kg/ml; give with calibrated syringe pump.

■ Intravenous Induction

Intravenous induction agents offer a practical means of achieving rapid induction of anesthesia in the neonate and infant, and of reducing psychological trauma in older children who refuse the mask. Thiopental requirements are increased in the infant under 12 months (ED_{50} 6 to 7 mg/kg), but the onset of unconsciousness appears more rapidly in infants because of their greater brain blood flow. The considerations involved in using ketamine in infants and children are the same as in adults.

■ Other Methods of Induction

Other methods of inducing anesthesia include rectal methohexital (20 to 30 mg/kg), a method particularly suitable for children 6 to 36 months old. Induction times with this method range from 4 to 22 minutes, averaging 8 minutes. However, 8 percent of patients are not asleep 15 minutes after administering the drug, and 8 to 13 percent of the patients defecate, producing unknown and sometimes inadequate absorption of the drug.

■ Airway Management

Managing the pediatric upper airway and ventilating the lungs by mask require different techniques than in the adult. Unintentional pressure from the third and fourth fingers can force the tongue against the palate. The fingertips of the hand holding the mask must be kept on bony surfaces. The second finger, applied to the posterior surface of the symphysis menti, applies anterior pressure to pull the mandible forward. Similarly, the third or fourth finger, applied to the posterior aspect of the mandibular ramus, pushes the mandible forward, lifting the tongue off the posterior pharynx.

Tracheal intubation demands technical finesse, especially in the infant. The minimal working space in the infant's oropharynx requires precise technique: the tongue is swept well to the left by the laryngoscope blade with the handle of the laryngoscope at 45 degrees to the ceiling and suspending the head to keep the epiglottis behind the blade and to put the blade and larynx in the same axis.

Because of their greater rate of oxygen consumption and smaller functional residual capacity, infants develop arterial hemoglobin desaturation during apnea more readily than do adults. Prior ventilation of the lungs with 100% oxygen for 1 minute prevents desaturation during a subsequent 30- to 60-second period of apnea.

The appropriate endotracheal tube size varies with the patient's age; the recommendations in Table 25-7 represent averages. Once the calculated size reaches 6.5 mm internal diameter (ID), using a cuffed endotracheal tube 0.5 mm ID smaller than the calculated size avoids excessive tracheal gas leaks. An appropriately sized tube allows an air leak at 10 to 40 cmH_2O peak inflating pressure.

A history of prolonged tracheal intubation, tracheostomy, laryngeal stridor, or laryngotracheitis (croup)

Table 25-7

Age of Patient	Internal Diameter* (mm)	Connector† (mm)	Minimum Length,‡ oral (cm)
Preterm	2.0–2.5	3.0	10–11
0–3 mos	3.0	3.0	11–12
3–7 mos	3.5	4.0	13
7–15 mos	4.0	4.0	14
15–24 mos	4.5	4.5	15–21
2–10 yrs	4+ age/4	4 + age/4	
10–15 yrs	6.0–7.5, cuffed	6.0–8.0	21–23
Adults	7.5–9.0, cuffed	8.0–10.0	24–26

*Average uncuffed tube size for age. Occasionally a size 0.5 mm ID smaller or larger is required in normal patients. Tubes are labeled with internal and external diameters in millimeters.

†Tapered, 15-mm male at machine end. Size refers to internal diameter at tube end.

‡For nasal tubes, add 2 to 3 cm.

suggests the possibility of a narrowed subglottic tracheal diameter. These children require an endotracheal tube at least 0.5 mm ID smaller than usual.

Maintenance of Anesthesia

■ Inhalation Agents

The average minimum alveolar concentration (MAC) of halothane increases from 0.87 percent in the term newborn to 1.2 percent at 1 month, remains at that value until 6 months, and then decreases to approximately 0.95 percent at 12 months and 0.9 percent at 3 years of age (Fig. 25-5). The reasons for these alterations in potency with age remain unclear. In the younger infant, the 30 percent increase in dose requirement is accompanied by a greater susceptibility to systemic arterial hypotension at effective anesthetic levels of halothane (end-tidal concentrations of approximately 1.5 to 2.0 MAC). Whether these findings represent a hazard to the infant because of impaired blood flow to vital organs remains uncertain.

There are similar age-dependent variations in MAC for isoflurane and desflurane (see Fig. 25-5). At 1 MAC, heart rate and systolic blood pressure decrease similarly during halothane, isoflurane, and desflurane anesthesia.

■ Narcotics

Narcotic anesthesia, usually supplemented by muscle relaxants, nitrous oxide, and minimal concentrations (< 0.5 MAC) of a potent inhalational agent, offers special advantages to the sick infant whose cardiovascular system may be severely impaired by anesthetic concentrations of the potent volatile agents. The drug most often used is fentanyl, given by intermittent bolus injection of 1 to 2 µg/kg to a total dose of 10 to 20 µg/kg. Postoperative management includes short-term mechanical ventilation (4 to 24 hours) to ensure safe recovery from narcotic effects.

Pediatric patients apparently experience fewer problems with intraoperative awareness than do adults. In healthy patients, 70% to 75% N_2O in oxygen allows sufficient oxygen. Morphine in increments 0.05 to 0.10 mg/kg provides good intraoperative pain relief that extends into the postoperative period. Fentanyl in doses of 0.5 to 1.0 µg/kg also gives good intraoperative pain relief. Some pediatric

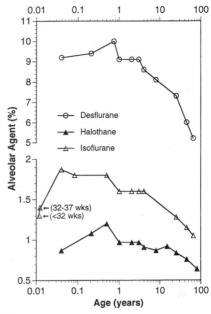

Figure 25-5

Effect of age on the MAC of inhaled anesthetics.
(Adapted with permission from Cameron CB, Robinson S, Gregory GA: The minimum alveolar concentration of isoflurane in children. Anesth Analg 1984;63:418-420; Gregory GA, Eger EI, Munson ES: The relationship between age and halothane requirements. Anesthesiology 1969;30:488-491; LeDaz KM, Lerman J: The minimum alveolar concentration (MAC) of isoflurane in preterm. Anesthesiology 1987;67:301-307; Lerman J, Robinson S, Willis MM, Gregor GA: Anesthetic requirements for halothane in children 0 to 1 month and 1 to 6 months of ages. Anesthesiology 1983;59:421-424; Rampil IJ, Lockhart SH, Zwass MS, et al: Clinical characteristics of desflurane in surgical minimal alveolar concentration. Anesthesiology 1991;76:975-979; Stevens WC, Dolan WM, Gibbons RT, et al: Minimum alveolar concentrations (MAC) with and without nitrous oxide in patients of various ages. Anesthesiology 1990;42:)

anesthesiologists avoid narcotics in infants less than 6 to 12 months old, especially if they have a history of prematurity or apnea and bradycardia.

Narcotic antagonists, though effective immediately in many of these infants, have not eliminated the need for mechanical support of ventilation. Thus narcotic anesthesia is reserved for infants undergoing major procedures who are expected to be candidates for intensive observation for up to 24 hours after anesthesia. This caveat does not apply to the use of narcotics to supplement inhalation agents, as in the use of fentanyl in doses of 1 to 3 µg/kg or morphine in doses of 0.1 to 0.2 mg/kg. The elimination half-life of morphine in neonates (13 hours) and presumably in younger infants greatly exceeds that of older children and adults (2 hours).

■ Relaxants

In healthy term and older infants, nondepolarizing muscle relaxants can be given in the usual doses adjusted for body weight, but variability in duration of effect seems to be greater and onset of action appears to be more rapid. The greater sensitivity of the immature myoneural junction of the infant to nondepolarizing relaxants is offset by the larger volume of distribution of the drugs. Infants require intravenous doses (in milligrams per kilogram) similar to those for adults when atropine and neostigmine are used for reversal of neuromuscular blockade. The effective intravenous dose of succinylcholine is 2 mg/kg in infants and 1 mg/kg in older children.

■ Monitoring

Minimum monitoring guidelines call for the same monitors in infants and children as in adults (see Chap. 6), although interpretation of these monitors may vary with age. For example, normal blood pressure is different in neonates and young infants than in adults (see Table 25-3).

Rectal or esophageal temperature monitoring readily detects hypothermia in infants. In malignant hyperthermia, axillary temperature may increase earlier than does core temperature.

Most neonates and young infants undergoing major procedures benefit from an intraarterial catheter for monitoring of blood pressure and changes in blood electrolytes. The radial artery of the full-term newborn accepts a 22-gauge catheter inserted either percutaneously or by cutdown (without ligating the artery). Aggressive flushing of a radial arterial catheter must be avoided because this can cause cerebral emboli. Less accessible, but perhaps safer, are the dorsalis pedis and posterior tibial arteries in the foot. The temporal and, in the newborn, umbilical arteries can be used but are associated with cerebral emboli and renal hypertension, respectively.

A central venous pressure catheter in the right atrium can be useful for evaluating adequacy of blood replacement in patients experiencing major blood loss. Pulmonary artery catheters are seldom indicated because right and left heart functions are rarely dissociated in pediatric patients undergoing noncar-

diac operations. Urine output in the infant can be measured accurately in a small collection bottle. Similarly, surgical suction lines used in infants are short and flow into calibrated traps.

■ Temperature Control

The environmental temperature of many operating rooms is between 20 and 22°C. This temperature is at the margin of the healthy newborn infant's ability to maintain its body temperature, requiring a two- to threefold increase in oxygen consumption. Thermal stress also increases plasma catecholamines, causing pulmonary and systemic vasoconstriction and metabolic acidemia that may precipitate a return to a fetal circulatory pattern, especially if the neonate cannot increase cardiopulmonary function to meet the raised metabolic demand.

Maintaining the body temperatures of neonates and young infants, even for short superficial procedures, requires a multifaceted approach. An overhead radiant warmer during induction and emergence, increasing the operating room temperature, placing a plastic sheet or bag between the patient and the operating room table sheets, placing the patient's head and limbs in plastic sandwich bags, and covering the remainder of the patient with an adhesive plastic drape, a circulating warm air blanket, or a reflective blanket all serve to reduce the patient's loss of heat to the environment. A servo-controlled circulating water blanket and heated and humidified anesthetic gases provide the heat needed to maintain an infant's core temperature, even when a body cavity is open.

■ Intraoperative Fluid Therapy

The daily requirements of neonates and children for fluids and nutrition were established in 1957 (Tables 25-8 and 25-9). Of the commercially available intravenous fluids, one-quarter normal (0.2%) saline most closely resembles the obligatory fluid losses of the neonate. Anesthesiologists and surgeons have tended to use this hypotonic maintenance fluid for third-space replacement and postoperative treatment, but this can produce hyponatremia. Because neonates readily handle the added sodium, most pediatric anesthesiologists now use lactated Ringer's solution for maintenance fluid replacement. We seek to administer 8 hours of maintenance fluids to ambulatory surgery patients in the operating room and postanes-

Table 25-8

Maintenance Fluid Requirements (Oral or Parenteral)		
Weight (kg)	ml/kg/h	ml/kg/24 h
<10	4	100
10–20	40 + 2 ml/kg > 10 kg	1000 + 50 ml/kg > 10 kg
>20	60 + 1 ml/kg > 20 kg	1500 + 20 ml/kg > 20 kg

Note: Requirements increase with fever or other causes of increased metabolism.

thetic care unit so that they are not required to drink shortly after anesthesia.

Third-space losses in the pediatric patient resemble those in adults (see Table 25-9). However, preterm infants or neonates with conditions such as diaphragra-

Table 25-9

Fluid Replacement Therapy

Third-space replacement
  Lactated Ringer's solution 3–10 ml/kg/h during operation depending on operative site; reevaluate when total dose reaches 40 ml/kg
Colloid replacement in lieu of blood if hematocrit ≥36 (newborn) or ≥30 (older infant, child)
  Fresh frozen plasma and/or 5% albumin in lactated Ringer's (10–20 ml/kg)
Blood replacement
  Estimated blood volume (EBV)
    90–100 ml/kg premature newborn
    90 ml/kg newborn
    80 ml/kg infant
    70 ml/kg child, adult male
    65 ml/kg adult female
  Acceptable arterial hematocrit (Hct_a)
    ≥36% if <52 weeks postconception
    ≥30% if ≥52 weeks postconception
  Allowable blood loss (ABL) calculation:
    Initial $Hgb = Hgb_i$
    Target $Hgb = Hgb_t$
    $ABL \leq EBV \times (Hgb_i - Hgb_t)/Hgb_i$
  Replace ABL ≤10 ml/kg with lactated Ringer's
  Replace ABL > 10 ml/kg with 5% albumin in lactated Ringer's or fresh frozen plasma
  Replace blood losses > ABL with blood to maintain acceptable Hgb
Technique
  Warm fluids and blood
  Use calibrated syringe pump for maintenance fluids
  Use manual syringe injection for colloid and blood

Adapted with permission from Holliday MA, Segar WI: Maintenance need for water in parenteral fluid therapy. *Pediatrics* 1957;19:823–828; Furman EB: Intraoperative fluid therapy. *Int Anesthesiol Clin* 1975;13(3):133–147; Grogono AW: Albumin extravasation during surgery. *Br J Anaesth* 1976;48:929–930; Gross JB: Estimating allowable blood loss: Corrected for dilution. *Anesthesiology* 1983;58:277–280.

matic hernia or congenital heart disease may not tolerate large volumes of third-space fluid replacement without developing interstitial pulmonary edema. The normal pediatric cardiovascular system handles acute variations in blood volume of up to 10 percent. This permits "priming" neonates and young infants with up to 10 ml/kg of blood immediately before a surgical procedure associated with major blood loss, especially when the blood loss will be difficult to measure, such as in craniectomies for craniosynostosis. All the problems of multiple blood volume transfusions appear to occur earlier in neonates and young infants, perhaps because the relative rate of infusion of blood is so great. Hyperkalemia and hypocalcemia often develop during rapid transfusion in infants and children, whereas dilutional coagulopathies occur less frequently.

Emergence from Anesthesia

Emergence ordinarily occurs more rapidly in neonates and young infants than in adults for the same reasons that induction is more rapid. As in adults, tracheal extubation during the excitement stage of emergence may result in laryngospasm. The initial treatment of laryngospasm consists of constant positive airway pressure with forward mandibular thrust and extension of the occipitoatlantal joint to relieve residual supraglottic soft tissue obstruction. For hypoxemia with an oxyhemoglobin saturation below 85 percent but before the onset of cyanosis or bradycardia, we advocate intravenous succinylcholine, 0.1 to 1.0 mg/kg. Rapid relief of obstruction is important because inspiratory efforts against a closed glottis can cause severe pulmonary edema in an otherwise healthy patient.

Because young infants cannot cooperate or follow verbal commands, alternative means of assessing recovery from neuromuscular blockade are used. One common sign, the flexion of the hips with the raising of one or both legs from the operating table, corresponds to an inspiratory pressure of −35 cmH$_2$O. Since hypothermia delays recovery of neuromuscular function following reversal of nondepolarizing muscle relaxants, reversal of the effects of neuromuscular blockers is not attempted unless the patient's core temperature is at least 35°C.

Postanesthetic Care

The special problems of pediatric patients recovering from anesthesia require a recovery room staffed with nurses who are experienced in dealing with children. Children require more psychological care than do adults because they are not capable of understanding the strange new environment. Even experienced nurses occasionally have difficulty determining if patients are crying because they are in pain, are hungry, or want their parents.

Postanesthetic prolonged apnea (≥15 s) occurs on average in 37 percent of infants born at less than 37 weeks gestation because of immaturity of respiratory control. This apnea, often with bradycardia and hypoxemia, may occur at up to 60 weeks of gestational age, but it is most common and severe in the infant under 44 weeks postconceptual age.

Mild hypoxemia presents the most common problem observed in the pediatric acute care unit, yet delivering increased inspired oxygen to the child is frequently complicated by the child's lack of cooperation. Therefore, it is best to monitor all patients in the recovery room with pulse oximeters. Because neonates and young infants are more at risk for apnea and bradycardia than older children, patients less than 6 months of age are also monitored with an electrocardiogram and impedance apnea alarm system.

Postextubation subglottic edema (croup) occurs occasionally in patients between 1 and 8 years of age. Humidity, aerosolized racemic epinephrine by mask every 0.5 to 2 hours, and intravenous hydration usually relieve the partial airway obstruction. The value of corticosteroids in the treatment of this entity remains unproven, but data indicate efficacy in viral tracheitis. Thus we and others favor the use of a single intravenous dose of dexamethasone (0.4 mg/kg).

In neonates and young infants, hypothermia frequently causes apnea, intense peripheral vasoconstriction, and metabolic acidosis from the metabolism of free fatty acids liberated during nonshivering ther-

mogenesis. The pediatric recovery room must be equipped to rewarm cold patients and maintain the body temperatures of small infants. Overhead radiant warmers or circulating warm air blankets are effective.

Regional Anesthesia

Regional anesthesia in infants and children provides the advantages of reduced requirements for other anesthetic agents and postoperative analgesia. It also exposes patients to the risks of both a general anesthetic and a regional technique because infants and children usually will not hold still if awake during an operation under regional block.

Local anesthetic agents, given in usual doses by body weight, exhibit efficacy and toxicity in neonates and infants similar to those seen in older children and adults. Because of small body mass, it is often necessary to use dilute solutions of local anesthetics to avoid overdose.

Pediatric axillary nerve blocks are administered under general anesthesia without the guidance of paresthesias for placement. Arterial puncture (25-gauge needle) or response to electrical nerve stimulation signal correct placement. Local anesthetics include lidocaine (7 mg/kg maximum) or bupivacaine (2.5 mg/kg maximum) with 1:200,000 epinephrine.

The absence of fat over the sacrum of infants and children makes caudal anesthesia technically easy. However, in the infant, the dural membrane may be as close as 1 cm to the sacrococcygeal ligament. Therefore, in pediatric caudal blocks, the needle is not advanced into the sacral canal; rather, the caudal canal is approached as if it were the lumbar epidural space, using loss of resistance. Caudal anesthesia is appropriate for most operations below the umbilicus. A dose of 1 ml/kg of 0.25% bupivacaine with 1:200,00 epinephrine produces a T10 level. Decreasing the concentration to 0.125% bupivacaine decreases the incidence of motor block and is particularly appropriate for ambulatory patients. Children may be discharged home after caudal anesthesia, provided no motor block is present and they can walk without assistance and without postural hypotension. Voiding prior to discharge is not required.

For herniorrhaphies, wound infiltration or ilioinguinal and iliohypogastric nerve blocks with 1 mg/kg (maximum 10 ml) per side of either 0.25% or 0.125%

bupivacaine provides effective postoperative pain relief. The block is performed by inserting a 22-gauge needle perpendicular to the skin one child's fingerbreadth from the anterior iliac spine along a line connecting the spine and the umbilicus. The needle is advanced until the internal and external oblique fascial planes have been pierced or until the needle strikes the inner table of the iliac crest (withdraw needle from the periosteum before injecting). Twothirds of the local anesthetic is injected here, and the remainder is injected as the needle is withdrawn, leaving a skin wheal to block the perforating branches of T11 and T12.

The neonatal spinal cord ends at L3; by the end of the first year of life, the end of the cord is found at the adult position of L1. Similarly, the neonatal dural sac ends at S3, rising to S1 by 1 year. Therefore, lumbar epidural blocks are done at L4-5 or L5-S1, using pediatric epidural kits. We use a dose of 0.5 to 0.75 ml/kg of 0.25% bupivacaine with 1:200,000 epinephrine. Preservative-free narcotics also can be instilled via this route.

Penile nerve blocks provide postoperative pain relief after circumcision and hypospadias repair. Inject 1 mg/kg of bupivacaine (the total dose diluted to a volume appropriate to the child's anatomy) without epinephrine in the midline just caudad to the symphysis pubis. The needle is inserted in the midline at the base of the penis and advanced off the symphysis in increments, similar to "walking off" a rib in an intercostal nerve block.

Spinal anesthesia is increasingly popular for the preterm infant requiring herniorrhaphy who is at risk for postoperative apnea. Because the spinal cord extends to L3 in neonates, the lumbar puncture is performed at L4-5 or L5-S1. Placing the patient in the sitting position makes the block technically easier. Spinal anesthesia produces very little hemodynamic change in neonates, so the intravenous cannula may be placed in the lower extremity after the block is established. Because extreme flexion of the neonatal neck produces airway obstruction, the neonate's head must be supported while the block is being introduced.

The dose of tetracaine for spinal anesthesia is 0.4 mg/kg in 0.04 ml/kg of 10% dextrose. Epinephrine increases the duration of the block from 60 to 95 minutes. Because the doses are so small, the dead space volume of the spinal needle must be measured and that volume (0.05 to 0.10 ml) must be considered in the volume the patient receives.

Anesthesia for the Neonate

The details of the anesthetic management of a neonate (0 to 28 days of age) lie beyond the scope of this text. The common lesions threatening the life of a neonate and their major associated clinical problems are outlined in Table 25-10.

The anesthesiologist who does not specialize in neonatal care may be required to prepare a newborn for emergency transport or for anesthesia and operation. Preparation of a sick neonate for transfer to a referral center or to an operating room aims at stabilizing the cardiopulmonary system, body temperature, and metabolic functions (including correction of birth asphyxia) and providing energy substrates to meet immediate metabolic needs. A protocol for this is outlined in Table 25-11, and appropriate drug doses are given in Table 25-6.

Anesthetic Management of Ambulatory Pediatric Patients

Pediatric patients are particularly good candidates for ambulatory procedures because they are generally healthy, because children emerge from anesthesia more rapidly than do adults, and because they benefit greatly from the psychological support of a familiar environment. Stable ASA physical status 3 patients are also suitable, even if they have a tracheostomy in place and are mechanically ventilated at home, provided that the family is capable of providing the special needs of these children.

Healthy full-term infants born at 37 weeks gestation or later are suitable ambulatory surgery patients if they are at least 4 weeks postnatal and 44 weeks postconception at the time of their anesthetic. Prematurely born infants become suitable candidates after they attain 60 weeks of postconceptual age and have not required an apnea monitor for 1 month.

Complications of Anesthesia

Over the past 40 years, the anesthesia-related mortality for infants and children has decreased from 1 in 600 cases to less than 1 in 1000 cases when all types of patients are included and to approximately 2 in 100,000 cases for elective anes-

Table 25-10

Surgical Lesions of the Neonate and Their Anesthetic Problems

Lesion	Problems

Airway obstruction
  Choanal atresia
  Pierre Robin syndrome
  Neoplasm
  Laryngeal stenosis
	Asphyxia, arrest, aspiration pneumothorax

Diaphragmatic hernia and eventration	Asphyxia, shock, hypoplastic lungs, pulmonary vascular hypertension, gastric distension, congenital heart disease, pneumothorax, small abdomen
Esophageal atresia and tracheoesophageal fistula (TEF)	Pneumonitis, gastric distension (TEF), airways secretions, congenital heart disease, possible inability to ventilate lungs after gastrostomy (TEF)
Lobar emphysema	Air trapping, mediastinal shift
Congenital heart disease	Asphyxia, cardiac failure, shock, pulmonary vascular hypoperfusion, pulmonary edema
Omphalocele, gastroschisis	Hypothermia, acidosis, shock, asphyxia, hypovolemia, congenital heart disease
Intestinal atresia	Regurgitation
Pyloric stenosis	Dehydration, aspiration, electrolyte derangement
Gastrointestinal perforation, peritonitis, other obstruction (volvulus, intussusception)	Hypovolemia, distension, shock aspiration, sepsis, hypoventilation
Incarcerated hernia, imperforate anus, megacolon	Fluid deficit/loss, occult blood loss
Sacrococcygeal teratoma	Massive blood loss, prone position during operation, hypothermia

Table 25-11

Stabilization of Vital Systems in the Neonate

Clear airway
Oxygen to achieve PaO_2 50–70 mmHg
Decompress stomach
Warm to 37°C (core), 36°C (skin over liver)
Establish intravenous route
  Plastic cannula (24-gauge or larger)
  Percutaneous, cutdown, umbilical vein
Correct acidosis of pHa < 7.30
Ventilate if $PaCO_2$ > 50 mmHg
Correct dehydration
  Insensible losses
  Gastrointestinal losses
  Other losses
Correct hypovolemia: Ringer's lactate, albumin, plasma; packed RBCs or whole blood if Hct < 36%
Correct hypoglycemia (< 40 mg/dl): 15% dextrose in water, 1 ml/kg IV
Arterial cannula—radial, temporal, umbilical

thesia in ASA physical status 1 or 2 patients in major pediatric centers. In an excellent prospective, multi-institutional study in France of 40,240 anesthetics administered to children under age 15 years (of whom 5 percent were infants under 1 year), only 1 death occurred, which resulted from unrecognized postanesthetic respiratory depression. The incidence of cardiac arrest overall was 3 in 10,000 cases; in the infants, the incidence was 2 in 1000 cases, whereas that in children age 1 to 14 years was 2 in 10,000 cases, a 10-fold difference. The overall incidence of major complications possibly caused by anesthesia was 7 in 10,000 cases.

Pain is the most frequent problem following anesthesia and operation; it is best treated by narcotics given before emergence from anesthesia or by a regional anesthetic. Prevention of pain usually requires less total drug than does treatment once pain becomes intense.

Emergence delirium occurs frequently in pediatric patients over 2 years of age, with a peak incidence of 13 percent between the ages of 3 and 9 years. Scopolamine premedication increases the incidence of emergence delirium, as does the lack of narcotics. Morphine, 0.05 to 0.10 mg/kg, or fentanyl, 0.5 to 1.0 µg/kg, effectively treats emergence delirium.

Nausea and vomiting affect 10 to 20 percent of children recovering from anesthesia. Challenging the patient postoperatively with clear liquids increases the incidence of postoperative nausea and vomiting; encouraging patients to wait until they are hungry (not just thirsty) decreases the incidence of postoperative nausea and vomiting. We no longer require children to drink and retain clear liquids as a condition for discharge home but encourage them to ingest clear liquids up to 2 hours prior to anesthesia induction. Combined with the administration of intravenous fluids, this ensures adequate hydration. This approach has reduced the incidence of nausea and vomiting by more than half compared with forced postoperative drinking. Ondansetron (0.05 mg/kg, maximum 4 mg) and granisetron (10 µg/kg) are the most effective antiemetics available to control persistent vomiting (more that three episodes). We routinely administer ondansetron prior to emergence in patients who have received intravenous narcotics as part of their anesthetic.

Postintubation subglottic edema, a potentially serious complication, has been discussed previously (see "Postanesthetic Care").

Nightmares, enuresis, and recall of separation from parents or of anesthesia induction by mask as terrifying events were reported over 30 years ago as sequelae of anesthesia and operations in children. Comparable data describing the sequelae of modern pediatric anesthesia practice with the type of preparations and sedation discussed above have not been published. Investing time and understanding in the preanesthetic relationship with the child and parents reduces to a minimum the incidence and severity of this psychic trauma.

BIBLIOGRAPHY

Cook DR, Marcy JH. *Neonatal Anesthesia*. Pasadena, Calif: Appleton Davies, 1988.

Coté CJ, Ryan JF, Todres ID, Goudsouzian NG. *A Practice of Anesthesia for Infants and Children,* 2nd ed. Philadelphia: WB Saunders, 1993.

Gregory G, ed. *Pediatric Anesthesia,* 2nd ed. New York: Churchill-Livingstone, 1989.

Kurth CD, Spitzer AR, Broennle AM, Downes JJ. Postoperative apnea in preterm infants. *Anesthesiology* 1987;64:483-488.

Motoyama EK, Davis PJ, eds. *Smith's Anesthesia for Infants and Children,* 5th ed. St Louis: CV Mosby, 1990.

Scarpelli EM, ed. *Pulmonary Physiology: Fetus, Newborn, Child, Adolescent*. Philadelphia: Lea and Febiger, 1990.

Schecter NL, ed. Acute pain in children. *Pediatr Clin North Am* 1989;36:781-1052.

Tiret L, Nivoche Y, Hutton F, et al. Complications related to anesthesia in infants and children. *Br J Anaesth* 1988;61: 263-269.

26

Obstetric Anesthesia and Perinatology

Brett B. Gutsche and Theodore G. Cheek

General Considerations

Anesthesia care for parturients entails issues beyond those involved in caring for surgical patients. Because almost all anesthetic drugs cross the placenta, they must be given in minimal effective doses that achieve effect but avoid deleterious effects on the fetus or the progress of labor.

Physiologic Alterations of Pregnancy: Implications for Anesthesia

Although pregnancy is not a pathologic state, it is associated with marked physiologic changes.

■ Respiration

In pregnancy, generalized swelling and capillary engorgement of the upper airway, larynx, and trachobronchial tree make airway obstruction more likely; the potential for further edema from laryngoscopy and tracheal intubation is also increased. Placement of a nasal airway in the engorged nasal passage can result in nosebleed. Because of laryngeal edema, endotracheal tubes one size smaller than usual are appropriate, especially in teenage mothers and those with preeclampsia or eclampsia.

In the normal mother at term, vital capacity is unchanged and total lung capacity is decreased by 5 percent owing to elevation of the diaphragm. Functional residual capacity is reduced by 15 percent, which speeds the uptake of the inhalation anesthetics. At term, minute ventilation is increased approximately 40 percent. During labor without adequate pain relief, minute ventilation may reach three times normal, hastening the uptake of inhalation anesthetics. Hyperventilation leads to respiratory alkalosis and compensating metabolic acidosis. At term, basal metabolic rate is increased by 15 percent and oxygen consumption by 20 percent or more. Increased oxygen consumption, combined with diminished functional residual capacity, adds to the risk of maternal hypoxia and speeds its onset.

■ Circulation

Maternal blood volume at term is increased by 35 to 40 percent, 1200 to 1500 ml; approximately half this increase is contained in the uterus but returns to the circulation when the uterus contracts at delivery. Since the average blood loss in vaginal delivery or cesarean section seldom exceeds 500 or 1000 ml, respectively, transfusion with blood or colloid solutions is rarely necessary for an uncomplicated delivery. Although the total red blood cell mass is increased in normal pregnancy, the increase in plasma volume is much greater, resulting in the diminished hematocrit of pregnancy. With proper diet, the hematocrit rarely decreases below 35 percent.

Measured in the lateral decubitus position, maternal cardiac output (CO) reaches 140 percent of normal at the end of the first trimester and decreases only slightly by term. The heart rate increases by approximately 10 to 15 beats per minute. With onset of labor, cardiac output again increases 40 percent or more and does not return to normal until 2 weeks postpartum.

Maternal vasodilation maintains normal blood pressure in uncomplicated pregnancy. During uterine contractions, cardiac output and blood pressure both increase; blood pressure is best measured in the interval between contractions. Effective analgesia decreases but does not eliminate the circulatory responses to contractions. Elevation of the diaphragm causes the heart to appear enlarged on both physical examination and chest x-ray. Benign systolic heart murmurs and left-axis shift by electrocardiography are common as pregnancy progresses.

In the supine position, even as early as 18 weeks of gestation, the gravid uterus can produce partial or complete obstruction of the vena cava and aorta, decreasing maternal venous return and cardiac output and reducing uterine and placental blood flow. Even in the absence of maternal symptoms, decreased uteroplacental perfusion may cause fetal compromise. Women who do not show signs of caval compression compensate by means of collateral circulation and vasoconstriction in the lower extremi-

ties. The engorged perivertebral veins are more easily entered during epidural block, making accidental intravenous injection of local anesthetics more likely.

Because of caval compression, the sympathetic blockade induced by spinal or epidural analgesia can result in severe cardiovascular compromise. In 80 percent of supine gravidae, spinal anesthesia with sensory levels at T8 or higher reduces the blood pressure enough to compromise uteroplacental circulation (systolic pressure decreased by 30 percent or to a value less than 100 mmHg). Prophylaxis and therapy for caval obstruction consist of left uterine displacement, accomplished by placing the patient in the left lateral decubitus position, by displacing the uterus to the left manually, or by placing a wedge or inflatable device beneath the patient's right flank (Fig. 26-1). From the end of the first trimester, it is best for the patient to avoid the supine position; during labor and delivery or cesarean section, left uterine displacement is maintained until birth.

■ Gastrointestinal

Both the volume and the acidity of the contents of the stomach are increased during pregnancy. Gastric emptying time is prolonged by labor, apprehension, pain, and displacement of the stomach by the uterus, which repositions both the gastroduodenal junction

Figure 26-1

Lateral and cross-sectional views of uterine aortocaval compression in the supine position and its resolution by lateral positioning of the pregnant woman.

(Reprinted by permission from Bonica JJ: Obstetric Analgesia and Anesthesia. Amsterdam: World Federation of Societies of Anaesthesiologists, 1980.)

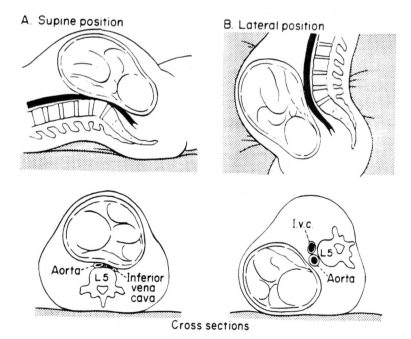

and the gastroesophageal junction, creating a functional hiatal hernia. Also, the enlarged uterus and the lithotomy position increase intragastric pressure. Together, these changes subject the sedated or unconscious parturient to increased risk of pulmonary aspiration of gastric contents. The interval from the last meal to induction of general anesthesia is of little value in determining the risk of aspiration in the gravid patient.

Acid aspiration pneumonia (Mendelson's syndrome), is a major risk of general anesthesia or sedation in the gravid patient. This occurs when the aspirate has a pH of less than 2.5. Reducing the acidity of stomach contents can decrease the pulmonary damage following aspiration. Clear antacids such as sodium citrate are preferred because the insoluble antacids, such as magnesium or aluminum salts, cause lung damage when aspirated. Thirty milliliters of a clear antacid given only minutes before induction usually increases gastric pH to greater than 4.0 for over an hour. H_2 blockers, such as cimetidine or ranitidine, decrease both gastric acidity and volume but require 60 to 90 minutes after oral intake for optimal effect. For elective operations under general anesthesia, these medications are given orally the night preceding and 2 hours before induction of general anesthesia. In an emergency, they can be given parenterally along with oral antacids. Metoclopramide is often used in conjunction with the H_2 blockers.

Reducing gastric acidity provides no protection against aspiration of solid material, which can be even more devastating than acid aspiration. If consciousness is lost or laryngeal reflexes are compromised, the lungs must be protected by cricoid compression of the esophagus, followed by prompt tracheal intubation. Induction of general anesthesia in patients in the lithotomy position is best avoided because of pressure exerted on the stomach by the gravid uterus. Perhaps the best protection against aspiration in the parturient is to ensure consciousness with intact protective airway reflexes.

The Parturient

■ Pain During Labor and Delivery

The pain of labor and delivery includes two components (Fig. 26-2). Visceral pain is caused by dilation and effacement of the cervix during uterine contrac-

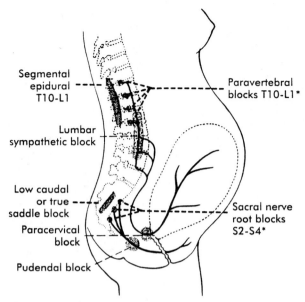

Figure 26-2

Sensory pathways and sites of injection for obstetrical regional anesthesia. Visceral pain from the cervix and uterus is blocked with bilateral paracervical blocks, bilateral lumbar sympathetic blocks at L2, and segmental epidural block from T10 to L1. Somatic pain from the perineum is blocked with bilateral pudendal nerve blocks, saddle (subarachnoid) block, or low caudal epidural block. All labor pain is abolished by a modified saddle (subarachnoid), lumbar epidural, or caudal epidural block extending from T10 to L5.

(Modified from Bonica JJ: Principles and Practice of Obstetric Analgesia and Anesthesia. *Philadelphia: FA Davis Co, 1967, p 492.)*

tions, and possibly by uterine ischemia. Somatic pain represents stretching of the vagina and perineum during descent of the fetus. Although visceral pain dominates the first stage of labor and somatic pain the second, there is considerable overlap.

The pain of cervical dilation and effacement is referred to the lower abdomen, between the umbilicus and pubis, and to the lower back. Early in labor, this may be perceived as pressure; as contractions strengthen, the pain intensifies and is referred to hips and thighs. These sensations are mediated by small, unmyelinated nerve fibers that pass from the cervix through the pelvis and hypogastric plexuses to enter the sympathetic chain at L3 to L5, reaching the dorsal root ganglia and spinal cord via the white rami communicantes of T10 to L1.

Somatic or vaginal pain characterizes the second stage of labor and begins as the presenting part starts its descent through the vagina, usually at about 8 cm of cervical dilation in a primigravida. Initially, this is perceived as a need to defecate, but with further descent, the mother has an uncontrollable urge to bear down, thus activating accessory forces of labor. Somatic pain is conveyed primarily via the pudendal nerves to dorsal nerve roots S2 to S4. Interrupting somatic pain with conduction anesthesia eliminates the urge to bear down.

Contractions produce pain when intrauterine pressure exceeds 30 mmHg, but the perception of pain varies greatly among parturients. Prenatal education, a supportive partner, and the helpful attitudes of nurses and physicians can reduce the discomfort considerably.

■ Providing Pain Relief

Ideal analgesia for labor and delivery embraces several goals:

1. Satisfactory pain relief for the mother.
2. No interference with the progress of labor.
3. Minimal risks to either mother or fetus.
4. Provision of satisfactory conditions for delivery.
5. Early interaction between mother and newborn, preferably at the time of delivery.

No single technique meets all these criteria in all instances. Modifications and combinations of various techniques are tailored to the needs of the parturient and the well-being of the fetus and vary depending on the type of delivery.

■ Nonpharmacologic Methods of Analgesia

Nonpharmacologic methods of maternal analgesia include acupuncture, hypnosis, and "prepared childbirth." Acupuncture is not used by classic Chinese practitioners for labor and delivery because it provides only limited and unpredictable analgesia. Likewise, hypnosis results in variable analgesia, ranging from none to complete, because patients differ greatly in their abilities to achieve a state of trance. Natural or prepared childbirth is based on the premise that prenatal education, encouragement by spouse and labor-floor personnel, and the use of breathing and relaxation exercises will reduce or eliminate the need for medication. Success is unpredictable, and many women require some form of pharmacologic analgesia as labor progresses.

■ Pharmacologic Methods of Analgesia

Pharmacologic techniques for pain relief include systemic medication with opioids, tranquilizers, or ketamine; subanesthetic concentrations of inhalation drugs; general anesthesia; and regional anesthetic techniques.

All patients receiving drugs for pain relief require monitoring of vital signs throughout labor, delivery, and during postpartum recovery. Trained nurses can perform these functions, but assistance from anesthesia personnel is essential. Parturients given analgesics or anesthetics also require intravenous access to provide for hydration, transfusion, or the rapid administration of anesthetics or drugs as needed.

■ Systemic Medications

Parenterally administered opioids, given initially to control pain in the first stage of labor, may suffice throughout uncomplicated labors. Meperidine, previously the most frequently used opioid in obstetrics, is being replaced by mixed agonists-antagonists, such as butorphanol, or by fentanyl. Frequent intravenous administration of small doses is preferred because of predictable pharmacokinetics; patient-controlled intravenous analgesia also is gaining popularity for this purpose.

Although careful testing reveals some impairment of neonatal neurobehavioral function after even small doses of opioids, deficiencies persist only for a day or two and do not affect subsequent neonatal feeding, weight gain, or development. Opioid-induced respiratory depression is antagonized rapidly by naloxone in both mother and newborn. Because naloxone given before delivery may cause hyperventilation, vomiting, hypertension, and extreme discomfort, it should be given only to depressed parturients and is reserved for the newborn. If the mother is a chronic opioid user, her habituated newborn may suffer opioid withdrawal if naloxone is given either to the parturient or directly to the newborn.

Ketamine is a potent analgesic for somatic pain. Small intravenous doses (0.25 mg/kg) yield profound analgesia and brief amnesia; with such small doses, consciousness is retained, and hallucinations and unpleasant dreams are uncommon. Ketamine is most useful in providing rapid onset of analgesia of a short duration for spontaneous vaginal delivery, vacuum extraction, or forceps delivery. Total doses larger than 1 mg/kg may cause loss of consciousness and increased uterine tone in the mother and respiratory depression and muscle rigidity in the newborn.

■ Inhalation Analgesia

The inhalation of subanesthetic concentrations of anesthetics provides effective analgesia for vaginal delivery. Advantages include rapid onset of analgesia, maintenance of protective airway reflexes, absence of significant maternal and neonatal depression regardless of duration of administration, little effect on uterine activity or the urge to bear down, and rapid maternal recovery. These advantages are obtained only when the mother remains awake and responsive to command. Drawbacks of the technique include the potential for delirium and excitement (second stage of anesthesia) and the need for constant supervision to avoid unconsciousness. Self-administered inhalation analgesia has been abandoned in the United States because of the hazards of unsupervised use of anesthetics. Continuous administration of 30% to 50% nitrous oxide usually provides effective analgesia for the latter part of labor, delivery, and postpartum examination. Forceps delivery is often possible if supplements such as small doses of ketamine, local anesthetic infiltration of the perineum, or preferably pudendal block are added.

■ General Anesthesia

General anesthesia is rarely needed for vaginal delivery. Because it results in loss of maternal bearing down, induction must be delayed until birth is imminent. General anesthesia increases the likelihood of pulmonary aspiration, forceps or vacuum extraction deliveries, and newborn depression. It denies the mother the birth experience and delays bonding. In the past, deep general anesthesia (halothane 1.5% to 2%) was used to inhibit uterine contractions and to terminate tetanic contractions or allow intrauterine manipulation for removal of a retained placenta. Now uterine relaxation is more rapidly and safely produced with intravenous tocolytics, such as nitroglycerin, beta-2 agonists, or magnesium sulfate, or with inhalation of amyl nitrite.

■ Regional Anesthesia

Of the many techniques of regional anesthesia described for labor and delivery, only local infiltration of the perineum, bilateral pudendal nerve block, subarachnoid block, and epidural block, including both the lumbar and caudal approaches, are now in common use. Paracervical block has been abandoned because of the unpredictable occurrence of fetal bradycardia accompanied by fetal acidosis and even death, resulting from both rapid uptake of large amounts of local anesthetic and uterine artery vasospasm. In the vaginal delivery of a dead fetus, paracervical block is useful in eliminating pain arising from cervical dilation and uterine contraction. It also provides excellent analgesia for postpartum curettage or repair of a cervical laceration.

Bilateral Pudendal Nerve Blocks

These blocks are usually performed before delivery using a transvaginal or a transcutaneous approach, with the mother in the lithotomy position. Most of the somatic pain associated with stretching of the vagina and perineum is eliminated, but because of the overlapping innervation of the perineum by the ilioinguinal nerve and the genital branch of the genitofemoral nerve, the urge to bear down is not abolished. Each block requires 8 to 10 ml of 1% lidocaine or the equivalent local anesthetic. Onset usually occurs within 5 minutes. The block provides complete anesthesia for episiotomy and repair and is usually sufficient for low forceps delivery; supplementation with inhalation analgesia is required for midforceps application. A properly performed pudendal block is not associated with maternal or fetal side effects, nor does it impede the progress of labor.

Subarachnoid Block

Either a true saddle block (L5 to S5) or a modified saddle block (T10 to S5) is useful for delivery. Saddle blocks are usually performed with the subject sitting as the hyperbaric local anesthetic is administered. For true saddle block, dural puncture is performed at the L4-5 or the L5-S1 interspace, with injection of 3 to 4 mg tetracaine, 4 to 5 mg bupivacaine, or 25 to 30 mg lidocaine. The patient remains sitting for 2 to 3 minutes after the injection. Adequate anesthesia is provided for forceps application and episiotomy without abolishing uterine pain.

Modified saddle block (T10) is accomplished by injecting 5 to 6 mg tetracaine, 6 to 8 mg bupivacaine, or 40 to 50 mg lidocaine at L3-4 and keeping the patient sitting for only 30 seconds. Not only does this block yield profound perineal analgesia, but the resultant T10 sensory level gives complete uterine pain relief, allowing cervical and uterine manipulation. The addition of 0.2 to 0.3 mg epinephrine or 2 to 3 mg phenylephrine prolongs tetracaine analgesia to 3 hours or more, which makes this block useful for analgesia for the latter part of the first stage of labor.

Severe hypotension may appear within a minute following injection; it is best prevented by left uterine displacement and rapid intravenous infusion of a balanced salt solution that does not contain dextrose. Treatment includes these measures and the intravenous injection of 5 to 15 mg ephedrine or mephentermine. Vasopressors with primarily alpha-agonist effects have been avoided because animal studies showed that they decreased uterine artery flow. Recently, small doses of phenylephrine (20 to 40 mg) given intravenously to parturients have been found to produce no adverse effects on the fetus.

Although subarachnoid block abolishes the mother's bearing-down reflex, this can be overcome by coaching her to push during contractions. In occiput transverse or posterior presentations, saddle block allows manual, forceps, or vacuum rotation or simply delivery in the posterior presentation over a large episiotomy.

Gravid women experience the greatest incidence of postspinal headache. The rate of this complication is reduced to 5 to 10 percent by using a 25- or 26-gauge needle and facing the bevel to the side so as to part and not sever dural fibers. Recently introduced "pencil point" needles of 24-gauge or smaller reduce the rate of headache to less than 2 percent. Adequate postpartum fluids (at least 3000 ml/day) and a tight abdominal binder may further reduce the incidence and severity of headache. Keeping the patient supine in bed after lumbar puncture is of no benefit.

Continuous Lumbar Epidural Analgesia

Continuous lumbar epidural analgesia is the standard for vaginal delivery because it provides a pain-free labor and delivery without measurable neonatal depression. Epidural block is begun during the active phase of labor when pain occurs, usually at 5 to 6 cm cervical dilation in the primigravida or at 4 to 5 cm in the multipara; anesthesia may begin earlier if the patient experiences severe pain.

Epidural block also is useful for trial of labor, as for an attempted vaginal birth after prior cesarean section (VBACS). An epidural to a T10 sensory level does not block signs of uterine dehiscence but provides excellent analgesia for the trial of labor. Should the trial fail,

the level of anesthesia can be raised quickly to the required T4 level needed for cesarean section.

After the epidural catheter has been inserted at L2-3 or L3-4 and a small test dose has been administered (see Chap. 18), analgesia is begun with a total of 10 to 12 ml of 0.125% to 0.25% bupivacaine, 1% to 1.5% lidocaine, or 2% chloroprocaine. This produces the T10 sensory level required to block visceral pain from the cervix and uterus, with only minimal motor block.

Anesthesia is maintained by repeated injections or continuous infusion of a dilute local anesthetic solution, such as 0.125% bupivacaine, at a rate of 10 to 12 ml/h. Later, the somatic pain of vaginal stretching is alleviated by injecting 10 to 14 ml of an anesthetic solution of the same or greater concentration. This injection provides a pain-free second stage as well as satisfactory conditions for delivery and episiotomy repair. As does spinal anesthesia, epidural anesthesia abolishes the urge to bear down.

Lumbar epidural block for labor is a major anesthetic, requiring frequent monitoring of maternal vital signs, fetal heart rate, and uterine contractions. Because the mother loses the sensation of uterine contraction, continuous monitoring of those contractions is required when labor is being induced or augmented with oxytocin. While hypotension after epidural block is slower in onset than that following subarachnoid block, it can be just as severe and is treated similarly.

Continuous Caudal Epidural Block

This approach, another form of epidural block, has largely been replaced by continuous lumbar epidural block, which is more reliable, easier to perform, requires only about one-half to two-thirds the amount of local anesthetic, and can be extended reliably to permit cesarean section. The caudal approach may be useful in patients in whom a lumbar epidural access is not feasible, usually due to anatomic considerations.

Combined Subarachnoid and Epidural Blocks

Recently, the combination of spinal and epidural anesthesia has gained popularity for obstetrical anesthesia. The epidural space is entered as usual with a Tuohy or Hustead needle. A longer pencil point needle is inserted through the epidural needle and into the subarachnoid space. After a subarachnoid injection, usually of an opioid to provide analgesia for labor without motor or sympathetic block, the spinal needle is removed, and an epidural catheter is placed. The epidural block is begun when the subarachnoid analgesia dissipates or for the delivery itself.

Intraspinal Opioids

Subarachnoid injection of 25 to 30 mg fentanyl or 7.5 mg sufentanil produces immediate analgesia that lasts 90 to 120 minutes without motor or sympathetic block. Patients may walk about during the first stage of labor yet experience no pain with contractions. Minimal decreases in blood pressure follow pain relief. Side effects include pruritus, occasional nausea and vomiting, and urinary retention. If morphine 0.25 mg is used, the onset of analgesia requires 30 minutes or longer, but the duration may exceed 4 hours. Combining fentanyl or sufentanil with morphine produces both rapid onset and a long duration of analgesia, although the side effects may be greater. The analgesia obtained with subarachnoid opioids is not satisfactory for the second stage of labor, especially if forceps or an episiotomy repair is needed. This limitation can be overcome by using a pudendal block or an epidural block, as in the combined technique.

Unlike subarachnoid opioids, epidural opioids alone do not produce adequate analgesia for even the first stage of labor. However, the addition of 50 mg fentanyl or 10 mg sufentanil to the local anesthetic solution decreases the latency and markedly prolongs the duration of the block. Continuous epidural infusion of 0.0625% bupivacaine containing 2 µg/ml of fentanyl, at 10 to 14 ml/h, provides excellent analgesia with essentially no motor block for labor and delivery, including repair of an episiotomy. A total of 200 µg or less of epidural fentanyl is not associated with depression of neonatal neuroadaptive capacity scores (NACS); doses up to and exceeding 400 µg before delivery may modestly decrease NACS at 15 minutes and 2 hours, but the scores are normal by 24 hours.

■ Effects of Conduction Analgesia on Labor

Some obstetricians fear that major conduction anesthesia, such as spinal or epidural anesthesia, may prolong labor and lead to cesarean section. There is little evidence to document that conduction anesthesia slows the first stage of labor; indeed, alleviation of severe pain may speed cervical dilation. Rapid infusion of 500 ml or more of intravenous fluid before the conduction block may decrease the frequency and amplitude of uterine contractions, but the effect is transient. Conduction anesthesia often eliminates maternal appreciation of contractions and the urge to bear down, which may prolong the second stage of labor somewhat, but without ill effects on the newborn or mother. This is overcome by coaching the mother.

Several earlier retrospective or poorly controlled studies reported that mothers who had continuous lumbar epidural blocks had an increased incidence of cesarean section as compared with mothers who received opioids and sedatives only. Recent studies contradict these findings; early administration of epidural analgesia to a mother having significant pain in labor probably does not increase the risk of abdominal delivery.

The pain of labor is stressful for both the mother and the fetus. It has been shown to result in maternal hyperventilation, maternal and fetal metabolic acidosis, increased maternal oxygen consumption, and increased maternal circulating catecholamines. Providing effective epidural analgesia markedly attenuates these responses and protects against the stress response to painful labor.

■ Anesthesia for Cesarean Section

The incidence of cesarean delivery has increased over the past two decades from less than 10 percent to nearly 20 percent of all deliveries in the United States. Cesarean section may be performed as an elective procedure, as an urgent procedure (10 to 15 minutes) when progress of labor ceases or when there is evidence of a deteriorating intrauterine environment, or as an emergency procedure that permits no delay because of extreme fetal compromise, such as a prolapsed umbilical cord or maternal hemorrhage. Anesthetic techniques for cesarean section include spinal or epidural block, general anesthesia, and local infiltration.

Spinal or Epidural Anesthesia

Regional anesthesia is usually preferred for cesarean delivery because of freedom from neonatal depression and decreased risk of maternal pulmonary aspiration. In addition, the mother remains awake and can share in the birth experience. Although regional techniques take time to perform (making them more suitable to elective cesarean section), they are also feasible for urgent operations in the hands of a skilled operator. Contraindications to regional anesthesia include uncorrected maternal hypovolemia, infection at or near the site of injection, septicemia, neurologic abnormality, severe coagulopathies, or the mother's refusal.

Subarachnoid or epidural block to at least the T4 sensory level provides satisfactory conditions for cesarean section. In the past, T6 sensory levels were considered adequate for cesarean section, but briefer operations through a high classic uterine incision were the rule. The low cervical incision now popular requires additional time, more abdominal retraction, and extraabdominal repair of the uterus, necessitating a high sensory level (T4 to T2) to decrease the visceral pain associated with these maneuvers. Subarachnoid block with hyperbaric tetracaine, 8 to 11 mg (or hyperbaric bupivacaine, 12 to 15 mg, or hyperbaric lidocaine, 65 to 80 mg), usually provides these levels. The addition of fentanyl, 25 μg, to the solution helps block visceral discomfort, and morphine, 0.25 mg, provides effective postoperative analgesia for as long as 24 hours.

Severe maternal hypotension follows such high subarachnoid blocks almost immediately unless left uterine displacement and intravenous administration of at least 15 ml/kg of balanced salt solution (without dextrose) precede the block. Prophylactic ephedrine, either 50 mg intramuscularly 10 minutes before the block or 10 to 25 mg intravenously immediately after subarachnoid injection, is also effective. Hypotension is treated with additional left uterine displacement, fluids, and ephedrine in 10- to 15-mg intravenous doses.

Continuous lumbar epidural block also is used for cesarean section. Onset of complete analgesia requires approximately 15 minutes, depending on the local anesthetic solution, but this need not hinder skin preparation or draping and rarely delays skin incision. From 20 to 25 ml of 1.5% to 2% lidocaine (or 0.5% bupivacaine or 3.0% chloroprocaine) containing epinephrine 1:200,000 plus $NaHCO_3$ (0.1 mEq/ml) usually produces rapid onset of a T4 sensory level. Fentanyl, 50 μg, and morphine, 5 mg, provide the benefits of immediate and long-acting analgesia, just as in spinal anesthesia.

Because large doses of local anesthetic are required, the total dose is given in increments, pausing between each 5- to 6-ml dose to observe for signs and symptoms of toxicity. Because maternal deaths have followed accidental intravascular injection of 0.75% bupivacaine, this concentration is no longer used in obstetric patients. However, maternal deaths have resulted from the inadvertent intravenous injection of equivalent amounts of 0.5% and 0.25% bupivacaine.

If the operation is not required for fetal compromise and the mother's oxygenation and circulatory status are satisfactory, delays between the induction of spinal or epidural anesthesia and delivery of the fetus do not harm the newborn, and careful surgical technique is possible. Haste is needed only after uterine incision, since a delay of more than 3 minutes between uterine incision and delivery may be produce neonatal depression and acidosis.

General Anesthesia

General anesthesia is used in true emergencies to reduce delay, when the mother refuses subarachnoid or epidural block, or when regional anesthesia is contraindicated. Several aspects of management require emphasis.

The minimum alveolar concentration (MAC) of inhalation anesthetics is decreased by 25 to 40 percent beginning at the middle of the first trimester in gravid women, perhaps because of increased circulating levels of progesterone and endorphins. Similarly, local anesthetic requirements for epidural and subarachnoid block are decreased by 25 to 30 percent. Return toward normal sensitivity for both inhalation anesthetics and local anesthetics occurs within a day following delivery.

Parturients are at special risk for aspiration pneumonitis; clear antacids, metoclopramide, and H_2 blockers are used to decrease this risk, and rapid-sequence induction and immediate intubation are required unless the patient's airway anatomy is such as to require awake intubation. Except in the most unusual circumstances, present standards of practice preclude general anesthesia without tracheal intubation at any time after the first trimester. Maternal death due to anesthesia is usually associated with either aspiration of gastric contents or inability to intubate or ventilate the patient.

When general anesthesia is used, neonatal depression is worsened by delays between induction and delivery and by delays between uterine incision and delivery. Nothing is gained by delaying delivery to allow redistribution of drugs in fetal tissues. The condition of the infant is also improved by maintaining left uterine displacement and by providing the mother with an inspired oxygen concentration of at least 60 percent before delivery, which appreciably increases neonatal oxygenation at birth.

Only a minimal depth of general anesthesia is necessary to provide sufficient analgesia and amnesia before delivery. Anesthesia is induced with 4 mg/kg thiopental or 1.0 mg/kg ketamine, usually not exceeding a total dose of 250 or 75 mg, respectively. Maternal awareness is prevented by maintaining the end-tidal concentrations of potent vapors at approximately two-thirds of the MAC (e.g., 0.5% halothane, 0.75% isoflurane, or 1.0% enflurane) with or without 40% nitrous oxide. Following delivery, the nitrous oxide concentration can be increased to 70%, and small amounts of narcotics may be given intravenously, while the volatile anesthetic is continued in the preceding concentrations. This ensures unconsciousness without impairment of uterine contractions.

Both depolarizing and nondepolarizing neuromuscular blockers cross the placenta to varying extents depending on the specific drug. Full blocking doses of nondepolarizing neuromuscular blockers given before birth may cause neonatal weakness; the required doses are reduced by the presence of inhalation anesthetics such as isoflurane.

Local Infiltration

Local infiltration is rarely employed today, except when competent anesthetic care is not available. It is time-consuming and requires large amounts of local anesthetic. Often it does not produce complete analgesia, and the patient may require heavy sedation or narcotics, particularly after delivery.

■ Preeclampsia and Eclampsia

Preeclampsia-eclampsia is a common complication of pregnancy that strongly affects the plan for anesthesia. The syndrome involves decreased placental perfusion; excesses of angiotensin, renin, and aldosterone; and increased general capillary permeability, perhaps due to release of polypeptides such as fibronectin. Usually it becomes evident in the second half of pregnancy. Proteinuria, hypertension, and generalized edema characterize preeclampsia, which progresses to eclampsia when convulsions occur. Other findings include depressed renal function, coagulopathy, hyperreflexia, and fetal compromise.

Although these hypertensive patients retain water and gain excessive weight, they suffer contracted intravascular volumes and may manifest severe hypotension in response to general, spinal, or epidural anesthesia. Preeclamptic parturients exhibit exaggerated hypertensive responses to painful stimuli, tracheal intubation, or vasoconstrictors. Epidural anesthesia blocks these sympathetic responses to pain with no ill effects on the fetus or placental blood flow. Special precautions are required for safety when employing epidural anesthesia in a preeclamptic patient. Significantly impaired coagulation must be ruled out to avoid epidural hematoma. Generous intravenous fluids help prevent hypotension, but a decreased colloid oncotic pressure and altered capillary permeability make pulmonary edema a hazard. A central venous or pulmonary artery catheter may be needed to guide fluid replacement. Because placental perfusion is already compromised, even small decreases in blood pressure may not be tolerated, and close maternal and fetal monitoring is required. These patients may overreact to vasopressors, so small doses are used initially.

When administering general anesthesia, as for an emergency cesarean section, the use of muscle relaxants is complicated by magnesium sulfate therapy. Magnesium potentates depolarizing and especially nondepolarizing muscle relaxants. If the latter are used, they should be given in reduced doses with continuous monitoring using a nerve stimulator.

■ Drugs Used in Obstetrics that Affect Anesthetic Management

Drugs used to enhance or retard labor or to treat preeclampsia or eclampsia have important systemic effects that must be considered when planning anesthesia management. These drugs and their important effects are summarized in Table 26-1.

Perinatology

The anesthesiologist must be familiar with perinatal medicine in order to manage the mother's anesthetic and to resuscitate the newborn when needed. Close observation of the fetus before and during labor permits early diagnosis of asphyxia and expeditious delivery. Fetal monitoring takes two forms: physical monitoring (fetal heart rate) and, less often, biochemical monitoring (fetal blood pH).

■ Biophysical Monitoring

Recent studies of neonatal outcome have raised questions about the value of electronic fetal heart rate monitoring, although the technique is still commonly employed in managing high-risk pregnancies. Fetal heart rate is determined either from the fetal electro-

Table 26-1

Drugs Used in Obstetrics that Affect Anesthetic Management

Drug and Dose	Use	Side Effects	Avoiding/Treating Side Effects
Oxytocin (synthetic) (10–30 units/liter IV)	Induce/augment labor Minimize postpartum blood loss by inducing uterine contraction	Vasodilation, decreased blood pressure, sinus tachycardia, increased cardiac output, antidiuresis, water retention	Avoid concentrated bolus; instead mix 10–30 units in IV bag and infuse rapidly
Ergot derivatives (ergotamine, methyl ergonovine) (0.2 mg IM)	Stimulate uterine contractions, postpartum only	Hypertension, nausea, agitation; severe hypertensive interaction with vasopressors; may exacerbate asthma	Avoid IV injection or give slowly; prefer IM injection
Prostaglandins (F2 alpha: 250 mg IM q20min)	Stimulate uterine contraction, for postpartum uterine atony	Bronchoconstriction; may exacerbate asthma, hypertension, uterine rupture, DIC, nausea, vomiting, fever	Administer IM or subcutaneously; avoid intrauterine injections
Beta-2 agonists (ritodrine, terbutaline)	Inhibit or arrest preterm labor, relax uterus for external version, treat hyperactive or tetanic uterine contractions	Maternal or fetal tachycardia, hypotension, increased cardiac output, nausea and vomiting, tremor, postpartum uterine atony, cardiac arrhythmia, maternal hypokalemia, hyperglycemia, pulmonary edema associated with rapid hydration, risk of arrhythmia during general anesthesia	Some suggest discontinuing 1 h if possible before proceeding to anesthesia for cesarean; in an emergency, isoflurane is preferred over halothane; hypokalemia and hyperglycemia do not require therapy but resolve quickly on stopping drug
Magnesium	Preeclampsia and preterm labor inhibition	Competes with calcium at the neuromuscular junction; may result in muscle weakness, respiratory embarrassment, or rarely, cardiac arrest; additive effect on all neuromuscular blockers	After full induction dose of succinylcholine, use nondepolarizers sparingly if at all; nerve stimulator; monitor for postoperative hypoventilation, weakness
Calcium channel blockers (nifedipine)	Preterm labor inhibition	Flushing, tachycardia, headache, dizziness, transient decrease in uterine blood flow; maternal hypokalemia and hyperglycemia less than with beta-2 agonist	May be continued until operation; postpartum uterine atony treated with prostaglandins

cardiogram (ECG) obtained from an electrode placed on the presenting part of the baby or from an ultrasound Doppler device placed on the mother's abdomen. Uterine contractions are monitored either directly, via a catheter or pressure-sensing device inserted into the uterine cavity through the cervix, or indirectly via a tocodynamometer, a pressure-recording instrument placed on the abdomen. A continuous, simultaneous tracing of fetal heart rate and uterine contractions is recorded on paper (Fig. 26-3).

The normal fetal heart rate of 120 to 160 beats per minute includes both short-term variability (5 to 10 beats per minute) and long-term variability (up to 15 beats per minute variation over a 15-second period of time) (see Fig. 26-3*A*). Absence of this variability is ominous and indicates fetal acidosis unless it can be attributed to other causes, such as prematurity, maternal fever, or the use of drugs such as opioids, tranquilizers, anticholinergics, magnesium, and some local anesthetics, particularly lidocaine and mepivacaine.

Decreases of fetal heart rate (called *decelerations* by obstetricians) and their relation to uterine contractions provide clues to fetal health. Three basic types have been described:

1. Early uniform deceleration is the mirror image of uterine contraction. It begins and ends with contraction, and the nadir of the fetal heart rate corresponds to peak contraction (see Fig. 26-3*B*). Compression of the head, not acidosis or fetal compromise, produces these changes. Although abolished by anticholinergics, early uniform deceleration does not require treatment.

2. Late uniform deceleration resembles early deceleration but is out of phase with contractions. The fetal heart rate does not begin to decrease until after the start of the contraction, reaches its slowest rate after the peak of intrauterine pressure has passed, and does not return to baseline until the contraction has ceased (see Fig. 26-3*C*). This pattern implies uteroplacental insufficiency associated with fetal acidosis and hypoxia and indicates the need for expeditious delivery. Circulatory insufficiency may result from aortocaval compression, maternal hypotension, or rapid or prolonged uterine contractions that can be corrected, with the resulting improvement in fetal health reflected in the tracing.

3. Variable deceleration is the most common type, occurring in over 50 percent of labors. Although associated with uterine contractions, bradycardia is irregular and occurs at various times throughout contractions (see Fig. 26-3*D*). These decelerations accompany umbilical cord compression and stimulation of baroreceptor reflexes and are thought to represent increases in vagal tone. Unless they are prolonged beyond 30 seconds, are associated with bradycardia of less than 70 beats per minute, show loss of fetal heart rate variability, or have an increased baseline heart rate, they are usually benign. Changing the maternal position often lessens or abolishes this pattern.

More sophisticated evaluation of the fetus includes assessment of fetal heart rate after oxytocin-induced contractions and physical findings such as breathing movements, body movements, and muscle tone or ultrasonic estimation of amniotic fluid volume. These more comprehensive approaches can indicate the need for prompt delivery without invasive testing.

■ Biochemical Monitoring

Biochemical monitoring of the fetal blood pH during labor often complements electronic fetal heart rate monitoring. A sample of fetal capillary blood is taken from the presenting part via an endoscope inserted through the vagina into the cervix. A capillary blood pH of greater than 7.25 is considered normal, whereas values of 7.21 to 7.25 are considered

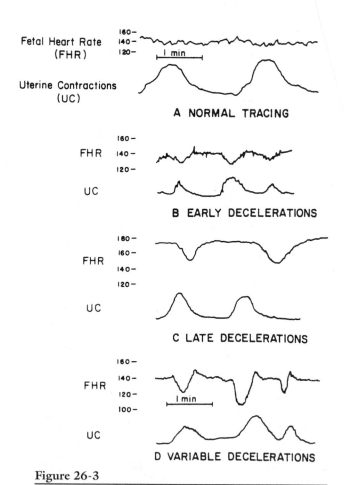

Figure 26-3

Bioelectronic monitoring of fetal heart rate (FHR) and uterine contractions (UC).

Table 26-2

The Apgar Score*

		Score		
Sign	0	1	2
Heart rate	Absent	<100 beats/minute	>100 beats/minute
Respiratory effort	Absent	Irregular, slow, gasping	Regular, rhythmic
Muscle tone	Limp	Some flexion of extremities	Active motion
Reflex response to stimulation	None	Grimace	Vigorous cry
Color	Pale, completely cyanotic	Body pink, extremities cyanotic	Completely pink

*The Apgar score at 1 minute is indicative of the degree of depression at birth. A score of 7 to 10 indicates minimal or no depression, 3 to 6 indicates moderate depression, and 0 to 2 indicates severe depression requiring vigorous resuscitation. The 5-minute Apgar score suggests the severity of depression and the effectiveness of resuscitation.

equivocal and described as preacidotic, and those below 7.21 are considered acidotic, signaling fetal compromise.

■ Care of the Newborn in the Delivery Rroom

Birth is associated with transient neonatal asphyxia, which is overcome spontaneously by most newborns. Normal newborns cry spontaneously, have good muscle tone, and cry in response to stimuli such as nasal suction. Heart rate is normally 120 to 160 beats per minute, and systolic blood pressure lies in the range of 55 to 70 mmHg. Moderately or severely depressed neonates require prompt and effective therapy to aid in rapid adaptation to extrauterine life and to prevent neurologic, circulatory, respiratory, and gastrointestinal problems.

From birth until the upper airway is cleared, the newborn's head is maintained below the level of the torso, in the sniffing position. The mouth and posterior pharynx are quickly cleared of secretions. Nasal suction and aspiration of gastric contents, often associated with bradycardia and further depression, are delayed until adequate respiration, circulation, and reflex activity are present. With the airway ensured, normal respiration usually appears. Gently slapping the soles of the feet encourages breathing, crying, and lung expansion; more vigorous forms of stimulation are traumatic, dangerous, and not effective. Should the neonate remain dusky or cyanotic despite normal respirations, oxygen is given via a tight-fitting face mask until color improves. Gentle assistance to breathing may prove helpful.

Immediate evaluation of a newborn is accomplished by assessing the Apgar score at 1 and 5 minutes (Table 26-2). If required, resuscitation is begun before the 1-minute score is obtained. If the neonate does not respond to initial routine treatment, or if the 1-minute score is less than 7, resuscitation is begun by following established guidelines of cardiopulmonary resuscitation (see Chap. 33).

Neonates who remain apneic, gasping, or with inadequate respirations require positive-pressure ventilation. With the head in a sniffing position and an oral airway in place, ventilation is immediately attempted with oxygen, using a mask and breathing bag, at 25 to 40 breaths per minute. Adequacy of ventilation is assessed by auscultation of the lungs. Although pressures up to 60 cmH$_2$O may be required initially to expand the newborn's lungs, lesser pressures usually provoke gasping followed by a normal breathing pattern. If the lungs cannot be expanded, or if the fetal heart rate remains below 100 beats per minute beyond 30 seconds, the trachea is intubated, followed by positive-pressure breathing with oxygen. Unless pulmonary aspiration of meconium is suspected or heart sounds are absent, bag and mask ventilation precedes intubation, since this is frequently successful in initiating respirations. Ventilation is continued until breathing becomes regular and respiratory exchange adequate.

The fetus may aspirate meconium in utero, but more frequently aspiration occurs just after birth, causing mechanical obstruction, chemical pneumonitis, and even death. When the fetus is delivered through thick meconium in a vertex presentation, the obstetrician thoroughly clears the baby's oral and nasal pharynx by suction before delivery of the shoulders. If, at birth, the neonate does not breathe at once, or if signs of respiratory obstruction are evident, tracheal intubation is performed immediately, but no attempt is made to begin positive-pressure ventilation. Instead, meconium is aspirated by applying negative pressure directly to the tracheal tube. Tracheal suction may be required several times before adequate ventilation is possible.

A neonate born through meconium who begins breathing immediately is first given oxygen. Although it was taught in the past that laryngoscopy and intubation must immediately follow birth to determine whether meconium is present below the cords, it now appears that this is only required for thick meconium observed in the mouth near the vocal cords. If meconium is found in the trachea, the cycle of oxygenation by mask, laryngoscopy, and tracheal suction via the endotracheal tube is repeated until no more meconium can be removed. If meconium is aspirated from the trachea, the baby is transferred to a neonatal intensive care unit for appropriate intensive care under the direction of a neonatologist.

The newborn's heart rate rarely fails to increase to over 100 beats per minute when ventilation and oxygenation are established. Should cardiac arrest occur or the heart rate remain less than 100 beats per minute after adequate ventilation, closed chest cardiac compression at 120 per minute is begun, and the trachea intubated. Positive-pressure breathing is at the rate of one breath for every fifth chest compression. The sternum is compressed 1.5 to 2 cm at its midpoint, as illustrated in Figure 26-4; compression continues until a heart rate above 100 beats per minute is maintained. Elevation of the legs may improve venous return.

Severely depressed neonates inevitably suffer marked metabolic acidosis, requiring correction before the transition to neonatal circulation occurs. This is accomplished with 2 mEq/kg of sodium bicarbonate solution prepared by diluting the usual bicarbonate solution (7.5% or 8.4%) with an equal volume of preservative-free water. The solution is injected into the umbilical vein over a 2-minute period and is repeated in 3 to 5 minutes if there is no improvement. Further doses of bicarbonate are not given without first ascertaining serum electrolyte values, osmolality, and acid-base status. Bicarbonate administration causes an increase in $PaCO_2$, which requires enhanced ventilation. Hyperosmolar bicarbonate solutions have been implicated in the development of intracerebral hemorrhages, especially in the premature neonate. The doses recommended present little risk compared with the hazard of untreated metabolic acidosis.

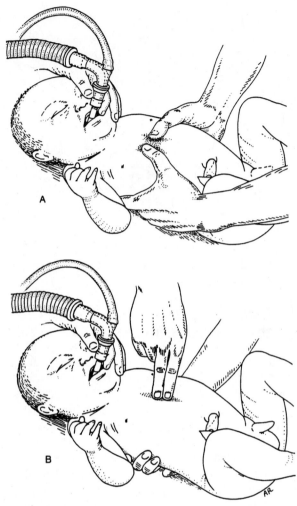

Figure 26-4

Two methods of closed chest cardiac compression of the neonate. (*A*) The two-thumb technique, in which the remainder of the fingers are interlocked behind the upper back. Note that the pressure is applied on the upper sternum just above the midline. Also note the continued ventilation of the neonate via an endotracheal tube. (*B*) The two-finger technique using the index and middle fingers of one hand. The other hand of the resuscitator is placed under the upper back to serve as a hard surface.

A poor response to therapy suggests an intravascular fluid deficit, which can be treated with 10 ml/kg of balanced salt solution or lesser amounts of 5% albumin, packed red blood cells, or whole blood, depending on the hematocrit. Failure of the heart rate to respond to these measures prompts the use of cardiac stimulants such as epinephrine (0.2 ml/kg of a 1:10,000 solution), calcium gluconate (1 to 2 ml/kg of a 10% concentration), or both, given through an umbilical venous catheter and not by direct cardiac injection. Until vascular access is established, epinephrine can be given through the endotracheal tube.

If opioids given to the mother have depressed the newborn's respiration, naloxone, 10 µg/kg, is given intravenously or intramuscularly. Because depression can recur when the effect of the naloxone dissipates, close observation is required. If respiratory depression does not respond to naloxone, there must be a cause other than opioids. If chronic maternal narcotic abuse is suspected, naloxone must be withheld from the neonate because it may cause sudden and disastrous withdrawal.

Its relatively large body surface area and inability to shiver render the neonate particularly vulnerable to cooling. To prevent hypothermia, the infant is dried immediately after bith and then placed fully exposed under a suitable warmer, protected from drafts. A newborn must never be placed directly on a metal surface, which causes rapid loss of heat.

Moderately or severely depressed neonates require pediatric evaluation and care in an intensive care facility. These babies frequently experience apneic episodes, respiratory distress, convulsions, and hypothermia and may be unable to accept oral feedings. They may require monitored oxygen supplementation and ventilatory support.

BIBLIOGRAPHY

Abboud TK, Shakuntala N, Murakawa K, et al. Comparison of the effects of general and regional anesthesia for Cesarean section on neonatal neurologic and adaptive capacity scores. *Anesth Analg* 1985;64:996-1000.

Chestnut DH. *Obstetric Anesthesia: Principles and Practice.* St. Louis: Mosby, 1994.

James FW III, Wheeler AS, Dewan DM. *Obstetric Anesthesia: The Complicated Patient,* 2nd Ed. Philadelphia: FA Davis, 1988:

Ramanathan J, Coleman P, Sibai BM. Anesthetic modifications of hemodynamic and neuroendocrine stress responses to cesarean delivery in women with severe preeclampsia. *Anesth Analg* 1991;73:772-779.

Shnider SM, Levinson G. *Anesthesia for Obstetrics,* 3rd Ed. Baltimore: Williams & Wilkins, 1993.

27

Geriatric Patients

Stanley Muravchick

Elderly Americans, already numbering more than 20 million, are the fastest growing component of our society. With aging comes age-related disease, much of it responsive to surgical treatment and requiring perioperative evaluation and care by an anesthesiologist. Typically, 25 percent or more of patients undergoing operation are 65 years of age or older. This chapter introduces the physiology of aging, the essentials of age-related disease, and their relevance to the design, execution, and outcome of anesthetic management.

Definition of Aging

Determining the chronologic age at which people become "elderly" has always been an inexact process. Aging is currently defined only in conceptual terms; the mechanisms responsible for this phenomenon at biochemical or cellular levels remain undiscovered. Whatever the underlying explanation may be, aging is a universal, progressive process that changes both the structure and function of tissues and organs during the adult and later years of the life span. Age-related changes that are not universal, or those in which severity or magnitude do not increase with advancing age, probably represent age-related disease rather than the physiologic process of aging.

Although at one time aging was thought to produce a simple, linear decline of all capacities with advancing years, the actual function of integrated organ systems changes in a surprisingly complex manner (Fig. 27-1). The peak of physical (somatic) maturation and organ system functional capacity

occurs not in the second decade of life but nearer the age of 30 years. In addition, most organ system functions appear to be well maintained in health throughout the middle adult years. Functional reserve begins to decline rapidly in the eighth decade and beyond. The rate of change of organ system function with age varies greatly even in the absence of disease. Those elderly patients who maintain functional capacities greater than usual are said to be "physiologically young." In contrast, when function declines early, patients are referred to as "physiologically old."

Estimating the relative physiologic age of geriatric patients during their preanesthetic evaluation assists both in predicting outcome and in designing the anesthetic plan, which includes not only the choice of drugs and technique but also selection of monitoring, development of a plan for managing postoperative pain, and consideration of the suitability for same-day discharge from the hospital or the need for intensive postoperative observation. The difference between maximal capacity and basal levels of function represents functional reserve, used to meet the demands imposed by trauma, disease, operation, and convalescence. Objectively assessed using various exercise or stress tests, functional reserve is progressively and significantly impaired in elderly patients (Fig. 27-2).

■ Cardiopulmonary Function

Throughout life, cardiopulmonary function responds automatically to physical activity and metabolic demands. The modest decreases in resting cardiac index seen in most elderly subjects, largely

% ORGAN FUNCTION

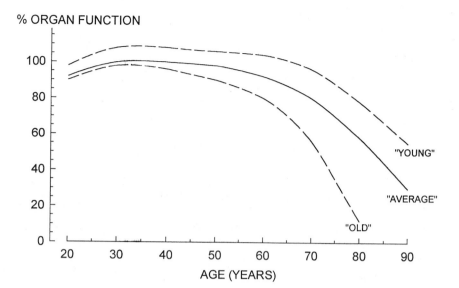

Figure 27-1

Variability (*broken lines*) in the rate at which organ system function changes with increasing age (*solid line*) explains the presentation of patients as physiologically "young" or "old." As with virtually all physiologic functions, variability itself increases with age.

resulting from a lower resting heart rate, are appropriate responses to the decreased metabolic requirements for oxygen that age imposes through the loss of skeletal muscle mass and the atrophy of major organs, such as the liver, that have high metabolic rates. Classic data suggesting that aging produces an irreversible and relentless primary reduction of resting cardiac output are not supported by recent studies of fit and active elderly subjects, in whom metabolic demands are maintained and readily met by changes in cardiopulmonary function.

However, aging does impose progressive limits on maximal heart rate and the inotropic response to

beta-adrenergic stimulation. Consequently, short-term demands for increased cardiac output appear to be met in the elderly largely by increased left ventricular end-diastolic volume and augmented stroke volume (Fig. 27-3), with little change in ejection fraction, and by slower maximal heart rates than are seen in younger subjects. Cardiopulmonary functional reserve, as determined by maximal sustainable aerobic capacity, is clearly less in older than in younger adults, but in the absence of disease, there are no age-related changes in myocardial function itself that compromise ventricular function. The maximal velocity of myocardial shortening (V_{max}) and the rate of ventricular

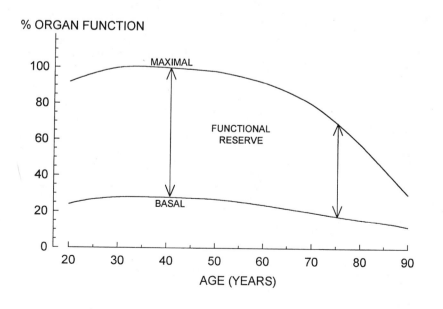

Figure 27-2

The age-related decline in organ system reserve is due to the progressive narrowing of the difference between basal and maximal levels of organ function.

pressure generation (dP/dT), two standard indices of myocardial contractility, remain uncompromised in healthy elderly subjects under conditions of submaximal demand.

Aging is associated with structural changes in the cardiovascular system that result in altered hemodynamics. Progressive increases in connective tissue cross-linking and loss of elastic fibers in the walls of the cardiac chambers make the aged heart stiffer and less compliant. Ventricular filling during the early passive phase of diastole is therefore compromised, increasing dependence on atrial contraction to achieve complete ventricular preloading at the end of diastole. As a result, the elderly patient is particularly susceptible to sudden hypotension if sinus rhythm is disrupted by a cardiac dysrhythmia. The reduced compliance of the aged ventricle implies that even healthy elderly patients have a narrowed range of acceptable filling pressures between the undesirable extremes of inadequate venous return or volume overload.

Aging also causes loss of arterial elasticity. Progressive stiffening of the arterial vasculature reduces the ability of the aorta and large arteries to store hydraulic energy, thereby increasing impedance to stroke volume ejection and requiring greater cardiac work. As a consequence, there is significant age-related concentric hypertrophy of the left ventricular wall. This loss of elasticity also acts to widen arterial pulse pressure (Fig. 27-4). Finally, the increased reflection of high-velocity pressure waves by a less elastic arterial tree produces the ringing or overshoot seen on radial artery waveform tracings and increases the discrepancy between invasive and cuff blood pressures. Although it is even more exaggerated in elderly patients with superimposed atherosclerotic disease, widening of arterial pulse pressures appears to be a manifestation of aging itself. It is seen even in nonindustrialized societies where overt hypertensive vascular disease is virtually unknown.

Loss of tissue elasticity also appears to be the primary mechanism by which age exerts its effect on pulmonary function, since elastic lung recoil decreases with age. Even without definable disease, elderly patients experience emphysema-like increases in lung compliance; residual volume and functional residual capacity (FRC) increase as a fraction of total lung capacity, markedly reducing vital capacity (Fig. 27-5). The changes in the elasticity and quality of the lung parenchyma are not uniform, however, so they compromise the normal intrapulmonary matching of ventilation ($\dot{V}$) and perfusion ($\dot{Q}$). Consequently, aging produces progressive increases in venous admixture, especially when hypoxic pulmonary vasoconstriction is depressed during general anesthesia (Fig. 27-6). In addition, loss of parenchymal tissue and elastin produces breakdown of alveolar septa, a process that results in a progressive reduction in the surface area available for gas exchange. Finally, age-related loss of the normal tethering of small airways by lung elastic recoil appears to allow closing capacity,

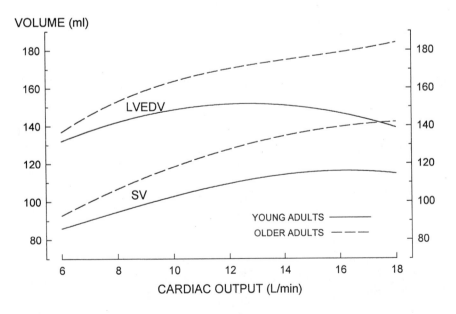

Figure 27-3

In healthy older subjects (*broken lines*), unlike young adults (*solid lines*), increased demand for cardiac output is met by an increased stroke volume (SV), which compensates for age-related decreases in maximum attainable heart rate. Lessened responsiveness to beta-adrenergic inotropy also may be responsible for increasing left ventricular end-diastolic volume (LVEDV) and lack of improved ejection fraction.

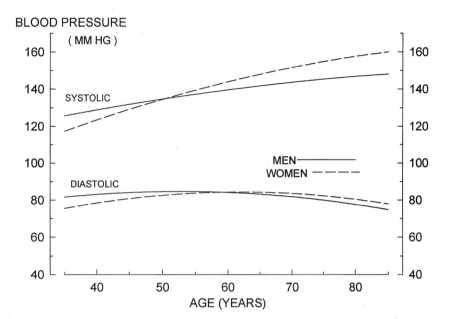

Figure 27-4

Data from the Framingham longitudinal study confirm that even in healthy elderly subjects, aging is associated with widening pulse pressure and relative systolic hypertension, especially in women (*broken lines*).

the lung volume at which small airway closure occurs, to increase into the range of lung volumes normally associated with tidal breathing.

Pulmonary functional reserve is adequate to maintain full oxygen saturation in most aged patients, but PaO_2 is significantly reduced in elderly patients be-

fore, during, and after operation (Fig. 27-7). Supplemental oxygen is sufficient treatment. Elderly individuals have diminished ventilatory responses to hypoxia or hypercarbia and therefore require closer monitoring than do younger patients until completely recovered from anesthetics, analgesics, and other

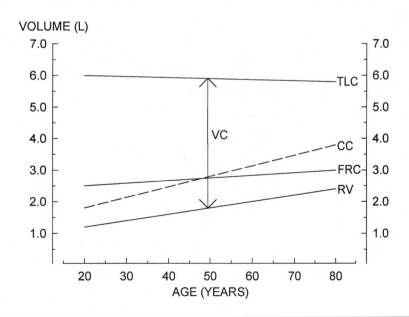

Figure 27-5

Age-related changes in the mechanical properties of the lung and chest wall are responsible for a progressive increase in residual lung volume (RV) and loss of vital capacity (VC), although total lung capacity (TLC) is relatively unchanged. By middle age, supine closing capacity (CC, *broken lines*), the lung volume at which there is small airway closure, increases markedly and begins to overlap functional residual capacity (FRC), the volume of the lung at rest, which increases only slightly.

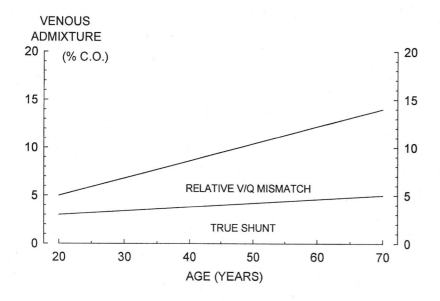

Figure 27-6

During general anesthesia with spontaneous breathing, older subjects have a higher fraction of venous admixture, due largely to age-related disruption of ventilation-perfusion (V/Q) matching within the lung parenchyma.
(Data courtesy of Dr. G. Hedenstierna.)

depressants. Aging produces a twofold increase in the risk of airway obstruction, hypoxemia, or carbon dioxide retention in patients recovering from general anesthesia in the postanesthesia care unit.

■ Hepatorenal Function

The primary effects of aging on hepatic physiology appear to be quantitative rather than qualitative. Hepatic microsomal enzyme activity in elderly subjects is comparable with that of young adults, but there is a one-third reduction in liver size and splanchnic blood flow by age 80. Perfusion is adequate for normal metabolic functions, but liver blood flow is significantly less in older subjects. In effect, age redistributes cardiac output away from the splanchnic and hepatic beds.

Consequently, bromsulfophthalein (BSP) retention test results usually approach the upper limit of "normal" by the seventh decade of life, and thereafter this test of overall hepatocellular capacity generally remains slightly abnormal even in healthy older patients. Serum albumin, however, is essentially age-independent. As they age, women are better able than men to maintain near-normal rates of hepatic clearance for drugs such as the benzodiazepines, although there is great individual variability. Although adequate for normal demands, hepatic function may be

Figure 27-7

Preoperative, intraoperative, and postoperative arterial oxygen tension (PaO_2) declines in a virtually linear fashion with advancing age.

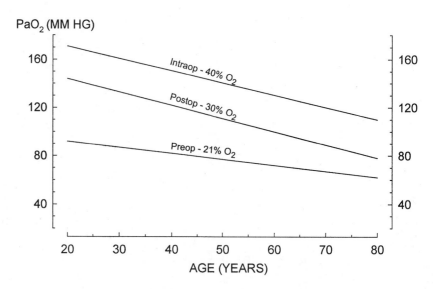

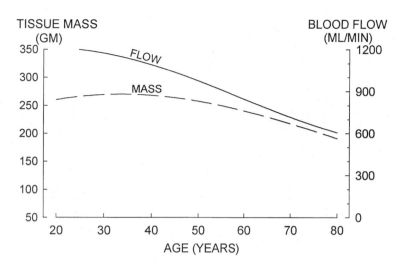

Figure 27-8

Total blood flow to the kidney (*solid line*) is compromised to a greater degree than would be expected from the relatively mild atrophy of renal tissue mass (*broken line*) seen in elderly subjects because of marked loss of renal tissue vascularity.

overwhelmed under conditions of stress or hemodynamic instability. The efficiency of hepatic biotransformation of drugs in elderly patients is extremely difficult to predict.

With increasing age, there is some atrophy of renal cortical tissue and a disproportionate reduction in the perfusion of renal tissue (Fig. 27-8). Glomerular filtration rate (GFR) decreases linearly by about 8 ml/min per 1.73 m² during each decade of the middle-adult years, a decrease somewhat more modest than that of renal plasma flow because of compensatory increases in filtration fraction.

Aging reduces skeletal muscle mass and creatinine load so that the serum creatinine level in elderly patients may be normal, even though GFR is decreased. Renal functional reserve needed to handle salt or water loading is reduced, and responsiveness to antidiuretic hormone (ADH) and aldosterone-mediated sodium conservation both are impaired. Diminished thirst, poor diets, and the widespread use of diuretics make dehydration likely. Consequently, elderly patients require careful preoperative evaluation and intraoperative fluid management.

■ Metabolism and Body Composition

The progressive loss of skeletal muscle mass and selective atrophy of intensely metabolically active tissues in brain, liver, kidney, and other vital organs steadily reduce the caloric requirements, basal oxygen consumption, total-body potassium, and total-body water of healthy aging subjects (Fig. 27-9). Resting body heat production decreases by about 15 percent

between young adulthood and senescence. More severe central hypothermia is required in older patients to trigger autonomic thermoregulatory responses during anesthesia, and those responses are less vigorous. During general anesthesia, the core body temperature of an elderly patient decreases more than twice as fast as that of a young adult.

Elderly patients also are less able to respond to an intravenous glucose challenge. Insulin secretion itself appears to remain normal, so age-related glucose intolerance probably reflects either impairment of insulin function or antagonism of its effects by other substances. Age-related muscle loss also contributes because skeletal muscle is insulin-sensitive tissue that normally provides storage for carbohydrates. After moderate increases due to fat gain through the sixth decade of life, total body weight decreases rapidly, because of continuing loss of skeletal muscle mass.

Despite the impression that aging produces hypovolemia, healthy elderly subjects maintain normal plasma and extracellular fluid volumes, although total-body water decreases with lean tissue mass. Aging increases the ratio of total-body lipid to total-body water in both sexes, a change that influences the pharmacokinetics of anesthetics and other lipid-soluble molecules.

■ Central Nervous System Function

Age-related changes in the nervous system have direct consequences for the planning of anesthetics for elderly patients. Among the most important changes is the selective attrition of cerebral and

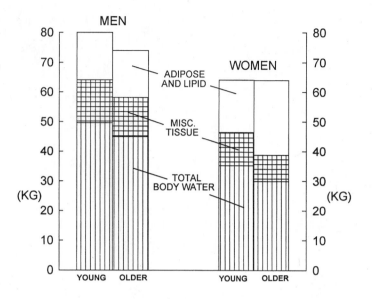

Figure 27-9

Changes in body composition are both age- and gender-sensitive. Men lose total-body mass, largely from contraction of total-body water. Women maintain body weight, losing water and bone but increasing adipose tissue.

cerebellar cortical neurons, including exaggerated loss of neurons involved in the synthesis of dopamine, catecholamines, serotonin, and other brain neurotransmitters. The enhanced side effects in the aged of drugs such as droperidol and scopolamine may reflect depletion of essential brain neurotransmitters.

The intrinsic mechanisms by which the brain closely couples regional neuronal electrical activity, cellular metabolism, and blood flow are intact in the healthy elderly subject. Autoregulation of cerebral blood and cerebrovascular responsiveness to carbon dioxide remain active. Total brain mass and cerebral blood flow are both reduced by 30 percent or more (Fig. 27-10). This decrease in cerebral blood flow is proportional to decreased metabolic requirements and is not the cause of age-related cerebral atrophy and dysfunction. Cerebrovascular accident is a surprisingly rare perioperative complication in elderly subjects, despite the wide fluctuations in blood pressure inevitably experienced during anesthesia and surgery.

Aging produces marked simplification of synaptic interconnections between neurons in cortical and some subcortical areas, producing deterioration of

Figure 27-10

With age, brain tissue mass (*solid lines*), especially grey matter, undergoes selective attrition and loss of neuronal density, producing a marked decline in total cerebral blood flow (CBF) requirements (*broken line*).

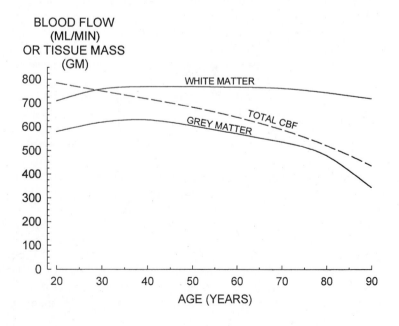

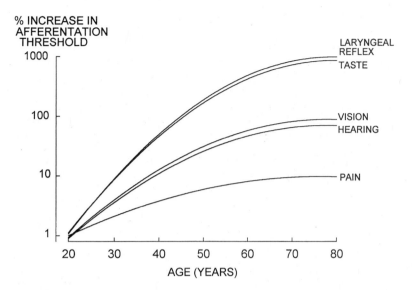

Figure 27-11

Central and peripheral degeneration within the nervous system leads to age-related increases in afferentation thresholds that vary greatly in magnitude (note logarithmic vertical axis).

complex mental functions that rely on short-term memory, visual and auditory reaction time, and other manifestations of "fluid intelligence." Even minimal perioperative sedation may produce amnesia or disorientation for long periods of time, a special problem in those scheduled for outpatient surgery. Elderly patients more often suffer short-term psychological abnormalities after cardiopulmonary bypass as well.

Aging also markedly increases thresholds for virtually all forms of perception, including vision, hearing, touch, joint position, smell, and temperature (Fig. 27-11). These changes are so consistent that objective measurements of summed sensory deficits may have value as biologic markers of aging. Nevertheless, complex afferent information such as pain continues to undergo extensive processing and modification within the central nervous system, so age-related changes do not guarantee the elderly patient reduced postoperative pain. The more imminent threat of death or incapacitation can worsen an elderly patient's responses. It is inappropriate to routinely reduce or withhold from aged patients treatment for pain and anxiety to avoid drug-induced complications. As for all other patients, therapy must be adjusted individually.

■ Peripheral Nervous System

Aging produces a loss of peripheral nerve fibers. Both afferent and efferent nerve conduction velocities decrease progressively, and corticospinal transmission is slowed, contributing to the delay between thought, intention, and movement. Reduced protoplasmic transport within motor nerve axons deprives aging skeletal muscle of essential myotrophic support. Muscle mass decreases and motor endplate structures proliferate, perhaps accounting for reduced effectiveness of nondepolarizing neuromuscular blockers.

Overall, the effect of aging on peripheral nerve and skeletal muscle is one of progressive disseminated atrophy. Fine skeletal muscle control and the ability to maintain postural steadiness decline by age 80. However, strength can be maintained by consistent physical activity, since use maintains the motor nerve–skeletal muscle unit.

With age, sympathoadrenal pathways also are subject to neuronal attrition and fibrosis. Adrenal tissue mass decreases about 15 percent by age 80, but plasma concentrations of epinephrine and norepinephrine are actually greater in the elderly both at rest and during exercise. Because age impairs beta-adrenoceptor responsiveness, increased levels of plasma catecholamines are usually not apparent unless abruptly suppressed. In effect, a generalized hyperadrenergic state counterbalances the reduced responses of aging vascular smooth muscle and other autonomic effectors. This compensatory mechanism partially restores the effectiveness of autonomic homeostasis.

Reduced autonomic end-organ responsiveness probably reflects a change in the quality rather than a reduction in the quantity of adrenoceptors. Receptor affinity for both beta-adrenergic (but not alpha-adrenergic) agonists and antagonists declines with

Table 27-1

Implications of Age-Related Physiologic Changes

Physiologic Change	Anesthetic Implications
Reduced central nervous system reserve	Decreased anesthetic requirement, prolonged residual depression
Neuronal atrophy in peripheral nervous system	Impaired autonomic responsiveness, slight increase in nondepolarizer dose requirements
Reduced renal blood flow; tissue loss	Reduced ability to handle salt and water loads, delayed excretion of many drugs
Reduced hepatic blood flow; tissue loss	Reduced rates of hepatic drug biotransformation
Decreased cardiac reserve, reduced ventricular compliance	Limitation of maximal cardiac output, intolerance of rapid changes in preload
Loss of pulmonary elasticity	Impaired matching of ventilation and perfusion, increased oxygen gradient
Decreased immune responsiveness	Susceptibility to stress-related infection and sepsis
Reduced skeletal muscle mass	Decreased heat production, relative glucose intolerance, increase in body lipid fraction

increasing age so that there are diminished increases in heart rate following isoproterenol, epinephrine, or atropine, yet greater doses of propranolol or esmolol are required, too. Reduced adenylate cyclase activity within the cell itself further impairs adrenoceptor function.

Whatever the precise mechanism, age-related limits on autonomic responsiveness impair an elderly subject's ability to maintain stable arterial blood pressures during anesthesia and operation. Baroreflexes, vasoconstrictor responses to cold, and postural changes in heart rate in elderly subjects are slowed, diminished, and less effective. Intraoperative and postoperative arterial hypotension and hypertension are more frequent, more severe, and more often require treatment than in younger adults (Table 27-1).

■ Clinical Pharmacology

Elderly patients often require lesser doses of anesthetic drugs than do the young, but the explanations for this are often unclear. Drug interactions and side effects do occur more often in elderly patients (Fig. 27-12). Chronic disease also encourages polypharmacy, further aggravating the chance for drug-induced complications (Table 27-2).

The changes in organ function and body compo-

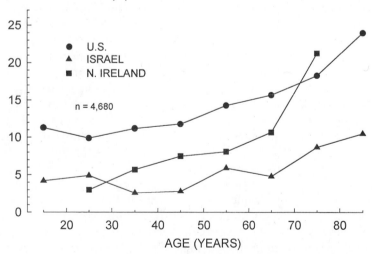

INCIDENCE OF ADVERSE
DRUG REACTIONS (%)

- ● U.S.
- ▲ ISRAEL
- ■ N. IRELAND

n = 4,680

AGE (YEARS)

Figure 27-12

Data from three different countries consistently demonstrate a progressive increase in the percentage of patients reporting adverse drug reactions in older patient groups.

Table 27-2

Adjustments of Anesthetic and Adjuvant Drugs in Elderly Patients

Drug Group	Adjustment Needed
Potent inhalational agents	Decrease end-tidal concentration, allow more time for emergence
Barbiturates, etomidate, propofol	Small to moderate decrease in initial dose, smaller maintenance doses
Narcotics	Marked decrease in initial dose, anticipate increased duration of effect (except fentanyl)
Local anesthetics for spinal or epidural anesthesia	Small to moderate decrease in segmental dose requirement, anticipate prolonged effect and urinary retention
Benzodiazepines	Modest decrease in initial dose, anticipate marked increase in duration (except midazolam)
Succinylcholine	None
Nondepolarizing relaxants	Same or slight increase in initial dose, anticipate increased duration (except atracurium)
Neostigmine, edrophonium	No change in dose, prolonged effect
Atropine	Increased dose requirement, anticipate central anticholinergic syndrome
Adrenergic agonists	Increased dose requirement

sition alter both the pharmacokinetics and the pharmacodynamics of drugs used in anesthesia. Elderly patients, especially those who are ill or hospitalized, also vary more in cardiac output and organ blood flows than do young adults. It is difficult to determine whether age-related increases in apparent drug potency represent actual enhanced tissue sensitivity to drug effects (pharmacodynamics) or the predictable consequences of plasma drug concentrations that are simply greater than expected (pharmacokinetics). It is clear that short-term or early-phase redistribution of an injected drug, rather than the ultimate elimination of all drug molecules, determines the duration of effect of intravenous anesthetic drugs in the elderly as well as in young adults.

Because it is determined under steady-state conditions, avoiding uncertainties about pharmacokinetics, minimum alveolar concentrations (MAC) for inhalational anesthetics reflect the effects of age on pharmacodynamics. For a wide variety of inhalational agents, anesthetic requirement decreases by about 30 percent from age 20 to age 80 (Fig. 27-13).

Unfortunately, the data for narcotics, barbiturates, and benzodiazepines are much less consistent. Their apparently enhanced potency in the aged may be real, or it may result from poor drug mixing within the central circulation or delayed redistribution to peripheral compartments. Interpretation of data is confounded by difficulty in defining anesthetic endpoints other than MAC. Analysis of the electroencephalo-

gram suggests that aging increases brain sensitivity to narcotics but not to barbiturates or to etomidate. Whatever the mechanism, older patients require lesser doses of virtually all drugs that depress the central nervous system.

The pharmacokinetic profiles of most drugs used in anesthesia are nevertheless dramatically altered by age. Elimination half-life $(t_{1/2\beta})$, the time required for a 50 percent reduction of plasma drug concentration, is inversely proportional to the rate of drug clearance and directly proportional to the volumes in which the drug is distributed. Aging impairs the clearance of virtually all drugs requiring hepatic or renal elimination and also increases the fraction of total body weight that is lipid, increasing the relative distribution volume for lipid-soluble molecules. The elimination half-lives for the ultimate disposition of almost all intravenous anesthetics, narcotics, and adjuvants are therefore prolonged in the elderly, although these values may not necessarily predict the durations of their primary clinical effects, since those appear to be determined by rapid redistribution between various compartments. With the possible exception of meperidine, reduced drug binding to plasma and tissue proteins reported to occur with advancing age is probably not pharmacokinetically important.

Slightly impaired mobilization of acetylcholine at the neuromuscular junction in elderly patients is offset by increases in number of endplate cholinergic receptors. Consequently, the initial doses to produce

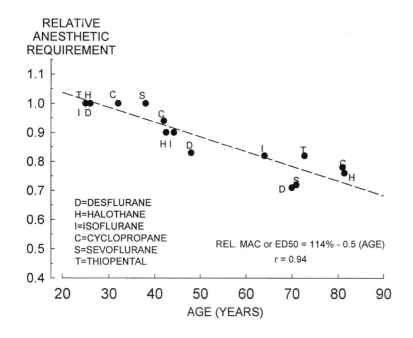

RELATIVE
ANESTHETIC
REQUIREMENT

D=DESFLURANE
H=HALOTHANE
I=ISOFLURANE
C=CYCLOPROPANE
S=SEVOFLURANE
T=THIOPENTAL

REL. MAC or ED50 = 114% - 0.5 (AGE)
r = 0.94

AGE (YEARS)

Figure 27-13

Linear regression analysis of data from many studies indicates that anesthetic requirement (MAC or ED_{50}) for all inhalational agents and for thiopental declines linearly with age.

nondepolarizing neuromuscular blockade with pancuronium, vecuronium, curare, or atracurium are either unchanged or increased only slightly. Pharmacokinetic factors in the elderly often prolong the duration of action of these drugs, but the choice of reversal agents, not patient age, determines the speed and completeness of return of neuromuscular function after a given level of blockade. The duration and the efficacy of antagonism by neostigmine or edrophonium are also unchanged.

Anesthetic Management and Outcome

Overall perioperative mortality increases with advancing age, beginning in the third decade of life. Epidemiologic data suggest that with the exception of very old or sick patients, anesthetic outcome and the incidence of major complications largely reflect the physical status, and not the age, of the patient (Fig. 27-14). Age-related disease, not age itself, is primarily responsible for morbidity and mortality among elderly patients. However, aging and loss of organ system function eventually become dominant risk factors for patients over age 80, especially if there is multiple organ system dysfunction.

Perioperative outcome also depends on the site of operation and the urgency of the procedure. Adequate time for diagnosis, treatment, and preparation wards off complications. Two-thirds of a geriatric surgical population demonstrate mild to severe hemodynamic and metabolic deficits when evaluated with invasive monitoring, and less than 15 percent of these patients are physiologically normal. One-third of the deficits discovered represent profound abnormalities such as congestive heart failure and marked hypoxemia, factors known to predict subsequent complications.

There is no single best anesthetic for elderly patients, but specific complications may be associated more commonly with one form of anesthesia than with another. For example, thromboembolism is more common with general anesthesia than with regional techniques in patients undergoing repair of hip fractures or major urologic operations. The risk of headache following dural puncture, closely related to needle size in young adults, is substantially less and relatively constant in older adults. Spinal or epidural anesthesia results in slight increases in dermatomal spread and duration in older patients for a given dose of local anesthetic and produces hypotension more often.

When overall outcome is determined over a period that encompasses both immediate and delayed sequelae (at least 30 to 60 days), the choice of anesthetic agent or technique per se does not appear to determine outcome; numerous retrospective and prospective clinical studies have concluded that there are no significant differences in perioperative survival or major morbidity attributable specifically to the anesthetic selected. Neither regional nor general anesthesia has yet been shown to provide the safest anesthetic for an elderly patient, although there is some evidence that the pain relief and sympathectomy produced by prolonged epidural analgesia may improve outcome by avoiding a sustained stress response.

The design of the anesthetic plan for elderly patients includes principles based on geriatric physiology. Prompt and complete recovery of mental function, a major concern in elderly patients who may already suffer deteriorating mental abilities, is compromised by polypharmacy. Fewer drugs are usually better. Hypothermia also delays awakening, perhaps because of the direct depressant effects of hypothermia or the reduced rates of drug clearance. Even when anesthetic management is appropriate and surgical convalescence uncomplicated, the return to preoperative mental status may require 5 to 10 days.

All the mechanisms responsible for this prolonged awakening remain unknown. The most common cause is the use of too much or too many anesthetic agents. Intravenous sedation delays rapid recovery of mental function otherwise expected after spinal or epidural anesthetic and may lead to prolonged disorientation or aggravate a preexisting situational psycho-

sis. Although "sundowning" and other types of abnormal mentation are often attributed to age, these problems also arise from deficient care. To remain oriented, elderly patients require increased sensory input and environmental cues that are often absent in a hospital setting. Feelings of dependency, loss of self-confidence, and despair for the future may worsen matters further.

Even the physical management of elderly patients requires some specific adjustments. Aged skin and bones are fragile. Joints are stiff, and the range of motion is limited, requiring gentle and expert care if traumatic injury from improper positioning, bandaging, or enforced inactivity is to be avoided. In elderly surgical patients, bleeding diatheses, hypercoagulable states, and a predisposition to bacterial infection appear more likely than in younger adults, especially if sustained sympathoadrenal stress responses occur during protracted recovery. Intraoperative hypothermia may produce postoperative vasoconstriction and shivering, precipitating myocardial ischemia.

An anesthetic plan that includes postoperative epidural analgesia may be of special value, eliminating the long periods of inadequate relief of postoperative pain sometimes imposed on geriatric patients because of fears of narcotic side effects. Perioperative management of fluids, metabolic state, electrolytes, and temperature must be meticulous. Aged patients do not require fundamentally different anesthetic management than do younger patients. They do require a higher standard of preparation, sensitivity, and vigilance.

Figure 27-14

Recent multicenter outcome data indicate that the probability a surgical patient will have a major complication (heart failure, arrhythmia, pneumonia) is increased slightly by age 50 in relatively healthy patients (ASA physical status II) but increases more sharply if elderly patients are seriously ill (ASA physical status IV). A physical status category of ASA I had no predictive value for serious complications.

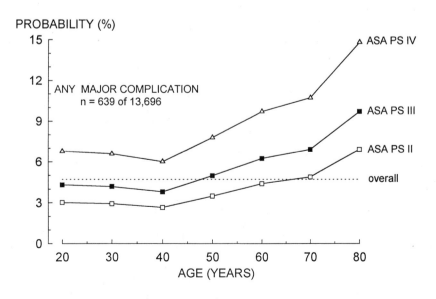

BIBLIOGRAPHY

Abrams WB, Beers MH, Berkow R, eds. *The Merck Manual of Geriatrics*. 2nd ed. Whitehouse Station, NJ: Merck and Co, 1995.

Avram MJ, Krejcie TC, Henthorn TK. The relationship of age to the pharmacokinetics of early drug distribution: The concurrent disposition of thiopental and indocyanine green. *Anesthesiology* 1990;72:403-411.

Creasey H, Rapoport S. The aging human brain. *Ann Neurol* 1985;17:2-10.

DelGuercio LRN, Cohn JD. Monitoring operative risk in the elderly. *JAMA* 1980;243:1350-1355.

Forrest JB, Rehder K, Cahalan MK, Goldsmith CH. Multicenter study of general anesthesia: III. Predictors of severe perioperative adverse outcomes. *Anesthesiology* 1992;76:3-15.

Geokas MC, Lakatta EG, Makinodan T, Timiras PS. The aging process. *Ann Intern Med* 1990;113:455-466.

Hanowell LH, Boyle WA III. Perioperative care of the hemodynamically unstable geriatric patient. *Int Anesthesiol Clin* 1988; 26:156-168.

Krechel SW, ed. *Anesthesia and the Geriatric Patient*. Orlando, Fla: Grune and Stratton, 1984.

Morrison RC. Hypothermia in the elderly. *Int Anesthesiol Clin* 1988;26:124-133.

Pfeifer MA, Weinberg CR, Cook D, et al. Differential changes of autonomic nervous system function with age in man. *Am J Med* 1983;75:249-258.

Scheff S. Morphological aspects of CNS aging: Human and experimental animal studies. *Rev Biol Res Aging* 1985;2:197-210.

Shock NW. Aging of physiological systems. *J Chron Dis* 1983;36: 137-142.

Wahba WM. Influence of aging on lung function: Clinical significance of changes from age twenty. *Anesth Analg* 1983; 62:764-776.

CHAPTER 28

Outpatient Anesthesia

Thomas J. Conahan and Marie L. Young

Outpatient procedures account for more than half the operations performed in the United States. They have become popular because patients believe it allows them greater control over their business and personal lives and because third-party payers find it reduces costs. The evolution of same-day surgery units has in many instances placed anesthesiologists in the role of gatekeeper for surgical outpatients, because they are in the best position to determine whether a patient is an acceptable candidate for an outpatient procedure. This chapter discusses patient selection and preoperative preparation, intraoperative anesthetic management, postanesthetic care, and follow-up for those undergoing outpatient surgery.

Patient Selection and Evaluation

The range of surgical procedures performed on outpatients now includes almost any that do not involve opening the cranium, chest, or abdomen; that do not produce major physiologic changes; and that do not require intense postoperative care. Discharge after outpatient surgery depends primarily on recovery from anesthesia rather than from the operation; the anesthesiologist often determines whether an outpatient surgical procedure is appropriate for an individual patient. Such patients are usually classified as ASA physical status I or II, but in many instances patients of ASA physical status III with stable systemic diseases are excellent candidates. On occasion, patients classified as ASA physical status IV, with appropriate preoperative evaluation and preparation, are candidates for outpatient operations. Other factors that affect the decision regarding outpatient surgery are included in Table 28-1.

Morbid obesity raises concerns about ventilation and airway management, pain management, and the patient's ability to walk postoperatively. Asthma is often cited as a contraindication to outpatient anesthesia and operation, but a patient with well-controlled asthma may undergo general anesthesia and operation as an outpatient. Both the patient and the surgeon must understand that hospitalization may be required if an acute asthma attack occurs. Physical or mental handicaps may make it impossible for a patient to receive adequate perioperative care outside of a skilled nursing facility. In general, the deciding question is whether the patient could be cared for more safely in a hospital than at home after the operation.

Some operations are not appropriate for outpatient care. Extensive blood loss or administration of large volumes of fluid require prolonged postoperative observation and continued treatment. When postoperative pain requires parenteral narcotics, special arrangements must be made to administer them safely at home. In recent years, free-standing recovery centers, nursing homes, and home nursing services have offered longer-term (24 to 48 hours) postoperative recovery care. The incidence and severity of complications that are due to the operation also may require inpatient management. Surgical procedures likely to produce postoperative bleeding, airway compromise, or vertigo are best performed where postoperative hospitalization is available.

Even if the patient and the procedure are amenable to outpatient management, the discharge environ-

Table 28-1

Outpatient Anesthesia: Patient Selection

Patient

1. ASA physical status (I, II, possibly III, rarely IV): There must be no substantial risk of a postoperative complication (MI, respiratory failure) that could be ameliorated by care in the hospital.
2. Reliability, compliance: The patient and partner must follow directions for postoperative care.
3. Discharge situation: A capable person must watch and help the patient at home after operation. The place in which the patient will live, whether apartment, hotel room, or nursing home, must be suitable for the care prescribed.
4. Age: Only specific health problems, not age itself, rule out same-day surgery for the elderly. Premature infants at risk of apneic episodes are not candidates for discharge on the day of surgery; infants born at term must be older than 4 weeks' postnatal and older than 44 weeks' gestation to undergo same-day surgery.

Procedure

1. Physiologic derangements produced by the operation itself must not require hospital care.
2. Blood loss must not be so great as to require transfusion (although autologous transfusion has been used for outpatient plastic surgery procedures).
3. Postoperative pain must be controlled with safe doses of opioids. These may be administered intravenously in the recovery area, but postoperative pain must be amenable to oral analgesics after discharge.
4. There must be no risk of postoperative airway obstruction.
5. The potential complications of the procedure must not immobilize the patient.

---

ment must be appropriate to provide adequate postoperative care. Patients who have received even a brief anesthetic suffer impairments in cognitive and motor functions. They need assistance in traveling home and must be accompanied by a responsible adult after the operation.

Preoperative evaluation before an outpatient operation is identical to that preceding any operation, but the patient may not be available in person for the preanesthetic visit, and the anesthesiologist must ensure that both the patient and the operation are appropriate for outpatient care (see Table 28-1). Necessary laboratory studies and basic information about the patient's medical and anesthetic history are best obtained prior to the day of operation so that significant abnormalities may be investigated, additional data may be obtained from consulting physicians, and wasted time is avoided for both the patient and the facility. Healthy patients may need to com-

plete a screening questionnaire (or respond to questions put by a health evaluation computer program) only, deferring the physical examination until the day of admission. Alternatively, the patient scheduled for an outpatient procedure may visit a preanesthetic evaluation clinic, as described in Chapter 2. An interview by the anesthesiologist in person or by telephone can clarify the available options for anesthetic management, allay anxiety, and provide realistic expectations regarding the day of operation and postoperative recovery.

The laboratory tests required for a given patient are determined by the patient's health and the proposed operation (see Chap. 2) and whether the patient is scheduled to go home on the day of operation or to stay overnight. The goal is appropriate testing only, in an effort to eliminate costly and unnecessary tests that do not modify care or outcome; thus "routine tests" are rarely appropriate.

Patients scheduled for outpatient procedures receive special preoperative instructions. They are advised as to when they can eat before operation and the medications they can take on the day of operation. There must be a clear understanding of arrangements for transportation home, the need for an adult to care for the patient after the operation, the degree of pain and immobility to be expected, the pain medication that will be prescribed, and any other measures needed postoperatively. Written instructions and an agreement signed by the patient and the person briefing the patient improve compliance.

Anesthetic Management

■ Preoperative Preparation

Patients who require medication daily, particularly for cardiac or pulmonary disease, are directed to take their prescribed doses on the morning of operation. Scheduling insulin-dependent diabetics early in the morning simplifies their care. Those receiving long-acting insulin receive one-third to one-half their usual dose, along with a glucose-containing intravenous solution. When the patient has recovered from anesthesia and can retain solid food without nausea or vomiting, the remainder of the morning dose of insulin may be administered. An alternative method of managing insulin requirements is useful when anesthesia and operation are unlikely to cause nausea. The patient takes no insulin before operation and treats the postoperative period as if he had just arisen in the morning, administering the normal dose of insulin postoperatively and resuming a normal meal schedule.

Before outpatient operations, patients are asked to abstain from food and liquids for several hours, but prolonged preoperative fasting is unnecessary, particularly for fluids. When risk factors are absent (e.g., impaired gastric emptying caused by pain, diabetes, opioids, pregnancy, obesity, or hiatal hernia), aspiration of gastric contents is a rare complication, the incidence of which probably is not reduced by prolonged fasting. A conservative recommendation is that healthy adult patients scheduled for elective outpatient operations should fast for 6 hours before anesthesia.

Although results vary among studies, more outpatients than inpatients arrive in the operating room with stomach contents of pH less than 2.5 or volume greater than 25 ml and thus are considered to be at risk for acid aspiration pneumonitis. These findings might suggest the routine preoperative prescription of histamine-2 (H_2) blockers, soluble antacids, or metoclopramide to reduce gastric acidity and volume before outpatient operation. However, this practice has not become popular, and there is no evidence that it would decrease the already small incidence of aspiration pneumonitis in these patients. The rare adverse side effects of H_2 blockers and metoclopramide also make it inadvisable to prescribe these drugs routinely for healthy outpatients who do not suffer the risk factors listed previously.

Premedication of outpatients varies widely; some centers use no premedication, while others premedicate patients routinely. Midazolam in small doses seems to delay discharge from the recovery room little, but usually premedicants are withheld to reduce the chance of delayed awakening. Factors influencing this decision include patient age, type and duration of operation, patient expectations, and the availability of a preoperative area to accommodate and monitor sedated patients. Those facilities where patients are admitted to a bed and observed for 2 hours preoperatively and at least 4 hours postoperatively are more likely to administer routine premedication than are the units where patients walk to the operating room shortly after arrival and are discharged as soon as possible postoperatively.

Pediatric patients often benefit from preanesthetic medication designed to allay anxiety, induce drowsiness, and minimize secretions, particularly when an inhalation induction is planned. Some physicians prescribe oral premedication for children, eliminating dreaded preoperative injections (see Chap. 25); emergence and postoperative recovery do not appear to be affected adversely by its use.

Anesthetic Agents and Techniques

Any anesthetic or technique may be used safely for outpatient operations, but some techniques are favored for efficiency and convenience. Determining factors include patient choice, surgical requirements, patient age and physical status, duration of drug action, and requirements for postoperative care (Table 28-2). The principal intent is to provide rapid recovery from the immobilizing effects of anesthesia and operation while leaving the patient as comfortable as possible for the transition from immediate postoperative recovery to recovery at home. This condition is often described as "street fitness," a misnomer that implies greater cognitive and motor ability than usually exist in the postoperative period.

More important than the choice of drugs in achieving this goal is the judgment of the person administering the anesthetic. Even agents soluble in tissue or with long durations of action allow early recovery if they are used in small doses and are discontinued early enough. Nevertheless, for outpatients, the best drugs are those with pharmacokinetic properties that provide a rapid offset of effect.

■ Local Anesthesia and Monitored Anesthesia Care

The combination of local anesthesia and monitored anesthesia care with sedation offers safety and early discharge for those outpatient surgical procedures and patients suited to these techniques. Local anesthetic may be administered by the anesthesiologist in the form of local infiltration of the operative site or field block, or it may be administered by the surgeon at the sterile field. The physical and the emotional comfort of the patient is attended to by the anesthesiologist (Table 28-3). Patients respond quite favorably to such attention and often voice their appreciation in the postoperative follow-up evaluation.

Patients' responses to sedative drugs are variable. Each administration is a titration, with respiratory depression and airway obstruction indicating that too

Table 28-2

Anesthetic Techniques for Ambulatory Surgery

General anesthesia
Advantages — Speed, guaranteed unconsciousness, intraoperative patient comfort

Disadvantages — Loss of protective airway reflexes, cardiovascular depression, delayed recovery, postoperative nausea and vomiting

Spinal or epidural anesthesia
Advantages — Patient awake, airway reflexes maintained, patient comfort, less physiologic disruption

Disadvantages — Time to do block, unpredictability of block, uncontrollable recovery time, difficulty voiding, back pain, post-dural puncture headache

Monitored anesthesia care
Advantages — Maintenance of protective airway reflexes, rapid recovery, patient participation in procedure (patient awareness)

Disadvantages — Patient awareness, potential for pain from inadequate local anesthesia, side effects of sedative drugs (e.g., nausea and vomiting), lack of patient cooperation

Regional or field block
Advantages — Anesthesia in area of incision, immediate readiness for discharge, patient awareness, less physiologic disruption

Disadvantages — Time to do block, potential for failed or inadequate block, patient awareness

much drug has been given and the patient's anxiety indicating too little drug. Adequate sedation may be identified by a patient's calm demeanor, slurred speech, slowed heart rate, or reduced blood pressure. The benzodiazepines, particularly midazolam, have assumed a major role in intraoperative sedation of outpatients. These drugs allay anxiety and produce some degree of amnesia. Individual responses vary widely: 1 to 10 mg midazolam may be needed for a 70-kg patient. Repeated administration of 0.5 to 1 mg intravenously every 2 to 5 minutes until the patient's eyes close spontaneously usually provides adequate anxiolysis and amnesia. When the patient asks to remain more aware, or when the patient must remain more alert because of bleeding in the airway or to cooperate with the surgeon, smaller doses of sedative are used and the patient is provided more constant verbal assurance.

The rapid onset, short half-life, and prompt recovery characteristics of propofol have made it a popular sedative for monitored anesthesia care. An infusion of propofol (50 to 150 μg/kg per minute) may be more expensive than other approaches, but it is easily controlled, and the shorter recovery period may offset cost of the drug alone.

Short-acting opioids such as fentanyl, sufentanil, and alfentanil are commonly part of monitored anesthesia care also. Narcotic analgesics administered prior to the injection of local anesthesia (e.g., 50 to 100 μg fentanyl 5 to 7 minutes before injection) often increase the patient's comfort. Infusions of short-acting narcotics allow precise control of depth of sedation and permit rapid recovery but also carry the risk of overdose if constant attention to the delivery of the drug lapses. Larger doses of opioids increase the likelihood of postoperative nausea and vomiting. Ultra short acting opioids, such as remifentanil, offer the possibility of greater control and safety and shorter duration of unwanted side effects. Meperidine in small doses (12 to 50 mg) controls shivering and provides postoperative analgesia.

Ultra short acting sedative-hypnotic drugs are sometimes employed in larger doses to provide hypnosis and sleep. A 25- to 100-mg dose of thiopental infused 2 minutes prior to a brief major stimulus (injection of local anesthetic, dilatation of the uterine cervix) effectively blunts patient discomfort during this period. However, sleep doses of barbiturates potentiate the respiratory depressant effects of opioids and other sedatives and must be administered with great care to avoid apnea or upper airway obstruction.

Table 28-3

Features of Monitored Anesthesia Care (MAC)

1. Minimize patient exposure prior to and during prepping and draping.
2. Arrange pillows and warm blankets for comfortable positioning.
3. Administer appropriate drugs in small increments to allay anxiety, reduce perception of pain, and produce amnesia without causing the patient to lose consciousness (conscious sedation).
4. Converse with the patient, offering reassurance and asking about patient's needs.

Propofol, 10 to 30 mg intravenously, can achieve the same effect as thiopental, but with faster recovery. Small doses of ketamine (0.1 to 0.5 mg/kg) can be used in place of opioids to supplement benzodiazepines with less risk of ventilatory depression, but at an increased risk of dysphoria.

Continuous intravenous sedation should not be administered in dilute solutions that require large infusion volumes for effect. The volume of intravenous fluid administered to a patient undergoing monitored anesthesia care with sedation must provide minimally adequate hydration only, to avoid the likelihood of an uncomfortably full bladder.

■ General Anesthesia

General anesthesia in outpatients must meet all the requirements of any successful general anesthetic, yet allow the patient to go home promptly after the surgical procedure. Less soluble inhaled anesthetics, intravenous agents with short durations of action, or those for which pharmacologic antagonists are available are popular. Inhalation induction of anesthesia may be employed (primarily in children) to avoid intravenous cannulation while the patient is awake. For most patients, anesthesia begins with propofol, thiopental, or methohexital, although large doses of either of the barbiturates contribute to postoperative lethargy. Consequently, propofol has gained popularity as both an induction and a maintenance agent for brief outpatient surgical procedures, although large doses (>1 g in adults) negate its short-acting characteristics. Use of etomidate as an induction agent has been limited because of its association with postoperative nausea, as well as concerns about suppression of adrenal function.

Indications for endotracheal intubation are identical in outpatients and in hospitalized surgical patients. One must weigh the risks of airway obstruction, hypoventilation, or passive regurgitation and subsequent aspiration against the risks of hypertension, tachycardia, sore throat, hoarseness, or dental or laryngeal damage attributable to intubation. The laryngeal mask airway (LMA) has become a popular airway adjunct for outpatient procedures because it reduces the need for tracheal intubation. Many cases that required tracheal intubation to remove the face mask from the surgical field are now managed with the LMA.

The choice of agents for maintenance of general anesthesia in outpatients is determined by patient factors, surgical requirements, and the preference of the anesthesiologist. The proponents of balanced anesthesia argue that the use of relatively large doses of narcotic analgesics and muscle relaxants and small doses of inhalation anesthetics allows a more rapid return to consciousness. Others believe that the administration of narcotic analgesics to patients who are expected to walk within a few hours of their operations increases the incidence of postoperative nausea and vomiting. As a rule, compared with those receiving opioids as part of the anesthetic, patients who receive greater concentrations of inhaled agents instead can be expected to awaken somewhat more slowly but to make a better recovery of cognitive function by several hours after operation if they have not received narcotic analgesics in the recovery room. Desflurane and sevoflurane are significantly less soluble in blood than the older inhalational agents, making them attractive in the ambulatory setting. This insolubility allows both rapid deepening and awakening, with the potential for early recovery and discharge home. Many clinicians advocate the administration of antisialagogues to decrease secretions if desflurane is used, for salivation is common with this drug. Somnolence is often not the limiting factor in determining discharge; instead, pain, nausea and vomiting, or complications of the surgical procedure delay recovery.

Total intravenous anesthesia (TIVA) is used sometimes for ambulatory patients. Infusions of propofol and an opioid with a rapid elimination profile (alfentanil, sufentanil) are supplemented with an amnesic (midazolam) and muscle relaxants. Inadequate anesthesia is difficult to detect with this technique, and some anesthesiologists are concerned about awareness. Awakening is typically rapid, but discharge may be delayed by persistent sedation, nausea, or pain.

Many outpatient procedures are superficial and require no muscle relaxation, so muscle relaxants may be required for intubation of the trachea only. Succinylcholine remains a good choice for this purpose because of its brief action. In cases where tracheal intubation is necessary and relaxation may be required for the surgical procedure, rocuronium, vecuronium, atracurium, or mivacurium may be suitable. Succinylcholine is associated with more postoperative myalgias, but nondepolarizing muscle relaxants may not be appropriate for many short procedures because of the duration of paralysis associated with intubating doses of these drugs.

■ Spinal and Epidural Anesthesia

Spinal or epidural anesthesia is sometimes used in ambulatory surgical patients. However, postural hypotension from residual sympathetic blockade and slow return of sensory and motor function may delay discharge. Spinal or epidural anesthesia may contribute to difficulty voiding also, and the ability to urinate is a criterion for discharge from most outpatient surgical units.

Subarachnoid anesthesia may be used, but it has not achieved significant popularity for outpatient surgery. The incidence of incapacitating post-dural puncture headache has been reported to be as great as 18 percent in ambulatory surgical patients. Such a complication rate may be accepted if choosing spinal anesthesia avoids some other more serious complication, but these situations are uncommon. Short-acting local anesthetics, such as procaine or lidocaine without epinephrine, are appropriate for brief procedures if subarachnoid anesthesia is selected.

Epidural anesthesia has been proposed as an effective alternative to spinal anesthesia. However, should dural puncture occur, the likelihood of headache is great because of the size of the needle used. Commonly used agents for epidural anesthesia in outpatients include 2-chloroprocaine, procaine, lidocaine, and mepivacaine.

Spinal or epidural anesthesia with minimal or no sedation may be advantageous in the elderly, in whom residual effects of general anesthesia or heavy sedation may last for days. However, a brief general anesthetic that employs only the least amounts required of the shortest-acting agents can produce nearly as prompt recovery as that after a regional anesthetic with modest sedation.

■ Regional Nerve Block

Regional nerve block or field block provides profound analgesia with minimal physiologic derangement. Periorbital and retrobulbar blocks are performed for ophthalmologic surgery. The brachial plexus may be blocked using either the axillary or interscalene approach, but the supraclavicular approach is less suitable because of possible pneumothorax. Intravenous perfusion blocks (Bier blocks) are easily performed and provide adequate analgesia for many brief procedures on the hand and wrist. The potential for sudden release of large amounts of local anesthetic into the systemic circulation detracts from the popularity of this technique. Blocks of the inguinal region for hernia repair and blocks at the wrist or ankle for operations on the hand or foot are accepted by most patients. Prolonged motor and sensory blockade impair postoperative mobility and increase the risk of inadvertent injury but may provide prolonged analgesia after particularly painful operations, such as orthopedic procedures. Because of the potential for side effects, prolonged regional anesthesia is used selectively, and not routinely, after outpatient procedures.

Postanesthetic Course

Ambulatory surgical patients remain in the care of skilled medical personnel for a much shorter time than do inpatients who progress from a recovery room to a surgical ward. Whereas the complications after anesthesia are the same in outpatients and inpatients, otherwise minor complications for inpatients may delay or prevent discharge of outpatients. Such complications are best avoided, and special efforts must be made to identify postoperative problems and reduce their impact.

Nausea, vomiting, and postoperative pain are the most common management problems in the outpatient recovery room. Nausea or vomiting occurs in 10 to 60 percent of postoperative patients. In addition to the physical discomfort, retching and vomiting may pose a risk to suture lines, thus increasing the risk of postoperative bleeding and hematoma. Many factors contribute to postoperative nausea, including narcotic analgesics, patient movement with subsequent motion sickness, middle ear disturbances, inhalational anesthetics, the surgical procedure, and postoperative pain. A variety of drugs, including anticholinergics (atropine), vasopressors (ephedrine), and tranquilizers, have been used to decrease nausea (Table 28-4). Other drugs (nitrous oxide, alfentanil) are sometimes avoided, with the same goal. Given the multitude of factors contributing to nausea and vomiting postoperatively and the sedative or dysphoric side effects of most antiemetics, it is not surprising that no single drug regimen has been effective invariably. Ondansetron and metoclopramide now offer the possibility of relief from postoperative nausea and vomiting while not adding to the level of sedation.

Patients may be surprised to experience significant pain after so-called minor operations. Pain management for these patients begins with preoperative education by the surgeon, anesthesiologist, and nurs-

Table 28-4

Antiemetic Agents for Outpatients

Drug	Dose (IV)	Potential Problems
Dopamine receptor antagonists		
Phenothiazines		Sedation, dystonic reactions
Prochlorperazine	2.5–10 mg	
Promethazine	6.25–25 mg	
Droperidol	0.625–1.25 mg	Sedation, dysphoria
Metoclopramide	5–10 mg	Agitation, dysphoria
Anticholinergics		
Atropine	0.5–1.0 mg	Tachycardia, dry mouth
Serotonin receptor antagonist		
Ondansetron	4 mg	Cost

ing staff so that the patient can anticipate the potential for discomfort and the plans for its relief (Table 28-5).

Life-threatening complications of anesthesia are most commonly related to the airway or the cardiovascular system. Airway or respiratory problems may develop over several hours postoperatively, especially when the operation has been in the airway or when airway injury has occurred during the course of the anesthetic; prolonged periods of postoperative observation are required when airway compromise is possible. Perioperative cardiovascular disturbances (hypertension, hypotension, myocardial ischemia, arrhythmias, or bradycardia) are becoming more common as older and less healthy patients are managed as outpatients. Consultation with specialists in other disciplines may be needed to determine the potential

severity of a perioperative incident and whether the patient must be observed overnight in the hospital.

Most symptoms that occur during the recovery room stay are part of the normal recovery process and require only reassurance. Careful preoperative preparation combined with gentle and caring reassurance postoperatively is preferable to pharmacologic treatments that might delay the return home.

Discharge from the Outpatient Recovery Suite

Before discharge, outpatients are expected to reach a level of function that includes return of vital signs to

Table 28-5

Postoperative Analgesics for Ambulatory Surgery Patients

Analgesia	Initial Dose	Potential Problems
Parenteral opioids		All: Respiratory depression, nausea, vomiting
Fentanyl	12.5–50 µg IV	
Meperidine	12.5–25 mg IV	
Morphine	2–5 mg IV	
Oral opioids		
Codeine	15–30 mg	Nausea, vomiting, sedation
Nonsteroidal analgesics		
Ketorolac	30–60 mg IM or IV	Potential platelet dysfunction
Oral analgesics		
Acetaminophen	300–600 mg PO	
Ibuprofen	300–600 mg PO	
Local anesthesia		
Wound infiltration	Bupivacaine 0.25%	
Joint perfusion	Bupivacaine 0.25% 10 ml	
	Morphine 1–10 mg	

baseline and, in most cases, walking, voiding, and tolerating oral fluids. Some patients are ready for discharge when they arrive in the recovery room; others may require several hours of care before they can go home safely. Duration of recovery may be affected by both anesthesia and operation. Factors considered in assessing readiness for discharge are listed in Table 28-6.

Assessment of respiratory function includes depth and frequency of respiration, as well as patency of the airway. There must be no residual effects of muscle relaxants, and the respiratory depression associated with narcotics must be acceptable. The complications of airway instrumentation such as sore throat, hoarseness, and lip, tooth, and gum injury also must be assessed and recorded.

The term *stable vital signs* is jargon for adequate cardiovascular and pulmonary function. In the postoperative period, patients ready for discharge must exhibit blood pressures and pulse rates similar to the preoperative values. Arrhythmias, chest pain, or other evidence of myocardial ischemia must be resolved and must be determined not to pose a threat to the patient's well-being. Attention to adequate hydration is particularly important in the ambulatory surgical patient to avoid hypovolemia and hypotension.

The surgical outpatient accompanied by an appropriate companion must be oriented to the surroundings, but need not be remarkably alert at the time of discharge, particularly if postoperative pain has required narcotic analgesics.

The rare patient who remains hypothermic in the recovery room is not a candidate for discharge. Most outpatient procedures are brief enough that the patient's body temperature does not decrease more than 1.5 to 2.5°C. Persistent hypothermia delays recovery, provokes shivering, and increases myocardial oxygen demand; it must be treated successfully before discharge.

Mobility, rather than the ability to walk per se, is required for discharge. The patient may not be able to walk because of the operation but must be able to move from wheelchair to car and from car to a comfortable place within the home.

Postoperative bladder distension is an inconvenient and uncomfortable complication of operation and anesthesia. Patients who can urinate prior to leaving the recovery room are less likely to experience this complication at home. Most patients who receive adequate fluids in the perioperative period experience an urge to void prior to meeting other criteria for discharge. Those patients who have received adequate intravenous fluids, those who have not had an operation likely to interfere with their ability to urinate, and those who have felt no need to do so may be released with specific instructions to seek care for urinary retention if they have not voided within 6 hours of the end of the operation.

Prior to discharge, patients and their escorts are again reminded of what to expect in terms of postoperative limitation of activity, pain management, and potential for delayed complications of anesthesia and operation. Postanesthetic follow-up, usually via a telephone call or postcard questionnaire, provides a means of identifying problems, documenting safe recovery, and monitoring the quality of the care provided.

In summary, successful outpatient anesthesia requires an appropriate patient undergoing a surgical procedure that allows recovery at home, with minimal risk of life-threatening complications. The recovery and return home are aided by choice of anesthetic techniques and agents that reduce postanesthesia

Table 28-6

Discharging Outpatients after Operation
Respiration
Maintains patent airway unassisted
Acceptable degree of respiratory depression
No threat of swelling or hematoma in airway
Cardiovascular
Heart rate and blood pressure near preoperative values
Hypovolemia corrected with IV fluids
Central nervous system
Orientated to person, place, and time
May doze but must awaken easily
Adequate vision
Surgical site
No more than expected swelling and drainage
No more than expected pain
Temperature
No hypothermia or unexplained fever
Nausea
Acceptable severity of vomiting
No threat of dehydration
Evening follow-up phone call scheduled
Mobility
Able to sit
Transfer bed-to-chair and back with one assistant
Walks, unless prevented by the operation
Bladder
Voids or is asked to call if has not voided in 6 hours

complications to the minimum and by careful preoperative preparation of the patient and the person who accompanies the patient home.

BIBLIOGRAPHY

McGoldrick K, ed. *Ambulatory Anesthesia: A Problem-Oriented Approach.* Baltimore: Williams & Wilkins, 1995.

Patel RI, Hannallah RS. Anesthetic complications following pediatric ambulatory surgery: A 3-year study. *Anesthesiology* 1988;69:1009-1012.

Wetchler BV. *Anesthesia for Ambulatory Surgery,* 2nd ed. Philadelphia: JB Lippincott, 1991.

White PF, ed. *Outpatient Anesthesia.* New York: Churchill-Livingstone, 1990.

Twersky RS. *The Ambulatory Anesthesia Handbook.* St. Louis: Mosby-Year Book, 1995.

Young ML, Conahan TJ. Complications of outpatient anesthesia. *Semin Anesth* 1990;9:62-68.

CHAPTER 29

Managing the Desperately Ill Patient

C. William Hanson, III

Managing the Desperately Ill Patient: Trauma and Shock

One of the most difficult medical tasks is the acute operative management of the critically ill patient. Advances in the technology of medicine and blurring of the distinctions between the operating room and the intensive care unit have made care of the critically ill an important part of anesthesia practice. Patients whose operative mortality would once have been considered prohibitive, such as the octogenarian cardiac surgical patient, the septic liver transplant patient, or the multiply injured accident victim, now undergo operations with a reasonable expectation of survival.

These patients present several challenges. They arrive for emergency operations at unusual hours, with full stomachs, and often in shock. Underlying physiologic processes differ, but the principles of anesthetic management are similar for all desperately ill patients. Successful treatment requires expertise in physiology, familiarity with a wide variety of drugs, technical dexterity, and the ability to react quickly to rapidly changing circumstances.

Shock

The common endpoint in many critically ill patients is *shock*, in which the metabolic needs of the body's tissues are not met by the circulation. This definition intentionally avoids reference to normal or abnormal hemodynamics or tissue metabolism. Shock occurs in the presence of normal, increased, or decreased cardiac output or blood pressure and may be absent with profound decreases in blood pressure or cardiac output (as during cardiopulmonary bypass with hypothermia).

Traditional definitions have differentiated between warm and cold shock, with sepsis or anaphylaxis representing the former and hemorrhage, trauma, or cardiogenic shock representing the latter. Characteristic hemodynamic patterns have been described for each of these syndromes. The term *warm shock* implies an increased cardiac output and reduced peripheral resistance. *Cold shock* suggests impaired cardiac output and increased peripheral resistance. A problem with the use of such terms is the tendency for shock patterns to overlap or change over time. Myocardial depressant substance is a circulating factor found in septic shock that can depress cardiac output even in the presence of decreased systemic vascular resistance (Table 29-1).

Lactic acidosis from anaerobic metabolism, decreasing urine output due to renal hypoperfusion, and respiratory failure are early indicators of shock. Adult respiratory distress syndrome (ARDS), disseminated intravascular coagulation (DIC), acute tubular necrosis (ATN), and multisystem organ failure (MSOF) are later sequelae of sustained tissue hypoxemia.

Table 29-1

Differential Diagnosis of Shock

Type	Etiology	Manifestations
Septic	Disseminated infection	Vasodilation, ↑ cardiac output,* fever
Spinal	Cervical cord lesion, spinal anesthesia	Vasodilation, neurologic deficits
Anaphylactic	Hypersensitivity (toxin, sting, drug)	Vasodilation, bronchospasm
Cardiogenic	Cardiomyopathy, ischemia, valvular lesion	Vasoconstriction, ↓ cardiac output
Hypovolemic	Dehydration (diuretics, sweating)	Vasoconstriction, ↓ urine output, ↓ skin turgor
Hemorrhagic	Blood loss	Hypovolemic shock with bleeding, internal or external
Traumatic	Tissue and organ injury, blood loss	Traumatic injuries
Endocrine	Adrenal, thyroid, pituitary insufficiency	Variable depending on hormone deficiency
Vascular	Pulmonary emboli, venous or arterial thrombosis	↓ Cardiac output

*In the initial stages; output may decrease in late sepsis.

An understanding of the balance among oxygen demand, oxygen consumption, and oxygen delivery in shock is critical to management. *Oxygen demand* is the volume of oxygen required by the tissues to supply metabolic needs. *Oxygen consumption* refers to the actual oxygen uptake by the tissues. There may be a discrepancy between demand and consumption. In cyanide toxicity, for example, cellular oxygen consumption is quite reduced, despite normal demand, because cyanide poisons the mitochondria and blocks oxidative phosphorylation. If oxygen demand is greater than oxygen consumption, anaerobic metabolism and lactic acidosis result. *Oxygen delivery* is the product of arterial oxygen content and cardiac output. It represents the blood-borne oxygen that is available for consumption by the body (Table 29-2).

Decreases in hemoglobin concentration, arterial oxygen saturation, or cardiac output proportionately decrease oxygen delivery. Note that decreases in arterial oxygen saturation, rather than in the partial pressure of oxygen in arterial blood, affect delivery. Hemoglobin is 100 percent saturated and oxygen delivery is essentially unaffected whether the PaO_2 is 90 or 500 mmHg (except in cases of severe anemia, when plasma-borne oxygen becomes significant). Changes in patient temperature or activity, acid-base balance, stress, injury, or the development of sepsis can change oxygen demand and consumption. The balance between supply and demand determines the patient's response to shock. The goal of supportive therapy in shock is to provide sufficient oxygen delivery to allow maximal tissue oxygen consumption, meeting tissue oxygen needs and thereby improving survival.

Anesthetic management of critically ill patients is complicated by the complex interplay between the primary disease and the operative and anesthetic interventions used in its treatment. Thiopental was termed the "ideal form of euthanasia" after its use as a sole anesthetic agent at Pearl Harbor resulted in deaths among the wounded. The profound hemodynamic alterations in these patients were unrecognized, as was the fact that the usual thiopental dose can be lethal in a bleeding casualty patient.

Table 29-2

Oxygen Delivery and Consumption

Oxygen delivery	= blood O_2 content (ml O_2/dl blood) × cardiac output (dl/min)
	= $(1.34 × Hb\ g/dl × 10 × SaO_2)$ × cardiac output (liters/min)
	= 1000 ml/min*
Oxygen consumption	= (oxygen delivered by arteries) − (oxygen returned by veins)
	= $1.34\ (SaO_2 − SvO_2) × Hb\ g/dl × 10$ × cardiac output (liters/min)
	= 250 ml/min*

*Values for a typical resting adult.

Hemorrhage and Shock

Hemorrhage produces the form of shock most familiar to the anesthesiologist. Its recognition and management are intrinsic to anesthetic practice. Acute loss of 15 percent of the blood volume of a healthy unanesthetized adult (class I hemorrhage) is well tolerated and may produce only a slight tachycardia. Class II hemorrhage, or the loss of 15 to 30 percent of the blood volume, can be diagnosed by the presence of tachycardia, a narrow pulse pressure, anxiety, and abnormal capillary refill. The diastolic component of the blood pressure often increases because of an increase in circulating catecholamines. Class III hemorrhage, or the acute loss of 30 to 40 percent of the blood volume, is accompanied by tachycardia, tachypnea, anxiety, and systolic hypotension. Any blood loss greater than 40 percent represents immediately life-threatening class IV hemorrhage; signs include marked tachycardia, hypotension with a narrow pulse pressure, depressed mental status, and profound oliguria (Table 29-3).

The anesthesiologist must recognize that the patient has lost blood and determine either that hypovolemia can be corrected before beginning anesthesia (always the preferable course) or that the rate of hemorrhage is so fast that correction is not possible without immediate operation to control bleeding. Once one of these two strategies has been chosen, decisions about the timing and route of volume resuscitation, appropriate hemodynamic monitors, preparation and use of blood products, and choices of agents for induction and maintenance of anesthesia can be made.

Bleeding patients usually appear pale, with cool or clammy extremities. Agitation, confusion, and combativeness are signs of inadequate cerebral perfusion. One can estimate the extent of intravascular volume depletion by seeking to provoke orthostatic hypotension in the patient on the operating table (using the "tilt test"). In this test, the blood pressure and the pulse are recorded in the supine position and after 1 minute in the 45-degree head-up position. If the systolic blood pressure decreases by more than 10 mmHg or the pulse increases by 10 or more beats per minute, the patient suffers from orthostatic hypotension, indicating an intravascular volume deficit exceeding 1 liter in a normal adult. In a volume-depleted patient with both hypotension and tachycardia, this test is unnecessary and may delay definitive management of active bleeding.

Patients with volume depletion from bleeding have increased sympathetic nervous system activity, with tachycardia, vasoconstriction, and myocardial stimulation. The most pressing concern in their treatment is the prompt repletion of intravascular volume. The placement of large, short intravenous cannulas (16 or 14 gauge or even no. 8 French) permits rapid administration of replacement solution. Each lost milliliter of blood requires 3 to 4 ml of crystalloid solutions, 1 to 2 ml of colloid solutions, or 1 ml of blood for replacement (see Chap. 15). Although the choice of colloid or crystalloid solution still generates controversy, crystalloid solutions are inexpensive, give satisfactory results in healthy patients, and may have beneficial effects on renal perfusion. Red cell transfusions are necessary in class III or IV hemorrhage, where oxygen delivery is seriously impaired by the loss of hemoglobin.

Patients with moderate blood loss (10 to 20 percent), who may appear to be in little distress before anesthesia, may suffer catastrophic cardiovascular collapse after receiving spinal or epidural anesthesia or a standard dose of an intravenous or an inhaled anes-

Table 29-3

Hemorrhagic Shock		
Class	**Signs and Symptoms**	**Treatment**
Class I hemorrhage (loss of <15%); EBL = 750 ml	Minimal tachycardia; normal BP, capillary refill	Crystalloid
Class II hemorrhage (loss of 15–30%); EBL = 750–1500 ml	Tachycardia, narrowed pulse pressure, delayed capillary refill, orthostatic hypotension	Crystalloid
Class III hemorrhage (loss of 30–40%); EBL = 1500–2000 ml	Tachycardia, change in mental status, decreased systolic pressure, hypotension	Crystalloid
Class IV hemorrhage (loss of >40%); EBL > 2000 ml	Marked tachycardia, very narrow pulse pressure, depressed mental status, hypotension	Crystalloid and blood

Modified with permission from Beecher HK, Simeone FA, Burnett CH, et al: The internal state of the severely wounded man on entry to the most forward hospital. *Surgery* 1947;22:642.

Table 29-4

Induction Drugs in Shock

Drug	Dose Range*	Side Effects
Thiopental	0.5–3.0 mg/kg	Myocardial depression, vasodilation, lowered ICP
Ketamine	0.5–2.0 mg/kg	Sympathomimetic, minimal respiratory depression, may enhance O_2 uptake
Etomidate	0.1–0.3 mg/kg	Hemodynamic stability, lowers ICP, adrenal suppression
Midazolam	0.05–0.4 mg/kg	Good amnestic, may decrease SVR and cause tachycardia
Propofol	0.5–4.0 mg/kg	Myocardial depression, decreases SVR
Fentanyl	1–25 µg/kg	No myocardial depression; loss of pain may diminish sympathetic activity
Sufentanil	0.1–5.0 µg/kg	Profound analgesia
Alfentanil	10–100 µg/kg	Respiratory depression

*Appropriate dose varies widely, but the lesser doses are recommended in critically ill or hypovolemic patients.

thetic. Anesthetic agents often depress the heart directly, but the abolition of compensatory reflex responses to hypovolemia is the major cause of hypotension after anesthesia in these patients. Positive-pressure ventilation impedes venous return, particularly when venous pressure is already decreased. Fluid resuscitation prior to induction of anesthesia is essential to prevent profound decreases in cardiac output and blood pressure.

Rapid-sequence induction of anesthesia with intravenous agents is often needed for bleeding patients, since they are presumed to be at risk for aspiration of stomach contents (Table 29-4). Diminished blood volume and the greater fraction of the total cardiac output directed to the brain and heart both accentuate the effect of intravenous anesthesia. Thiopental, despite its mild depressant effects on the heart, may be used safely in greatly reduced doses (0.5 to 1.5 mg/kg, depending on the patient's condition). Propofol causes hypotension, probably through a decrease in vascular resistance. Midazolam is used infrequently in this country for hemodynamically compromised patients but is a preferred agent in Europe. It is a mild myocardial depressant when used alone. Two drugs often used in hypotensive patients are etomidate and ketamine. Etomidate causes minimal myocardial depression and virtually no change in heart rate, preload, or afterload. Its major drawback lies in its ability to suppress the adrenal axis and therefore the endocrine response to stress.

Ketamine is the only induction agent with stimu-

latory effects on the cardiovascular system; it causes an increase in heart rate and central sympathetic output. There is also some recent laboratory evidence that ketamine can improve survival in hemorrhagic shock, possibly by improving capillary perfusion in regional tissue beds. Patients in severe shock, however, can still become severely hypotensive after even small doses of ketamine.

The potent inhalational agents can be used for the maintenance of anesthesia. They cause dose-related myocardial depression and impair sympathetic reflexes as well; patients tolerate only small amounts of anesthetic until intravascular volume is returned to normal. Isoflurane may be preferable to halothane or enflurane because it is associated with vasodilation and tachycardia and might favor oxygen delivery to the peripheral tissues. Nitrous oxide may be used provided oxygen saturation is not diminished.

The cardiovascular actions of the nondepolarizing muscle relaxants determine their use in these patients. Curare and atracurium cause the release of histamine and can produce hypotension when given rapidly in large doses in the presence of hypovolemia. Vecuronium has little effect on hemodynamics and is often preferred for this reason. Pancuronium is inexpensive and vagolytic and can be used if tachycardia is acceptable.

Pressors such as phenylephrine or ephedrine may be used to support the circulation during volume replacement. The goal of volume replacement is adequate oxygen delivery; pressors increase blood pressure and maintain flow to heart and brain at the expense of blood flow to the skin, muscles, splanchnic circulation, and kidneys as well.

In the awake patient, vital signs and mental status are monitors of organ perfusion, while in the anesthetized patient, invasive monitors are often appropriate. Urinary output of greater than 0.5 ml/kg per hour is consistent with adequate renal perfusion (when diuretics have not been administered). In uncomplicated cases, good urinary output generally indicates an adequate cardiac output.

An arterial catheter is helpful but not mandatory in the management of pure hemorrhagic hypotension. While it permits immediate monitoring of the blood pressure during induction, difficulties in obtaining access to the arterial circulation must not delay surgical intervention. The shape, respiratory variation, and amplitude of the arterial waveform provide information about the patient's intravascular volume, vascular resistance, and cardiac ejection. An arterial catheter also provides ready vascular access for monitoring of hemoglobin, electrolytes, blood gases, and pH, all of which may be abnormal during shock and resuscitation (Table 29-5).

Central venous catheters are used in the bleeding patient to monitor central venous pressure (CVP), to infuse vasoactive agents into the central circulation, or for volume infusion. Although the CVP best reflects filling of the right side of the heart and is a poor estimate of left ventricular preload, trends in the CVP can guide volume replacement.

The pulmonary artery catheter allows measurement of left-sided filling pressures and cardiac output and calculation of systemic vascular resistance. Placement and interpretation of data from a pulmonary artery catheter require more time than central venous access, and the incidence of complications is greater. Central venous monitoring is preferred to pulmonary artery monitoring in hemorrhagic shock in the absence of coexistent cardiac disease or the need for vasoactive infusions. Volume resuscitation is adequately monitored by trends in the CVP. Changing the CVP catheter to a Swan-Ganz catheter is appropriate if the CVP is greater than 15 mmHg and the blood pressure remains inadequate, in which case some degree of cardiogenic shock should be suspected.

Cardiogenic Shock

Like hemorrhagic shock, cardiogenic shock is a variant of cold shock (low cardiac output). The lesion, however, is not that of insufficient intravascular volume (preload) but of inadequate stroke volume. Anesthesiologists care for these patients after acute myocardial infarction and during emergency cardiac transplantation, repair of acute valvular rupture, or cardiac revascularization (Table 29-6).

Patients in cardiogenic shock are cool, clammy, and tachypneic. They prefer the head-up position (because of excess lung water) and are often unable to assist in positioning themselves on the operating room table. Having no myocardial reserve, they tolerate myocardial depressants poorly, including inhaled or intravenous anesthetics. All normal compensatory responses to poor cardiac performance,

Table 29-5

Monitoring in Shock		
Monitor	**Indication**	**Use in Shock**
ECG	Standard OR monitor	Arrhythmia, ischemia
End-tidal CO_2	Standard OR monitor	Adequacy of ventilation
Pulse oximetry	Standard OR monitor	Arterial O_2 saturation
Urinary catheter	All forms of shock	Indicates renal perfusion
Arterial catheter	All forms of shock	Immediate blood pressure measurement; blood gas analysis; Hb, electrolyte analysis
Central venous catheter	Uncomplicated hemorrhage, dehydration, trauma	Cardiac preload monitoring; vasoactive infusions; volume repletion
Pulmonary arterial catheter	Cardiogenic shock, septic shock, anaphylaxis	Indirect indicator of LV preload, measures cardiac output, SVR
Mixed venous oximetry	All forms of shock	Indicates balance between O_2 supply and demand

Table 29-6

Cardiogenic Shock

Types	Signs and Symptoms	Treatment
Cardiomyopathy	Fatigue, congestive failure, increased SVR, decreased CO	Diuretics, afterload reduction, inotropic support
Cardiac ischemia	Angina, reversible ECG changes	Nitrates, decrease heart rate, sedation
Aortic stenosis	Syncope, angina, congestive failure, increased SVR, decreased CO	Maintain SVR, increase preload, maintain or decrease heart rate
Aortic regurgitation	Congestive failure, angina, decreased SVR	Increase heart rate, preload; decrease SVR; maintain contractile state
Mitral stenosis	Atrial fibrillation, pulmonary edema, pulmonary hypertension	Increase heart rate, increase preload, maintain SVR
Mitral regurgitation	Congestive failure, pulmonary hypertension	Maintain or raise heart rate, increase SVR, maintain preload

including vasoconstriction and tachycardia, are maximally invoked. Drugs that depress the heart, decrease heart rate, or dilate blood vessels all have adverse consequences. Of the intravenous sedative-hypnotic agents, midazolam and etomidate are the least likely to have significant hemodynamic effects. Ketamine has been used, but it increases myocardial oxygen demand.

Combinations of large doses of narcotics, muscle relaxants, and oxygen have emerged as the anesthetic regimen of choice where myocardial compromise exists. The synthetic narcotics, such as fentanyl and sufentanil, cause no histamine release, minimal changes in myocardial contractility, myocardial oxygen consumption, and vascular resistance, and provide the greatest stability during the induction and maintenance of anesthesia.

Nitrous oxide and the potent inhaled anesthetics cause myocardial depression in a dose-related manner. They are unsuitable as sole anesthetics in cardiogenic shock but may be used cautiously as components of balanced anesthesia. Isoflurane depresses cardiac output less than enflurane or halothane because of vasodilation associated with its use.

There are a variety of ways in which the anesthesiologist can alter blood pressure, pulse, and cardiac output. Each approach produces characteristic effects on coronary perfusion and myocardial oxygen consumption (Table 29-7).

Drugs are employed to improve cardiac performance by modifying the reflex responses to decreased cardiac output. Tachycardia and volume retention (which increases preload) are compensatory responses that support cardiac output in the failing

Table 29-7

Myocardial Oxygen Consumption ($M\dot{V}O_2$) after Hemodynamic Interventions

Intervention	Effect on Cardiac Output	Effect on MVO_2	Effect on Coronary Perfusion
Increase afterload (vasoconstrictor)	↓	↑	Increased perfusion pressure
Increased preload (volume)	↑	↑	Variable
Increased heart rate (pacing, beta-1 agonist)	↑	↑	Decreased, due to ↓ diastolic flow
Inotropic support (Ca^{2+}, beta-2 agonist)	↑	↑*	Variable
Decreased afterload (vasodilator)	↑	↓	Decreased

*Phosphodiesterase inhibitors have inotropic properties but do not change myocardial oxygen consumption.

Table 29-8

Inotropic Agents and Vasopressors

Agent	Dose (Adults)	Agonist Effect
Endogenous catecholamines		
Dopamine (DA)	1–3 µg/kg/min	Renal, splanchnic
	3–10 µg/kg/min	Beta
	>10 µg/kg/min	Alpha
Norepinephrine (NE)	2–20 µg/min	Mixed alpha and beta
Epinephrine (EPI)	1–2 µg/min	Beta
	2–10 µg/min	Mixed alpha and beta
	>10 µg/min	Alpha
Synthetic catecholamines		
Dobutamine (DB)	2–20 µg/kg/min	Beta
Isoproterenol (ISO)	0.5–20 µg/min	Beta
Noncatecholamines		
Calcium	0.25–1 g	Increase inotropy
Ephedrine	5–10 mg	Releases NE
Phenylephrine	10–500 µg/min	Alpha
Metaraminol	20–500 µg/min	Releases NE
Methoxamine	1–5 mg	Alpha
Digoxin	0.5-mg increments	Inhibits Na^+/K^+ pump
Amrinone	0.75–3 mg/kg (load)	Phosphodiesterase inhibitor
	5–10 mg/kg/min infusion	Increases cAMP
Glucagon	1–5 mg	Increases cAMP

heart. Arterial vasoconstriction, however, preserves blood pressure at the expense of cardiac output. Judicious afterload reduction with agents such as sodium nitroprusside and trimethaphan allows the heart to function on a more favorable Starling curve and can enhance stroke volume without decreasing blood pressure.

Afterload reduction is not tolerated in severely ill patients, and intraoperative inotropic support is often necessary. Dopamine, epinephrine, dobutamine, and amrinone are common choices. The first two are endogenous sympathetic hormones, the third is a synthetic sympathomimetic, and the last inhibits intracellular phosphodiesterase (Table 29-8).

At lesser rates (2 to 5 µg/kg per minute), dopamine infusions act primarily on renal and splanchnic dopaminergic receptors to increase organ perfusion. In the middle range (5 to 10 µg/kg per minute), beta-adrenergic effects predominate, primarily affecting cardiac stimulation. Alpha-adrenergic receptors are stimulated at rates greater than 10 µg/kg per minute, causing peripheral vasoconstriction. Epinephrine also has markedly different effects at different infusion rates. At 1 to 2 µg/min it is primarily a beta-adrenergic agent, between 2 to 10 µg/min it affects alpha and beta receptors, and above 10 µg/min alpha-adrenergic effects predominate. Dobutamine is a synthetic beta-1 and beta-2 agent, causing both increased inotropy and peripheral vasodilation. Each of these agents binds to specific cellular receptors and causes increased cyclic adenosine monophosphate (cAMP), which modulates intracellular calcium movement. Amrinone increases cAMP by inhibiting phosphodiesterase. It has positive inotropic effects and causes peripheral vasodilation. Dobutamine and amrinone decrease myocardial oxygen consumption and pulmonary artery pressure, unlike dopamine and epinephrine, and may be preferred for this reason.

The intraaortic balloon pump (IABP) provides a mechanical means of supporting the failing heart both by enhancing coronary perfusion and by decreasing left ventricular afterload. The IABP acts sequentially with the left ventricle. The left ventricular assist device (LVAD) and the mechanical heart are alternatives that are employed occasionally as bridging devices while awaiting a suitable heart for transplantation. They act in parallel with the failing left ventricle.

The monitoring devices routinely used for intraoperative management of patients in cardiogenic shock vary among institutions, depending on available technology and expertise. The use of a urinary catheter is routine as a general measure of organ perfusion. Temperature is monitored with rectal, esophageal, nasal, or intravesicular probes intrinsic to the urinary catheter.

Patients in cardiogenic shock are monitored with arterial and pulmonary artery catheters. The performance of the failing left ventricle is evaluated with serial cardiac output determinations and pulmonary artery diastolic (PAD) or occlusion pressures (PAOP). Pulmonary artery catheters are available that continuously monitor right ventricular ejection fraction, cardiac output, and mixed venous oxygen saturation. Therapy is titrated to enhance oxygen delivery by following trends in the cardiac output, arterial oxygen saturation, and hemoglobin.

A cardiac index greater than 2.0 to 2.2 liters/min per square meter is usually consistent with adequate systemic perfusion. The index is determined by averaging several successive output determinations and dividing the result by the body surface area. Consistent technique, with the output measurement at the end of exhalation, will reduce error. Although thermodilution cardiac output values are inaccurate in the presence of significant tricuspid regurgitation, shunts, or inaccuracies in injectate temperature or volume, reproducible results are the rule. The systemic vascular resistance (SVR) is derived by calculation (see Chap. 6). The value of the pulmonary artery catheter in management of the patient in shock is in the titration of volume therapy, inotropic state, and afterload to obtain a desirable balance of cardiac output, blood pressure, SVR, and oxygenation.

The oxygen saturation of mixed venous blood ($S\overline{v}O_2$) obtained from the distal port of the pulmonary artery catheter is a measure of systemic oxygen balance. $S\overline{v}O_2$ decreases with anemia, decreased cardiac output, arterial oxygen desaturation, or increased oxygen consumption. Normal $S\overline{v}O_2$ is between 60 and 75 percent. Values greater than 75 percent are consistent with error due to obtaining a sample from a PA catheter in the wedged position, hypothermia, left-to-right shunt, sepsis, or cell poisoning from cyanide. Values less than 60 percent are consistent with cardiac decompensation; those less than 50 percent, with lactic acidosis; and those less than 20 percent, with permanent cellular damage owing to asphyxia. Continuous monitoring of mixed venous oxygen saturation is possible with fiberoptic catheters and is used in some institutions for all cardiac surgical cases.

The newest technological advance is the transesophageal echocardiogram. Use of this device allows visualization of the left ventricle, regional wall motion, and evaluation of valvular function. It can assist in directing volume therapy, in diagnosing regional ischemia, or in inotropic support for patients in cardiogenic shock.

Septic Shock

Septic shock typifies warm shock; there is peripheral vasodilation with decreased systemic vascular resistance. In the initial phase of septic shock, heart rate and cardiac index increase, and the blood pressure decreases. Recent research has shown that despite the increase in cardiac index, the ventricle dilates, stroke volume remains the same, and as a result, ejection fraction decreases. The dilated, compliant left ventricle responds well to increases in preload, and volume therapy is generally the first step in treatment of septic shock. Some patients develop a progressively decreasing cardiac index owing to myocardial depression, while others continue to show a hyperdynamic pattern (Table 29-9).

Sepsis is not purely a disturbance in cardiovascular physiology; virtually all organ systems suffer from some derangement in blood flow or function. Central

Table 29-9

Septic Shock		
Phase	Signs and Symptoms	Treatment
Early: increased cardiac outut	Peripheral vasodilation, tachypnea, fever, hypotension, decreased resistance, high output	Antibiotics and drainage, maintain intravascular volume, vasopressors
Late: decreased cardiac output	Vasoconstriction, myocardial depression, multisystem organ failure (ARDS, renal failure, CNS), lactic acidosis	Vasodilators, inotropic agents, ventilator support

nervous system effects are manifested by confusion, lethargy, or obtundation. Adult respiratory distress syndrome (ARDS) can develop from sepsis, and hyperpnea with respiratory alkalosis is an early manifestation. Decreases or redistribution in renal blood flow can cause oliguria or anuria. Cholestasis and increased transaminase values indicate hepatic dysfunction.

Although early treatment of the primary disorder with antibiotics or an operation to eliminate the infection is of paramount importance, sepsis is a toxic process that often takes 48 to 72 hours to respond to treatment. During those hours, support of vital organ perfusion is the goal of therapy.

The coincident development of sepsis and ARDS was recognized as early as 1950. Owing to concerns about exacerbating ARDS, physicians were reluctant to infuse fluids to support blood pressure in hypotension. As a result, many septic patients were given inadequate volume support. Routine use of invasive monitoring has led to recognition of the characteristic capillary leak, systemic vasodilation, and reduced left ventricular preload of untreated sepsis. Aggressive volume support governed by measurement of pulmonary artery occlusion pressure and cardiac output is the foundation of resuscitation of the hypotensive septic patient. Some patients require alpha-adrenergic agonists such as norepinephrine or phenylephrine when SVR is decreased; others need beta-adrenergic inotropic support in the later stages of the sepsis syndrome.

The pulmonary effects of sepsis include increases in vascular permeability and shunting. Increased inspired oxygen concentrations or positive end-expiratory pressure (PEEP) is often necessary. The minute ventilation of a spontaneously breathing patient can increase dramatically at the onset of sepsis, probably due to an increase in alveolar dead space. Under anesthesia, these patients often require increased minute volumes.

Recent studies have shown that ARDS involves the lung in a heterogeneous fashion and that there are areas of normal lung adjacent to consolidated lung. Traditional ventilatory management, with large tidal volumes and large peak airway pressures, causes additional injury to normal lung and exacerbates the ARDS lesion. Current management approaches emphasize limiting peak airway pressures, inverse-ratio ventilation (inspiratory-to-expiratory ratios of 1 : 1 or greater), and permissive hypercapnia. It may be nec-

essary to use a microprocessor-controlled (intensive care) ventilator in the operating room in order to ventilate and oxygenate adequately a critically ill ARDS patient. This requires the use of an intravenous anesthetic.

Patients in septic shock who require emergency operations usually have an abscess, ischemic viscera, or gas gangrene. They come to the operating room on short notice and are desperately ill.

The approach to anesthesia in the patient with sepsis and shock is similar to that used in hemorrhagic and cardiogenic shock. Drugs and doses for induction and maintenance of anesthesia are chosen for their lack of hemodynamic effects. Early and continuing fluid therapy is important. The pulmonary arterial catheter is preferable to central venous pressure monitoring because septic shock affects preload, cardiac contractility, and afterload. Arterial and urinary catheters are used to monitor perfusion. Trends in left ventricular filling pressures guide fluid and inotropic therapy (Table 29-10).

Appropriate antibiotics are continued throughout the operation on schedule. Neuromuscular blockade is monitored carefully because many of the antibiotics used in septic patients potentiate nondepolarizing muscle relaxants.

In some cases, regional anesthesia is appropriate. The amputation of a septic limb or drainage of a perirectal abscess are two examples of procedures that can be done with a regional anesthetic. Some anesthesiologists are concerned about seeding the epidural space or the cerebrospinal fluid (CSF) in a bacteremic patient while performing a spinal or an epidural injection and avoid these procedures in such patients. Other practitioners feel that the benefits of regional anesthesia outweigh the risks. Animal studies suggest that there is little risk of such seeding if appropriate antibiotics can be given before performing the spinal or epidural anesthetic.

An interesting and not uncommon observation is that some patients improve dramatically with drainage of an abscess or amputation of a septic extremity. Typically, however, there is a period of hours to days before all evidence of organ dysfunction disappears.

A number of animal and human studies have shown that overwhelming infections are accompanied by systemic cytokine release, and many investigators believe that it is uncontrolled, nonspecific immune activation that results in many of the manifestations of sepsis.

Table 29-10

Cardiovascular Support for Septic Shock

Mean Arterial Pressure <60 mm Hg			
Cardiac Index Decreased*		**Cardiac Index Normal or Increased***	
PCWP <10 CVP <10 ↓ Intravascular volume	PCWP >15 CVP >15 ↓ Inotropic support ↓ Dopamine Dobutamine Epinephrine	PCWP <10 CVP <10 ↓ Intravascular volume	PCWP >15 CVP >15 ↓ Drugs with mixed inotropic and vasoconstrictor effects ↓ Large doses of Dopamine Epinephrine Norepinephrine

*Some authors suggest an index of 2.1 or above as normal; others, who advocate the use of supranormal values in septic shock, suggest an index of 4.5 or greater.

Shock and Trauma

Management of the patient who has suffered massive trauma is similar to management of hemorrhagic shock but is complicated by a variety of confounding factors. Blood loss is accompanied by intracranial, intrathoracic, intraabdominal, and skeletal injuries. Hypotension can be due to hypovolemia from blood loss, to cervical spine and cord injury, to pericardial tamponade, or in the 12 to 24 hours after injury, to undiagnosed fecal contamination of the peritoneal cavity with resulting sepsis. A systematic approach to the diagnosis and management of trauma patients is necessary to direct appropriate therapy (Table 29-11).

In the many areas that have organized trauma systems, emergency medical personnel transport injured patients by ground or air to a regional trauma center, where the patient is evaluated and treated according to established protocols. Assessment of the patient's airway, breathing, circulation, and neurologic status occurs immediately. All clothing is removed, and the extent of injuries is ascertained. Oxygen therapy and blood pressure, pulse, and electrocardiographic monitoring are begun. At least two large-bore intravenous catheters are inserted.

Early control of the patient's airway is of major value in the management of critically injured patients. Indications for tracheal intubation include airway obstruction, obtundation, combativeness, hemodynamic lability, or to allow hyperventilation in the

Table 29-11

Trauma and Shock

Type of Injury	Signs and Symptoms	Anesthetic Management
Injured with intoxication	Combative, uncooperative, alcohol on breath	Paralysis and intubation may be necessary for staff and patient safety
Exsanguination	Tachycardia, hypotension, vasoconstriction	Volume and hemoglobin replacement, hemostasis
Cervical spine	Mechanism of injury, cervical spine collar, neurologic examination	In-line stabilization during intubation, collar on during surgery
Closed head injury	Mechanism of injury, obtundation, low Glasgow Coma Scale	Airway control, hyperventilation, ICP monitoring
Burn/inhalation	Facial burns, hoarseness, carbonaceous sputum, unconscious at scene	May need hyperbaric O_2, intubate early while stable

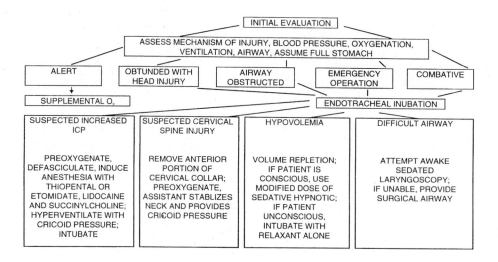

Figure 29-1

Airway management in the injured patient.

event of increased intracranial pressure. Tracheal intubation in trauma patients is complicated by the coexistence of hypovolemia, injuries that distort the airway, suspected cervical spine injury, intracranial hypertension, or a full stomach (Fig. 29-1).

Hypotensive patients require volume repletion and modified doses of induction agents. Pericardial tamponade and tension pneumothorax must be considered.

Patients with suspected cervical spine injuries often require endotracheal intubation before radiologic examination is available. The trachea is intubated while the neck is stabilized, without extending the neck. Neck stabilization is distinguished from cervical traction (which was once recommended) and implies prevention of rotational or anteroposterior movement. It is appropriate to remove the cervical spine collar during intubation to allow simultaneous application of cricoid pressure and cervical spine stabilization by an assistant.

Tracheal intubation in an injured patient suspected to have increased intracranial pressure (ICP) and assumed to have a full stomach involves a compromise among competing goals. Whereas patients with increased ICP usually undergo hyperventilation prior to intubation, patients with full stomachs are preoxygenated and then allowed to be apneic (to prevent any stimulus that might cause vomiting or regurgitation). Elective induction of anesthesia in patients with intracranial hypertension generally involves slow, titrated administration of drugs, whereas rapid-sequence induction to prevent gastric aspiration re-

quires the use of induction regimens that can precipitate significant changes in blood pressure or ICP. Succinylcholine is an ideal muscle relaxant for rapid-sequence induction because of its speed of onset, although it can cause brief increases in intracranial pressure. The approach to the head-injured trauma patient used at many trauma centers includes preoxygenation, the administration of a defasciculating dose of a nondepolarizing muscle relaxant followed by judicious doses of thiopental and succinylcholine, hyperventilation while cricoid pressure is applied, and prompt intubation of the trachea (see Chap. 30).

The Advanced Trauma Life Support Protocol recommends blind nasotracheal intubation for unconscious, spontaneously breathing patients and patients in whom there is strong suspicion or proof of cervical spine injury because it is less likely to require movement of the spine. Despite this recommendation, the vast majority of such patients can be intubated safely via the oral route by experienced practitioners. Nasal intubation risks injury to patients with basilar skull fractures, and it can provoke bleeding in the pharynx, resulting in airway compromise. In the hands of experienced individuals, oral intubation with cervical stabilization is safe, with few complications.

Paramedics are now trained to institute early, aggressive airway management at the scene of an accident. They are experienced at nasal or oral intubation. Initial evaluation of the airway includes verifying proper position of a previously placed endotracheal tube. Esophageal or pharyngeal airways are replaced by an endotracheal tube as soon as possible.

Hypotension often follows endotracheal intubation and positive-pressure ventilation. It can be due to drugs, hypovolemia, pericardial tamponade, tension pneumothorax, or a combination of these. A normal dose of a sedative, analgesic, or induction agent can precipitate hypotension in a volume-depleted patient. The decrease in venous return with positive-pressure ventilation in a hypovolemic patient can cause a decrease in cardiac output. Positive-pressure ventilation can convert a pneumothorax to a tension pneumothorax. Venous air embolism, a vasovagal response, and air trapping are other unusual causes of hypotension after intubation. Prompt diagnosis and treatment of each of these problems are critical.

Poor capillary refill, tachycardia, and hypotension are seen with most trauma patients and indicate a decrease in cardiac output. Successful resuscitation depends on differentiation between hypovolemia and impaired venous return. Blood loss can be obvious, as with major vascular lacerations and head wounds, or occult, as in the case of hemothorax, abdominal bleeding, and pelvic fractures. Impaired venous return, by way of contrast, can cause hypotension and decreased output even when circulating blood volume is adequate. Pericardial tamponade, tension pneumothorax, and positive intrathoracic pressure (with PEEP, intrinsic PEEP, or overzealous ventilation) are causes of impaired venous return that must be recognized promptly and treated appropriately.

Anesthesia care depends on a fundamental understanding of the implications of the mechanisms of injury in the trauma patient. Blunt injuries (motor vehicle accident, falls from height), penetrating wounds (stabbings, shootings), burns (thermal, electrical, chemical), and mixed injuries produce different effects, requiring different care.

Blunt injuries result from the combination of several forces; direct impact, contrecoup, shearing, and rotary forces all contribute. Shearing injuries go beyond those sustained from direct contact. Blood vessels, nerves, and the musculoskeletal system are disrupted. Patients with blunt injuries are at risk for cervical spine injury, intracranial injuries, respiratory insufficiency (from lung contusion, thoracic injury), and aortic damage, each of which requires special management.

Penetrating injuries are more localized, although a high-velocity projectile also produces blunt injury. Stab wounds injure along the path of the blade.

Bullets and shotgun pellets are less predictable; they do not necessarily follow straight lines through tissue. These patients can develop occult pneumothorax, hemopneumothorax, and pericardial tamponade. These problems must be suspected in injured patients who develop otherwise unexplained hypotension or hypoxemia intraoperatively.

Burns produce a heterogeneous group of injuries, including chemical, thermal, or mixed insults to the airway and skin. Toxic chemical gases such as carbon monoxide, carbon dioxide, nitrogen dioxide, hydrogen chloride, hydrogen cyanide, benzene, aldehydes, and ammonia are released from combustion. Carbon monoxide and cyanide interfere with cellular respiration. Thermal burns from heated gases or steam cause upper airway swelling and possible obstruction. Early endotracheal intubation is appropriate, since it is easier to intubate before edema affects the pharynx, vocal cords, and tracheal mucosa.

Immediate operative intervention for burn patients is seldom necessary in the absence of other injuries or a constricting eschar that interferes with respiration or circulation. Carbon monoxide inhalation is treated with oxygen therapy. Indications for hyperbaric therapy after carbon monoxide inhalation include loss of consciousness at the scene of injury, angina, or increased carboxyhemoglobin concentration (see Chap. 12).

After initial treatment in the emergency room, trauma victims come to the operating room. Unlike other areas of anesthetic management, anesthesia for trauma requires preparedness for any degree of injury, type and duration of operation, and the ability to proceed despite limited information. An organized regional trauma system ensures the immediate availability of surgical subspecialists at trauma centers, and the trauma anesthesiologist must be prepared to manage orthopedic, intraabdominal, cardiac, and neurosurgical emergencies on an instant's notice.

Successful care depends on adequate preparation. A specific operating room is designated for trauma cases and equipped for major procedures. Ideally, the room is large enough to accommodate more than one operating team, as well as fluoroscopy, perfusionists, and cardiopulmonary bypass equipment. The room temperature is maintained at 80°F because trauma patients are often cold on arrival, and they become more so during the operation.

Anesthetic management is dictated by the nature of the patient's injuries and prior treatment. For example, the patient may have been sedated and paralyzed and the trachea intubated in the trauma area, in which case airway management in the operating room is simplified (although the position of the endotracheal tube must be verified). In many cases, the trachea has not been intubated, and the choice between regional and general anesthesia must be made. Regional anesthesia offers the advantage of retained protective airway reflexes in a patient with a full stomach. It improves perfusion to limbs with compromised blood flow, and it provides good postoperative analgesia. Disadvantages in trauma patients are that the airway remains unprotected should the patient lose consciousness or the condition worsen. The sympathectomy may compromise the circulation, and the anxious, possibly uncooperative patient remains awake.

Most critically ill patients receive general anesthesia and intubation. In rare cases, when massive intraabdominal blood loss is present, intubation is deferred until the patient is draped so as to reduce the delay between the induction of anesthesia and operative control of bleeding.

The choice of drugs to induce anesthesia in the trauma patient is similar to that for any hemodynamically unstable patient. Succinylcholine deserves special consideration because it can provoke lethal hyperkalemia in patients after burns or crush injuries, but this response requires at least 48 hours to appear after injury. Succinylcholine is safe and appropriate in the immediate management of an injured patient but must be avoided 2 days or more after major burns, massive crush injuries, or spinal cord injuries.

Invasive monitoring for operations after major trauma usually includes an arterial and central venous catheter, temperature measurement, and a urinary catheter. Timing the placement of intravascular cannulas requires judgment. The use of an arterial catheter during induction can be quite helpful, and central venous routes are reliable paths by which to administer drugs in patients with circulatory impairment. However, delays in establishing vascular access must not prevent definitive surgical intervention. A radial arterial catheter can be placed after induction of anesthesia, for example, while draping or the operation proceeds.

Temperature monitoring is important. Coagulopathy, arrhythmias, and shivering result from hypothermia and are life-threatening to the critically ill patient. Injured patients are draped so as to allow easy access to the trunk and extremities. Large incisions are the rule and further decrease body temperature. A warm operating room, humidifier or artificial nose, and minimal flows in the anesthetic circuit prevent heat loss from the respiratory system. Intravenous fluids must be warmed. In cases of major blood loss, a rapid-infusion device can be used, whereby large volumes of warmed blood products are given by a perfusionist (freeing the hands of the anesthesiologist). Standard blood warmers are an alternative.

The management of multiply-injured trauma patients requires assessment of the extent and severity of injuries and a schedule of treatment. The stabilization of a bleeding pelvic fracture takes precedence over the repair of a small intimal tear in the aorta, for example. Several surgical teams operate simultaneously in certain circumstances; an intracranial hematoma can be evacuated while a ruptured spleen is removed.

Operations for traumatic injuries are by their nature long and attended by hemodynamic and respiratory instability. The anesthesiologist must function as an intensivist, attending to critical organ systems while aware of the nature and implication of each of the patient's injuries.

Neurologic injuries are seen frequently with blunt trauma and gunshot wounds. Preoperative neurologic examination and radiographic studies are preferred, but when neurologic evaluation is deferred owing to the severity of coexisting injuries, it is appropriate to hyperventilate a patient who might have head injuries. In some circumstances, early intracranial pressure monitoring is instituted to improve management during long surgical procedures and in anticipation of prolonged ICU care.

Renal hypoperfusion or direct injuries to the kidney and urinary tract are frequent causes of decreased urine output during anesthesia for trauma. Rhabdomyolysis with crush injuries can injure renal tubules. Some clinicians advocate the use of osmotic diuretics such as mannitol to increase urinary blood flow during the posttraumatic period. Alternatively, a loop diuretic can be used to differentiate renal from prerenal failure; the conversion from oliguria to polyuria is consistent with prerenal causes and a better prognosis.

Conclusion

Success in managing anesthesia for the critically ill patient depends on applying simultaneously two apparently contradictory philosophies. First, protocols, routines, and highly practiced skills must be employed to save time and ensure that nothing is overlooked. Second, analysis and imagination are required to resolve diagnostic dilemmas and treat multiple disorders successfully, especially when therapeutic goals conflict.

BIBLIOGRAPHY

American College of Surgeons. *Advanced Trauma Life Support Course for Physicians.* New York: American College of Surgeons, 1984.

Grande CM, ed. *Trauma Anesthesia and Critical Care, Critical Care Clinics.* Philadelphia: WB Saunders, 1990.

Parillo JE. Septic shock in humans: Clinical evaluation, pathogenesis, and therapeutic approach. In Shoemaker WC, Ayres S, Grenvik A, et al, eds: *Textbook of Critical Care.* Philadelphia: WB Saunders, 1989, p 1008.

Shoemaker WC. Physiologic monitoring of the critically ill patient. In Shoemaker WC, Ayres S, Grenvik A, et al, eds: *Textbook of Critical Care.* Philadelphia: WB Saunders, 1989, p 145.

30

Neuroanesthesia and Neurologic Diseases

Harry S. Seifert and David S. Smith

This chapter begins with a brief review of relevant biochemistry and physiology, followed by a discussion of the anesthesia management of patients undergoing neurosurgical procedures and of patients who have incidental neurologic diseases but who are undergoing nonneurosurgical operations.

Brain Biochemistry and Physiology

■ Intracranial Pressure

Cerebral perfusion pressure (PP) is the net blood pressure supplying the brain (Table 30-1). Normal cerebral PP is 80 to 90 mmHg and normal intracranial pressure (ICP) is 0 to 10 mmHg. Acute increases in ICP above 20 mmHg warrant treatment.

The brain tissue shares the intracranial space with interstitial fluid, blood, and cerebrospinal fluid (CSF). Because these intracranial contents are liquid, and therefore largely incompressible, and the dura and cranium are rigid, the relationship between ICP and the volume added to the intracranial contents can be described by the curve shown in Figure 30-1. Examination of this idealized curve indicates that an increase in the volume of any one component will initially cause no change in ICP. This is so because the increased volume of one intracranial component can be compensated for by displacement of an equal volume of another component (usually CSF) to an extracranial site. However, once the limit of compen-

sation is reached, further small increases in volume may cause dramatic increases in ICP. In reality, most clinical situations are not described by this idealized ICP curve, since the relationship of ICP to volume depends on the rate at which the volume is added. More gradually added volume such as from a slowly growing tumor is better tolerated than more rapid additions, for example, an acute subdural hematoma. In addition to foreign bodies, tumor, or hemorrhage, the volume of the intracranial contents can be increased rapidly by obstructing CSF outflow or jugular venous drainage, increasing arterial CO_2, inducing profound hypoxemia, or administering certain anesthetic drugs. Increased ICP is significant when it interferes with brain oxygenation by reducing PP or causes mechanical compression by herniation of brain tissue.

Table 30-1

Cerebral Perfusion Pressure
PP = MABP − ICP
or
PP = MABP − CVP
when
CVP > ICP
where MABP = mean arterial blood pressure
ICP = intracranial pressure
CVP = central venous pressure
PP = cerebral perfusion pressure

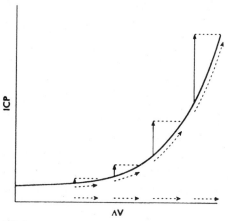

Figure 30-1

An idealized curve of the relationship between the volume of intracranial compartments (ΔV) and intracranial pressure (ICP). The upward, solid arrows reflect the changes in ICP obtained with additional increments of volume (*dashed arrows* along the abscissa). Note that equal increases in volume have markedly different effects on the increase in ICP depending on the position along the volume pressure curve. This idealized model assumes a single distribution curve relating pressure and volume, which is a conceptually useful oversimplification.

(Used with permission from JS Schweitzer et al: Intracranial pressure monitoring. In Cottrell JE, Smith DS, eds: Anesthesia and Neurosurgery. St Louis: Mosby–Year Book, 1994, p 119.)

Brain Oxygen Demand

Relative to other organs, the brain has a large metabolic requirement, about 50 percent of which is used to maintain the electrochemical gradients required for neurologic activity. The cerebral metabolic rate for oxygen ($CMRO_2$) averages 3 ml per 100 g of brain per minute. The brain cannot meet its metabolic requirements though anaerobic glycolysis. As CBF decreases below a critical value, oxygen extraction from arterial blood increases. The conversion of glucose to lactate also increases, but $CMRO_2$ remains unchanged until oxygen delivery is severely compromised.

Cerebral Blood Flow

Whole brain cerebral blood flow (CBF) in unanesthetized, normothermic humans is about 54 ml per 100 g of brain per minute. Cortical CBF less than about 20 ml per 100 g per minute in anesthetized patients is associated with decreased electroencephalogram (EEG) activity, and at CBFs of less than about

15 ml per 100 g per minute, EEG activity ceases. Brain damage may occur if CBF decreases further (the CBF threshold for neuronal depolarization due to energy depletion is about 10 ml per 100 g per minute). Normally, the brain can tolerate a 50 percent reduction in CBF before there is a significant risk of irreversible brain damage. This margin is decreased in patients with hypertension, carotid occlusion, or increased ICP.

Autoregulation of CBF

Through autoregulation, cerebral vascular resistance changes in response to changing blood pressure so that CBF remains nearly constant despite large changes in PP. In a normal adult, CBF is autoregulated over a PP of about 50 to 150 mmHg, or a mean arterial blood pressure (MABP) of 60 to 160 mmHg (Fig. 30-2). Below a PP of 50 mmHg, CBF decreases as PP decreases. As PP exceeds 150 mmHg, cerebral vessels dilate and CBF increases dramatically. There is significant individual variation with respect to the upper and lower limits of autoregulation.

In hypertensive patients, the blood pressure limits for autoregulation are shifted to the right so that compared with a normotensive person, autoregulation and CBF might fail at a greater MABP. With

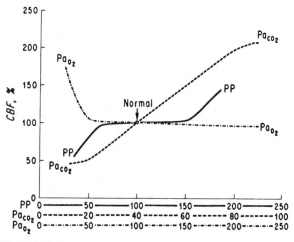

Figure 30-2

The relationship of cerebral blood flow (CBF) to cerebral perfusion pressure (PP), $PaCO_2$, and PaO_2. Units on the abscissa are in millimeters of mercury (mmHg).

(Reproduced with permission from Michenfelder JD: Anesthesia and the Brain. New York: Churchill-Livingston, 1988, p 6).

therapy, the hypertensive patient's autoregulation curve returns toward normal. In the elderly, autoregulation may be compromised because of occlusive vascular disease or loss of vessel distensibility. Autoregulation is lost after hypoxic or ischemic insults and in brain tissue near tumors. With impaired autoregulation, CBF depends more directly on the MABP. Because autoregulation is not instantaneous, a rapid increase in MABP may result in transient increases in CBF.

Within the range of 20 to 60 mmHg, changes in $PaCO_2$ directly affect CBF (see Fig. 30-2). Increases in $PaCO_2$ tend to increase brain vascular volume, thereby increasing ICP. Decreases in $PaCO_2$ have the opposite effect. In patients with brain swelling or increased ICP, hyperventilation is the most effective initial treatment to decrease ICP. With continued hyperventilation, vasoconstriction diminishes over 8 to 24 hours because of compensatory changes in serum bicarbonate. Rapid return to normocarbia after prolonged hyperventilation may increase cerebrovascular volume and ICP.

Changes in arterial oxygen tension between values of 50 and 250 mmHg have little effect on CBF. As PaO_2 decreases below 50 mmHg, CBF increases dramatically (see Fig. 30-2). Decreases in brain temperature decrease CBF and reduce $CMRO_2$ about 5 percent for each 1°C.

■ Effects of Drugs Used During Anesthesia on CBF, ICP, and $CMRO_2$

Anesthetic drugs alter cerebrovascular volume. Intravenous anesthetic drugs, except ketamine, acutely produce cerebral vasoconstriction, reduce cerebrovascular volume, and decrease ICP (Table 30-2). Inhalational anesthetics produce acute cerebral vasodilation and may increase ICP. In patients

Table 30-2

Effects of Drugs on Brain Oxygen Consumption, Blood Flow, and ICP

Drugs	$CMRO_2$	CBF	ICP
Inhalational drugs			
N_2O	↑	↑	↑
Halothane	↓↓	↑↑↑	↑↑↑
Enflurane	↓↓	↑↑	↑↑
Isoflurane	↓↓↓	↑	↑
Desflurane	↓↓	?	↑↑
Intravenous induction drugs			
Barbiturates	↓↓↓	↓↓↓	↓↓↓
Etomidate	↓↓	↓↓	↓↓
Propofol	↓↓	↓↓	↓↓
Midazolam	↓	↓	↓
Ketamine	↑↑	↑↑	↑↑
Narcotics			
Morphine	±	±	↑
Fentanyl	±	±	0
Sufentanil	±	↑	↑
Alfentanil	?	↑	↑
Muscle relaxants			
Atracurium	0	?	0
Doxacurium	0	0	0
Pancuronium	0	0	0
Pipecuronium	0	0	0
Rocuronium	0	0	0
Tubocurarine	0	?	0
Vecuronium	0	0	0
Succinylcholine	↑	↑	↑↑

These data have been compiled from a variety of sources, primarily human but also animal, to serve as an initial guide. This table does not show changes in which PP is a function of both ICP and MABP; any drug that tends to decrease MABP may produce a decrease in PP. $CMRO_2$, cerebral metabolic rate for oxygen; CBF, cerebral blood flow; ICP, intracranial pressure; PP, cerebral perfusion pressure; MABP, mean arterial blood pressure.

with cerebral edema, intracranial masses, or obstructive hydrocephalus, drugs that increase brain volume may increase ICP enough to compromise cerebral perfusion or produce herniation. In contrast, drugs that reduce brain volume and ICP may improve cerebral perfusion, and the decreased brain volume may allow better surgical access.

Nitrous oxide (N_2O), 50% to 70%, produces a 36 percent increase in CBF and $CMRO_2$ in human volunteers and increases ICP by 100 to 200 percent in patients with brain masses. However, the effect of N_2O on ICP can be attenuated by the administration of other anesthetic drugs such as thiopental. Increased ICP after dural closure in sitting patients occurs occasionally, presumably due to N_2O diffusing into entrapped air. Nitrous oxide is useful during neurosurgery because of its analgesic effects, rapid elimination, and lack of significant effects on blood pressure.

At less than 1 minimum alveolar concentration (MAC), isoflurane has minimal effects on ICP; an increase in ICP from isoflurane appears to be prevented by hyperventilation. Isoflurane and other halogenated drugs also may decrease MABP, producing a significant decrease in cerebral perfusion. In patients with brain tumors, both sufentanil and alfentanil have been associated with increases in ICP that are usually clinically insignificant.

Succinylcholine increases ICP under many conditions, but this may be attenuated by blocking fasciculations. This intracranial hypertension may be produced by an afferent stimulus generated by mass activation of muscle spindle fibers during the initial depolarization, which produces a central arousal response accompanied by increases in CBF and cerebrovascular volume. Although many practitioners avoid succinylcholine for patients at risk for intracranial hypertension, it may be used with defasciculating doses of nondepolarizing relaxant when rapid tracheal intubation is required. The nondepolarizing muscle relaxants pancuronium, vecuronium, and atracurium do not increase ICP. Histamine release with D-tubocurarine administration may cause cerebral vasodilatation that increases ICP or it may produce hypotension that decreases perfusion pressure and thus reduces ICP.

Drugs used to control blood pressure also may alter ICP. In general, adrenergic receptor agonists such as ephedrine, dopamine, and phenylephrine or adrenergic antagonists such as propranolol, labetalol, or esmolol have no direct effect on ICP, nor does the ganglionic blocking drug trimethaphan. Direct-acting vasodilator drugs such as hydralazine, sodium nitroprusside, nitroglycerine, and adenosine increase cerebrovascular volume, as do calcium antagonists, which act on the cerebral vasculature (e.g., nimodipine).

Diuretics also alter ICP. Mannitol (0.25 to 1 g/kg) increases plasma osmotic pressure relative to brain osmotic pressure. The movement of water from brain to blood reduces brain volume. Initially, rapid infusion of mannitol may increase vascular volume and ICP. Furosemide appears to be a less effective means of decreasing brain size, but it enhances the diuretic effect of mannitol and may inhibit mannitol-induced intracranial hypertension.

The effect of a drug on ICP is an important consideration for its use during neurosurgery; however, effects on blood pressure and postoperative alertness are also important. Anesthetics alter brain volume in varying degrees, and these effects may be modified by other drugs or by hyperventilation. Thus medications have proved useful during neurosurgery despite the fact that they can increase ICP. Hyperventilation, steroids, diuretics, and other drugs may lessen or abolish the tendency of an anesthetic drug to increase ICP. To choose anesthetic drugs only by their effects on ICP may eliminate some that have unique benefits for a particular patient.

■ Electrophysiologic Monitoring

Electroencephalogram (EEG) electrodes reflect localized cortical electrical activity and provide useful information about brain function and possible ischemia. With compromise of cerebral perfusion, the EEG shows a loss of high-frequency activity (>14 Hz), possibly an increase in low-frequency activity (2 to 4 Hz), and eventually loss of all activity. The EEG is sensitive to perfusion pressure, $PaCO_2$, anesthetic drugs, and electrocautery. In anesthesia practice, the EEG is most commonly used to monitor brain activity during carotid endarterectomy or to monitor efficacy of barbiturate-induced metabolic suppression.

The interpretation of the EEG can be eased by computer processing, which emphasizes frequency changes and compresses the data in a digital format. However, all the current approaches to EEG processing sacrifice information that may be necessary. Many clinicians still consider the 16-channel analog EEG to be the standard approach.

Sensory evoked potentials (SEPs) are cortical electric signals triggered by electrical stimulation of a sensory nerve. Commonly used nerves are the median, ulnar, posterior tibial, and auditory nerves; the resulting signals are detected by repeated stimulation and signal averaging and are sensitive to ischemia, anesthetics, and electrocautery. Sensory evoked potentials indicate only the integrity of the sensory pathways and not motor pathways that might be independently compromised. During major spine operations, SEP monitoring may detect compromise in sensory pathway integrity; during operations near the brainstem, monitoring the function of the facial or auditory nerve is useful.

The function of the motor system can be assessed by motor evoked potentials (MEPs). MEPs can be produced by stimulation of the cerebral cortex directly or through the intact skull or by transcranial magnetic stimulation. The responses are measured as compound action potentials along the lateral columns of the spinal cord, the peripheral nerves, or the muscles. MEPs are extremely sensitive to depression by most anesthetic drugs. Although not nearly as commonly used as SEPs, MEPs may be helpful in situations where the motor tracts are endangered, such as during operations on the thoracic aorta or brainstem. Because of the arrangement of the blood supply to the spinal cord, motor pathways may be at greater risk of compromise than many of the sensory pathways.

■ Brain Ischemic Damage, Protection, and Resuscitation

Complete loss of cerebral perfusion, such as during cardiac arrest, produces unconsciousness within 6 to 7 seconds in normothermic subjects, loss of EEG activity within 15 to 25 seconds, and almost complete loss of brain high-energy metabolites such as adenosine triphosphate within 2 minutes. The disappearance of high-energy metabolites appears to set into motion a series of events that makes neuronal loss irreversible. The transition to irreversible damage occurs more slowly when regional CBF is compromised (e.g., by focal ischemia or stroke), perhaps because of collateral flow.

Considerable research has produced neither a mechanism to explain ischemic neuronal damage nor generally accepted approaches to increasing tolerance to an ischemic insult (protection) or for treatment

after ischemia (resuscitation). In the operating room, decreasing the oxygen demand may be a useful strategy. Profound hypothermia (18°C) slows cerebral metabolism enough to allow periods of circulatory arrest during cardiac operations. Recent animal data suggest that moderate hypothermia (30 to 34°C) also may reduce neurologic damage during less severe compromises in oxygen delivery.

Thiopental in doses that abolish EEG activity or produce EEG patterns of burst suppression decreases neurobehavioral deficits after normothermic cardiopulmonary bypass. Although the use of intraoperative barbiturates during carotid endarterectomy or cerebral aneurysmectomy has been advocated, there are no prospective studies to demonstrate efficacy. Etomidate also has been suggested but remains unproven. Isoflurane (about 1.5%) decreases the level of regional CBF at which EEG changes occur. In addition, during carotid endarterectomy, the incidence of EEG changes suggestive of ischemia appears to decrease with use of isoflurane instead of halothane.

A large number of animal studies suggest that hyperglycemia superimposed on an ischemic insult increases the neurologic damage. Because withholding glucose does not appear to produce hypoglycemia, this has become common practice during neurosurgical operations.

Anesthesia for Patients with Intracranial Masses

■ Acute Intracranial Hypertension

Patients with rapidly increasing ICP require emergency treatment to secure the airway, to provide oxygenation and ventilation, and to reduce ICP. Patients with subdural, epidural, or subarachnoid hemorrhage, severe head injury, or large tumors may present with acute loss of consciousness, seizures, and decorticate or decerebrate posturing.

The management of these patients for emergency neurosurgery begins by establishing oxygenation and hyperventilation by mask (Table 30-3). If vascular volume appears adequate and a rapid examination of the airway does not suggest difficulty, induce anesthesia. Treat transient increases in blood pressure with additional thiopental or another similar drug such as propofol. Begin mannitol therapy before or after

Table 30-3

Priorities in Emergency Craniotomy

1. Ensure oxygenation and ventilation by mask.
2. Rapidly assess airway, cardiovascular status, associated injuries, and coexisting pathology.
3. If airway appears normal, induce anesthesia with thiopental (2–5 mg/kg) or etomidate (0.2–0.3 mg/kg), administer vecuronium (0.1–0.2 mg/kg) or rocuronium (1 mg/kg), and intubate. Patients with head trauma are assumed to have spinal cord injury and are managed accordingly (see section on spinal cord injury).
4. If neurologic examination is to be required after intubation, use succinylcholine with a defasciculating dose of a nondepolarizer.
5. Continue hyperventilation after intubation.
6. Assume that arterial hypertension, especially when accompanied by bradycardia, results from increases in intracranial pressure. Treat with additional doses of thiopental or propofol.
7. Administer mannitol and/or furosemide.
8. Do not allow the placement of invasive monitors to delay decompression.

tracheal intubation; hyperventilation and thiopental have more immediate effects. If the need for continued neurologic evaluation rules out a nondepolarizing relaxant, succinylcholine may be used. Invasive monitoring is helpful but must not delay surgical decompression of a treatable lesion. Anesthesia may be maintained with additional thiopental or narcotic and, after decompression, with small doses of isoflurane (< 0.5 MAC).

■ Intracranial Masses

The etiology of an intracranial mass is not as important as its volume, speed of formation, and anatomic location. Thus tumors or accumulations of blood may have similar effects, although rapidly expanding masses create greater neurologic impairment than do more slowly progressing lesions. The goals of anesthetic management include maintaining cerebral perfusion without increasing intracranial volume.

Preoperative Evaluation

Drowsiness, obtundation, unconsciousness, nausea, vomiting, and papilledema all indicate increased ICP and a patient at significant risk for herniation or cerebral ischemia. The preoperative computed tomo-

graphic (CT) scan or magnetic resonance image (MRI) can help identify patients at special risk for intraoperative intracranial hypertension, as indicated by cerebral edema, obliterated, small, or massively dilated lateral ventricles, and a 5-mm or more midline shift. Narcotic or heavy sedative premedications are avoided because they may depress ventilation and increase ICP.

Monitoring for most intracranial neurosurgical procedures includes capnography, pulse oximetry, electrocardiogram, temperature, and urine output. An arterial catheter allows accurate assessment of blood pressure and sampling for $PaCO_2$, serum electrolytes, and serum osmotic pressure. Central pressure monitoring guides fluid management if significant blood loss is expected.

Elevating the head of the table 10 to 15 degrees promotes venous drainage to avoid brain engorgement. Excessive rotation of the head or flexion of the neck may interfere with venous drainage, as may pressure on the anterior neck.

Induction of Anesthesia

Prior to induction of anesthesia, a brief period of voluntary hyperventilation may decrease brain volume. Induction of anesthesia with intravenous drugs that decrease cerebrovascular volume and ICP is followed immediately by hyperventilation, avoiding hypercapnia, hypoxia, coughing, or excessive peak inspiratory pressures, all to prevent increases in brain volume. Because abrupt increases in MABP may increase ICP, fentanyl (5 µg/kg in divided doses) may be given to obtund the response to tracheal intubation and other stimuli; this does not prevent rapid emergence after a 3- to 4-hour operation. Local anesthetics injected subcutaneously before the skin incision or placement of head fixation devices ameliorates hypertensive responses.

Vecuronium, rocuronium, or cis-atracurium are appropriate choices to ensure immobility. Not only do they have minimal cardiovascular effects, but the short duration of action limits residual neuromuscular blockade, even though these patients must often be kept paralyzed until the surgical dressing is in place.

Many of these patients have decreased intravascular volumes that may contribute to intraoperative hypotension. In adults, maintaining fluid replacement at rates of 1 to 1.5 ml/kg per hour with an isosmotic crystalloid or colloid solution causes minimal additional brain swelling. Maintaining hemoglobin concentrations between 8 and 10 g/dl further decreases the risk of increased ICP or brain swelling. Glucose-containing solutions are avoided, as described earlier.

Intraoperative Management

Nitrous oxide combined with amnestic doses of isoflurane (much less than MAC) and hyperventilation produce, at worst, minimal brain swelling. For massive brain swelling or severe intracranial hypertension, it may be best to avoid the halogenated anesthetics, substituting thiopental (intermittent injection of 50 to 100 mg or an infusion at 0.02 to 0.2 mg/kg per minute), propofol (50 to 150 µg/kg per minute), or etomidate (20 to 200 µg/kg per minute). The major risks of barbiturate and propofol are hypotension. Excessive postoperative sedation is most likely with a barbiturate.

Because the concentration of inhalational anesthetic must be held to a minimum, hypertension occurring at the time of the incision is treated with narcotic, additional thiopental or propofol, or esmolol. During the operation, hypertension responds to labetalol, usually in 5- to 10-mg increments. The mixed alpha- and beta-adrenergic antagonist action of this drug has no effect on ICP and may allow better control of MABP with less bradycardia than pure beta-adrenergic antagonists do.

Brain Volume

Surgical manipulation of the brain may produce swelling, treatable by hyperventilation ($PaCO_2$ of 25 mmHg) and osmotic or loop diuretics. Mannitol given at the time of skin incision will take effect in the 45 minutes the surgeon usually requires to reach the dura. Brain swelling can be treated by elevating the head, giving thiopental (50 to 200 mg), propofol, (25 to 50 mg), or etomidate (2 to 4 mg), and discontinuing any inhalational anesthetics.

Emergence from Anesthesia

Large doses of sedatives or narcotics or large concentrations of halogenated anesthetics may delay emergence from anesthesia and interfere with the prompt recognition of intracranial bleeding or other causes of increased ICP. During emergence, hypertension is best controlled with antihypertensive drugs rather than by adding anesthetic. Esmolol does not increase CBF or ICP and is useful in this situation.

Usually, the endotracheal tube is removed while the patient is still in the operating room. Exceptions include patients with preoperative obtundation or severe intraoperative brain swelling or ischemia. Changes in neurologic status that may indicate postoperative problems such as bleeding can best be detected in alert patients. As the patient emerges from anesthesia, coughing may increase ICP or cause intracranial bleeding. Early signs of reaction to tracheal stimulation, such as swallowing or irregular ventilation, may be treated with small doses of additional narcotic or lidocaine (20 to 40 mg intravenously).

■ Pituitary Tumors

Pituitary tumors tend not to increase ICP. Patients with acromegaly have increased jaw size, enlarged tongues, and overgrowth of laryngeal soft tissue, often requiring awake sedated intubation.

The most common surgical approach to pituitary tumors is a sublabial transsphenoidal route. A right-angle oral or wire spiral tracheal tube allows surgical access without compromise of airway control.

■ Posterior Fossa

Anesthesia for operations in or near the posterior fossa requires managing the specific risks associated with the surgical position, increased ICP, brainstem compression, and brainstem stimulation. Operations include removal of cerebellar or brainstem tumors, removal of acoustic neurinomas, microvascular decompression for pain, and decompression of the brainstem. Preoperative considerations, induction, and maintenance of anesthetic are similar to those described for other intracranial tumors.

A variety of operative positions may be used, including supine with the head turned, lateral, partial lateral (park bench), prone, or sitting. The management of these positions is described in Chapter 16.

Intraoperative Monitoring

Monitoring is similar to that for intracranial tumors. The sitting position increases the risk of air embolism, requiring special monitoring. Resection of acoustic neurinoma and other procedures may require evoked potential monitoring, possibly limiting the use of greater concentrations of N_2O or halogenated anesthetics.

Air Embolism

When the surgical site is above the heart, there is a risk of air entry into the venous system. Air embolism occurs in about 40 percent of posterior fossa operations performed in the sitting position and less often in the prone position. Patients placed in the sitting position are monitored for air embolism by a precordial Doppler device and continuous capnography. End-tidal nitrogen detected by mass spectrometry appears to be a less sensitive monitor. Transesophageal echocardiography is the most sensitive detector of intracardiac air. It also can detect air movement from the right to the left side of the heart but is not used routinely because of expense and complexity. Hypotension, murmurs, and hypoxemia are late signs of air embolism.

In order to remove air from the heart, many anesthesiologists place a right atrial catheter in these patients, using changes in the P wave of the ECG (monitored through a saline- or bicarbonate-filled catheter) as a guide. Saline may not provide adequate conductance for some monitoring systems; sodium bicarbonate usually does in standard clinical concentrations. Optimal position of the catheter is just above the right atrium. Multiorifice catheters are more efficient than single-orifice catheters for capturing intravascular air, including that trapped in the superior vena cava.

Maintaining adequate intravascular volume may decrease the incidence of air embolism. If air embolism occurs, the surgeon occludes open vessels or sinuses and covers the surgical field with saline. The anesthesia team discontinues nitrous oxide, aspirates air via the right atrial catheter, and supports blood pressure with vasopressors and fluids. Persistent air entry or hypotension may require lowering the patient's head.

Intraoperative Management

When muscle relaxants cannot be used, such as when the facial nerve is monitored, the dose of anesthetic is increased to prevent patient movement. This may produce hypotension, requiring vasopressors to maintain blood pressure and cerebral perfusion.

During posterior fossa operations, nitrous oxide may increase the size of air emboli. Because of its other favorable features, one may choose to use N_2O until an air embolus occurs or until the dura is closed, which creates a circumstance in which air might be trapped beneath the dura.

Cerebrovascular Operations

■ Carotid Endarterectomy

This operation is done to remove plaque that has produced a critical decrease in the diameter of the carotid artery or which may be a source of cerebral emboli. The carotid artery is exposed near its bifurcation, cross-clamped above and below the lesion, and opened so that the plaque can be removed. Patients may have hypertension, coronary artery disease, or chronic obstructive pulmonary disease. Common complications include postoperative stroke and myocardial infarction.

Anesthetic choice may depend on local preference. Under regional anesthesia, the awake patient may provide information about mental function, and intraoperative hemodynamic instability may be lessened. Patient comfort and control of the airway are guaranteed with general anesthesia. Outcomes are similar. The majority of carotid endarterectomies are done using general anesthesia.

General anesthesia must be managed to allow smooth, rapid emergence with minimal postoperative sedation and close control of cardiovascular responses. For this reason, monitoring usually includes an arterial cannula. Infiltration of the carotid body with local anesthetic under direct vision can decrease intraoperative fluctuations in heart rate and blood pressure. The decrease in CBF that accompanies hyperventilation is avoided by maintaining $PaCO_2$ between 35 to 40 mmHg.

During the period of carotid artery cross-clamping, systemic blood pressure is maintained at the upper end of the patient's normal range to facilitate cerebral perfusion. Three approaches are used to maintain cerebral perfusion: relying on collateral circulation, routinely placing a plastic shunt to carry blood from the common carotid artery to the internal carotid artery, and selective shunting based on some measure of cerebral perfusion adequacy. Complications of shunting include embolization and increased operating time.

Cerebral perfusion in awake patients can be monitored by asking the patient to follow commands or answer questions, although untested pathways may suffer unrecognized compromise. Changes often occur within 30 seconds of cross-clamping if collateral circulation is inadequate. Other measures of cerebral perfusion have included jugular venous oxygen saturation, carotid artery stump pressure, oculoplethys-mography, Doppler ultrasound, and intraoperative arteriography. Many of these techniques are intermittent, and some are inaccurate. Cerebral blood flow measurements have been used, but the EEG is the most commonly used monitor.

■ Cerebral Aneurysms and Arteriovenous Malformations

Cerebral aneurysms occur most commonly at bifurcations of vessels, most frequently along the anterior and posterior communicating arteries, as well as the anterior and middle cerebral arteries. Patients who bleed from an aneurysm have a significant risk of bleeding again. They also suffer hypertension and cerebral vasospasm (thought to be related to extravascular hemoglobin decomposition), which reduces blood flow to the local tissue. Initial therapy consists of sedatives, anticonvulsants, and antihypertensive drugs. The calcium channel blocker nimodipine has been shown to reduce the incidence of neurologic complications from vasospasm. The antifibrinolytic drug aminocaproic acid can retard clot lysis and potentially reduce the risk of further bleeding, but it also increases cerebral ischemia, so its use is declining.

The risk of rebleeding is greatest during the first 72 hours, and operation within this period has become increasingly common. Most aneurysms are attached to the parent vessel by a narrow neck, across which the surgeon places a metal clip to isolate the aneurysm. Postoperative problems include cerebral vasospasm resulting in stroke, stroke from clip placement, continued hypertension, seizures, brain swelling, and bleeding because of clip dislodgment.

Arteriovenous malformations (AVM) are masses of abnormal vessels that may present with bleeding, seizures, headache, or focal neurologic deficits. These lesions can be treated with invasive neuroradiologic techniques or operations. The operation involves isolation and ligation of the arterial supply and venous drainage followed by resection of the malformation. The risk of sudden intraoperative bleeding is considerably less than for aneurysms. The anesthetic management of AVMs is more like that of brain tumors than aneurysms.

Anesthetic Considerations

The anesthetic goals during operations for cerebral aneurysms are listed in Table 30-4. In some patients, blood accumulation and edema from the initial aneurysmal bleeding may create a mass effect,

Table 30-4

Goals of Anesthesia Management for Operation for Cerebral Aneurysm

1. Induction of anesthesia and tracheal intubation without hypotension that might compromise cerebral perfusion or hypertension that might cause bleeding
2. Brain relaxation to allow surgical exposure
3. Occasional use of intraoperative hypotension to facilitate exposure or to control bleeding
4. Maintenance of vascular volume to decrease the effects of vasospasm
5. Emergence from anesthesia and extubation in the operating room, allowing early assessment of neurologic state

and considerations similar to patients with brain tumors apply.

Many regimens have been used to avoid hypertension during induction and intubation; each has its advocates. The plan described for patients with intracranial mass lesions works well. Body temperature often is allowed to decrease to about 33°C to decrease $CMRO_2$. In addition to the usual measures to prevent brain swelling, a lumbar drain may be used to allow removal of CSF during the operation.

To ease exposure of the aneurysm, the surgeon may temporarily clip the vessels feeding the aneurysm or request reduction in arterial blood pressure. These maneuvers create extra risks of brain ischemia. The period of clipping must be as brief as possible, less than 4 minutes. Pharmacologic measures (e.g., thiopental) to improve tolerance of inadequate oxygen delivery have not yet proven effective in this situation.

Deliberate hypotension has been used in some institutions to reduce wall tension in the aneurysm and to decrease the rate of blood loss from ruptured aneurysms and from arteriovenous malformations or vascular tumors. As described in the section on brain physiology, normotensive patients tolerate decreases in MABP to 50 to 60 mmHg; hypertensive patients tolerate decreases in MABP to 55 to 65 percent of the preoperative MABP. Isoflurane, sodium nitroprusside, or nicardipine with beta-adrenergic blockers for reflex tachycardia, provide controllable hypotension.

After the aneurysm is clipped, MABP is increased to values greater than the patient's normal MABP to overcome vasospasm. Decreasing the depth of anesthesia and infusing fluids usually suffice, but a vasopressor may be needed. This moderate hypertension is continued into the immediate postoperative period, but during emergence from extubation, excessive hypertension must be prevented.

Anesthesia for Neuroradiologic Procedures

Patients may require anesthesia or sedation for radiologic diagnostic procedures. Planning must take into account the degree of neurologic compromise and diminished intracranial compliance. Sedation may be contraindicated if increased ICP is present. Tracheal intubation and controlled ventilation may be required.

Magnetic resonance imaging (MRI) is unique because of the strong magnetic field. Ferrous objects can be drawn toward the magnet, damaging equipment and people. Standard noninvasive blood pressure monitors, sidestream capnographs, and ECG oscilloscopes may be usable if placed sufficiently far from the magnet. However, monitoring equipment and infusion pumps designed to function safely near these magnetic fields are becoming increasingly available, thus easing the anesthetic management of patients. Because there is no ionizing radiation, the anesthesiologist can be near the patient to provide sedation and reassurance, which are often sufficient. If needed, the induction of anesthesia and tracheal intubation take place outside the magnet area. Although MRI-compatible anesthesia machines have been described, many practitioners have found them unnecessary for adult patients. Oxygen and intravenous drugs such as propofol, narcotics, and muscle relaxants provide adequate maintenance of anesthesia.

Neurologic Disease

Patients who require any sort of operation may suffer from neurologic or muscular diseases that produce impaired consciousness, weakness, or autonomic nervous system dysfunction.

■ Loss of Consciousness

Coma usually results from a diffuse insult to both cerebral hemispheres because, except for brainstem lesions involving the reticular activating system, isolated focal lesions do not impair consciousness. Preoperative sedation for comatose patients is usually unnecessary and may be harmful; hypoventilation may increase ICP. If intracranial compliance is decreased, induction and tracheal intubation are conducted as described for patients with intracranial masses. Because the comatose patient's ability to protect the airway may be impaired, careful evaluation is needed before extubation.

■ Seizures

The patient with seizures that recur without recovery (status epilepticus) is at risk for hypoxic injury and pulmonary edema from increases in systemic and pulmonary vascular resistance. Neuromuscular blocking drugs halt the motor activity and permit airway control but do not stop seizure activity, which is treated with barbiturates, phenytoin, or benzodiazepines. General anesthesia has been used to stop seizures that are refractory to other therapies.

For the patient with a known seizure disorder, important preoperative information includes the nature and frequency of the seizures, the etiology of the seizures, if known, and current medication. Blood concentrations of antiepileptic drugs can be determined (most can be increased to therapeutic values within 24 to 48 hours). Antiepileptics are continued through the operation; unexpected recurrence of seizures is not a common problem. The effects of anesthetic drugs are summarized in Table 30-5.

Table 30-5

Pro- and Anticonvulsant Effects of Anesthetic Drugs

Proconvulsants
    Methohexital (in complex partial seizures only)
    Etomidate
    Enflurane (in greater concentrations with hypocapnia)
    Meperidine and its metabolite, normeperidine
    Ketamine
    Local anesthetics*
    Laudanosine (metabolite of atracurium)
Questionable
    Fentanyl (myoclonic activity; minimal evidence for convulsive activity in humans)
Anticonvulsants
    Barbiturates
    Benzodiazepines
    Propofol
    Halothane
    Isoflurane
    Local anesthetics*

*Rapidly increasing blood levels of local anesthetics tend to suppress inhibitory neurons and promote seizures, but intravenous infusions of local anesthetics have been employed for their anticonvulsant effects.

■ Head Injury

The Glasgow Coma Score (GCS) is used to characterize neurologic impairment after head injury (Table 30-6). The GCS does not substitute for a minute-to-minute record of neurologic function because it does not include signs of lower brainstem function such as respiratory rate, pattern and depth, and blood pressure. Coma corresponds to a GCS of 8 or less; these patients do not open their eyes, speak, or respond to commands.

The first step in the care of the patient with head injury is airway control, which is often complicated by facial or cervical spine injuries, bleeding into the mouth, a full stomach, or hypovolemia. Neck flexion or hyperextension must be prevented throughout, unless there is an unequivocal radiologic diagnosis of cervical spine stability.

Blind nasotracheal intubation without muscle relaxants offers minimal neck movement but also carries the risk of failure, blind passage into the cranial vault in the presence of a basilar skull fracture, epistaxis, and paranasal sinusitis with prolonged intubation. Orotracheal intubation after anesthesia and paralysis is often successful and carries other advantages as well. Movement, coughing, and hypertension in response to laryngoscopy and tracheal intubation can be prevented. Hyperventilation and rapid-sequence induction with thiopental, propofol or etomidate, and vecuronium allow prompt intubation while reducing the risk of aspiration or of increasing ICP. In the absence of brainstem injury, hypotension does not result from the head injury; decreased blood pressure prompts a search for bleeding or spinal cord injury.

Patients with head injury may present for craniotomy or other operations. Anesthetic management depends on ICP. If ICP is normal, simply avoiding measures that increase ICP is adequate. Management of brain swelling or intracranial hypertension is the same as that employed with intracranial masses.

The patient with diffuse bihemispheric cerebral impairment may be at risk for a lethal hyperkalemic response to succinylcholine beginning 24 to 48 hours after injury. Brain injury also can produce ECG changes, such as QT prolongation or T-wave and ST-segment changes, despite the absence of myocardial ischemia.

■ Brain Death

Brain death is the irreversible absence of cortical and brainstem function; cardiac death usually follows within 48 to 72 hours. Management of the brain-dead organ donor includes supporting the cardiopulmonary system after loss of central control and protecting the organs to be donated from hypertension and tachycardia provoked by surgical stimuli (Table 30-7).

■ Weakness

It is useful to group disorders of motor function by the location of the lesion. Chronic upper motor neuron deficits (i.e., above the level of the anterior horn cell) present with spastic paresis with hyperreflexia and pathologic reflexes (upgoing toe). Interruption of neuromuscular transmission at the lower motor neuron or the peripheral nerve causes flaccid paralysis and hyperreflexia. Interference with transmission at the neuromuscular junction produces fatigue and weakness that may improve with anticholinesterase therapy. Finally, weakness may result from dystrophic changes within the muscle cell.

■ Spinal Cord Injury

Injured patients can have significant vertebral column instability without neurologic damage. Definitive cervical spine films are difficult to obtain; when

Table 30-6

Glasgow Coma Scale		
Response	**Characteristics**	**Score**
Eye opening	Spontaneous	4
	To speech	3
	To pain	2
	Nil	1
Verbal response	Oriented	5
	Confused conversation	4
	Inappropriate words	3
	Incomprehensible sounds	2
	Nil	1
Best motor response	Obeys	6
	Localizes	5
	Withdraws (flexion)	4
	Abnormal flexion	3
	Extensor response	2
	Nil	1

Reproduced with permission from Teasdale G, Jennett B: Glasgow Coma Score formulation. *Lancet* 1974;2:81.

Table 30-7

Perioperative Management for the Brain-Dead Organ Donor

Problem	Recommended Treatment
Hypotension due to neurogenic shock and hypovolemia	Copious fluid therapy Vasopressors if needed
Bradycardia	Atropine
Hypoxemia due to atelectasis or neurogenic pulmonary edema	Oxygen PEEP (positive end-expiratory pressure)
Diabetes insipidus	Replace water as needed
Organ hypoperfusion	Maintain perfusion pressure and cardiac output Treat reflex vasopressor responses with appropriate vasodilators

results are equivocal, the patient's neck is splinted against movement. Neck flexion appears to increase the risk of further damage, whereas minimal neck extension may be tolerated. Hard and soft collars do not restrict the neck's range of motion adequately; a combination of a hard collar and bilateral sandbags joined with wide tape across the forehead most effectively controls neck motion. Excessive traction may cause vertebral dislocation, as can excessive cricoid pressure. Muscle relaxants, intravenous induction agents, and adjuvant drugs are used as dictated by the clinical situation. For patients with unstable necks in traction who require elective operations, fiberoptic intubation with adequate sedation and topical anesthesia is preferred.

Methylprednisolone (30 mg/kg intravenously over 15 minutes followed by a 24-hour infusion at 5.4 mg/kg per hour) is begun within 8 hours of spinal cord injury. This improves neurologic recovery with no additional morbidity.

The early autonomic response to spinal cord injury is called *spinal shock* and is the result of depression of neurons below the level of injury. The acute clinical manifestations depend on the level of injury and include hypotension, bladder and bowel paralyses, and gastric dilation. Pulmonary edema may result from aggressive fluid loading. Hypotension is corrected by a combination of fluid and vasopressors such as dopamine. In addition, many advocate the use of pulmonary artery catheters as a guide to fluid replacement.

After recovery from spinal shock, autonomic hyperreflexia may follow with injuries above T5. This mass reflex response to noxious stimuli includes vasoconstriction with resulting relative intravascular volume overload and extreme hypertension. Bladder irrigation, childbirth, defecation, surgical anal dilation, and intraabdominal procedures are potent stimuli that provoke the response. A few patients respond to cutaneous stimulation, and a small minority develop the reflex spontaneously, requiring chronic treatment with ganglionic blocking drugs. Intraoperatively, autonomic hyperreflexia occurs with local anesthesia, sedation, and light nitrous oxide-narcotic techniques but not usually with sufficiently deep general anesthesia using halogenated anesthetics or spinal anesthesia of adequate extent. Episodes of hypertension can be treated with deeper anesthesia, direct-acting vasodilators, or ganglionic blocking drugs.

Denervation produces changes in the muscle membrane that alter the response to neuromuscular blocking drugs, as described in Chapter 11. Severe hyperkalemia, ventricular arrhythmias, and cardiac arrest have been reported after succinylcholine as early as 3 days after spinal cord injury; the risk persists for 6 months to a year. Succinylcholine has been used within the first 24 to 36 hours after injury without untoward response. Other management issues arising from spinal cord injury are listed in Table 30-8.

■ Myasthenia Gravis

Myasthenia gravis causes a functional decrease in acetylcholine receptors of the neuromuscular junction. Weakness affecting muscles of the airway, the chest wall, and the diaphragm and the concomitant risks of postoperative respiratory failure are of first concern in anesthesia management. Tests of muscle strength, such as the vital capacity or the maximal inspiratory pressure, warn of impending ventilatory failure before dyspnea, hypercarbia, or hypoxia oc-

Table 30-8

Problems Caused by Spinal Cord Injury	
Pathologic Process	**Etiology**
Impaired temperature regulation	Increased cutaneous blood flow due to sympathectomy
Atelectasis	Acutely due to pulmonary contusion; later, due to hypoventilation, decreased vital capacity, and inadequate cough
Pulmonary emboli	Dilated veins, immobility
Urinary tract infections	Bladder dysfunction
Nephrolithiasis, hypercalcemia	Immobility, calcium wasting
Decubital ulcers	Immobility, muscle atrophy

curs. Preoperative medical management to improve respiratory muscle function has been shown to reduce the need for postoperative mechanical ventilation.

There is no consensus on whether the anticholinesterase drugs used to treat myasthenia are best withheld or given just before operation; management has been successful with both approaches. Withholding anticholinesterase drugs for a prolonged period risks respiratory failure. Excessive doses of anticholinesterase drugs can cause cholinergic crisis, which is marked by weakness and muscarinic symptoms such as salivation, bradycardia, and miosis.

Drugs that affect the neuromuscular junction, such as the type Ia antiarrhythmic drugs (procainamide, quinidine) and the aminoglycoside antibiotics, may worsen myasthenia. Intravenous lidocaine accentuates the neuromuscular blocking properties of other anesthetic drugs, but the use of lidocaine for regional or local anesthesia does not seem to exacerbate myasthenia.

Patients with myasthenia gravis respond variably to succinylcholine and tend to develop phase II block. Myasthenic patients are sensitive to competitive neuromuscular blocking drugs and require doses only 20 to 50 percent of those required by healthy patients. Elimination pharmacokinetics are normal; the prolonged drug effect results from relative overdoses. Administration of small increments of short-acting muscle relaxants, guided by monitoring of the response to a nerve stimulator, yields appropriate doses for each patient.

Myasthenic patients also can be managed with regional anesthesia or general anesthesia without relaxants. Regardless of the anesthetic employed, these patients require extra vigilance at the end of the procedure because, even if they meet conventional criteria of adequate strength and ventilatory function, fatigue may occur later, rapidly and unexpectedly.

■ Myopathies

Patients afflicted with one of the progressive muscular dystrophies that present in childhood, most commonly Duchenne's, require operations for diagnostic biopsy as well as for orthopedic procedures such as Achilles tendon transfer and Harrington rod placement for scoliosis. Endomyocardial fibrosis with conduction abnormalities and other cardiac abnormalities are common. Restrictive respiratory disease results from weakness and kyphoscoliosis. Life-threatening gastric dilation under anesthesia has been described, suggesting use of a nasogastric tube.

Case reports and in vitro contracture testing indicate that many patients with myopathies, particularly of the Duchenne type, are susceptible to malignant hyperpyrexia, but the magnitude of this risk is unknown. An anesthetic plan for a myopathic patient might well include capnography, close temperature monitoring, and avoiding drugs known to trigger malignant hyperthermia. Prophylaxis with dantrolene is not indicated and may be harmful, since it exacerbates weakness.

■ Dysautonomia and Mixed Disorders

Movement disorders can involve deterioration of central dopaminergic or cholinergic pathways, which can cause diminished movement (bradykinesia), as with Parkinson's disease, or increased movement, as in Huntington's chorea. Cerebellar degeneration causing ataxia may involve other organ systems, as in the cardiomyopathy seen with Friedreich's ataxia.

Other degenerative conditions may impair protective airway reflexes.

Initially, Parkinson's disease responds to oral L-dopa combined with carbidopa to block the systemic effects of dopamine. Butyrophenones and phenothiazines exacerbate parkinsonism. Both droperidol and metoclopramide have been reported to cause severe rigidity that requires postoperative respiratory support. Parkinsonism can cause dyskinesias of airway musculature and functional airway obstruction.

Multiple sclerosis is a demyelinating disease characterized by exacerbation and remission. Exacerbations occur spontaneously and with systemic stress, particularly fever. Because of these unpredictable exacerbations, and because of possible direct neurotoxic effects of local anesthetics, it may be prudent to avoid regional anesthesia in patients with demyelinating diseases.

Disorders of the autonomic system can be congenital or acquired and often are characterized as central or peripheral. Diseases associated with autonomic neuropathy are listed in Table 30-9. Autonomic neuropathy may produce orthostatic hypotension or syncope. Other clinical features include a relatively fixed heart rate, gastroesophageal reflux, disturbances in intestinal motility, and episodic hypertension. The cardiac output depends on preload, and the systemic vascular resistance is typically decreased. With a peripheral autonomic neuropathy, denervation hypersensitivity may cause an abnormal response to direct-acting sympathomimetic drugs.

Case reports of patients with significant autonomic neuropathy have identified possible approaches to anesthetic management based on known pathophysiology. Preoperative intravenous hydration and premedication with metoclopramide and cimetidine seem reasonable. Elastic stockings may be useful,

especially for surgical positions that cause venous pooling. Gastroparesis may warrant rapid-sequence induction of general anesthesia. When dysautonomia is also associated with a peripheral neuropathy that produces significant motor denervation (such as Guillain-Barré syndrome), succinylcholine may cause hyperkalemia. Doses of direct-acting vasopressors must be reduced to avoid severe hypertension, and indirect-acting vasopressors may be unreliable in peripheral dysautonomias. General anesthesia with halogenated anesthetics, narcotics, or ketamine has been reported to be safe. Regional anesthesia has been rejected by some because hypotension may be difficult to treat.

■ Overall Management of Patients with Neurologic Disease

Many neurologic diseases are rare, therefore limiting experience to case reports or small series of patients. Furthermore, many conditions, particularly degenerative disorders, are characterized by relapsing and remitting courses that make it difficult to draw inferences based on a small group of patients. Thus detailed recommendations for the anesthesia management of these patients are likely to be based on personal preference as much as on scientific data. For example, regional anesthesia is often cited as contraindicated, but there is little direct evidence for such a recommendation, which may reflect primarily medicolegal concerns. Successful anesthesia management of patients with neurologic diseases depends on a thorough appreciation of the pathophysiology of the disease and a cautious approach more than it does on adherence to absolute caveats.

Table 30-9

Diseases Associated with Autonomic Neuropathy

Congenital (Riley-Day syndrome)
Idiopathic (Shy-Drager syndrome or multisystem atrophy)
Peripheral neuropathies
  Guillian-Barré syndrome (acute idiopathic polyneuritis)
  Diabetes mellitus
  Alcohol abuse
  Vitamin B_{12} deficiency
  Heavy metal toxicity

BIBLIOGRAPHY

Azar I. The response of patients with neuromuscular disorders to muscle relaxants: A review. *Anesthesiology* 1984;61:173-187.

Bedford RF, Morris L, Jane JA. Intracranial hypertension during surgery for supratentorial tumor: Correlation with preoperative computed tomographic scans. *Anesth Analg* 1982;61:430-433.

Bracken MB, Shepard MJ, Collins WF, et al. A randomized, controlled trial of methylprednisolone or naloxone in the treatment of acute spinal-cord injury: Results of the Second National Acute Spinal Cord Injury Study. *N Engl J Med* 1990;322:1405-1411.

Cottrell JE, Smith DS, eds. *Anesthesia and Neurosurgery*. St Louis: Mosby, 1994.

Drummond JC. Brain protection during anesthesia: A reader's guide. *Anesthesiology* 1993;79:877-880.

Martz DG, Schreibman DL, Matjasko MJ. Neurological diseases. In Katz J, Benumof JL, Kadis LB, eds: *Anesthesia and Uncommon Diseases*. Philadelphia: WB Saunders, 1990, pp 560-589.

Modica PA, Templehoff R, White P. Pro- and anticonvulsant effects of anesthetics, part I. *Anesth Analg* 1990;70:303-315.

Modica PA, Templehoff R, White P. Pro- and anticonvulsant effects of anesthetics, part II. *Anesth Analg* 1990;70:433-444.

Schonwald G, Fish KJ, Perkash I. Cardiovascular complications during anesthesia in chronic spinal cord injured patients. *Anesthesiology* 1981;55:550-558.

Schurr A, Rigor BM, eds. *Cerebral Ischemia and Resuscitation*. Boca Raton, Fla: CRC Press, 1990.

Sieber FE, Smith DS, Traystman RJ, Wollman H. Glucose: A reevaluation of its intraoperative use. *Anesthesiology* 1987;67:72-81.

Working Group on Status Epilepticus. Treatment of convulsive status epilepticus. *JAMA* 1993;270:854-859.

Young WL, Pile-Spellman J. Anesthetic considerations for interventional neuroradiology. *Anesthesiology* 1994;80:427-456.

31

Management of Anesthesia for Specialty Procedures

Angelina D. Castro

Unique problems arise when operative procedures involve the airway or when patients undergo special procedures in remote locations such as lithotripsy facilities, radiology suites, and catheterization laboratories. This chapter describes the special concerns involved in managing anesthesia for these patients.

Otorhinolaryngology

Procedures in otorhinolaryngology (ORL) are unique because the anesthesiologist and the surgeon share the airway. Management of anesthesia in these patients centers on control of the airway. Preoperative airway assessment is as described in Chapter 13, with emphasis on a review of prior airway operations, airway management during these procedures, radiation treatment, and progression of the disease. If any uncertainty remains after these data have been evaluated, it is mandatory to pursue study of the anatomy of the patient's airway in consultation with the surgeon until all the information is on hand to plan the induction of anesthesia and airway management. Indirect laryngoscopy, conventional x-rays, computed tomographic (CT) scans, and magnetic resonance imaging (MRI) provide information on impingement of the airways by tumors, infection, or foreign bodies.

■ Managing the Compromised Airway

Cooperation with the surgeon is essential so that plans for airway management are clear to all caring for the patient.

Four rules apply in all cases. First, the patient with a compromised airway must not be given muscle relaxants unless control of the airway is ensured. Second, almost all these patients benefit from premedication to provide a dry mouth, which simplifies airway management by avoiding one stimulus to laryngospasm and by facilitating the effect of topical anesthetics. Third, pulse oximetry is essential to provide warning that airway obstruction is producing hypoxemia; efforts to intubate the trachea must stop from time to time to allow for ventilation and oxygenation. Fourth, supplemental oxygen given by insufflation can prevent hypoxemia during laryngoscopy (see Chap. 13).

In the management of ORL patients with compromised airway anatomy, the available airway management schemes may be arranged in a hierarchy, from those designed for normal anatomy to those which cope best with airways distorted or obstructed by disease.

■ Conventional Intravenous Induction of Anesthesia

Conventional techniques of inducing anesthesia are appropriate when airway anatomy is normal, with no bleeding, abscess, friable tumor, or area of tracheomalacia that might produce obstruction after anesthesia or paralysis.

Small-Dose Intravenous Induction

When the airway is likely to be adequate and the patient is free of cardiopulmonary disease and has a normal functional residual capacity (FRC), preoxygenation is followed by very small doses of thiopental (1 to 2 mg/kg), given so as to just cause the patient to lose consciousness. If the airway is obstructed, preoxygenation allows time for the patient to recover before becoming hypoxemic. If the airway can be maintained, anesthesia may be deepened with injectable anesthetics or gases. Also, a small dose of succinylcholine can be given and laryngoscopy performed; if the prospects for intubation are favorable, additional anesthetic and relaxant are given before passing the endotracheal tube. This strategy is appropriate only under limited circumstances: There must be no systemic illness, and the anesthesiologist must be nearly certain of an intact airway. Gentle technique is required to manipulate the airway of such lightly anesthetized patients.

Gas Induction

Induction of anesthesia by breathing a mixture of oxygen and a potent anesthetic offers the prospect of an induction that automatically reverses itself when the airway becomes obstructed. Halothane is not unpleasant to smell and does not irritate the upper or lower airway, in contrast to enflurane, isoflurane, and desflurane. Despite the theoretical kinetic advantages offered by the less soluble agents, in practice, the greater concentrations possible with halothane make it easier to perform smooth induction of anesthesia. Nitrous oxide is usually not used for gas induction of anesthesia in patients with compromised airways so that the maximum amount of oxygen may be used. This technique is applied to the same patients as are the two intravenous techniques described previously but may be somewhat safer

because inadvertent overdoses are less likely. The scheme works best in the hands of an experienced individual.

Awake Laryngoscopy

For patients with even more distortion of the airway, one may begin the sequence of an awake intubation with opioids, sedatives, topical anesthetics, and supplemental oxygen given so as to produce a responsive but calm and spontaneously breathing patient. If direct laryngoscopy demonstrates that intubation is possible, the laryngoscope may be withdrawn and the anesthetic completed before proceeding with intubation. If it does not seem possible to intubate with direct laryngoscopy, one may proceed with one of the techniques described below. This technique amounts to completing the preoperative evaluation by performing a sedated laryngoscopy.

Awake Fiberoptic Laryngoscopy

When poor mouth opening, a large tongue, or other distortions of normal anatomy make it evident that direct laryngoscopy will fail, one may begin with fiberoptic laryngoscopy through the nose or mouth, depending on anatomy, and proceed to intubation by passing the tube over the fiberscope (see Chap. 13).

Blind Nasal Intubation

This technique, also described in Chapter 13, is less popular since the advent of fiberoptic techniques. It is applicable to the same patients—those in whom conventional laryngoscopy is impossible. When secretions and bleeding make fiberoptic laryngoscopy difficult, blind nasal intubation may be preferred.

Operative Laryngoscopy or Bronchoscopy

Experienced surgeons can sometimes identify the glottic opening with an operating laryngoscope or intubate the trachea with a rigid bronchoscope when swelling or a mass in the airway makes it otherwise impossible to see the larynx or to pass a tube blindly.

Transtracheal Needle Ventilation

This temporizing measure applies when unexpected airway obstruction cannot be resolved and rarely is needed in the ORL setting if the patient has been evaluated well preoperatively and the surgeon is present to assist with a difficult airway. See Chapter 13 for details of this technique.

Tracheotomy Under Local Anesthesia

When upper airway distortion is severe, or when swelling, bleeding, or a friable tumor threatens complete obstruction if the airway is manipulated, planned tracheotomy under local anesthesia as the first part of the operative procedure is the safest course.

Although patient comfort is a concern in managing these patients, airway obstruction and death can result from the abrupt induction of anesthesia or paralysis, from excessive manipulation of swelling tissue, and from persisting inappropriately with efforts to intubate.

■ Pharyngoscopy, Laryngoscopy, and Bronchoscopy

Pharyngoscopy, laryngoscopy, and bronchoscopy are diagnostic procedures that require direct visualization and frequently biopsies. Anesthetic considerations include thorough airway assessment for pathology; suppression of secretions, cough, gag, and laryngeal reflexes; protection of teeth and relaxation of jaw muscles; rapid return of protective airway reflexes; and airway management.

Premedication with an anticholinergic drug helps to minimize oral secretions. With proper patient selection and surgical skill, some of the endoscopic and minor airway procedures such as biopsies, vocal cord stripping, and Teflon injections can be accomplished under local anesthesia. This can be administered topically by means of sprays, nebulizers, or soaked applicators, by regional block, and by the transtracheal route. Lidocaine is the most commonly used local anesthetic; because of rapid absorption from the trachea, doses must be limited to prevent toxic reactions.

General anesthesia is used when a protected and controlled airway is essential, for the patient's comfort, in extended procedures, or because of the surgeon's preference. Volatile anesthetics provide adequate suppression of upper airway reflexes and allow increased concentrations of oxygen. In specific cases, such as foreign-body removal, when positive-pressure ventilation may be harmful, spontaneous ventilation may be required. For endoscopy and laryngoscopy, a small endotracheal tube (5 mm inside diameter) protects the trachea, facilitates ventilation, and allows for extended surgical time. Muscle relaxation for these procedures can be accomplished with succinylcholine

infusion or intermediate-acting muscle relaxants such as atracurium or vecuronium.

When the endotracheal tube interferes with the operation, methods of airway management without an endotracheal tube are used. One method is to allow the patient to breathe spontaneously a mixture of oxygen and a potent inhaled anesthetic, insufflated into the pharynx through a port on the laryngoscope or via a plastic tube lying in the pharynx. It can be difficult to control the depth of anesthesia with this technique because the patient entrains room air with each breath. Also, the surgeon and others in the operating room breathe the anesthetic too.

Another method is jet ventilation via a port on the laryngoscope or by means of a metal cannula. It is essential that the vocal cords be fully relaxed and no airway obstruction exists so that there may be proper inflow and egress of the gas. Oxygen, mixed with anesthetic if necessary, is delivered intermittently at 50 lb/in^2, with a rate of 6 breaths per minute. This method also contaminates the operating room atmosphere and entrains room air, but it does allow the use of muscle relaxants. Oxygenation is good, but carbon dioxide sometimes accumulates, especially in patients who are difficult to ventilate.

Another method is apneic oxygenation with insufflation of oxygen and anesthetic gas through a small catheter that is placed between the vocal cords just above the carina. This does not isolate the trachea, nor does it allow for positive-pressure ventilation or carbon dioxide elimination. Apneic times are limited to 10 or 15 minutes because of hypercarbia. See Chapter 13 for details of this technique.

Bronchoscopes most commonly used are the flexible fiberoptic and rigid ventilating types. The flexible fiberoptic scope is placed through a large (8.0 mm inside diameter) endotracheal tube, permitting reliable ventilation during the procedure. With rigid bronchoscopy, oxygen flows in through a sideport of the bronchoscope; when the proximal end of the bronchoscope is occluded by a window or by the surgeon's thumb, ventilation through the sideport is possible. Jet ventilation also can be used. Because patient movement can result in a tracheal tear, complete paralysis with a muscle relaxant is appropriate.

■ Laser Surgery of Structures in the Airway

Lasers produce intense monochromatic beams of light that can be focused to vaporize tissue. In addition to the usual considerations described above, anesthetic management includes measures to protect the patient and operating room personnel from misdirected laser beams and to lessen the probability of fire during laser surgery. Laser beams, through reflection or scatter, can burn unprotected skin and mucous membrane. The patient's eyes are taped shut and covered with moist gauze, and operating room personnel wear protective goggles that absorb the radiation frequency of the laser in use.

Fire is the most serious danger during laser surgery. Endotracheal tubes made of flammable polyvinylchloride are avoided for this procedure. Special tracheal tubes made of rubber, silicone, or metal have been designed to afford protection by harmlessly absorbing the energy and providing a nonflammable airway. Wrapping an endotracheal tube in reflective aluminum tape reduces its vulnerability to the laser beam, but the cuff of the endotracheal tube may still be punctured. Inflating the cuff with saline enables it to absorb more energy, and the escaping fluid will alert the surgeon to cuff perforation and may extinguish a fire. The atmosphere the patient breathes can be made less combustible by eliminating nitrous oxide, substituting nitrogen or helium, and by decreasing the concentration of oxygen to the minimum safe for the patient.

■ Tonsillectomy

In cooperative patients, tonsillectomy can be accomplished under local anesthesia. General anesthesia provides reliable control of the airway and suppression of laryngeal reflexes and avoids reflex-induced hypertension, tachycardia, and arrhythmias. Extreme care is taken with the endotracheal tube as it is moved from side-to-side during the procedure. Rapid recovery with a return of the airway reflexes prior to extubation is desirable. Postoperatively, these patients are placed in the head-down lateral position to allow drainage of blood through the mouth.

The most common complication is postoperative bleeding, occurring most often within 8 hours after operation and sometimes requiring reoperation. Unsuspected hypovolemia from hidden blood loss, a full stomach, and airway obstruction are problems encountered during reoperation.

■ Endoscopic Sinus Surgery

Recent advances in endoscopic technology allow sinus instrumentation, visualization, and operation.

Anesthetic management in the cooperative patient consists of infiltration by the surgeon of local anesthetic in combination with sedation. There is less bleeding associated with local anesthesia, and the surgeon can evaluate the patient for neurologic damage, since the periorbital tissues and dura are not infiltrated with local anesthesia. Injury to the orbit, optic nerve, or skull can be recognized immediately. Sedation techniques must avoid obtundation with respiratory depression and airway obstruction, inadequate sedation with anxiety, or disinhibition with agitation.

■ Pharyngeal Abscess

An abscess in the mouth or pharynx can cause severe pain, trismus, and respiratory obstruction. Sometimes, the abscess can be drained or decompressed by aspiration under local anesthesia. General anesthesia must address respiratory obstruction, difficult endotracheal intubation because of distorted anatomy and trismus, and the danger of rupture of the abscess with pus entering an unprotected airway. Any of the hierarchy of airway management plans described may be applied, but gentle technique is required to avoid rupturing the abscess. If the glottis cannot be seen, tracheostomy under local anesthesia may be the safest means of securing the airway.

■ Tracheostomy

Tracheostomy is most easily performed in the operating room. By intubating the trachea first, the airway may be protected from bleeding and the tracheostomy performed in a meticulous fashion. When the surgeon places the tracheostomy tube, the endotracheal tube is withdrawn so that the tip remains in the larynx, just above the tracheal incision. In case of difficulty in passing the tracheostomy tube, the orotracheal or nasotracheal tube can be advanced to secure the airway again.

■ Head and Neck Operations

Patients undergoing head and neck operations for carcinoma often have a history of cigarette smoking and chronic obstructive pulmonary disease. The airway may present a problem owing to distortion of normal structures by the tumor, by inflammation and edema, or by fibrosis caused by radiation therapy. The hierarchy of airway management described previously applies in these cases. Tracheostomy under local anesthesia may be required if the tumor is extremely friable or exophytic to avoid dislodging cancerous tissue into the tracheobronchial tree or provoking bleeding.

Several intraoperative complications are specific to head and neck operations. Manipulation around the carotid sinus may cause vagal responses such as hypotension and bradycardia; this is treatable with atropine or by infiltration of local anesthetic around the carotid sinus. Cardiac dysrhythmia and prolonged QT interval occur during right radical neck dissection because of damage to the cervical sympathetic system. Venous air embolism may occur through open neck veins. Laryngectomy and radical neck dissection are prolonged procedures (6 to 8 hours) involving substantial blood loss. Careful fluid management and prevention of hypothermia are required.

■ Otologic Surgery

Most otologic procedures involve the middle ear and the mastoid air cells and are performed for hearing loss resulting from scarring and fibrosis of the tympanic membrane, cholesteatoma of the ossicular chain, and occasional involvement of the labyrinth and the facial nerve.

The middle ear represents an air-filled noncompliant space; pressure is vented by the eustachian tube under normal conditions. As it does in other closed spaces, nitrous oxide can accumulate in the middle ear. Tympanic membrane rupture and dislodgment of tympanic grafts have occurred during nitrous oxide use. Until the surgeon begins to close the middle ear, there is no closed space, and nitrous oxide use does not present a problem; discontinuing nitrous oxide 30 minutes before the tympanic membrane graft is placed ensures that there will be neither ingress or egress of nitrous oxide after the graft is placed.

The facial nerve is adjacent to structures of the ear, and it may be injured during ear operations. If muscle relaxants are used, some skeletal muscle response to direct nerve stimulation must be allowed to remain so that the surgeon can use mechanical or electrical stimulation to help identify and preserve the facial nerve.

A bloodless operating field is essential for microsurgery of the ear. To achieve this, many surgeons infiltrate the area with epinephrine solutions. This may produce hypertension and dysrhythmia, particularly with halothane, less so with isoflurane and enflurane. Other measures are controversial. Raising the head above the level of the heart aids in venous drainage and reduces cerebral venous pressure but increases the risk of venous air embolism. Induced hypotension reduces bleeding but may introduce additional morbidity.

Volatile inhalation anesthetics are logical choices for ear operations because they produce adequate levels of anesthesia without the use of nitrous oxide, muscle relaxants, or narcotics. Nausea and dizziness are postoperative problems common to patients undergoing ear operations. Avoiding opioids and prophylactic administration of antiemetics (e.g., droperidol) are helpful measures to decrease the incidence of nausea and vomiting.

■ Nasal Surgery

During operations on the nose, the surgeon uses topical vasoconstrictors to minimize bleeding, most often cocaine, neosynephrine, or epinephrine. Cocaine is used widely as a local anesthetic in intranasal operations because it blocks reuptake of norepinephrine and serves as a vasoconstrictor; the safe dose is 3 mg/kg. Equally as effective and not a controlled substance is 4% lidocaine with phenylephrine added as a vasoconstrictor.

Pharyngeal packs aid in absorption of blood intraoperatively, and nasal packs are used for hemostasis postoperatively. It is important to verify that all pharyngeal packs have been removed and that the pharynx is cleaned by suction before the endotracheal tube is removed.

Extracorporeal Shock Wave Lithotripsy

During extracorporeal shock wave lithotripsy (ESWL), high-energy waves are focused on kidney and ureteral stones. The R wave of the electrocardiogram (ECG) triggers each shock wave. The stone location and the state of stone disintegration are confirmed by fluoroscopy. Newer versions of the lithotripter require no water bath and inflict less pain than do the older models, so analgesia can be provided by short-acting narcotics such as fentanyl and alfentanil.

In other models of the device, the shock wave is transmitted through water and human tissue that have similar acoustic impedances, thus allowing its propagation without dissipation of energy. The shock wave produces cutaneous pain at the entry and exit points and visceral pain at the peritoneum and the renal capsule. A single shock wave can be tolerated, but 2000 shocks may be necessary to pulverize the stone, requiring some form of analgesia for the procedure.

Access to the patient who is secured to a frame in a water bath is difficult, and it can be impossible to hear heart and breath sounds because the noise made by the machine is in the range of 90 to 100 dB. Monitoring consists of ECG, automated blood pressure, pulse oximetry, and during general anesthesia, capnography.

Hemodynamic changes occur with immersion. Cardiac preload is increased as a result of compression of peripheral vessels by hydrostatic pressure, which shifts blood into the central vascular compartment. In healthy volunteers immersed to the clavicles, an increase of up to 700 ml in central blood volume, an increase in stroke volume of 30 to 79 percent, and an increase in cardiac output of 30 to 62 percent with no change in heart rate are noted. Increases in central venous pressure and pulmonary artery pressure are directly related to the degree of immersion. Patients with cardiovascular compromise are immersed gradually and only partially for the treatment.

Hydrostatic pressure on the chest decreases functional residual capacity by 30 to 36 percent and vital capacity by 20 percent. Intrapulmonary pressure and the work of breathing increase as a result of the altered compliance.

Patients may require procedures such as retrograde catheterization to aid in visualization of the stone or manipulation of a stent. Continuous epidural anesthesia allows for safe transfer of these patients from the cystoscopy room to the ESWL room and is the preferred anesthetic for many of these patients. The epidural catheter site is protected with a simple waterproof dressing because bulkier dressings can absorb and attenuate the shock wave.

When regional anesthesia is contraindicated, a general anesthetic is administered. High-frequency jet ventilation or high-frequency (20 to 25 breaths per minute), small-volume (300 ml) positive-pressure ventilation minimizes movement of the diaphragm and the stone.

Transurethral Resection of the Prostate (TURP)

Prostate resection by the resectoscope requires continuous irrigation with glycine-containing fluid.

The absorption of this irrigant through open venous sinuses may lead to volume overload and the classic TURP syndrome of acute dilutional hyponatremia that produces central nervous system and cardiovascular signs of water intoxication. Central nervous system signs and symptoms include disorientation, headache, visual impairment, seizures, and even a coma-like state. Cardiovascular signs are manifested as dysrhythmias, hypotension, and pulmonary edema. Therapy requires aggressive diuresis with furosemide to facilitate excretion of water. Hypertonic saline is reserved for life-threatening hyponatremia because the additional salt load may aggravate pulmonary edema and congestive heart failure. Too rapid correction of brain sodium also can cause neurologic injury.

Spinal or epidural anesthesia not only improves patients' ability to tolerate the increase in blood volume but also permits prompt diagnosis and immediate treatment of the TURP syndrome at the earliest signs of altered mental state. Bladder perforation by the resectoscope is also communicated as intense visceral pain, the onset of hiccups, or referred shoulder pain caused by diaphragmatic irritation.

Radiology

Anesthesia may be required to allow patients to tolerate the increasingly complex procedures performed by radiologists. The same operating conditions may be required as during open surgical procedures, but the setting is remote and unfamiliar. The anesthesia requirements focus on the special needs for each procedure. Position changes are integral to many procedures, allowing movement of the contrast material for better radiologic visualization. Radiation hazards require that the anesthesiologist wear protective lead shields. Most procedures are not particularly painful, and many can be accomplished with local infiltration, sedation, and a minimum of opioids; some interventional procedures involve visceral stimulation as well.

Most procedures are done in dark rooms to allow fluoroscopy and imaging. The radiology procedure room is a confined area with bulky equipment that limits access to the patient. Frequently, there are no piped gases, wall suction, or isolated power supplies. The anesthesiologist therefore must plan carefully to ensure the availability of all the features of a safe anesthetizing location: oxygen, suction, means for positive-pressure ventilation, airway equipment, anesthetics, pulse oximetry, blood pressure and ECG monitoring, capnography, resuscitative drugs, and assistance. The intravascular injection of radiocontrast dye not only produces hyperosmolar hypervolemia but also may provoke adverse immunologic reactions in 2 to 3 percent of patients. The prevention and management of these reactions are described in Chapter 4.

Anesthetic management for most radiology procedures is limited to monitoring and sedation because discomfort is experienced only transiently during placement of a cannula, injection of the contrast material, or balloon dilation of a vessel or hollow viscus. Regional anesthesia may be indicated for visceral pain, such as occurs during nephrostomy, nephrolithotomy, cholecystostomy, or biliary duct drainage and cannulation. Often, epidural analgesia for the segments involved, peripheral nerve blocks, intercostal blocks, or celiac plexus blocks are ideal. Sensory analgesia without motor involvement is preferred so that position changes can be accomplished with the patient's help. General anesthesia may be needed for patients with movement disorders or when communication and cooperation are a problem.

Electroconvulsive Therapy

Electroconvulsive therapy (ECT) is used to treat depression in patients who have not responded to antidepressant drugs. Generalized electrically induced seizures have a therapeutic effect for patients suffering from depression, with biochemical changes at the regional, cellular, and subcellular levels as possible mechanisms of action. The treatment results in seizures lasting 30 to 60 seconds and is administered two or three times weekly for a total aggregate of 210 to 1000 seconds. No benefits occur at lesser doses, and more side effects (memory loss, confusion) are noted beyond it.

The electrical stimulus, consisting of 500 to 800 mA of bidirectional square-wave current applied with scalp electrodes to the nondominant hemisphere, causes a grand mal seizure with increased cerebral blood flow and cerebral oxygen consumption. The autonomic nervous system is activated with a transient parasympathetic outflow followed by sympathetic effects such as hypertension and tachycardia.

The most common cardiac changes noted are sinus and ventricular tachycardia with a rate increase of 20 to 115 percent, bradycardia (especially among patients taking beta blockers), premature atrial contractions, premature ventricular contractions, and ST-segment depression. These are self-limited and generally do not require treatment in most patients but may be harmful to those with cardiovascular disease.

The incidence of medical complications is 0.4 percent, and the mortality rate is 0.03 percent. Complications include myocardial ischemia, arrhythmias, laryngospasm, prolonged apnea, oral lacerations, and pulmonary aspiration. The most common causes of death are arrhythmia, infarction, and congestive heart failure occurring during the recovery period. Electroconvulsive therapy can be safe and effective with proper selection, pretreatment, and careful clinical management.

The anesthetic management starts with a thorough preoperative evaluation of the patient, with appropriate medical consultations as indicated. Drug interactions must be considered because patients often take drugs such as tricyclic antidepressants, monoamine oxidase inhibitors, benzodiazepines, and lithium.

The anesthetic requirements include rapid induction and rapid recovery, amnesia for the procedure, prevention of seizure sequelae such as long bone or vertebral fractures, injuries to tongue and lips, increased intraocular pressure, increased intragastric pressure, and attenuation of the hemodynamic effects of ECT. The combination of methohexital, succinylcholine, and ventilation with oxygen is widely used.

Short-acting intravenous induction drugs given in hypnotic doses satisfy the requirements of rapid onset and minimal recovery time. Increasing the dose of the drug to control hypertension and tachycardia also increases seizure threshold and shortens seizure time. Retrograde amnesia results from effective seizures, even without an anesthetic. Attenuation of the parasympathetic response to ECT by atropine or glycopyrrolate also provides a dry mouth. The table of intravenous hypnotics for ECT (Table 31-1) uses methohexital as the standard for induction and lists the dosages used and observations made by various investigators.

The dose of succinylcholine (0.25 to 0.75 mg/kg) is adjusted to attenuate the tonic-clonic motor responses that may result in fractures in susceptible patients and yet minimize the postictal apneic period. Routine intubation is not recommended because of increased drug requirements and cardiovascular responses provoked by intubation, but a protective device such as a bite block is used to prevent damage to teeth, lips, and tongue. Verification of seizures after complete neuromuscular blockade can best be ascertained by electroencephalographic (EEG) monitoring or, alternatively, by occlusion of arterial flow to a

Table 31-1

Effects of Induction Drugs Used for ECT		
Hypnotic	**Dosage (mg/kg)**	**Observations**
Methohexital	0.7–1.2	Minimal postictal side effects, hiccups, muscle twitches, some venous irritation
Thiopental	2.0–3.0	Longer sleep time, more ECG abnormalities, less K^+ elevation
Propofol	1.5–1.6	Less increase in heart rate and BP, decreased seizure time, pain on injection
Etomidate	0.2–0.3	Involuntary movements, increased muscle tone, pain on injection
Ketamine	1.0–2.2	Slow onset, increased duration of seizure, delayed recovery, nausea, ataxia, postoperative delirium and confusion
Diazepam	0.3–0.5	Slow onset, prolonged recovery, increased seizure threshold, decreased seizure time, more ECG abnormalities, venous irritation and phlebitis

limb prior to administering succinylcholine, allowing seizure activity in the unparalyzed extremity. Intermediate-acting nondepolarizing muscle relaxants such as vecuronium and atracurium are not recommended because of their longer durations of action.

Intense stimulation of the sympathetic nervous system and an increase in catecholamines result in tachycardia and hypertension, insignificant in most cases but catastrophic in a few, causing cardiovascular and cerebral injury. Sinus tachycardia and most arrhythmias are short-lived (10 minutes) and revert to normal as catecholamines subside. Pharmacologic intervention includes the use of beta-blocking agents (esmolol, propanolol, or labetalol), ganglionic blocking agents (trimethaphan), or vasodilating agents (nitroprusside or nitroglycerine) that are sufficiently short-acting to control increased blood pressure and heart rate but avoid undesirable hypotension later. Intravenous lidocaine is effective in preventing arrhythmias but suppresses or shortens beneficial seizure activity. Termination of a prolonged seizure (greater than 90 seconds' duration) may be accomplished by administering additional intravenous short-acting barbiturates.

Ophthalmology

Anesthesia for ophthalmic operations is based on a knowledge of ocular anatomy and physiology, an understanding of the factors influencing intraocular pressure and the interaction between ophthalmic drugs and perioperative medications, and an appreciation of the oculocardiac reflex. Patients represent extremes of age, with a preponderance of the elderly with coexisting medical conditions such as coronary artery disease, hypertension, diabetes, and chronic lung disease.

Normal intraocular pressure (IOP) is 10 to 22 mmHg. Aqueous humor is formed in the ciliary body by active filtration on the anterior surface of the iris and is eliminated via the canal of Schlemm at the episcleral venous network through connecting channels to the superior vena cava. Thus central venous pressure directly affects IOP, whereas arterial pressure has minimal influence because of autoregulation of the blood supply. Straining, coughing, vomiting, and the Valsalva maneuver can increase IOP as much as 40 mmHg. Another physiologic determinant of IOP is intraocular (choroidal) blood volume. Hypocarbia decreases IOP by vasoconstriction of the choroidal blood vessels and reduces formation of aqueous humor through diminished carbonic anhydrase activity. External pressure on the eye or contraction of the orbicularis oculi muscle also causes increased IOP.

Most anesthetics decrease IOP by relaxing extraocular muscle tone, improving outflow of the aqueous humor, and decreasing venous and arterial blood pressure. A summary of the effects of anesthesia drugs on IOP is outlined in Table 31-2. Succinylcholine and ketamine increase IOP. Anatomically, ocular muscles have multiple motor nerve endings that respond to succinylcholine by a sustained tonic contracture instead of flaccid paralysis as in skeletal muscle, resulting in ocular hypertension. Nystagmus and blepharospasm limit the use of ketamine for ophthalmic operations.

Ophthalmic drugs may produce systemic effects that must be accounted for in planning anesthesia. Concentrated topical medications are absorbed systemically by way of the conjunctiva or via the nasal mucosa following drainage through the nasolacrimal duct. Topical eye medications and systemic medications administered during eye operations that can cause systemic effects are listed in Table 31-3.

The oculocardiac reflex is a trigeminal-vagal reflex arc characterized by a 10 to 50 percent reduction in heart rate precipitated by pressure on the globe or traction on the extraocular muscles, especially the medial rectus. Other manifestations include junctional rhythm, A-V block, premature ventricular contractions, ventricular fibrillation, and asystole. The reflex occurs most often during strabismus operations, during the injection of a retrobulbar block, or when pressure is exerted on the eyeball. Premedication with atropine or glycopyrrolate reduces the incidence but does not abolish it. The treatment is removal of the stimulus and, if bradycardia persists, intravenous atropine (0.006 mg/kg).

General requirements of anesthesia for ophthalmic operations include an unmoving globe (akinesia), profound analgesia, minimal bleeding, and a smooth emergence. Specific clinical situations may dictate special anesthetic management.

Patients with glaucoma need special attention. Ophthalmic medications are continued to ensure miosis through the perioperative period. Anticholinergics used for premedication and for reversal of the effects of depolarizing muscle relaxants are safe because too little drug reaches the eye to dilate the pupil. However, topical application of mydriatics such as atropine and scopolamine is contraindicated.

A sulfur hexafluoride (SF_6) bubble is injected into the vitreal cavity during retinal reattachment; the bubble remains in place for 10 days, holding the retina in place. Newer gases may persist as long as 28 days. Nitrous oxide is 117 times more soluble than SF_6 and rapidly enters the bubble, causing it to expand and increasing IOP. Nitrous oxide is discontinued 20 minutes before SF_6 injection and is not employed in the anesthetic gas mixtures for 4 weeks after retinal operations.

Anesthesia for emergency treatment of penetrating eye injuries involves conflicting goals between prevention of aspiration of gastric contents and prevention of increases in IOP that may cause further eye damage and loss of vision. Succinylcholine is used in rapid-sequence induction of anesthesia to protect the airway, but it increases IOP and risks extrusion of ocular contents. A modified rapid-sequence induc-

Table 31-2

Effects of Medications on Intraocular Pressure

Anesthesia Drugs	Intraocular Pressure Effect
Inhalation agents	
Halothane	18–33% decrease
Enflurane	21–40% decrease
Isoflurane	Decrease, similar to halothane
Perioperative drugs	
Thiopental 3 mg/kg IV	Decrease, baseline after 6 minutes
Innovar 0.1 ml/kg IV	12% decrease
Ketamine 5 mg/kg IM	37% increase, normal after 30 minutes
Etomidate 20 µg/kg/min IV	Decrease 61%
Midazolam IV	Decrease similar to thiopental
Diazepam IV	Decrease
Muscle relaxants	
Succinylcholine bolus or IV infusion	Increase 33%, normal after 7 minutes
Succinylcholine IM	Increase IOP for 15 minutes
Pancuronium IV	70–84% decrease
Atracurium IV	No effect
Vecuronium IV	Slight decrease

Table 31-3

Anesthetic Implications of Ophthalmic Drugs

Medication	Ophthalmic Use	Anesthetic Implications
Topical drugs		
Acetylcholine	Miotic used after lens extraction	Bradycardia, hypotension, bronchospasm, salivation
Betaxolol	Beta-adrenergic blocker oculospecific for glaucoma	Additive effects with beta blockers
Cocaine	Analgesia, vasoconstriction in dacryo-cystorhinostomy	Triggers dysrhythmia
Cyclopentolate	Mydriatic	CNS toxicity; dysarthria, convulsions, psychosis
Echothiophate	Long-acting anticholinesterase miotic for glaucoma	Prolongs succinylcholine and local anesthetic ester action
Epinephrine	Mydriatic used for open angle glaucoma	Tachycardia, nervousness, PVCs, caution with halothane
Phenylephrine	Pupillary dilatation, capillary decongestion	Hypertension, headache, tremulousness
Timolol	Beta-adrenergic blocker (nonselective)	Bronchospasm, bradycardia, postoperative apnea in infants, exacerbation of myasthenia gravis
Systemic drugs		
Glycerol PO	Reduces IOP	Nausea, vomiting, risk of aspiration
Mannitol IV	Reduces IOP by decreasing aqueous humor formation	Cardiovascular and renal effects
Acetazolamide IV	Reduces IOP	Renal tubular effects, loss of HCO_3^- and K^+ ions

tion has been advocated that includes a dose of thiopental to ensure adequate depth, an intermediate-acting nondepolarizer in large doses (rocuronium or vecuronium), cricoid pressure, and intubation after profound muscle relaxation has occurred. Measures to blunt the cardiovascular and IOP responses to laryngoscopy and intubation are similar to those used to manage increased intracranial pressure and may include lidocaine, a beta-adrenergic blocking drug, and a short-acting narcotic.

Strabismus operations are the most common pediatric ocular operations. In addition to oculocardiac reflex, these patients seem to have an increased incidence of malignant hyperthermia. Forced duction testing (FDT) is often done to differentiate between a paretic muscle and a restriction preventing ocular motion. Succinylcholine administration affects the results of FDT for a time longer than the duration of skeletal muscle relaxation. If FDT is planned, it is best to avoid the drug completely or to perform the test before or at least 20 minutes after succinylcholine administration. Vomiting after strabismus operations is common (85 percent). Droperidol (0.075 mg/kg) given at induction of anesthesia before ma-

nipulation of the eye has decreased the incidence to 10 percent.

Cataract extraction is the most common ophthalmologic procedure done for the elderly, and anesthesia planning must address the presence of associated diseases. Analgesia and akinesia are provided by a retrobulbar block or general anesthesia. If general anesthesia is given, a smooth intraoperative course must occur with no coughing or straining to increase IOP. Extubation is accomplished under "deep" anesthesia, and coughing is attenuated by intravenous lidocaine administration. Prophylactic intravenous droperidol is helpful in minimizing the occurrence of postoperative nausea and vomiting.

Most cataract operations are performed with retrobulbar block, which provides local anesthesia and akinesia of the globe. Complications associated with the block include the oculocardiac reflex, hemorrhage, local anesthetic toxicity owing to intravascular injection, and inadvertent intraocular injection. An impressive record of safety is associated with local anesthesia, and available data do not demonstrate any difference in ocular morbidity between local and general anesthesia.

Cancer Chemotherapy

Multiple side effects, interactions, and complications are associated with chemotherapeutic agents. Anesthesiologists must be familiar with these side effects because they can complicate the management of anesthesia in cancer patients who have received these drugs. Table 31-4 lists cancer medications with the most commonly associated systemic effects. The immediate side effects are nausea and vomiting, chills and fevers, tissue necrosis, phlebitis, rash, renal failure, and hypocalcemia. Complications occurring later (days to weeks) are bone marrow depression, paralytic ileus, hypercalcemia, disseminated intravascular coagulation, pulmonary infiltrate, and fluid retention. Side effects delayed for months are anemia, hepatocellular damage, pulmonary fibrosis, inappropriate secretion of antidiuretic hormone, peripheral neuropathy, and cardiac necrosis. Secondary malignancies, hepatic fibrosis, and encephalopathy can occur years later.

Administration of chemotherapeutic agents to specific tumor sites by means of regional perfusion (a modification of cardiopulmonary bypass) is done to minimize systemic side effects. Regional perfusion represents a single operative chemotherapeutic exposure. The best responses have occurred with melanomas and soft tissue sarcomas of the limbs.

A variety of specific organ or system involvement occurs with cancer therapy. Myelosuppression caused by all the chemotherapeutic agents is usually resolved 6 weeks after termination of therapy. A complete blood count, including platelet count, may provide the guide for component replacement therapy during the perioperative period. Coagulation defects not associated with thrombocytopenia can occur with mechlorethamine, mithramycin, and L-asparaginase. Immunosuppression occurs with the alkylating agents and a majority of the chemotherapeutic agents. Thus meticulous aseptic technique must be observed to prevent infections.

The two types of cardiac effects noted with anthracycline antibiotic therapy (doxorubicin and daunorubicin) are the acute transient ECG abnormalities that occur during the course of therapy and chronic, cumulative, dose-related (greater than 500 mg/m^2) congestive heart failure. Loss of myocardial cells accounts for the cardiac effects. Cardiotoxicity is irreversible, and the fibrotic heart responds poorly to inotropes and digitalis. Within 3 weeks of onset of symptoms, mortality is 59 percent.

Pulmonary fibrosis and pneumonitis can be induced by alkylating agents, methotrexate, cytabrine, and bleomycin. Synergistic lung damage can occur when radiation therapy is combined with bleomycin. Case reports have suggested that the lung exposed to bleomycin is susceptible to oxygen toxicity and that the FiO_2 must be limited to 30 percent in these patients, but some of these patients may have suffered fluid overload. It is prudent to limit both oxygen and fluids in these patients to the doses required.

Hepatotoxicity occurs with the use of most antimetabolites, mithramycin, L-asparaginase, and the nitrosoureas. Relevant factors that can cause hepatic insult in cancer patients are multiple blood transfusions, immunosuppressive infection, and other drugs related to the chemotherapeutic protocol. The usual precautions for patients with compromised hepatocellular function are appropriate (see Chap. 23).

Nephrotoxic antineoplastic agents include cisplatin, streptozocin, vincristine, cyclophosphamide, and mithramycin. The nephrotoxic effects of these drugs are ameliorated by diuresis with saline and mannitol when urinary output is maintained at 100 ml/h. Hyponatremia can occur with cyclophosphamide and vincristine. Hypomagnesemia, hypokalemia, hypocalcemia, and hypophosphatemia are encountered often with cisplatin therapy. Potentially nephrotoxic anesthetics are withheld from these patients, and the anesthetic management includes perioperative monitoring of urinary output and central venous pressure to guide fluid and electrolyte replacement.

Neurotoxicity of chemotherapeutic agents must be considered when administering an anesthetic. Intrathecal methotrexate and cytosine have been reported to cause transient paraplegia and changes in sensorium. Peripheral neuropathy is caused by the plant alkaloids: vincristine, vinblastine, and vindesine and cisplatin, cytosine, and procarbazine. The earliest, most consistent sign is loss of Achilles tendon reflex, and the most common complaint is paresthesia of the hands and feet. Cranial nerve involvement, autonomic neuropathy, and ototoxicity are other effects of chemotherapy. Preoperative documentation of neurologic deficits provides a baseline for assessment of the patient postoperatively. Conduction anesthesia may be inadvisable in these patients with preexisting, possibly progressive neurologic defects.

Table 31-4

Side Effects of Chemotherapeutic Agents

Chemotherapeutic Agents	Side Effects
Alkylating agents (interfere with normal mitosis by alkylating DNA)	**General** Bone marrow suppression is dose-limiting factor, mild immuno-suppression Hemolytic anemia and increased skin pigmentation Inhibit pseudocholinesterase resulting in prolonged succinyl-choline action Pneumonitis and pulmonary fibrosis **Drug-specific**
Melphalan, (Alkeran, L-PAM)	Side effects as listed for alkylating agents
Thiotepa	Side effects as listed for alkylating agents
Mechlorethamine (nitrogen mustard)	CNS toxicity
Busulfan (Myleran)	Pulmonary toxicity, renal toxicity, minor GI effects like diarrhea and stomatitis
Chlorambucil (Leukeran)	Hepatic, CNS toxicity
Cyclophosphamide (Cytoxan)	Strong immunosuppression, hemorrhagic cystitis, inappropriate ADH secretion, stomatitis
Antimetabolites (inhibit enzymes thus producing aberrant, nonfunctioning molecule)	**General** Strong immunosuppressant Liver dysfunction, reversible with cessation of therapy **Drug-specific**
Methotrexate (MTX)	Severe GI effects: stomatitis, diarrhea, hemorrhagic enteritis; occasional renal tubular necrosis, mild pulmonary toxicity
Mercaptopurine (6-MP)	Severe hepatotoxicity, occasional renal toxicity, mild diarrhea and stomatitis
Thioguanine (6-TG)	Severe hepatotoxicity, mild GI effects: diarrhea and stomatitis
Fluorouracil (5-FU)	Severe GI symptoms: diarrhea and stomatitis; rare CNS effect: cerebral ataxia
Cytarabine	Mild pulmonary toxicity, mild GI symptoms
Plant alkaloids (bind to microtubule, arrest mitosis, affect protein synthesis)	**General** Major side effect: leukopenia Moderate immunosuppression Peripheral and autonomic neuropathy **Drug-specific**
Vincristine (VCR)	Mild CNS toxicity, renal toxicity, inappropriate ADH secretion
Vinblastine (Velban)	Moderate diarrhea; mild stomatitis
Anthracycline antibiotics (inhibit DNA and RNA formation by forming stable DNA complex)	**General** Moderate stomatitis; leukopenia, thrombocytopenia, and anemia **Drug-specific**
Doxorubicin (Adriamycin)	Moderate cardiotoxicity, mild hepatic toxicity, red urine
Daunorubicin (DNR)	Cardiotoxicity, mild immunosuppression and hepatic toxicity, red urine
Bleomycin (BLM)	Pulmonary toxicity, acts synergistically with radiation therapy in producing lung damage
Dactinomycin	Mild immunosuppression
Mithramycin	Moderate hepatic and renal toxicity; coagulation defects
Nitrosoureas (alkylation of nucleic acid and carboxylation)	**General** Moderate leukopenia, thrombocytopenia, and anemia **Drug-specific**
Streptozocin	Severe hepatic and renal toxicity, selective destruction of pancreatic beta cells causing hyperglycemia
Carmustine	Mild pulmonary, hepatic, renal, GI effects
Enzymes and random synthetics	
L-Asparaginase	Moderate hepatic dysfunction, mild immunosuppression, coagulopathy
Cisplatin	Severe renal tubular damage, myelosuppression, peripheral neuropathy, seizures, loss of sense of taste
Procarbazine	Moderate myelosuppression, weak MAO inhibitor, lethargy, depression, synergism with sedatives

Gastrointestinal effects such as nausea, vomiting, and diarrhea may cause fluid and electrolyte abnormalities that require correction. Stomatitis is caused by the antimetabolites and some of the alkylating agents and plant alkaloids. Trauma and excessive manipulation of the upper airway must be avoided.

Anticholinesterase effects of the alkylating agents, most notably thiotepa, mechlorethamine, and cyclophosphamide, may produce prolonged apnea after succinylcholine. Monoamine oxidase inhibition and synergistic action with barbiturates, antihistamines, and phenothiazines occur with procarbazine.

BIBLIOGRAPHY

Donlon JV. Anesthesia and eye, ear, nose and throat surgery. In Miller RD, ed: *Anesthesia*. New York: Churchill-Livingstone, 1990, pp 2001-2023.

Krementz ET. Regional perfusion, current sophistication, what next? *Cancer* 1986;57:416-432.

Muravchick S, Castro AD. Anesthetic considerations for urologic procedures. In Hanno PM, Wein AJ, eds: *Clinical Manual of Urology*. New York: McGraw-Hill, 1994, pp 815-833.

Murphy DF. Anesthesia and intraocular pressure. *Anesth Analg* 1985;64:520-530.

Selvin BL. Electroconvulsive therapy–1987. *Anesthesiology* 1987;67:367-385.

Selvin BL. Cancer chemotherapy: Implications for the anesthesiologist. *Anesth Analg* 1981;60:425-434.

Weber W, Madler C, Keil B, et al. Cardiovascular effects of ESWL. In Gravenstein JS, Peter K, eds: *Extracorporeal Shock Wave Lithotripsy for Renal Stone Disease*. Boston: Butterworth, 1986, pp 101-112.

Care Outside the Operating Room

CHAPTER 32

Postanesthesia Care

Elizabeth C. Behringer

Anesthesia care does not end at the conclusion of the operation but extends to include the initial emergence from anesthesia, the transport of the patient to the postanesthesia care unit (PACU), the management of recovery room problems, continued care of complications resulting from anesthesia, and a subsequent assessment called the *postoperative visit*. In the first few hours after operation, the patient suffers the effects of pain, blood loss, hypothermia, and other consequences of the operation, while responses are impaired by the residual effects of anesthesia. This phase of management is influenced by the anesthetic, the operation, and the patient's current condition and associated diseases; the management of emergence and recovery is part of the overall anesthesia plan.

Emergence from General Anesthesia

Patients awaken progressively by passing through the stages of general anesthesia. From the stage of surgical anesthesia, in which even sympathetic responses to pain are minimal, patients pass to the excitement stage, in which responses to stimuli may be exaggerated and harmful. To prevent complications, the duration of this period is kept to a minimum, pain is managed with opioids or regional anesthesia, and the patient receives close attention to prevent or manage the responses (hypertension, tachycardia, etc.) associated with hyperreflexia. There follows a period when patients follow orders and respond to questions but may not remember events, after which they appear to return to near their preoperative mental state. This sequence of events may occupy minutes or hours, depending on the

drugs and the doses used to maintain anesthesia. Even at this point, residual impairment in cognitive functions persists for days, due in part to residual concentrations of anesthetic drugs and the administration of postoperative drugs such as analgesics.

The apparent level of consciousness depends on the stimuli applied and the level of response desired. Patients who attempt to cough because the endotracheal tube is in place, yet who do not respond to commands, are awake only in the sense that they have recovered at least one reflex. In most cases, an adequate level of recovery from anesthesia implies that the patient breathes spontaneously, maintains a patent airway without assistance, and responds to simple commands and questions.

■ MAC Awake

By analogy with the minimum alveolar concentration (MAC) for anesthesia, *MAC awake* is the end-tidal concentration of anesthetic agent at which 50 percent of patients respond appropriately to a verbal command (open eyes on request). MAC awake is about 50 percent of MAC for inhalation anesthetics used alone. In most patients emerging from general anesthesia, responses to verbal commands do not occur until end-tidal concentrations of inhaled agents have decreased to 10 to 20 percent of MAC. This is accounted for by the presence of adjuvant drugs such as opioids and intravenous anesthetics and by differences between end-tidal concentrations and brain concentrations during rapid emergence. Hypothermia and the residual effects of sedatives and anticholinergic drugs also decrease the patient's responsiveness.

■ Managing Emergence

Emergence is begun by eliminating anesthetic gases from the inspired mixture and discontinuing intravenous administration of hypnotics, opioids, and relaxants. Depending on its pharmacokinetic properties and the need for its continued effects in the closing moments of the operation, each drug is discontinued individually based on the expected time of emergence. This may mean discontinuing a soluble anesthetic such as halothane 30 or more minutes before emergence but continuing nitrous oxide until the operation is completed. With experience, it is possible to maintain light anesthesia with analgesia, muscle relaxation, and amnesia just sufficient for the demands of the operation. This balancing permits a timely end to the anesthetic.

Other considerations affect speed of emergence as well. All those factors that make patients more sensitive to the effects of anesthetics also make them susceptible to relative anesthetic overdose and delayed emergence, including alterations in pharmacokinetics due to organ dysfunction, hypoproteinemia, or age. These influences need not delay emergence, provided that doses of anesthetics are used only according to need and not according to a standard protocol. Hypothermia delays emergence. Premedicants, as well as drugs not ordinarily thought of as sedatives, cross the blood-brain barrier and exert central sedative effects; these include some antihypertensives, beta blockers, and atropine, especially in the elderly. Some studies have shown that small doses of benzodiazepines used as premedicants need not delay emergence, but these results may not apply to sicker, older patients. The level of stimulation affects awakening. Usually the endotracheal tube is a potent stimulus for coughing, hypertension, and tachycardia, but even with an endotracheal tube in place, some patients lie quietly with eyes closed, yet respond to verbal stimuli.

■ Analgesia and Emergence

Unless the patient has received a regional anesthetic, as in combined epidural and general anesthesia, it is appropriate to administer opioids near the end of a general anesthetic so that the patient may awaken as comfortably as possible. This may delay emergence somewhat, but the benefits include reduced agitation and excitement on emergence and reduced cardiovascular responses to pain. A useful technique to avoid excessive narcosis involves allowing spontaneous ventilation before awakening the patient. If the respiratory rate is greater than 15 breaths per minute and the minute ventilation is appropriate for the patient, then intravenous morphine or fentanyl is given in small incremental doses that maintain the respiratory rate at 11 to 13 breaths per minute.

■ Timing of Emergence

Choosing the time for emergence from anesthesia depends on circumstances. At one extreme, a patient who has just undergone a minor outpatient procedure is awakened as rapidly and promptly as possible. At the other extreme, no measures at all may be taken to end anesthesia after a complex cardiac procedure because the patient will require analgesia, amnesia, muscle relaxation, and mechanical ventilation in the intensive care unit. The need to control intracranial pressure, intraocular pressure, coughing, or hypertensive responses modifies plans for the end of anesthesia. A slower, more controlled awakening may be preferable in these patients, even at the expense of delayed emergence. Patients with difficult airways or full stomachs, on the other hand, benefit from rapid, complete awakening to prevent airway obstruction or aspiration of gastric contents.

In most cases, it is best for the patient to pass through the excitement stage and awaken and for the endotracheal tube to be removed immediately at the end of the operation. This enhances safety, since the anesthesia team can manage these dangerous steps in the operating room with adequate monitoring and in a controlled fashion. This practice is not universal, for some fear that awakening patients in the operating room wastes time. However, to admit regularly to the PACU patients who are unconscious with endotracheal tubes in place is to neglect the management of critical phases of the anesthetic. With skill and attention, it is possible routinely to remove the endotracheal tube as the surgical dressing is applied.

■ Neurologic Abnormalities During Emergence

Abnormal neurologic findings are common among normal patients emerging from anesthesia. These signs must be distinguished from inadequate reversal of neuromuscular blockade and from neurologic conditions requiring intervention. Transient hyperreflexia, sustained ankle clonus, and upgoing plantar responses are all common, especially following the use of inhalation agents. Although these abnormal responses to neurologic examination can persist for 40 minutes or even longer after anesthesia, they disappear as the patient awakens, which distinguishes them from the signs of neurologic insult suffered during anesthesia.

Transporting the Patient

The journey from the operating room to the recovery room or the intensive care unit can be hazardous. Complications may be severe or life-threatening and include hypertension, hypotension, hypoventilation, vomiting, aspiration, airway obstruction, and hypoxemia. Managing the move from the operating table to the PACU or ICU is part of anesthesia care. As always, the level of care depends on the patient's condition. A healthy, wide awake outpatient may need little more than simple watchfulness during the trip to the recovery room. A gravely ill patient may require continuous invasive cardiovascular monitoring, positive-pressure ventilation, and infusions of cardiovascular drugs by battery-operated pumps.

For the usual patient who has undergone general anesthesia or regional anesthesia with sedation, safe transfer begins with the decision to move the patient from the operating table to the bed or litter. This requires that the airway, breathing, and circulation be satisfactory and unlikely to deteriorate in the next few minutes. The move from the operating table to the litter must be well organized, with enough assistants to prevent accidents. Once on the bed or litter, the patient is again evaluated and the results recorded in the anesthesia record (Table 32-1).

During transport to the recovery room, an assistant pulls the litter, while the anesthesiologist, positioned at the patient's head, monitors the patient as needed by giving simple commands, holding a conversation, watching the chest, feeling for exhaled gas at the mouth and nose, supporting the chin, or feeling a pulse. Additional monitoring and emergency drugs and supplies are provided to match the severity of the illness of the individual patient.

Hypoxemia is common in the immediate postoperative period. The use of battery-operated pulse oximeters has shown that patients who do not receive oxygen during transport to the PACU often suffer hypoxemia. All patients should receive oxygen during

Table 32-1

Checklist for Evaluating Patients Before Departing the Operating Room and After Arriving in the PACU

After the patient has been moved from the operating room table and before leaving the operating room, a careful evaluation ensures that no complications require treatment.

1. Airway patency
2. Breathing (rate and depth)
3. Arterial oxygenation (pulse oximeter)
4. Blood pressure
5. Heart rate, ECG
6. Level of spinal or epidural anesthesia
7. Level of consciousness

The same evaluation is carried out and recorded with the PACU nurse when the patient arrives there, with the addition of a measurement of body temperature.

the trip to the PACU, and some require the use of a pulse oximeter.

Care in the PACU

Patients who undergo minor operations under local anesthesia without significant sedation may be discharged directly to home or to a hospital room. Others, whose care includes general anesthesia, spinal or epidural anesthesia, or significant sedation, require a period of observation and care in a special nursing unit, usually a PACU. Their management may range from brief observation followed by discharge from the hospital to an overnight stay for intensive care in the PACU.

■ Admitting the Patient to the PACU

When the patient arrives in the PACU, supplemental oxygen is changed from the transport cart or bed to the wall supply, monitoring devices are attached, and the receiving nurse and the anesthesiologist together evaluate the patient. Routine monitors in the PACU include a pulse oximeter, electrocardiograph (ECG), temperature, and blood pressure by noninvasive cuff or arterial catheter. The evaluation is the same as that performed before the patient left the operating room, with the addition of body temperature (see Table 32-1). The results of the evaluation and the time of admission to the unit are recorded at

Table 32-2

Report on Admitting a Patient to the PACU

1. Patient's name
2. Brief medical history
   a. Significant concomitant diseases (e.g., asthma, angina)
   b. Drugs
   c. Allergies
3. The operation
   a. Site
   b. Bleeding
4. The anesthetic
   a. Anesthetic agents, sedatives, narcotics
   b. State of alertness
   c. Muscle relaxants, recovery
   d. Expected vital signs
5. Summary of fluid balance
   a. Blood and fluids given
   b. Urine output
   c. Blood loss
6. Expected problems and plans
   a. Oxygen required
   b. Fluid therapy
   c. Pain management
   d. Any alterations in usual PACU discharge criteria

the end of the anesthesia record and the beginning of the recovery room record. The anesthesiologist provides the receiving nurse with a complete report that describes the patient, the operation, and the anesthesia, along with plans for any further care that might be needed, such the administration of analgesics or the management of fluids (Table 32-2).

The anesthesiologist leaves the recovery room only when satisfied that the patient can be cared for by the receiving personnel. Many recovery rooms have an anesthesiologist in attendance, but the anesthesiologist who cared for the patient intraoperatively is notified as well when problems arise.

■ Problems Commonly Experienced by Patients in the PACU

As many as 20 percent of patients admitted to the PACU experience complications while recovering from the immediate effects of anesthesia and operation. Most common is nausea or vomiting (5 percent), unexpected alterations in mental state (5 percent), a requirement for upper airway support (3.6 percent), hypotension (3 percent), dysrhythmias (2 percent), and hypertension, myocardial ischemia, or a major cardiovascular complication (<1 percent each).

Persistent Somnolence

When a patient fails to emerge from anesthesia and remains obtunded, the possible diagnoses are similar to those of coma. A systematic approach begins by ensuring adequate cardiac output, oxygenation, and ventilation and then considers such metabolic derangements as hypoglycemia and electrolyte imbalances before moving to less urgent concerns such as hypothermia (Table 32-3). Appropriate antagonists of narcotics, anticholinergic agents, and benzodiazepines can be used, but doses must be small to avoid unwanted withdrawal effects. Even if an antagonist is successful, continued observation is needed because sedation may recur.

Agitation and Delirium

Although many patients pass through brief periods of excitement as they awaken from anesthesia, some remain agitated for a prolonged period. Delirium may be associated intermittently with postoperative somnolence (see Table 32-3), but it may result from other causes that are more likely to cause agitation (Table 32-4). Emergence delirium is common in healthy young patients, patients who are emotional or anxious

Table 32-3

Delayed Awakening After Anesthesia

The disorders that most often account for delayed awakening from anesthesia are listed here in the order of priority for diagnosis and treatment, not in the order of prevalence.

1. Acute metabolic disorders
   a. Hypoxia
   b. Hypercarbia
   c. Hypotension
   d. Hypoglycemia
   e. Other electrolyte disorders
   f. Water intoxication
2. Residual neuromuscular blockade
3. CNS disorders
   a. Stroke
   b. Post-anoxic encephalopathy
4. Residual effects of anesthetics, sedatives
5. Other medications
   a. Premedicants
   b. Central anticholinergic syndrome: scopolamine, atropine
   c. Illicit drugs
   d. Cimetidine
6. Hypothermia
7. Preexisting coma or obtundation
8. Interpatient variation in response to anesthetics

Table 32-4

Agitation and Delirium in the PACU

Possible causes of agitation or delirium among patients in the recovery room:

1. Hypoxemia or airway obstruction
2. Pain
3. Full bladder
4. Incomplete reversal of neuromuscular blockade
5. Withdrawal from alcohol or other drugs
6. Central anticholinergic syndrome (especially scopolamine)
7. Residual anesthetics or sedatives
8. Senile dementia

prior to induction of anesthesia, or patients who awaken restrained, as by large, immobilizing casts. Drugs such as scopolamine, barbiturates, ketamine, and phenothiazines can incite emergence delirium. Delirium is uncommon in patients who receive opiates perioperatively.

The cause of delirium is established before treating the patient because agitation may signal dangerous underlying disorders such as hypoxia, hypercarbia, or cerebral ischemia. After these problems have been addressed, opioids, benzodiazepines, or a combination of them usually will calm the patient. Physostigmine, 1 to 2 mg intravenously, is sometimes required as specific treatment for the central anticholinergic syndrome caused by atropine, scopolamine, tricyclic antidepressants, antihistamines, butyrophenones, or phenothiazines.

Pain

Before beginning empiric treatment of postoperative pain, causes of pain not directly related to the operation must be considered (Table 32-5). In addi-

Table 32-5

Causes of Postoperative Pain

1. Operative site
2. Muscle spasm
3. Bladder distension
4. Musculoskeletal
   a. Exacerbation of arthritis
   b. Injury from positioning
5. Tight cast or dressing
6. Phlebitis, infiltration of intravenous fluids
7. Angina
8. Corneal abrasion

tion, anxiety or drug-seeking behavior may present as pain in some patients. If the pain is the result of the operation, techniques of nerve block or epidural injection often are most effective. Intravenous opioids are an alternative. Small intravenous doses, such as 2 to 5 mg morphine for most adults, are given to produce the desired effect, following which patient-controlled analgesia may begin (see Chap. 34).

Nausea and Vomiting

Nausea and vomiting occur commonly after anesthesia and operation. Those most at risk for postoperative nausea and vomiting are described in Table 32-6. Young women may be at increased risk. Nitrous oxide has been proposed as a possible cause, perhaps because of accumulation of the agent in bowel or the middle ear, but recent studies refute this idea. Improving patients' comfort is reason enough to avoid this complication, but for those who have undergone ophthalmic or neurosurgical procedures or who are unable to open their mouths because of wires used to fix the mandible, it is essential.

Prophylaxis against nausea and vomiting includes avoiding distension of the stomach during mask ventilation. Should this occur, emptying the stomach with a gastric tube after intubation of the trachea may be helpful. Propofol may be associated with a lesser incidence of postoperative nausea and vomiting than is thiopental. The same drugs are used for both prophylaxis and treatment (see Chap. 4). Droperidol reduces the incidence of nausea and vomiting when used in small doses (0.625 mg intravenously) that do not prolong emergence. Larger doses seem to be no more effective as antiemetics and may even be less

Table 32-6

Contributing Factors for Postoperative Nausea or Vomiting

1. History of nausea or vomiting after previous operations
2. Gastric distension
   a. Ileus
   b. Bowel obstruction
   c. Prolonged or inept mask ventilation
3. Full stomach before operation
4. Opioids
5. Operation
   a. Ophthalmologic procedures
   b. Laparoscopy
   c. Otorhinologic procedures, especially inner ear
   d. Abdominal operations

effective, though studies differ. Prochlorperazine, 5 to 10 mg intravenously, is sedating and may produce dysphoria or hypotension. Metoclopramide, 10 to 20 mg intravenously, is well tolerated, but antiemetic efficacy in a number of studies has been inconsistent. Ondansetron, 4 to 8 mg intravenously, is effective and well tolerated and does not cause sedation; it is expensive, however.

Residual Neuromuscular Blockade

When examined closely for subtle signs of weakness, some patients who have undergone recent general anesthesia prove to have residual neuromuscular blockade despite receiving anticholinesterases. This weakness often goes unnoticed, even by the patients, and may dissipate relatively quickly if they have received modern muscle relaxants of intermediate duration of action. It has become apparent recently that even seemingly minor weakness may produce ill effects, since these patients may suffer upper airway obstruction due to loss of muscle tone in the neck and pharynx.

Occasionally, some patients become profoundly weak despite what appeared to be adequate recovery from nondepolarizing neuromuscular blockade in the operating room. This may be due to inadequate testing to verify return of strength or to potentiation of the remaining neuromuscular blocking drug by progressive respiratory acidosis that follows hypoventilation. These patients may suffer emotional distress, airway obstruction, hypoventilation, hypoxemia, hypercarbia, and brain damage if the problem is not recognized and treated. Any patient with unexplained upper airway obstruction, hypoventilation, or slow recovery after a general anesthetic should be evaluated for residual neuromuscular blockade. One of the more stringent tests of strength, such as lifting the head or legs for 5 seconds, rules out this diagnosis. Treatment with additional neostigmine or other anticholinesterase is usually effective.

Airway Obstruction

Airway obstruction and pulmonary aspiration are significant causes of morbidity or mortality after anesthesia. In several surveys, 0.1 to 0.2 percent of patients admitted to PACUs required emergency tracheal intubation, most within the first hour following extubation. Postoperative airway obstruction occurs more often with somnolence, residual weakness, obtunded airway reflexes, upper airway edema, sleep apnea, or obesity, as well as in those patients with partial airway obstruction preoperatively. When obstruction is complete, the initial paradoxical movements of the chest and other classic signs are followed rapidly by hypoxemia. The signs of partial upper airway obstruction in the PACU can be more subtle and difficult to recognize. Airway obstruction always must be considered when evaluating postoperative patients for somnolence, noisy breathing, dyspnea, cyanosis, hypoxemia, cardiovascular abnormalities, tracheal tug, nasal flaring, or rocking motions of the chest.

Treatment of upper airway obstruction is similar to the management of the problem during anesthesia. Beginning with repositioning the head and neck and administering oxygen, management progresses in an orderly fashion to include jaw thrust, nasal and oral airways, intubation of the trachea (with or without muscle relaxants, as appropriate), and (rarely) cricothyroidotomy or transtracheal jet ventilation.

Hypoxemia

Hypoxemia occurs commonly in patients in the PACU, so all receive supplemental oxygen on admission. The clinical signs of hypoxemia are not always obvious or specific, making the use of a pulse oximeter mandatory. Oxygen is discontinued only when the pulse oximeter verifies that it is no longer needed. In addition to the causes of hypoxemia listed in Table 32-7, depression of ventilatory responses to hypoxemia by residual anesthetic agents and of responses to hypercarbia by opioids play an important role. Inhalation anesthetics at 0.1 MAC significantly depress hypoxic ventilatory drive in humans. Intravenous agents such as thiopental, morphine, and midazolam also depress hypoxic ventilatory responses. Bilateral

Table 32-7

Causes of Hypoxemia Most Likely Among PACU Patients

1. Atelectasis
2. Aspiration pneumonitis
3. Decreased FRC
4. Pulmonary edema
5. Pneumothorax
6. Pneumonia
7. Splinting from incisional pain
8. Increased oxygen consumption (e.g., fever, shivering)
9. Decreased cardiac output

carotid endarterectomy can abolish hypoxic ventilatory drive entirely.

Treatment of hypoxemia addresses the specific causes listed in Table 32-7 (see also Chaps. 22 and 33).

Respiratory Depression

In general, hypoventilation implies failure of minute ventilation to match the production of CO_2 so that hypercarbia ensues (see Chap. 3). Among patients in the PACU, hypoventilation may be due to residual drug effects, airway obstruction, lung disease (COPD), or increased CO_2 production (shivering, fever). Because somnolence potentiates the effects of opioids on ventilatory responses, opioid-induced depression of ventilatory responses to CO_2 is prevalent among patients in the PACU. Immediate treatment begins with administering oxygen and arousing the patient; commands to breathe are often effective. Assisted or controlled positive-pressure ventilation by mask may be needed. These simple measures often suffice if respiratory depression follows the intravenous injection of an opioid, since ventilation improves with redistribution of the drug. If these steps fail, naloxone may be required. Using small doses (40 to 80 mg intravenously) can restore ventilatory drive without eliminating analgesia. If these are effective, then either intramuscular or continuous intravenous naloxone is required to prevent the return of excess opioid effect after these small doses (the effective duration of action of naloxone is only 1 hour even when administered in much larger doses that result in pain, agitation, and cardiovascular stimulation).

Hypertension

Hypertension is a common reaction after operations and may be a sign of other complications such as fluid overload, hypoxia, or hypercarbia. Management begins with seeking and treating these conditions (Table 32-8). Usually, however, no immediate explanation is apparent; postoperative hypertension occurs most often in hypertensive patients as a result of pain and the neurohumoral stress response to operation. Although the course of the hypertension is usually acute, beginning within an hour of the end of the operation and resolving within 4 hours, treatment is required to avoid pulmonary edema, myocardial ischemia, bleeding, disruption of vascular anastomoses, or stroke. Otherwise healthy patients who have under-

Table 32-8

Causes of Hypertension in the PACU

1. Preexisting hypertension
2. Antihypertensive medication not taken
3. Pain
4. Distended bladder
5. Volume overload
6. Emergence delirium
7. Hypoxemia, hypercarbia
8. Hypothermia with vasoconstriction

gone relatively minor procedures may tolerate mild hypertension without aggressive therapy. Patients with coronary artery disease or impaired left ventricular function or those who have undergone vascular, neurosurgical, cardiac, or ophthalmologic procedures may require immediate and effective treatment of even mild hypertension.

Adequate treatment for pain and anxiety are the first steps; these are often effective. If not, antihypertensive therapy should be chosen with the transient nature of the problem and the patient's special requirements in mind. If bronchoconstriction, bradycardia, and congestive heart failure are not problems, intravenous labetalol (5- to 10-mg increments at intervals of several minutes, to effect) offers the advantages of alpha- and beta-adrenergic blockade. Hydralazine, 10 to 20 mg intravenously, reaches peak effect in 10 to 20 minutes and does not require an intravenous infusion, but tachycardia may result. Sodium nitroprusside by infusion is effective; nitroglycerin may be preferred if hypertension is complicated by myocardial ischemia.

Hypotension

Among patients in the PACU, hypotension most often occurs in three settings. Hypovolemia may be due to unreplaced intraoperative losses or to continuing bleeding and third space losses. The residual effects of anesthesia, especially spinal or epidural anesthesia, may worsen hypotension by blunting sympathetic responses. Occult hypovolemia may produce hypotension when pain is relieved by effective analgesia from intravenous opioids or an epidural injection. Other less common causes of hypotension in PACU patients include left ventricular failure, sepsis, pulmonary embolus, tension pneumothorax, and others. After assessment, management is conventional, beginning with a fluid challenge and progressing eventually to invasive cardiovascular monitoring, vasopressors, and inotropes if required (see Chap. 29).

Hypothermia

Most patients come to the PACU with body temperatures less than 37°C. Of itself, hypothermia is uncomfortable for patients and does harm by slowing emergence and impairing organ function and coagulation. Harmful effects also result from physiologic efforts for natural rewarming. Vasoconstriction exacerbates hypertension. Increased oxygen consumption, due to shivering and nonshivering thermogenesis, not only worsens the effects of pulmonary shunt on arterial oxygen content but also demands increases in cardiac output that patients compromised by age or cardiac disease may not be able to achieve.

Management of hypothermia begins in the operating room with efforts to keep patients warm. These include warming the operating room to 26°C, employing warming blankets or active heating devices, warming intravenous fluids, and using low-flow breathing circuits where possible. However, these steps are usually employed to the fullest only for patients at special risk, including victims of major trauma, infants, or liver transplant patients.

When the patient is very ill or very cold (<33.5°C), treatment relies on blocking physiologic responses to hypothermia by delaying emergence and extubation and maintaining muscle relaxation until passive warming brings the patient's body temperature toward normal. This requires several hours of treatment, which may include warming lamps, hot air or hot water blankets, and the like. In less severe cases of hypothermia, simple measures to warm the patient usually suffice; these include heating lamps, warm blankets, active hot air blankets, and warmed intravenous fluids. Small amounts of intravenous meperidine (12.5 to 25 mg) may terminate shivering after general anesthesia.

Fever

Fever is far less common than hypothermia among patients in the PACU. As elsewhere, fever often is a sign of infection. Among postoperative patients, pulmonary atelectasis is a common cause of fever. Less common are febrile reactions to drugs and to transfused blood. Rare, but grave, is the onset of malignant hyperthermia in the PACU (see Chap. 36).

Table 32-9

Routine Criteria for Discharge from the PACU

1. Vital signs satisfactory and unchanging
2. Return to preoperative mental state
3. Adequate pain control
4. Immediate treatment of any complications completed
5. Adequate treatment of nausea or vomiting
6. Adequate function of all drains, tubes, catheters
7. Surgical bleeding stopped or treated
8. Postoperative orders reviewed, implemented as appropriate
9. Laboratory studies needed immediately obtained and results reviewed

■ Discharge from the PACU

Patients are ready for discharge from the PACU when they may be cared for safely elsewhere. If the patient is to go home, the discharge criteria are those used for outpatient surgery (see Chap. 28); these patients must be able to be cared for by family and friends only. If the patient is to be transferred to an ICU, the only criterion for discharge is that the patient be able to withstand the journey from the PACU to the ICU.

For most patients who will go to a hospital bed, discharge from the PACU is possible when the acute effects of anesthesia and operation have resolved, the patient no longer requires a nurse in the room, and the risk of abrupt catastrophes such as airway obstruction or profound hypotension is gone. The decision to discharge the patient from the PACU usually requires that a period of time elapses during which no special intervention is required. For a healthy patient after a minor procedure, this period may be as brief as 20 to 30 minutes; for a sick patient, a period of several hours may be required. A discharge protocol that sets an arbitrary period of observation for all patients is inappropriate. Routine discharge criteria appear in Table 32-9.

The Postanesthetic Visit

After anesthesia, good practice requires that a postoperative visit be performed and the results be recorded in the chart, just as with the preoperative visit. This serves several purposes. First, it alerts the anesthesiologist to complications that can be treated and must be followed, such as post-dural puncture

Table 32-10

Elements of the Postanesthetic Visit

1. Overall patient satisfaction. Did the perioperative course match expectations? What should be done differently next time?
2. What does the patient remember about the induction or about being in the operating room? (This question may reveal intraoperative awareness.)
3. Adequacy of pain relief.
4. Review of the outcome of any special problems identified in the preoperative visit, such as nausea and vomiting, hypertension, back pain.
5. Any other complaints. (This may uncover postsuccinylcholine myalgias, for example.)

headache, dental injuries, or backache. Indirect questioning can uncover tactfully such problems as intraoperative awareness (Table 32-10). Second, regularly evaluating the outcome of anesthetics and comparing it with the preoperative assessment improves care. Third, answering patients' questions can serve to correct misconceptions and misunderstandings that might otherwise lead to dissatisfaction or litigation. Indeed, if there has been a complication of anesthesia or the question of such a complication has been raised, then close contact with the patient must be maintained until the problem is resolved. Postoperative visits are difficult to arrange for patients who leave the hospital within hours of the end of the operation.

Sometimes, the postoperative visit can only be accomplished by a phone call or brief visit as the patient departs.

BIBLIOGRAPHY

Bidwai AV, Stanley TH, Rogers C, Riet EK. Reversal of diazepam-induced postanesthetic somnolence with physostigmine. *Anesthesiology* 1979;51:256.

Cooper JB, Cullen DJ, Nemeskal R, et al. Effects of information feedback and pulse oximetry on the incidence of anesthesia complications. *Anesthesiology* 1987;67:686.

Cullen DJ, Collee GG. Recovery from anesthesia. In Tinker J, Zapol W, eds: *Care of the Critically Ill Patient*, 2nd ed. London: Springer-Verlag, 1992.

Cullen DJ, Eichorn DH, Cooper JB, et al. Postanesthesia care unit standards for anesthesiologists. *J Postanesth Nurse* 1989;4:141.

Gewolb J, Hines R, Barash P. A survey of 3244 consecutive admissions to the PACU at a university teaching hospital. *Anesthesiology* 1987;67:A471.

Muir JDJ, Warner MA, Offord KP, et al. Role of nitrous oxide and other factors in postoperative nausea and vomiting: A randomized and blinded prospective study. *Anesthesiology* 1987;66:513.

Panza WS, Behringer EC. Intubation in the postanesthesia care unit. *Anesth Analg* 1993;76:S476.

Rosenberg H, Clofine R, Bialik O. Neurologic changes during awakening from anesthesia. *Anesthesiology* 1981;54:125.

Rosow CE, DiBiase PM, Zaslavsky A, Burch L. Propofol vs thiopental in in-patients: Comparison of recovery after general anesthesia. *Anesthesiology* 1993;78:A336.

Stoelting RK, Longnecker DE, Eger EI. Minimum alveolar concentrations on awakening from methoxyflurane, halothane, ether and fluroxene in man: MAC awake. *Anesthesiology* 1970;33:5.

CHAPTER **33**

Critical Care of the Surgical Patient

Ralph T. Geer

Critical care medicine has evolved during the past 30 years to provide care for patients in whom potentially reversible life-threatening changes in clinical condition may occur very quickly. The major indication for admission to the intensive care unit is potentially reversible cardiorespiratory instability, present or impending, that could cause death. Regardless of the underlying illness, all critically ill patients are susceptible to a number of common problems, including sepsis, renal failure, gastrointestinal bleeding, cardiovascular failure, and respiratory failure. Although intensive care of the surgical patient requires attention to all organ systems, altered pulmonary function occurs frequently (Table 33-1), and respiratory function is the major determinant of survival. Patients in respiratory failure requiring more than 24 hours of mechanical ventilation at inspired oxygen concentra-

tions exceeding 50% have a greater than 50 percent chance of in-hospital death. Thus this chapter emphasizes clinical management of respiratory failure in the surgical patient.

Transportation of the Critically Ill Surgical Patient

The critical care of the surgical patient begins in the operating room. During transport to the intensive care unit (ICU), the patient requires the same monitoring and support as in the operating room.

Portable mechanical ventilators have advantages when transportation time is prolonged or when end-expiratory pressure is required, but such equipment may malfunction. Self-inflating bags function even when the oxygen supply fails, but clinical assessment of oxygen delivery and ventilation are less certain than with a flaccid rebreathing bag because the sensation of the bag filling and emptying is obscured. During transportation, respiratory monitoring may be limited to patient observation, but battery-operated pulse oximeters are preferred for many of these patients.

The hemodynamic monitoring used during transportation depends on the patient's condition. Because movement often provokes hypotension or hypertension, those who need indwelling arterial pressure monitoring during operation require similar monitoring during transportation to and from the ICU. Likewise, the vasoactive drugs available to sup-

Table 33-1

Changes in Pulmonary Function in Postoperative Critically Ill Patients

1. Compromised lung volumes
   a. Functional residual capacity
   b. Residual volume
   c. Vital capacity
   d. Total lung capacity
2. Diminished flow rates
3. Decreased compliance
4. $\dot{V}/\dot{Q}$ mismatching
   a. Intrapulmonary shunting
   b. Dead space
5. Increased work of breathing
6. Increased demand for oxygen

port the circulation during anesthesia are brought with the patient during transportation to the ICU.

The anesthesiologist notifies the intensive care unit before moving the patient so that preparations can be made to continue uninterrupted care. On arrival in the ICU, greater minute ventilation and FIO_2 than are thought necessary are provided until proper monitoring provides data that justify lesser values. Endotracheal tube position is reconfirmed immediately by auscultation and chest x-ray.

Pulmonary Problems in Postoperative Patients

A number of pulmonary or systemic problems alter gas exchange in critically ill patients (Table 33-2).

■ Aspiration Pneumonia

In critically ill patients, general debility, neuromuscular dysfunction, and the blunting of airway reflexes from oversedation and from the presence of oropharyngeal tubes and airways all favor pulmonary aspiration of oropharyngeal contents. Despite precautions for prevention of aspiration of gastric contents, this problem causes significant morbidity and mortality in critically ill patients. Endotracheal tubes limit but do not eliminate the risk of aspiration of gastric or oropharyngeal contents. Further, during the 24 hours immediately following removal of endotracheal tubes, there persists residual laryngeal dysfunction.

Management of aspiration pneumonia includes meticulous removal of secretions, postural drainage, antibiotic treatment based on culture sensitivities, maintenance of fluid and nutritional balance, and therapy for ventilatory failure as needed. Acid aspiration may result in severe lung injury with massive extravasation of fluid into lung parenchyma and the need for intravascular fluid replenishment. Neither steroids nor prophylactic antibiotics appear to be of benefit.

■ Atelectasis

Atelectasis, the collapse of lung parenchyma that can be seen on chest x-ray, occurs commonly after major operations (50 percent of patients after abdominal procedures). In critically ill patients, it may

Table 33-2

Disease Processes Worsening Gas Exchange in Critically Ill Patients

Aspiration pneumonia
Atelectasis
Airway obstruction
Sepsis
Bacterial pneumonia
Obstructive pulmonary disease
Pulmonary embolism
Pulmonary edema
Neuromuscular dysfunction

impair oxygenation or lead to pneumonia and respiratory failure. The distinction between pneumonia and atelectasis is never clear. Fever in excess of 38°C with purulent sputum, intracellular bacteria on sputum Gram stain, radiographic evidence of infiltrates, and positive sputum cultures strongly suggest bacterial pneumonia.

A syndrome of progressive loss of lung volume and hypoxemia without x-ray evidence of atelectasis has been referred to as *microatelectasis*. In spontaneously breathing patients, a program of getting the patient out of bed and deep breathing exercises, with appropriate analgesics or regional anesthesia to reduce splinting, limits atelectasis. In mechanically ventilated patients, periodic sighing and clearing of the trachea by suction, along with ventilation with tidal volumes greater than 10 ml/kg of body weight, usually limit or reverse both types of atelectasis. Prophylactic positive end-expiratory pressure or bronchoscopy is not more effective than this simple regimen. When significant atelectasis fails to respond to conservative therapy, bronchoscopy may be effective in removing large mucus plugs or particulate material from major bronchi.

■ Acute Airway Obstruction

Obstruction of an endotracheal tube may present insidiously, often mimicking decreased lung compliance or bronchospasm. It is usually caused by inspissation of secretions, due to inadequate humidification of inspired gases or inadequate removal of secretions by suction. Mechanical causes include overinflation of the tracheal cuff, biting on the tube, kinking, or tracheobronchial disruption. Partial obstructions may produce increased airway pressures during inspiration (peak pressure) with normal static lung compliance (plateau pressure relative to tidal volume), calling attention to this possibility. Partial endotracheal tube obstruction sometimes can be differentiated from bronchospasm by the absence of wheezing, but expiratory wheezing also may be present with partial obstruction. Failure to pass easily a suction catheter or fiberoptic bronchoscope through the endotracheal tube is a strong indication for replacement or repositioning of the tube.

■ Sepsis

Sepsis both causes and complicates ventilatory failure. The diagnosis depends on signs of systemic infection such as fever, tachycardia, hemodynamic instability, leukocytosis, and altered mental status and on not positive blood cultures. Table 33-3 lists common sources for septic contamination in critically ill patients. Sepsis is the major cause of death among patients developing the adult respiratory distress syndrome (ARDS), described in a later section of this chapter.

Survival depends on rapid recognition and treatment of the infection with antibiotics, surgical drainage where possible, and fluid resuscitation to maintain renal function. Other supportive measures, including maintenance of hemodynamic function with inotropes and vasodilators, mechanical ventilation, and supplemental oxygenation, allow time for definitive therapy to be effective (see Chap. 29).

■ Bacterial Pneumonia

Bacterial pneumonia is the most common fatal hospital-acquired infection; more than 50 percent of critically ill patients with bacterial pneumonia do not survive to leave the hospital. In patients with ARDS and bacterial pneumonia, mortality approaches

Table 33-3

Common Causes of Sepsis in Critically Ill Surgical Patients
From known infection:
Pneumonia
Urinary tract infection
Postoperative infection (abscess, empyema)
Wound infection
Primary:
Intravascular cannulas
Implanted foreign material
Drainage tubes

90 percent. Common causes of bacterial pneumonia in the critically ill surgical patient include aspiration, atelectasis, hematogenous spread from extrapulmonary sources, and retention of secretions due to lack of an effective cough mechanism. Patients in whom tracheostomy or prolonged tracheal intubation is necessary are at increased risk for development of bacterial pneumonia through aspiration of secretions and loss of upper airway defense mechanisms. Clearing these secretions from the trachea with suction, postural drainage, and early treatment with antibiotics (often directed at gram-negative organisms) offer the best chance of success. In the presence of lobar pneumonia, positive end-expiratory pressure (PEEP) may worsen gas exchange (see later section on PEEP, CPAP).

Among ICU patients, sputum cultures usually reveal gram-negative organisms, even without clinical evidence of pneumonia. Treatment of this infestation leads to rapid appearance of antibiotic-resistant organisms, limiting therapeutic options should pneumonia occur later. It is important to withhold antibiotics unless other evidence of infection beyond positive sputum cultures is present, including fever, new pulmonary infiltrates, leukocytosis, and increased purulence of sputum. Early detection of bacterial pneumonia in a critically ill patient is required for successful treatment; any change in the patient's clinical condition, sputum quality or quantity, or chest physical findings is an indication for sputum culture and chest x-ray.

■ Chronic Obstructive Pulmonary Disease

Chronic obstructive pulmonary disease (COPD) consists of a spectrum of illnesses, the major types of which include chronic bronchitis, asthma, and emphysema. Although the severity of respiratory obstruction may be measured by pulmonary function testing, unless obstruction is severe, these tests do not correlate well with postoperative morbidity. Functional testing and exercise tolerance are more likely to give meaningful prognostic information regarding postoperative pulmonary complications (see Chap. 22).

The pathogenesis of these complications has its origin in the patient's reduced ventilatory ability, which may become severe enough postoperatively to produce CO_2 retention, requiring mechanical ventilation. In addition, inadequate cough associated with viscid pulmonary secretions results in progressive airway plugging and gas exchange abnormalities. The patient with COPD who suffers respiratory failure following operation presents a therapeutic dilemma. Often the respiratory muscles of the patient with severe obstructive disease are fully employed to support even minimal activities; subsequent mechanical ventilation results in disuse atrophy and alterations in respiratory control mechanisms. The return to spontaneous ventilation may require a prolonged period of reconditioning of both muscles and control systems. Thus complete mechanical support of ventilation may make the patient ventilator-dependent, whereas limited support may overburden an already compromised cardiovascular or pulmonary system.

The first choice is to avoid ventilatory support, treating pain with parenteral or epidural analgesics, controlling fluid excess with diuretics, relieving reversible airway obstruction with nebulized bronchodilators, limiting inspired oxygen concentration to the minimum so as to preserve hypoxic pulmonary drive, and ensuring adequate reversal of residual muscle relaxants. If these measures fail, then mechanical ventilation is limited to as short a time as is possible. Frequent brief intervals of maximal respiratory work, without allowing the development of fatigue, often will promote later weaning from mechanical ventilation. This may be accomplished by allowing the patient to breathe spontaneously without ventilatory assistance for short intervals. Newer modes of partial ventilatory support that provide graded exercise, such as intermittent mandatory ventilation or pressure-support ventilation, may maintain respiratory muscle strength if excessive fatigue is not allowed to develop. Weaning is discussed more fully later.

In patients with acute ventilatory decompensation imposed on COPD, there are several special considerations. First, many such patients compensate for their illness by increasing sympathetic tone to maintain cardiac output and by retaining bicarbonate to maintain a normal blood pH despite hypercarbia. Restoring normal CO_2 elimination by mechanical ventilation abruptly corrects respiratory acidosis without immediately affecting plasma bicarbonate concentrations, resulting in severe metabolic alkalosis. This may provoke dangerous hypokalemia and loss of sympathetic tone, leading to cardiovascular collapse. Deliberate initial underventilation and slow correction of the ventilatory disturbance over hours, with careful attention to maintenance of normal

blood hydrogen ion concentrations, create the least metabolic and hemodynamic disturbance.

Second, some of these patients have diminished ventilatory responses to carbon dioxide; ventilation may depend on blood oxygen tension ("hypoxic drive"). In these few patients, excessive oxygen, especially in combination with sedatives and narcotics, can decrease ventilatory drive and alter the effects of hypoxic pulmonary vasoconstriction on distribution of lung ventilation and perfusion, leading even to carbon dioxide narcosis and ventilatory arrest. Inadequate blood oxygenation in patients with COPD is usually due to maldistribution of ventilation and perfusion in the lung. Unless significant shunting is present due to some other process, adequate blood oxygenation can be attained with modest concentrations (usually < 50%) of inspired oxygen. In spontaneously breathing patients, the oxygen content of the inspired gas may be controlled by delivery through a Venturi mask at a concentration dilute enough to preserve hypoxic ventilatory drive.

■ Pulmonary Embolism

Critically ill surgical patients are at risk for pulmonary embolism because they are bedridden and because circulatory insufficiency leads to peripheral venous stasis. Common signs and symptoms include the sudden onset of dyspnea, wheezing, diaphoresis, tachycardia, and a feeling of impending doom. These nonspecific findings are often seen with acute cardiogenic pulmonary edema; objective tests, including pulmonary angiography or radioisotopic ventilation-perfusion lung scans, may be necessary to confirm the diagnosis. Small pulmonary emboli may produce dramatic changes in hemodynamics, with hypotension, tachycardia, and hypoxemia that do not readily respond to oxygen therapy; this diagnosis must be considered whenever these findings occur. The classic electrocardiographic (ECG) and radiographic findings (right ventricular strain and abrupt termination of pulmonary vasculature or wedge-shaped infiltrates) may be absent. Pulmonary function testing reveals increased dead space ventilation, but this finding also occurs in acute cardiogenic pulmonary edema.

Once pulmonary embolism has occurred, there is a significant likelihood of recurrent embolism and death. Unless contraindicated, prophylactic therapy with anticoagulants (usually heparin) and pneumatic stockings benefits all critically ill surgical patients. These measures failing, larger doses of heparin are required. If full anticoagulation fails to prevent recurrence or cannot be used, an intravenous filter or ligation of the inferior vena cava may prevent migration of large emboli to the lungs.

After large pulmonary emboli, mechanical ventilation combined with fluid therapy and inotropic support may allow time for more definitive therapies to be effective. In such circumstances, thrombolytic therapy must be considered despite the risks of serious hemorrhage. In severe cases, early operative pulmonary embolectomy may offer salvage rates of up to 50 percent.

■ Pulmonary Edema

The diagnosis of pulmonary edema is based on history, physical examination, blood gas analysis, and chest x-ray. Preexisting cardiac or renal dysfunction heightens suspicion, as does a history of prolonged illness or extensive intraoperative fluid resuscitation. When fluid and sodium are given in excess of patient requirements, virtually all critically ill patients retain fluid unless given diuretics. On physical examination, aside from the usual findings related to respiratory distress and decreased lung compliance, moist bibasilar rales and wheezing are present. Although blood carbon dioxide tensions may remain normal or decreased until severe respiratory failure supervenes, the gradient between alveolar and arterial oxygen tensions increases and does not respond readily to oxygen therapy.

The major physiologic causes of pulmonary edema include hydrostatic edema due to heart failure and fluid overload and permeability edema, in which the pulmonary vascular bed is damaged by toxic or inflammatory processes. The latter type is often called the *adult respiratory distress syndrome* (ARDS) or, more recently, *acute lung injury*. It may be difficult to distinguish between hydrostatic and permeability edema of the lung; both types are often present in critically ill patients. In hydrostatic edema, chest x-rays show characteristic central venous congestion with alveolar and interstitial infiltrates. In acute lung injury, central vascular congestion is absent. Although ARDS has many causes, the majority of cases are associated with intraabdominal sepsis or other major bacterial infections. Pulmonary edema associated with sepsis may occur without a clearly defined focus of infection, particularly when the patient is elderly or debilitated and malnourished.

The response to treatment may help differentiate forms of pulmonary edema. Permeability edema usually clears slowly as the inciting cause resolves. Hence rapid clinical improvement with treatment (within several hours) strongly supports a diagnosis of hydrostatic pulmonary edema. When the diagnosis is in doubt, measurement of cardiac output and pulmonary artery pressure may aid in both management and diagnosis. Normal left ventricular filling pressures are seen in permeability edema, but increased pressures characterize relative fluid overload and heart failure.

Despite the differences in course and causes of the two types of edema, management is similar and aims at maintaining gas exchange and cardiac output while decreasing pulmonary capillary hydrostatic pressure. Assisted ventilation, supplemental oxygen, and positive end-expiratory pressure support the patient while awaiting response to more definitive therapy. Since excessive sodium and water administration worsens pulmonary function in all forms of pulmonary edema, close control of fluid balance is required. In hydrostatic edema, narcotics, diuretics, sodium and fluid restriction, vasodilators, and inotropic support usually result in rapid improvement. In permeability edema, the course to recovery commonly lasts several weeks, with a mortality approaching 75 percent. Prognosis worsens as the course extends beyond several weeks.

Monitoring in the ICU

■ Respiratory Monitoring

Anticipated need for respiratory monitoring after operation depends on the predicted risk of pulmonary failure, according to factors outlined in Table 33-4. Although scoring systems have been established to predict the risk of respiratory difficulties, these have not been subjected to rigorous prospective evaluation. At one extreme, the alert patient without signs of respiratory distress may require no more than hourly assessment of vital signs. Patients with marginal ventilatory function or neuromuscular disease who are breathing spontaneously may suffer sudden respiratory collapse; such patients require constant observation or electronic apnea monitoring. At the other extreme, the desperately ill patient may require continuous monitoring of arterial oxygenation and carbon dioxide output, together with frequent monitoring of cardiovascular values, including cardiac output and pulmonary artery pressures.

Table 33-4

Respiratory Failure: Predisposing Factors

1. Diminished ventilatory reserve
   a. Advanced age
   b. Malnutrition
   c. Neuromuscular disorders
   d. Impaired cardiovascular function
   e. Pulmonary disease
2. Operation
   Limiting ventilatory reserve:
   a. Intraabdominal operations
   b. Thoracic operations
   Affecting control of ventilation: intracranial operations
3. Residual anesthetic effects
4. Relative overdose of analgesics
5. Pain limiting vital capacity and functional residual capacity
6. Relative fluid overload
7. Increased metabolic demands, due to pain, fever, response to hypothermia

■Physical Examination

The physical signs of pulmonary distress include dyspnea, tachypnea, restlessness, and increased sympathetic tone, but all these signs may be muted or missing due to effects of anesthetics, sedatives, narcotics, and neuromuscular disease. Physical examination of the chest may detect pneumothorax, pleural effusion, bronchospasm, major atelectasis, the accumulation of secretions, or incorrect placement of endotracheal tubes and is required at regular intervals or with any change in the patient's vital signs.

■Blood Gas Measurements

Definitive diagnosis of respiratory failure is based on abnormalities in arterial blood gas measurements, which are indicated whenever respiratory failure is suspected (see Chaps. 2 and 22). No reliable method now exists for continuous monitoring of arterial oxygen tensions in adults. For patients who require routine surveillance and for those whose peripheral oxygen saturations are less than 100 percent, pulse oximetry is valuable. It is of particular value in patients dependent on hypoxic drive, in whom careful adjustment of inspired oxygen concentrations is necessary to maintain saturation in the range of 88 to 90 percent, where hypoxic ventilatory drive is active. For critically ill patients in whom subtle changes in $(A-a)DO_2$ must be detected, especially when the PaO_2 exceeds 90 mmHg, pulse oximetry is inadequate.

In critically ill patients, capnography does not substitute for the measurement of arterial carbon dioxide tension. Airway obstruction, alterations in dead space, and changes in cardiac output all affect the apparent end-tidal CO_2. As acute airway obstruction develops, isolated values of "end-tidal" carbon dioxide tension measured by capnography may decrease as ventilation and mixing of dead space and alveolar gas worsen. Thus the end-tidal CO_2 value may suggest improvement as gas exchange deteriorates. The continuous monitoring of expired carbon dioxide (i.e., the waveform) may provide subtle additional information about respiratory function that is not evident by other simple means. For example, the failure to achieve a plateau on the expirogram suggests bronchoconstriction or another form of obstruction.

Balloon-tipped flow-directed pulmonary artery catheters monitor both cardiovascular and respiratory functions by providing mixed venous saturation and gas tension measurements. These values may be used to assess oxygen transport, derived from the Fick equation (Table 33-5). Each variable is changed so as

Table 33-5

Oxygen Consumption: the Fick Equation

Fick Equation:

$$O_2 \text{ consumption} = \text{cardiac output} \times \text{A-V } O_2 \text{ content difference}$$
$$\dot{Q} = CO \times K \times (SaO_2 - SvO_2)$$

where $K = 1.38 \text{ ml } O_2/\text{g Hgb} \times \text{Hgb g/dl}$

Mixed venous O_2 saturation:

$$SvO_2 = SaO_2 - \frac{\dot{Q}}{(CO \times K)}$$

Mixed venous oxygen saturation increases when arterial oxygen saturation, the hemoglobin concentration or cardiac output increase, or when total oxygen consumption decreases. Management of patients with inadequate total oxygen delivery begins with this relationship, but insight into the patient's overall physiology is essential. For example, mixed venous oxygen saturation can be improved in a febrile patient by reducing fever or in one moving about violently by sedation or paralysis to decrease oxygen consumption. Mixed venous oxygen saturation (approximately 75 percent normally) provides an index of oxygen extraction by the tissues but not by specific organs.

to keep to a minimum adverse effect while producing therapeutic benefit. Factors affecting this balance, including metabolic rate, cardiac output and its determinants, arterial oxygen-carrying capacity, and arterial oxygen saturation, all are reflected in changes in the mixed venous oxygen tension or saturation. This measurement can be made by sampling blood from the distal port of the pulmonary artery catheter or from direct measurement with a fiberoptic catheter. Mixed venous oxygen saturation is of particular value in determining the best positive end-expiratory pressure (PEEP) and in regulating cardiac output with volume replacement, inotropic agents, and vasodilators.

■ Ventilator Monitors

During mechanical ventilation in the ICU, monitoring of the ventilator and breathing circuit is even more necessary than in the operating room, where the anesthesia team is in constant attendance. All recent ventilators provide these monitoring capabilities, including inspired oxygen content, minute ventilation, and airway pressures. These monitors also detect airway obstruction or disconnection from the ventilator and are used whenever the patient is connected to the ventilator.

More sophisticated measurements derived from pressure and volume in the breathing circuit are of value in assessing the severity of pulmonary disease and the effects of treatment. These include static compliance, inspiratory-to-expiratory time ratio, and assessment of breath stacking (autoPEEP) to determine whether adequate time has been permitted during a ventilatory cycle for complete exhalation of each inspired breath. Many are included as part of the monitoring package provided with newer ventilators. Measurements of static compliance and peak inflation pressure are helpful in differentiating airway obstruction from changes in lung stiffness.

■ Monitoring Cardiovascular Function

The monitoring of cardiovascular function is described in Chapter 6. Heart and lung function are closely linked; to monitor cardiovascular function is to monitor respiratory function also. Although the uses of invasive cardiovascular monitors in the ICU are similar to those in the operating room, there are several special considerations.

In patients with severe ARDS, regulation within narrow limits of fluid balance, inotropes, and PEEP may be required to obtain satisfactory urine output, cardiac output, and oxygenation. Repeated measurement of pulmonary arterial pressures and cardiac output may be required to accomplish these goals. Long-term invasive arterial and venous monitoring presents special hazards including thrombosis, infection, bleeding, and misinterpretation of data. Thorough knowledge of waveforms and common artifacts, combined with sterile precautions, regular dressing changes, and replacement of indwelling cannulas (every 4 days), is required. These risks may be reduced with new noninvasive methods, including impedance cardiography and transcutaneous and transesophageal Doppler echocardiography. These have yet to find widespread use in the ICU because they still lack the precision and accuracy needed for long-term monitoring in this environment.

The Need for Tracheal Intubation

In critically ill surgical patients, intubation of the trachea serves the same functions as in patients under anesthesia. It preserves airway patency, prevents aspiration, allows removal of pulmonary secretions, and provides a route for mechanical ventilation. Prolonged tracheal intubation and mechanical ventilation are associated with significant morbidity, as listed in Table 33-6.

To avoid complications, the endotracheal tube is removed as soon as it is safe to do so. In general, intensive care patients who are awake with intact upper airway reflexes and who have no need for continued mechanical ventilatory support are candidates for tracheal extubation. If upper airway obstruction was related to an infection, resolution of the infection (as indicated by a lower white blood cell count and less pharyngeal inflammation and neck swelling) usually indicates that extubation is safe. If the upper airway obstruction is due to edema and hemorrhage following an operation, these usually resolve within 24 to 48 hours, permitting extubation. The precautions for extubation are described in Chapter 13 and include preparations for immediate reintubation if needed.

The complications associated with the use of prolonged intubation of the trachea have engendered

Table 33-6

Difficulties Related to Tracheal Intubation and Mechanical Ventilation

Related to intubation (58/354 Patients*)
  Damage to teeth
  Pharyngeal or laryngotracheal damage
  Nasal necrosis, sinusitis, or otitis media
  Tube obstruction (secretions, kinking)
  Right mainstem bronchus intubation
  Cuff leak or rupture
  Tracheal hemorrhage
  Infection (pneumonia, tracheostomy infection)
  Retained secretions
  Tube dislodgment
Related to mechanical ventilator (103/354 Patients*)
  Accidental disconnection of power source, gas supply, or patient from ventilator
  Tension pneumothorax, pneumomediastinum, pneumopericardium
  Inspissated secretions (inadequate humidification)
  Circuit leaks
  Air trapping or autoPEEP
  Fluid retention
  Overventilation or underventilation
  Ventilator patient's efforts not synchronous
  Hemodynamic instability due to hypovolemia
  Atelectasis

*Data on incidence from Zwillich CW: Complications of assisted ventilation: A prospective study of 354 consecutive episodes. *Am J Med* 1974;57:161-165.

controversies about the best route and permissible duration of endotracheal intubation. Endotracheal tubes with cuffs of large volume and minimal compliance have reduced the incidence of tracheal stenosis, allowing tubes to remain in place for 3 weeks or more. However, prolonged orotracheal intubation causes laryngeal damage and interferes with feeding, mouth care, and patient comfort. Tracheostomy allows oral feeding, easier mouth care and tracheal toilet, while reducing damage to the larynx. Adverse effects of tracheostomy include tracheomalacia and stenosis at the stoma site and stomal infection with seeding of the lungs. Nasal intubation is of value in managing the airway after certain operations and in some trauma patients (see Chaps. 13, 29, and 31). However, in patients requiring intensive care, nasotracheal tubes are best left in place for only a few days because of the prevalence of purulent sinusitis with their continued use. Computed tomographic (CT) scanning or sinus films may be the only clue that sinusitis is the source of sepsis in patients with nasotracheal tubes.

The Need for Mechanical Ventilation

Mechanical ventilators are used to enhance alveolar ventilation, decrease the work of breathing, and improve carbon dioxide elimination and oxygenation. The major indication for their use is acute or impending respiratory failure, usually manifested by changes in blood gas tensions and ventilatory fatigue. Table 33-7 lists criteria signaling the need for ventilatory assistance. Single measurements of pulmonary function are of less predictive value than trends involving multiple indices; abnormalities occur together. While one minor abnormality may be well tolerated, two or more signs of impending failure, none of which is as severe as suggested in Table 33-6, may still indicate the need for mechanical ventilation.

Although arterial blood gas values provide the major criteria for the diagnosis of respiratory failure, often mechanical ventilation is begun before significant abnormalities appear. In patients with neuromuscular disease or acute asthma, the margin between adequate gas exchange and total respiratory collapse is very small. The signs of fatigue listed in Table 33-7 or clinical signs of excessive sympathetic activity provide warning of respiratory failure in such patients and indicate the need for intervention even if blood gas values are still acceptable. Conversely, in some patients with significant hypoxemia or hypocarbia, every effort is made to avoid assisted ventilation because of predictable difficulties in weaning later. Patients with progressive respiratory failure despite optimal treatment are less likely to derive long-term benefits from mechanical ventilation than are patients in whom mechanical ventilation provides short-term support during which an acute derangement can be treated. Thus the patient with long-standing COPD who finally develops ventilatory failure with no acute precipitating cause (e.g., pneumonia or an abdominal operation) is unlikely to be weaned from mechanical ventilation, whereas a young patient with the sudden onset of asthma can expect to recover.

Mechanical ventilators subject the patient to life-threatening risks. Complications include mechanical malfunction and adverse physiologic effects; they occur in almost 30 percent of patients undergoing mechanical ventilation. New features added to mechanical ventilators also bring new possibilities for malfunction, requiring added vigilance in monitoring both patient and ventilator. Emergency equipment to

Table 33-7

Values Used to Assess Need for Mechanical Ventilation

Measurement	Normal	Mechanical Ventilation Indicated
Ventilatory reserve		
Tidal Volume, ml/kg	5–8	<5
Respiratory rate, breaths/min	12–20	>35
Ventilatory rate/tidal volume		
Ratio (breaths/min/liter)	35	>104
Vital capacity, ml/kg	65–75	<10–15
Arterial PCO_2, mmHg	35–45	>55
FEV_1, ml/kg	50–60	<10
Negative inspiratory pressure, cmH_2O	75–100	<25
Maximum voluntary ventilation, liters/min	150	$<2 \times \dot{V}_E$
V_D/V_T Ratio	0.25–0.40	>0.6
Resting $\dot{V}_E$, liters/min	6	>15
Blood oxygenation		
Intrapulmonary right-to-left shunt, %	<5	>20
$P_{(A-a)}O_2$, mmHg	25–65	>450
Arterial PO_2/alveolar PO_2	0.75	0.15
Clinical signs		
Fatigue		
Tachycardia		
Diaphoresis		
Accessory respiratory muscle activity		
Hemodynamic instability (hyper-, hypotension)		
Hypoxia		
Cyanosis		
Restlessness, confusion		
Hypercapnia		
Peripheral vasodilatation		
Headache, somnolence		

maintain artificial ventilation, including self-inflating bags, always must be available at the bedside in case of mechanical breakdown. Physiologic sequelae of mechanical positive-pressure ventilation include diminished venous return to the heart, mismatching of pulmonary blood flow with ventilation, fluid retention, electrolyte and blood acid-base disturbances, and pulmonary barotrauma.

It is sometimes necessary to use muscle relaxants to accomplish mechanical ventilation, especially in patients with poor compliance or increased airway resistance who require rapid respiratory rates and are unable to synchronize with mechanical support despite opioids and sedatives. Muscle relaxants also may reduce the patient's metabolic rate by decreasing muscle oxygen utilization. Muscle relaxants present well-recognized risks; it is difficult to communicate with the patient or assess the neurologic state, and ventilatory effort is lost. Also, prolonged use of nondepolarizing muscle relaxants, especially in large

doses without proper monitoring, may lead to prolonged weakness after the drug is stopped despite the absence of relaxants or metabolites in the patient's blood. This myopathy includes profound weakness, electromyographic evidence of muscle disease, and increased blood concentrations of muscle enzymes and is reported most commonly following relaxants whose structures contain a steroid nucleus, such as vecuronium and pancuronium. Muscle relaxants must be employed in minimally effective doses, with careful monitoring and only when absolutely necessary. Neuromuscular blockade does not substitute for adequate sedation or proper matching of ventilatory mode to patient effort.

During inspiration, positive-pressure ventilation increases intrathoracic pressure, limiting venous return to the right side of the heart and diminishing cardiac output. The magnitude of this effect depends on the fraction of the total respiratory cycle occupied by inspiration and on the plateau pressure. It is worsened by hypovolemia or airway obstruction that causes air trapping within the lung. In contrast, if the lungs are stiff and noncompliant, then only part of the airway pressure is transmitted to the intrathoracic space, and the effect will be lessened. Shortening inspiratory time diminishes the impairment of venous return. In adult patients with normal lungs, positive-pressure inspiration occupying less than half the total cycle causes minimal depression of cardiac output because of compensatory increases in right-sided heart output occurring during exhalation.

Mechanical ventilation increases physiologic and anatomic dead space by redistributing pulmonary blood flow away from well-ventilated areas of the lung and by distending airways with positive pressure. Airway obstruction or restrictive disease further alters distribution of gas flow to areas of lesser resistance or greater compliance. This augments collapse of alveoli distal to partially obstructed airways, causing atelectasis. This may be relieved by using large tidal volumes (>10 ml/kg) or periodic large breaths (sighs) to distribute gas back into those areas at risk for collapse.

Some patients who retain CO_2 as compensation for metabolic alkalosis due to diuretics or gastrointestinal drainage or who suffer chronic respiratory acidosis experience abrupt alkalosis as mechanical ventilation begins and minute ventilation increases. The ensuing derangements in oxyhemoglobin dissociation, electrolyte balance, and oxygen delivery to the brain may precipitate convulsions, cardiac arrhythmias, and death. To ameliorate these responses and to avoid hypotension, it is best to decrease $PaCO_2$ slowly, allowing time for metabolic adjustments.

After several days of positive-pressure ventilation, progressive fluid retention is likely, particularly when positive end-expiratory pressure (PEEP) is used or sodium and water are administered freely, as often occurs with intravenous hyperalimentation. Fluid retention sometimes produces clinical signs of pulmonary edema despite normal venous pressures and results from mechanical and humoral mechanisms, including renal retention of sodium and water, partial intrathoracic venous obstruction, and impaired pulmonary lymphatic clearance. Control of sodium and fluid intake, diuretics, and monitoring of patient weight help to avoid this complication.

In patients with decreased lung compliance or small airways obstruction, greater than normal airway pressures may be required to deliver adequate tidal volumes. These increased airway pressures, particularly peak inflation pressure, increase the risk of damage to the lung (pulmonary barotrauma), including subcutaneous emphysema, tension pneumothorax, and mediastinal and pericardial air accumulation, which occurs in 5 percent of mechanically ventilated patients and rapidly causes cardiovascular collapse. Limiting mean and peak airway pressures by reducing delivered tidal volumes, particularly in ARDS, may decrease the incidence of barotrauma, at the expense of reduced minute ventilation and carbon dioxide retention. This "permissive hypercapnia" is usually well tolerated, as long as the minute ventilation is reduced gradually to allow for metabolic and renal compensation for the ensuing respiratory acidosis. The clinical signs of tension pneumothorax are caused by accumulation of gas within the pleural space: increased airway pressures, hypoxemia, hypercapnia, diminished breath sounds, hyperresonance, pulsus paradoxus, and decreased cardiac output. Although these signs may be equivocal, impending cardiovascular collapse may not permit time to obtain a chest x-ray. Immediate placement of an interpleural catheter or chest tube is required whenever a patient in distress is suspected of having a tension pneumothorax.

Modes of Mechanical Ventilation

For prolonged use in critically ill surgical patients, a mechanical ventilator must maintain good exchange of warmed, humidified, oxygen-enriched gas despite airways obstruction or greatly decreased compliance. It must be capable of positive end-expiratory pressures up to 30 cmH_2O, peak inflation pressures up to 100 cmH_2O, and peak inspiratory flows up to 100 liter/min. It must provide alarms for disconnection from the patient, loss of power source, or loss of gas supply. It must monitor continuously inspired gas temperature, oxygen concentration, airway pressure, exhaled gas volumes, rate, tidal volume, and minute ventilation. Ventilators of different types deliver different patterns of ventilation, all of which may be appropriate for use in the ICU.

■ Ventilator Types

Today, the overwhelming majority of ventilators used for the prolonged ventilation of critically ill surgical patients produce positive airway pressures (positive-pressure ventilation). Positive-pressure ventilators are divided into three types, depending on the method used to stop inspiratory gas flow. Pressure-cycled machines end inspiration when a preset airway pressure is reached; time-cycled ventilators deliver a constant flow of gas during inspiration for a preset time interval; and volume-cycled ventilators deliver a preset volume of gas per breath regardless of the flow waveform, which may be altered independently. Many newer ventilators provide all three methods of operation and all the multiple modes of ventilatory support outlined below. Although each possesses advantages, with few exceptions, all ventilators now manufactured for continuous use can be adapted to the majority of ICU patients.

■Ventilatory Modes

Modern ventilators provide a wide variety of methods of augmenting minute ventilation in a graded fashion, most of which are reported to improve ease of use and patient comfort. However, there are no properly controlled studies to show differences in patient outcome. Table 33-8 outlines major features of these modes of ventilation.

Controlled Mechanical Ventilation

In controlled mechanical ventilation (CMV), the ventilator delivers a fixed tidal volume at a fixed respiratory rate regardless of the patient's efforts. This provides respiratory support when spontaneous ventilation is completely suppressed, as by muscle relaxants or other forms of paralysis of the respiratory musculature. It also provides a default mode during assisted ventilation, as discussed below. The disadvantage of CMV is that it allows no control by the patient, who may not synchronize respiratory efforts with the machine. Also, the ventilator settings must be adjusted as metabolic demands and pulmonary function change to prevent marked blood gas abnormalities.

Assisted Mechanical Ventilation

In assisted mechanical ventilation (AMV) mode, the machine determines the tidal volume, but the patient sets the ventilatory rate. Each inspiratory effort creates a negative pressure in the airway, triggering a breath from the ventilator. The patient's efforts are synchronized with the ventilator, usually without sedation or paralysis. If the patient's respiratory rate is inadequate, the ventilator reverts to timed control as a default mode. Assisted mechanical ventilation allows the patient with intact respiratory control mechanisms to regulate ventilation to satisfy metabolic demands. This mode of ventilation has been used for more than 30 years and is provided on nearly all ventilators manufactured for use in ICU settings.

To wean patients from AMV requires periodic cessation of ventilatory support while allowing the patient to breathe spontaneously. During weaning, intervals of ventilatory support are gradually shortened, while intervals of spontaneous ventilation are progressively lengthened, based on the patient's ability to maintain adequate gas exchange without fatigue. The major disadvantage of AMV is that some patients' native respiratory rates are rapid, leading to respiratory alkalosis. A second disadvantage is the increased complexity of weaning efforts, requiring careful monitoring to avoid unexpected ventilatory collapse during periods of spontaneous breathing.

Intermittent Mandatory Ventilation

Intermittent mandatory ventilation (IMV) provides breaths of fixed tidal volume at a (low) rate set by the operator. Between these breaths, the ventilator provides gas for the patient's spontaneous ventilation. In AMV, each of the patient's breaths is mechanically assisted, and the machine provides a fixed rate of breathing only if the patient becomes apneic. In IMV, the patient's breaths are unassisted, but the fixed breaths are automatic and occur regularly even if the patient continues to breathe. In newer ventilators, the fixed breaths are synchronized with the inspiratory effort of the patient (SIMV) to avoid conflict between a spontaneous breath and one delivered by the ventilator. Numerous theoretical advantages are cited for IMV, including less ventilator-induced depression of cardiac output, improved acid-base balance, ease of weaning, and reduced incidence of pulmonary barotrauma. Theoretical disadvantages include respiratory muscle fatigue and risk of hypoventilation (at the IMV default rate) should the patient receive muscle relaxants or ventilatory depressants. None of the studies of these advantages or disadvantages has been well enough controlled to provide definitive conclusions.

In older ventilators, the demand valves supplying inspiratory gas to the patient between IMV breaths were insensitive, slow to respond, and unable to match patient inspiratory flow requirements. The excessive work of breathing caused the rapid onset of fatigue during IMV. Newer inspiratory demand valves minimize these problems. Although IMV appears to

Table 33-8

Modes of Ventilation

	CMV, Continuous Mandatory Ventilation	AMV, Assisted Mechanical Ventilation	IMV, Intermittent Mandatory Ventilation	PSV, Pressure-Support Ventilation	HFJV, High-Frequency Jet Ventilation	IRV, Inverse-Ratio Ventilation	APRV, Airway Pressure-Release Ventilation	PCV, Pressure-Control Ventilation
Default on apnea	CMV	CMV	IMV rate	CMV	Controlled	CMV	CMV	CMV
Patient's spontaneous breath	Uncoordinated with machine	Assisted	Spontaneous + assisted	Assisted	Spontaneous	Not coordinated with machine	Not coordinated with machine	Assisted
Size of patient's breath	Fixed	Fixed	IMV fixed; variable sized spontaneous breath	Variable	Fixed	Depends on flow, pressure and I:E ratio settings	Variable size depending on patient effort	Variable, depending on set pressure, flow, inspiration time, lung compliance and patient effort
Response to need for increased ventilation	None	Increased rate	Increased rate and tidal volume, if patient strong enough	Increased rate and tidal volume, if patient strong enough	None	Usually fixed	None	Minute ventilation decreases to CMV default
Response to narcotics, neuromuscular blocker	None	Rate decreases to default	Minute ventilation decreases to IMV default	Minute ventilation decreases to CMV default	None	Rate decreases to default	None	Rate decreases to CMV default
Respiratory muscle deconditioning	Maximal deconditioning	Not as marked as CMV	Minimal deconditioning depending on IMV level	Minimal deconditioning depending on CMV level	None	Maximal	Minimal	Not as high as CMV
Respiratory muscle fatigue	None	Minimal	Fatigue likely	Fatigue likely	Minimal	Minimal	Fatigue likely	Depends on pressure control settings
Weaning	Abrupt	Abrupt	Graduated	Graduated	Graduated	Abrupt	Graduated	Graduated

have stood the test of time and provides an acceptable alternative to the older AMV mode, its superiority remains unproven.

Pressure-Support Ventilation

In pressure-support ventilation (PSV), with each breath the ventilator delivers a flow of gas to the patient's airway until a set pressure is reached. This pressure is maintained until inspiratory flow decreases to a predetermined level, at which point flow ceases and the expiratory phase begins. The patient initiates each breath when the ventilator senses negative airway pressure. Thus the patient sets both the tidal volume and the rate. Pressure-support ventilation supplements the patient's effort, allowing breathing at varying rates and volumes. Further, like IMV, PSV can be discontinued gradually as patient gas exchange and respiratory muscle strength improve. Also like IMV, PSV allows the patient to exercise respiratory musculature. Theoretical disadvantages include respiratory muscle fatigue and ventilatory failure if drugs are administered without changing the amount of assistance and lack of studies proving its efficacy.

Pressure-Control Ventilation

In pressure-control ventilation (PCV), the ventilator is set to generate a predefined airway pressure. Inspiration time is controlled in one of three ways: by setting the inspiration time, by adjusting the inspiratory-to-expiratory time ratio and the respiratory rate, or by regulating the tidal volume delivered. Minute ventilation is controlled by spontaneous patient triggering or by setting the respiratory rate. This ventilatory pattern is a refinement of the cycling pattern used on many of the early models of so-called pressure-cycled ventilators. On newer ventilator models, inspiration time and tidal volume are not determined primarily by the point in the inspiratory cycle at which the preset pressure is reached.

The theoretical advantage of this ventilator mode is that the decelerating flow wave pattern may improve ventilation distribution, resulting in improved oxygenation. Further, the limited peak inflation pressure may reduce the incidence of pulmonary barotrauma. However, there are also disadvantages. First, in some instances, inspiration time is prolonged to improve gas distribution and oxygenation, resulting in patient discomfort and the need for sedation and muscle relaxation. Second, unanticipated changes in lung compliance may cause unexpected changes in minute ventilation. Finally, as with most of the other newly developed modes of ventilation, there is no documentation of improved outcome with this mode.

High-Frequency Jet Ventilation

High-frequency jet ventilation (HFJV) provides high-pressure jet flow of gas at rapid respiratory rates, between 60 to 150 breaths per minute, using tidal volumes not much greater than the anatomic dead space of the lung. The small tidal volumes minimize peak airway pressure and the consequent adverse hemodynamic effects of pulmonary barotrauma. Although it is effective in some patients with bronchopleural fistulas, there is no consensus as to its use in other disorders. Disadvantages include difficulty in monitoring the ventilation it produces, the lack of alarms, and poor warming and humidification of inspired gases. High-frequency oscillation, a mode of ventilation related to HFJV, is used only experimentally.

Inverse-Ratio Ventilation (IRV)

Prolongation of inspiration time, produced by setting tidal volume, inspiratory pressure, or flow, may facilitate even pulmonary gas distribution while limiting inspiratory airway pressures. When the inspiratory time is longer than the time of exhalation, the normal I:E ratio is reversed, and the ventilatory mode is designated *inverse-ratio ventilation* (IRV). Although IRV can be superimposed on many ventilatory modes, it is used most often with those in which inflation pressure controls the ventilatory cycle, such as pressure-control ventilation. IRV may improve oxygenation in patients with stiff lungs while avoiding barotrauma. Sedation or paralysis is required, and the benefits of the technique have not been proven.

Airway Pressure-Release Ventilation (APRV)

Airway pressure-release ventilation (APRV) is used to improve oxygenation and assist ventilation in spontaneously breathing patients. It provides continuous positive airway pressure (CPAP) while periodically releasing pressure in the ventilatory circuit to improve ventilation and cardiac venous return. It avoids increased peak inflation pressures and does not require sedation. APRV, along with IMV and PSV, improves gas exchange in patients unable to tolerate depression of cardiac output. At present, it is not known whether this mode is superior to others for these purposes.

PEEP, CPAP

Limiting expiratory gas flow from the patient has long been considered as a method for minimizing airway collapse, improving distribution of ventilation and perfusion, and reducing intrapulmonary shunting. Unfortunately, reduction in venous return to the heart limits the use of this technique. Positive end-expiratory pressure (PEEP) has been the most successful variant, improving oxygenation with minimal hemodynamic disturbance. An adjustable valve allows control of pressure in the exhaled limb of the breathing circuits of all ventilators now manufactured for ICU use. The valve applies constant airway pressure through the full exhalation cycle. When used in conjunction with a mode of ventilation that never allows airway pressure to decrease to ambient levels, PEEP is designated as *continuous positive airway pressure* (CPAP).

PEEP is beneficial when arterial hypoxemia persists despite use of increased inspired oxygen concentrations and minimizes the risk of oxygen toxicity by allowing the patient to attain a given PaO_2 with a lesser FiO_2. It also may reduce bleeding following thoracotomy. Adverse effects include impaired cardiac venous return, pulmonary barotrauma, fluid retention, and difficulties in interpreting pressure data from pulmonary artery catheters. The most significant drawback is depression of cardiac output; as PEEP improves arterial oxygen tension, it may so depress cardiac output and diminish the total quantity of oxygen transported to the body. It is useful to evaluate the effects of PEEP by calculating oxygen transport (the product of cardiac output and arterial oxygen content) or by measuring the oxygen saturation of mixed venous blood.

Because its adverse effects are directly related to the pressure applied, PEEP is limited to that required to permit adequate tissue oxygen delivery while avoiding pulmonary oxygen toxicity. PEEP is best used to treat diffuse, homogeneous lung disease such as pulmonary edema. The salutary effect on arterial oxygenation is much less certain when disease in the lung is localized, as in atelectasis or lobar pneumonia. The lack of efficacy of PEEP in localized lung disease may be due to redistribution of pulmonary blood flow away from well-ventilated lung and into the impaired region.

Weaning the Patient from Mechanical Ventilation

Debility, acute illness, and prolonged need for ventilatory support all make weaning from mechanical ventilation more difficult. Prolonged maintenance of mechanical ventilation is expensive and exposes patients to increased risks that can be reduced by proceeding to weaning and extubation as soon as possible. Weaning young patients without lung disease from mechanical ventilation is usually simple. Normal arterial blood gas values, a vital capacity in excess of 15 ml/kg, and negative inspiratory pressures of greater than 20 cmH$_2$O usually predict that it will be safe to discontinue mechanical ventilation. This is the case in the majority of mechanically ventilated patients in the surgical ICU.

The longer mechanical ventilation is continued, the more difficult it is to stop. For this reason, progressive weaning from the ventilator must begin as soon as possible. Quantitative criteria for weaning are sparse and largely empirical. The clinical state of the patient, along with periodic measurement of arterial blood gas tensions and tests of ventilatory adequacy, usually provides enough information to assess effects of weaning efforts. Numerical indices of ventilatory adequacy are shown in Table 33-7. Because fatigue may limit weaning in elderly and debilitated patients who have been maintained on mechanical ventilation for even short periods of time, measurements of ventilatory performance are made during weaning trials. Failure due to respiratory muscle fatigue during weaning often leads to further deterioration, requiring prolonged rest. Although there is no single clinical sign or number diagnostic of fatigue, increased sympathetic tone and respiratory rates greater than 30 breaths per minute suggest impending failure.

The most common cause of continued ventilator dependence is persistence of the original pathophysiologic process that mandated mechanical ventilation. Failure of organ systems other than the lungs may forbid weaning. Neurologic depression and blunted airway reflexes threaten aspiration of pharyngeal contents. Weakened airway and respiratory muscles may be inadequate to maintain an unobstructed airway or adequate alveolar ventilation. Cardiovascular responses to discontinuing mechanical ventilation include increased venous return and increased cardiac output needed to support the work of breathing. In borderline congestive heart failure, these changes may precipitate pulmonary edema, making it important to adjust fluid balance, blood oxygen-carrying capacity, and cardiac performance with inotropic support and vasodilators prior to weaning. Increased sympathetic tone associated with increased work and inadequate gas exchange, as well as electrolyte abnormalities, may provoke life-threatening arrhythmias in some patients.

Patients with coexisting renal and respiratory failure are difficult to wean because stable fluid balance is difficult to maintain. Weaning of the patient in acute or chronic renal failure is best delayed until satisfactory fluid balance can be maintained for several days. Although poor nutrition and cachexia are associated with difficult weaning, no studies have demonstrated that acute nutritional support improves the likelihood of rapid weaning. Nevertheless, maintenance of respiratory muscle function, ventilatory drive mechanisms, and lung defense mechanisms against infection depend on maintenance of nutrition, particularly in critically ill patients with increased nitrogen catabolism and loss of lean body mass. Perversely, nutritional support also can impede weaning, owing to increased CO_2 production from glucose and amino acid loading and fluid retention.

The three factors ultimately determining the success of weaning are pulmonary oxygen exchange, ventilation, and fatigue. A timed trial of unassisted ventilation often helps to predict with certainty whether fatigue and deterioration in pulmonary gas exchange will occur following discontinuation of ventilation. Unless unassisted ventilation sustains a PaO_2 greater than 60 mmHg with an inspired oxygen concentration of 60% or less, successful weaning is unlikely for several reasons. First, it is quite difficult to maintain inspired oxygen concentrations above 60% without intubation. Second, unintentional discontinuation of the oxygen supply in patients requiring more than 60% oxygen can quickly lead to life-threatening hypoxia. Third, such patients may still suffer from the original disease that precipitated respiratory failure.

Assessment before weaning also must predict the likelihood of hypoventilation induced by fatigue. Avoiding fatigue may be accomplished in several ways. The first is to gradually decrease assistance until it is no longer required using IMV and PSV. Either the frequency of mandatory breaths or the amount of inspiratory pressure support can be reduced gradually while vital signs and arterial blood gas tensions are monitored. When signs of fatigue, including increased respiratory rate and hemodynamic signs of sympathetic nervous system activity, become pronounced, ventilatory assistance is increased until signs of fatigue diminish or are eliminated.

Another approach derives from the observation that patients with normal lung function can sustain one-half their maximal voluntary ventilation indefinitely. Based on this, the following method both assesses adequacy of ventilation and predicts likelihood of fatigue. The patient is allowed to breathe spontaneously humidified, oxygen-enriched gas for a period of 1 hour. During this time, clinical signs of hypoxia or hypercarbia, any marked increase in restlessness or sympathetic activity, or a respiratory rate above 30 breaths per minute is considered a sign of worsening respiratory failure or fatigue, indicating the need for measurement of arterial blood gas tensions and possible return to assisted ventilation. If all goes well for an hour, arterial blood gas tensions, minute ventilation, and maximal breathing capacity are measured. If the patient cannot cooperate, maximum voluntary ventilation can be estimated by measuring vital capacity and multiplying it by 35. If the minute ventilation required to maintain an acceptable PCO_2 during the trial is less than one-half the maximum voluntary ventilation, fatigue is unlikely to develop. If the patient cannot maintain adequate ventilation for the full hour, a shorter time period of unassisted ventilation during which unacceptable fatigue does not occur is interspersed with periods of rest, allowing adequate periods of time for sleep at night. As weaning progresses, the period of unassisted ventilation is progressively prolonged until there is no deterioration or fatigue.

Unfortunately, there are increasing numbers of patients who cannot be weaned after prolonged ventilatory support in critical care units. For these patients, the options for continued care are limited and extremely expensive. For some, there is the possibility of productive activity despite the need for chronic ventilatory support. For others, options are much more limited.

Such concerns are not limited to those who have required prolonged ventilatory or circulatory support. Critical care is expensive, and it is clear that society cannot afford to provide unlimited intensive care to all who might possibly benefit. Yet it is through such intensive care that high-risk patients can recover from major operations and severe illnesses. Selection of appropriate candidates for admission to critical care facilities and the dilemmas presented by patients who cannot be weaned from mechanical ventilatory support present medical, legal, and ethical problems that are not yet resolved.

BIBLIOGRAPHY

Goldenheim PD, Kazemi H. Cardiopulmonary monitoring of critically ill patients. *N Engl J Med* 1984;311:717-720, 776-780.

Morganroth ML, Grum CM. Weaning from mechanical ventilation. *J Intensive Care Med* 1988;3:109-119.

Norwood SH, Civetta JN. Ventilatory support in patients with ARDS. *Surg Clin North Am* 1985;65:895-916.

Perel A. Newer ventilation modes: Hazards and pitfalls. *Crit Care Med* 1987;15:707-709.

Ruark JE, Raffin TA, Stanford University Medical Center Committee on Ethics. Initiating and withdrawing life support: Principles and practice in adult medicine. *N Engl J Med* 1988;318:25-30.

Stauffer Jl, Olsen DE, Petty TL. Complications and consequences of endotracheal intubation and tracheostomy: A prospective study of 150 critically ill adult patients. *Am J Med* 1981;70:65-76.

Weisman IM, Rinaldo JE, Rogers RM. Positive end-expiratory pressure in adult respiratory failure. *N Engl J Med* 1982;307:1381-1384.

Yang KL, Tobin MJ. A prospective study of indexes predicting the outcome of trials of weaning from mechanical ventilation. *N Engl J Med* 1991;324:1445-1450.

CHAPTER 34

Management of Postoperative Pain

Timothy R. VadeBoncouer

Patients suffer pain after almost any operation. Until recently, anesthesia care for pain relief ended in the recovery room, and the recuperating patient received intermittent oral or parenteral narcotics, which often gave only partial relief. Recently, techniques such as patient-controlled intravenous narcotic infusions, spinal and epidural narcotics, and prolonged regional anesthetics have offered effective relief of postoperative pain, as well as the risk of new complications and requirements for closer supervision of patients.

Although convincing evidence that it improves patient outcome is lacking, there are well-recognized benefits from effective postoperative pain management. Effective analgesia significantly increases lung volumes and the ability to cough after major abdominal or thoracic operations. Tachycardia and hypertension resulting from pain may be alleviated by effective analgesia. Effective management of postoperative pain clearly relieves human suffering and may ameliorate some complications; provision for postoperative analgesia is part of any plan for anesthesia management.

Pain Pathways

The central nervous system includes interconnected neural circuits that provide information about noxious stimuli. At several points in this system the flow of information may be altered to produce analgesia.

Painful stimuli to somatic and visceral structures evoke response from two types of nerves. A-delta fibers are thinly myelinated neurons that respond primarily to intense mechanical stimulations. C fibers are unmyelinated neurons that respond to mechanical, thermal, and chemical irritation. A-delta and C fibers transmit information about noxious input through the dorsal spinal roots and into the dorsal horn of the spinal cord. At the level of the spinal roots, afferent pain impulses may be interrupted by local anesthetics administered via the epidural or spinal route.

From the dorsal horn, sensory information is transmitted through the dorsal columns and the spinothalamic tract, whose cells of origin arise from the laminae of the dorsal horn, including the substantia gelatinosa, which is richly populated with opioid receptors. Through a complex network involving brain to spinal cord descending systems and dorsal horn interneuron pools, information about painful stimuli arriving at the spinal cord is amplified or attenuated. The attenuation mechanisms, including opioid and adrenergic inhibition of noxious input, provide the basis for selective blockade of pain at the spinal level.

A specific neurotransmitter for nociception by primary afferent neurons terminating in the dorsal horn has not been identified. It has been shown that substance P, a small peptide neurotransmitter, is released in response to noxious stimuli. This release is blocked by application of opioids to the dorsal horn,

Figure 34-1

Sites of potential interruption of acute pain pathways. Descending inhibitory systems are simplified but are probably activated by central effects of parenteral opioids. Epidural local anesthetic-opioid mixtures act at dorsal horn and nerve root level. Adrenergic agonists (e.g., clonidine) also act at dorsal horn level. Nerve block includes various blocks described in text, as well as interpleural technique.

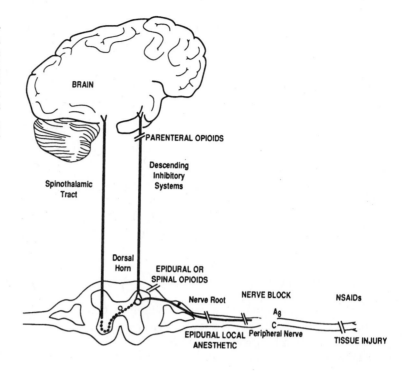

which may explain the action of opioids at the spinal level. Multiple opioid receptor subtypes are involved in this selective spinal analgesia, since different opioids produce qualitatively different effects when applied to the dorsal horn. Figure 34-1 summarizes these neural pathways and the sites where analgesia may be produced.

Patient-Controlled Analgesia

The intramuscular (IM) administration of narcotics for acute pain is standard practice because intravenous access is not needed and the tissue depot releases drug over 3 to 6 hours. Serious drawbacks limit the effectiveness of IM injections. Large depot doses of opioid (e.g., 75 mg meperidine or 10 mg morphine) often result initially in excessive blood levels of drug and corresponding side effects such as nausea, pruritus, or unwanted sedation. A few hours after IM injection, blood levels decrease to subtherapeutic values, and analgesia is inadequate. This cycle of side effects and pain results from the variable and erratic absorption of the drug from the depot (Fig. 34-2). The peaks and valleys of this cycle are accentuated by the time required to respond to the needs of the patient in pain.

To circumvent these difficulties, self-administration by patients of intravenous opioids was developed in the 1970s. These patient-controlled analgesia (PCA) devices overcome the drawbacks of intermittent IM injection techniques by administering opioids intravenously at the request of the patient, with limits set by the physician.

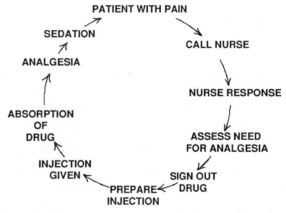

Figure 34-2

The cycle of conventional intramuscular (IM) opioid analgesia.

(Modified with permission from Graves DA, Foster TS, et al: Patient-controlled analgesia. Ann Intern Med *1983;99:360-366.)*

■PCA Devices and Indications for Use

Although the technology is new and designs differ according to manufacturer, a complete PCA device incorporates the design features shown in Table 34-1.

Nearly all patients in acute pain are candidates for PCA, including the old and the young, provided they understand the need to request drug themselves and are physically able to do so. Patients with histories of narcotic dependency may require large doses and may be managed more easily with epidural or spinal analgesic techniques in combination with baseline opioid therapy.

■ Management of PCA

Patient-controlled analgesia is best begun in the recovery room as soon as the patient is alert enough to use the demand button and while the patient is still comfortable, either from perioperative opioids or a regional anesthetic technique. Patients in severe pain usually do not obtain effective analgesia from demand doses alone and require an intravenous loading dose of opioid prior to starting PCA. Morphine, meperidine, and hydromorphone are the most common opioids used for PCA; Table 34-2 lists typical demand doses and lockout intervals for several different drugs.

Table 34-1

Features of a PCA Device

1. A programmable microprocessor that is set by the physician to determine drug doses, minimum intervals between doses ("lockout interval"), background constant infusion rate, and limits on maximum total dose.
2. An easily accessible control button by which the patient registers with the PCA device a request for drug.
3. A drug cartridge or syringe connected by tubing to the patient's intravenous site.
4. A drive mechanism controlled by the microprocessor.
5. A compact design that permits the patient to move about.
6. Simultaneous delivery of intermittent demand doses and a continuous infuson (background infusion) of small amounts of opioid.
7. A mechanism for caregivers to deliver loading doses for severe pain. The mechanism is locked or a code is required to prevent tampering.

Table 34-2

Guidelines for PCA Opioid Doses

Drug	Demand Dose	Lockout Interval (minutes)
Morphine	1–3 mg	5–15
Meperidine	10–30 mg	5–15
Methadone	0.5–3 mg	10–20
Fentanyl	15–75 μg	3–10
Hydromorphone	0.1–0.5 mg	5–15

■ Adjustments in PCA Therapy

Because opioid requirements vary among individuals, doses and lockout intervals (minimum interval between doses) must be adjusted when the patient complains of pain or side effects. If analgesia is inadequate, the demand dose may be increased or the lockout interval decreased to allow more drug in a given time. A background continuous infusion, for example, 0.5 mg morphine per hour, also may improve analgesia, especially for pain associated with movement such as walking, coughing, or physical therapy, but such continuous infusions may increase the incidence of opioid-related side effects. Ideally, one change in one PCA parameter is made at a time; the appropriate change must be tailored to the specific patient problem. Complete pain relief is unlikely in most patients; an appropriate goal is a tolerable amount of pain with no side effects. A suitable set of PCA orders is shown in Table 34-3.

Table 34-3

Typical Orders for Patients Receiving PCA Therapy

Opioid used, concentration:	Morphine, 1 mg/ml
Demand dose:	1.5 mg
Lockout interval:	7 minutes
Four-hour dose limit:	30 mg

Monitor respiratory rate every 2 hours.

Call pain treatment physician for
   Nausea
   Pruritus
   Respiratory rate less than 10 breaths per minute
   Somnolence
   Inadequate pain relief

Naloxone available at bedside at all times.

No other narcotics to be given unless ordered by pain treatment physician.

Table 34-4

Converting PCA to Oral Opioid Analgesia

Drug	Oral Dose Equivalent to 10 mg Parenteral Morphine
Morphine	30 mg
Codeine	200 mg
Hydromorphone	7.5 mg
Oxycodone	30 mg
Meperidine	300 mg
Methadone	30 mg

Side effects also require adjustments in dose schedule, since excess opioid delivery is nearly always the cause of untoward effects associated with PCA. Sedation, nausea, pruritus, urinary retention, and respiratory depression are the usual presenting problems. If side effects occur soon after each demand dose, then the dose is too great. If side effects are present continuously, then the background infusion rate likely is excessive. Severe side effects may require therapy beyond simply adjusting the doses. For nausea, an antiemetic may be prescribed. Also effective are small incremental intravenous doses of naloxone (0.05 to 0.1 mg) or partial agonist-antagonists such as butorphanol (0.25 to 0.5 mg) and nalbuphine (1 to 3 mg). These drugs must be given carefully so as to avoid reversal of adequate analgesia.

Patients on PCA therapy can experience side effects through overdose, because lockout intervals are often shorter than the time to maximum opioid effect following intravenous administration. For severe sedation or respiratory depression, PCA is discontinued temporarily and an intravenous infusion of naloxone begun. Although this phenomenon is the exception rather than the rule, it reinforces the need to tailor PCA therapy to the needs of the individual patient.

Patient-controlled analgesia is discontinued when pain is amenable to oral analgesic therapy, usually 1 to 3 days after operation. Orders for oral analgesics are based on PCA dose schedules (Table 34-4). After abdominal operations, PCA may continue until a liquid diet is tolerated.

Nonsteroidal Anti-Inflammatory Drugs

Nonsteroidal anti-inflammatory drugs (NSAIDs) produce analgesic and anti-inflammatory effects through blockade of prostaglandin synthesis. In the past, the lack of a parenteral preparation has limited the usefulness of these drugs for postoperative pain management. The recent development of ketorolac, a potent parenteral NSAID, allows for the treatment of moderate to severe postoperative pain without the side effects of opioids.

Ketorolac is given as an intramuscular or intravenous injection of 30 to 60 mg followed by 15 mg every 6 hours. Analgesic potency is similar to opioids, with 2 mg ketorolac equivalent to 1 mg morphine. Doses are reduced in patients who are over 65 years of age, weigh less than 60 kg, or have impaired renal function. Ketorolac may be inadequate for severe pain; small amounts of opioids may be needed in addition. Ketorolac is also useful as an adjuvant to PCA and epidural analgesic techniques.

Gastric ulceration can occur with prolonged ketorolac use. An increase in bleeding time is typical but does not result in increased postoperative bleeding. Renal toxicity may occur, especially in patients dependent on renin-angiotensin system activation for maintenance of renal blood flow.

Epidural Analgesia Techniques

Single doses or prolonged administration of local anesthetics or opioids to the epidural space provide excellent postoperative analgesia. The required techniques for epidural anesthesia appear in Chapter 18.

■ Epidural Opioids

Opioids applied to the dorsal horn of the spinal cord produce analgesia without loss of sensation or motor function. Because sympathetic nerve fibers are not affected, hypotension does not result. Thus selective analgesia is possible with epidural or subarachnoid administration of opioids. Although the epidural injection of local anesthetics produces more profound analgesia, hypotension, motor blockade, and sensory loss also follow. When early mobility is essential, or when even mild hypotension is unacceptable, opioids alone are given without local anesthetics. Epidural opioids may be unsuitable for patients in whom the risk of respiratory depression is greatest, such as those with severe chronic obstructive pulmonary disease or sleep apnea.

Although knowledge of epidural opioid pharmacokinetics and pharmacodynamics is incomplete, enough data exist to guide clinical applications.

Table 34-5

Commonly Used Epidural Opioids

Drug	Relative Lipid Solubility	Bolus Drug	Onset (minutes)	Duration (hours)	Infusion Rate (mg/h)
Morphine	1	2.5 mg	30–45	12–24	0.1–0.8
Meperidine	30	50–75 mg	5–10	5–8	10–30
Fentanyl	700	50–100 µg	5–10	5–8	0.030–0.100
Hydromorphone	1	1 mg	15	10–15	—
Methadone	80	5 mg	10–15	5–10	—
Sufentanil	1500	10–60 µg	5	2–4	0.005–0.025

Table 34-5 lists the properties of opioid drugs commonly used in the epidural space. The pharmacokinetics of epidural opioids are best predicted by their lipid solubilities. The lipid-soluble opioids fentanyl, sufentanil, and meperidine reach their sites of action rapidly and take effect in 5 to 30 minutes. Morphine, which is relatively insoluble in lipids, requires 30 to 60 minutes to act.

The duration of action of an epidural opioid is determined by movement of drug away from spinal cord receptors as the drug dissociates from opioid receptors and is carried away by blood flow. Lipid-soluble agents pass into blood vessels more easily than do lipid-insoluble drugs. Fentanyl, sufentanil, and meperidine have short or intermediate durations of action, and morphine has a more prolonged effect.

Lipid solubility accounts for another important clinical feature of epidural opioids: their cephalad migration in the cerebrospinal fluid (CSF). Less lipid-soluble opioids remain dissolved in CSF, migrating with CSF up the spinal fluid column. Thus drugs like morphine tend to produce analgesia over multiple dermatomes regardless of the site of epidural injection. Morphine given in the lumbar epidural space relieves thoracic pain, for example. The cephalad migration of lipid-insoluble drugs increases brain CSF opioid levels, thereby promoting nausea, pruritus, sedation, and respiratory depression.

■ Bolus versus Continuous Infusion

Epidural opioids may be given by bolus or continuous infusion. A single bolus is given either with the dose of epidural local anesthetic or at the end of the operation, the opioid chosen according to the duration of postoperative analgesia desired. Morphine reliably gives 10 to 24 hours of analgesia; fentanyl and meperidine give 4 to 6 hours. Subsequent doses given through an indwelling epidural catheter extend the period of analgesia, as does infusing opioids continuously.

Continuous administration of lipid-soluble opioids minimizes side effects expected with the more water-soluble drugs by limiting spread of the drug to distant dermatomes and avoiding cephalad spread in the CSF. This requires placing an epidural catheter as close as possible to the relevant nerve roots.

If the epidural catheter is distant from the critical nerve roots, or if the surgical incision is extensive, lipid-insoluble opioids are preferred because they produce effective and reliable pain relief at moderate doses. The large doses of lipid-soluble drugs required to produce analgesia in the same circumstance lead to excessive blood absorption and more side effects.

■ Complications of Epidural Opioids

Respiratory depression, nausea, sedation, and pruritus result from significant concentrations of opioid reaching the brainstem, usually by cephalad migration in CSF but also from excessive blood levels of drug after large epidural doses of opioid. They appear to be mediated by µ opioid receptor agonist activity, since µ-antagonist drugs reverse these effects. Carefully written orders and thorough nursing care are required for safe care of these patients (Table 34-6).

Respiratory depression may be fatal. The likelihood of ventilatory compromise is probably greatest for the lipid-insoluble drugs because of their propensity for cephalad spread to brainstem respiratory centers. A progressive decrease in respiratory rate to the range of 4 to 10 breaths per minute is the common clinical presentation. However, significant respiratory depression (increased arterial CO_2 tension and decreased tidal volume) may occur despite a normal respiratory rate. Other evidence of excessive brain

Table 34-6

Typical Orders for Patients Receiving Epidural Narcotics

Patient received (dose) mg epidural (opioid) at (time).

Measure respiratory rate, sedation level every hour for first 24 hours.

Call pain treatment physician for
    Nausea
    Pruritus
    Respiratory rate less than 10 breaths per minute
    Somnolence
    Inadequate pain relief

Naloxone available at bedside at all times.

Infuse (opioid) into epidural catheter at (mg or μg) per hour via pump.

No other narcotics to be given unless ordered by pain treatment physician.

CSF opioid, such as somnolence or pruritus, usually accompanies ventilatory depression.

Unless the epidural dose of opioid is excessive or accidental intrathecal injection has occurred, respiratory depression develops slowly and can be detected well before an emergency ensues. Respiratory depression after a single dose usually has an early and a late phase. The early phase occurs within an hour of injection and represents vascular uptake and delivery of opioid to the brain via the circulation. Later respiratory depression begins several hours after the epidural dose and occurs almost exclusively with the lipid-insoluble opioids. It results from the cephalad movement of drug in CSF and persists as long as brain CSF concentrations are substantial. Respiratory depression during continuous epidural opioid infusions may occur regardless of the drug used. With water-soluble drugs it is due to opioid in the CSF; with lipid-soluble drugs, to opioid in the circulation.

Moderate degrees of respiratory depression are dangerous for some patients but safe for many. Clearly, markedly decreased respiratory rates (less than 6 breaths per minute), apnea, and severe obtundation require immediate treatment in all patients. Healthy patients with moderate respiratory depression (i.e., 6 to 10 breaths per minute and arterial CO_2 tension of 45 to 55 mmHg) require only increased observation and supplemental oxygen. All patients who receive opioids require monitoring for respiratory depression, ranging in intensity from frequent determinations of respiratory rate to apnea detectors

or intensive care. The choice depends on the general condition of the patient and the presence of risk factors such as obesity, sleep apnea syndrome, lung disease, or advanced age. After conventional doses of epidural opioids, if there are no special risk factors, simple monitoring of breathing rate alone is safe for most patients.

Epidural opioid-induced respiratory depression is treated with narcotic μ-receptor antagonists, of which naloxone is the prototype. Small intravenous doses (0.05 to 0.1 mg) are given until the desired respiratory rate or level of alertness is achieved. In most cases, respiratory depression can be expected to recur, requiring an intravenous infusion of small amounts of naloxone (0.05 to 0.1 mg/h). This is adjusted according to the patient's respiratory rate and discontinued as the expected duration of action of the epidural opioid is exceeded. Small doses of opioid antagonists reverse most side effects without reducing pain relief, perhaps because of the relatively lesser opioid concentrations in the brainstem (respiratory depression) than in the spinal cord (analgesia).

Nausea also results from excessive brain CSF opioid, presumably stimulating the vomiting centers and chemoemetic trigger zone. Although antiemetics may be useful for treatment, small doses of intravenous naloxone readily eliminate nausea without affecting analgesia.

Pruritus occurs when opioid spreads over the spinal cord, perhaps owing to extensive alteration of sensory input. It is not due to histamine release, and it responds poorly to antihistamines. Naloxone, nalbuphine, and butorphanol all relieve pruritus.

Urinary retention resulting from opioid receptor-mediated inhibition of normal micturition mechanisms may require use of a bladder catheter after epidural opioids. Urinary retention is readily reversed by naloxone, but the necessary doses may be high enough to reverse analgesia.

Reactivation of oral herpes simplex can occur in women who receive epidural morphine following cesarean delivery. Neonates born to these women have not been similarly affected.

■ Intrathecal Opioids

Opioids injected directly into the CSF also produce analgesia. The implications of lipid solubility for duration of action are identical to those for epidural opioids, but lesser doses are required because opioids injected directly into the CSF are not lost to vascular and tissue absorption, as happens with epidural opioids. Intrathecal morphine in doses of 0.25 to 0.5 mg produces excellent pain relief of long duration. Doses of 1 mg or more produce long periods of analgesia but result in many side effects, especially respiratory depression. Subarachnoid catheters may be used for continuous treatment of postoperative pain.

The opioid-related side effects of respiratory depression, pruritus, nausea, and urinary retention also occur with intrathecal administration. Their etiologies and treatment are the same as those described for epidural opioids.

■ Epidural Anesthetics

Epidural anesthesia with lesser concentrations of local anesthetics provides good relief of postoperative pain. Bupivacaine 0.125% to 0.25% is chosen for its long duration of action and relatively selective sensory blockade. Continuous infusion rates of bupivacaine are usually between 5 and 10 ml/h in adults. Tachyphylaxis, the progressive reduction in effect seen when local anesthetics are given for prolonged periods, may make treatment difficult when local anesthetic is used alone and may require increased rates of infusion as therapy progresses. Hypotension, numbness, weakness, and urinary retention may all occur but are unusual when small concentrations of bupivacaine are used. As with epidural opioids, the catheter site is best placed as close as possible to the nerve roots innervating the surgical wound. This helps limit the extent of epidural blockade and attendant risks of hypotension. Table 34-7 gives typical orders.

Table 34-7

Typical Orders for Patients Receiving Epidural Local Anesthetics

Patient received (dose) ml (concentration) epidural (local anesthetic) at (time)

Infuse (concentration) epidural (local anesthetic) into epidural catheter at (ml) per hour via pump

No other analgesics to be given unless ordered by pain treatment physician

Measure blood pressure every hour

Patient may ambulate only with assistance

Call pain treatment physician for
   Inadequate pain relief
   Numbness of legs
   Weakness of legs
   Blood pressure less than _____ systolic

■ Combined Local Anesthetic and Opioid Epidural Infusions

Mixtures of subanalgesic doses of local anesthetics and opioids produce profound analgesia with minimal side effects. The two drugs act at different sites in the pain pathway (nerve roots and dorsal horn), raising the possibility of greater than additive effects. Synergy has been demonstrated in animals, but conclusive evidence in humans is lacking.

The usual mixtures consist of bupivacaine 0.05% to 0.1% and any of the several commonly used epidural opioids. Morphine 0.05 to 0.1 mg/ml, meperidine 1.0 to 2.5 mg/ml, and fentanyl 5 to 10 μg/ml have all been used effectively in this regimen. Typical infusion rates are from 4 to 12 ml/h, depending on the location of the epidural catheter (lesser rates for thoracic catheters) and the size of the surgical wound (greater rates for large incisions). Just as with opioid infusions, hourly doses of morphine in excess of 1 mg, fentanyl in excess of 100 μg, and meperidine in excess of 30 mg may result in excessive blood or CSF levels of drug, producing sedation or respiratory depression.

Although the lesser doses of local anesthetic and opioid do result in fewer side effects, complications related to each drug may occur. Opioid-induced side effects are treated as described earlier. Local anesthetics produce sympathetic blockade and hypotension, treated with intravenous fluids or vasoactive drugs. Motor and sensory blocks are unlikely unless bupivacaine concentrations of 0.25% or greater are used; nevertheless, these patients are not expected to walk or stand unassisted.

Epidural local anesthetic and opioid infusions are not used if mild hypotension is unacceptable or early mobility is essential for postoperative care. It may be difficult to achieve analgesia with these solutions when the epidural infusion site is distant from the nerve roots serving the surgical incision. In these instances, less lipid-soluble opioids without local anesthetic may be useful (see Table 34-5).

Peripheral Nerve Blocks for Acute Pain

Peripheral nerve blocks provide profound postoperative pain relief. These can be performed in the operating room or postoperatively as specific treatment for acute pain; they are particularly useful when epidural or spinal techniques are contraindicated or difficult to perform. Because these techniques are often used for patients who have undergone orthopedic procedures, special precautions are required. The profound analgesia and motor block may make it impossible for the surgeon to evaluate a limb after operation or for the patient to report pain; both increase the risk of compartment syndromes and nerve damage from tight casts. Nerve blocks of an extremity for postoperative pain relief are inappropriate when the limb is to be placed in a cast or when there is risk of neurovascular compromise. Directions for specific nerve blocks are found in Chapter 19.

Brachial Plexus Block

The simplest method of providing postoperative analgesia for operations on the upper extremity is to perform a brachial plexus block with an epinephrine-containing local anesthetic. When 0.5% bupivacaine with epinephrine is used for brachial plexus blockade, analgesia usually persists for 10 to 15 hours after the operation. The site of the operation determines the preferred approach to the brachial plexus.

If extended analgesia is needed, a brachial plexus catheter permits giving additional doses or a continuous infusion. This technique is not popular, perhaps because it is difficult to fix brachial plexus catheters in place. Continuous infusions of 0.25% bupivacaine at 6 to 12 ml/h maintain analgesia. In the axillary approach to the brachial plexus, it is best to place the catheter nearest the nerve or cord innervating the surgical site. Thus, for analgesia after reimplantation of the fifth finger, the catheter is placed near the medial cord and ulnar nerve.

Femoral Nerve Block

Blockade of the femoral nerve provides significant analgesia after operations on the knee or distal femur. A reliable method for easily locating the femoral nerve is with a peripheral nerve stimulator, as discussed in Chapter 19. Peripheral nerve stimulation is especially useful during or just after an operation, when the patient may be unable to report a paresthesia. This block provides useful but incomplete pain relief after knee operations because the obturator, lateral femoral cutaneous, and sciatic nerves also innervate the knee area.

Intercostal Nerve Block

Intercostal nerve blocks can provide excellent pain relief for areas served by the thoracic dermatomes; when 3 to 5 ml of 0.5% bupivacaine with epinephrine

are used for each nerve, analgesia persists for 6 to 12 hours. Because of the rich vasculature, local anesthetic toxicity is a risk, particularly when several nerves must be blocked repeatedly. Finally, pneumothorax is a risk, especially if multiple injections are performed. This complication is rare when blocks are performed by trained persons.

Interpleural Analgesia

A recent innovation is the interpleural injection of local anesthetics, which produces the equivalent of unilateral multiple intercostal blocks, thus giving analgesia after cholecystectomy, splenectomy, nephrectomy, or breast operations. Simple techniques allow placement of an interpleural catheter, through which intermittent injections or a continuous infusion of local anesthetic can be given (see below).

Even when efforts are made to ensure that local anesthetic is not lost through chest tube drainage, the analgesia obtained with this technique is often unsatisfactory after thoracotomy. Perhaps pleural reaction or dilution of drug by pleural fluid contributes to this problem.

Although pneumothorax is unusual, it must be considered if the patient develops dyspnea. Aspiration of air through the interpleural catheter is diagnostic. In severe cases, a chest tube may be necessary.

Interpleural analgesia may be preferred over epidural anesthesia when thoracic epidural puncture is difficult or when hypotension is to be avoided. Al-

Technique of Interpleural Block

An epidural needle filled with saline is advanced over the cephalad margin of the fifth, sixth, or seventh rib until it pierces the parietal pleura and the saline is drawn into the pleural cavity. This is analogous to the "hanging drop" method of epidural placement; do not substitute the loss of resistance technique, which may lead to puncture of the visceral pleura and pneumothorax. An epidural catheter is threaded 5 to 6 cm into the thoracic cavity, the needle is removed over the catheter, and the injection site covered with an adhesive sterile dressing.

Bupivacaine, 20 to 30 ml of 0.25% or 0.5%, is injected through the catheter, and the patient is placed supine or tilted slightly to the nonoperative side so that local anesthetic solutions are in contact with pleura where it is nearest the intercostal nerves. Analgesia reaches its maximum within 30 minutes. The block is maintained with injections repeated every 4 to 6 hours or an infusion of 0.25% bupivacaine at 10 to 12 ml/h.

Table 34-8

Techniques of Postoperative Pain Relief

Therapy	Indications	Contraindications	Advantages/Benefits	Disadvantages/Risks
Patient-controlled analgesia (PCA)	Postoperative pain that is severe, prolonged, not amenable to oral analgesics	Narcotic allergy; patient cannot activate PCA; history of drug abuse or drug-seeking behavior	Drugs given on time; dose titrated to need; patient satisfaction; little physician or nurse labor required	Opioid-related side effects, incomplete analgesia, overdose due to errors
Epidural and subarachnoid opioids	Pain relief after any major operation below shoulder girdle	Narcotic allergy; risks of respiratory depression especially in COPD, sleep apnea, obesity	Good analgesia; motor, sensory, sympathetic functions intact; continuous block	Nausea, pruritus, urinary retention, respiratory depression
Local anesthetic with or without opioids in epidural	Pain relief after any major operation below shoulder girdle	Narcotic allergy; risk of hypotension unacceptable	Most profound analgesia; less severe opioid-related side effects; continuous block	Hypotension, nausea, pruritus, urinary retention, respiratory depression
Peripheral nerve	Procedures on the extremities or in areas served by thoracic dermatomes	When early neurovascular evaluation of limb is required; circumferential cast	Most profound analgesia; possible improved blood flow to ischemic areas such as skin flaps	Motor and sensory deficits in distribution of block; continuous analgesia difficult
Interpleural analgesia	Unilateral incisions through areas served by thoracic dermatomes	Pleural effusion or fibrosis; pleural inflammation; continuous techniques possible	Technical simplicity; profound analgesia; avoids hypotension; frequent repeat injections	Pneumothorax, local anesthetic toxicity

though interpleural blocks can produce unilateral thoracic sympathetic or splanchnic nerve block, this has not been associated with hypotension.

Table 34-8 summarizes modern techniques for relief of postoperative pain.

Future Advances in Postoperative Pain Therapy

Current research on the physiology and pharmacology of pain is likely to have more impact on the treatment of postoperative pain than on anesthesia for surgical procedures. Potent receptor-specific opioids may produce powerful analgesia without depressing respiration. Alpha-2-adrenergic agonist drugs such as clonidine produce epidural analgesia and reduce minimum alveolar concentration (MAC) by affecting nonopioid receptors. The new amide local anesthetic ropivacaine may block sensory fibers without producing motor block in lesser concentrations, although it has yet to undergo clinical trials as a postoperative analgesic agent. Transcutaneous electrical nerve stimulation (TENS) is usually not effective when given alone for acute pain but has been shown to reduce narcotic requirements when used postoperatively.

The optimal combination of local anesthetics and opioids for epidural analgesia remains to be determined. A "balanced" analgesia approach, using techniques that interact at several of the sites shown in Figure 34-1, is one solution. Patient-controlled epidural analgesia may permit patients to achieve satisfactory pain relief with a minimum of side effects.

The Postoperative Pain Treatment Service

The treatment of postoperative pain with these newer techniques is appealing to both patients and anesthesiologists, but comprehensive acute pain services are not widely established. Favoring this approach are the clear opportunities to relieve human suffering, the physiologic benefits such as improved pulmonary function and reduced cardiovascular stress, and the potentially favorable effects on perioperative mortality. Against it are several factors. Third-party payers are reluctant to pay for new therapies, especially when routine methods of pain treatment are already reimbursed as part of postoperative care. The lack of definite improvements in outcome makes it more difficult to establish funding. Lastly, the risk of complications makes these procedures less appealing to some.

Nevertheless, when the environment and funding permit, an organized postoperative pain treatment service offers considerable benefits to patients. Anesthesiologists skilled in the techniques of epidural and peripheral nerve blockade and knowledgeable in the area of pharmacokinetics of narcotic drugs are logical choices to be physicians in charge of postoperative pain therapy, but the concurrent treatment of numerous patients is demanding and labor-intensive. Participation by surgeons, other consultants, pharmacists, and nurses is necessary for success, but these combined efforts can benefit patients greatly.

BIBLIOGRAPHY

Bridenbaugh LD. The upper extremity: Somatic blockade. In *Neural Blockade in Clinical Anesthesia and Management of Pain*, 2nd ed. Philadelphia: JB Lippincott, 1987, pp 387-416.

Bridenbaugh PO. The lower extremity: Somatic blockade. In *Neural Blockade in Clinical Anesthesia and Management of Pain*, 2nd ed. Philadelphia: JB Lippincott, 1987, pp 417-441.

Cousins MJ, Mather LE. Intrathecal and epidural administration of opioids. *Anesthesiology* 1984;61:276-310.

Mather LE, Owen H. The pharmacology of patient–administered opioids. In *Patient-Controlled Analgesia*. Boston: Blackwell Scientific Publications, 1990, pp 27-50.

Reiestad F, Stromskag KE. Intrapleural catheter in the management of postoperative pain: A preliminary report. *Reg Anesth* 1986;11:89.

Sjistrim S, Hartvig P, Persson MP, Tamsen A. Pharmocokinetics of epidural morphine and meperidine in humans. *Anesthesiology* 1987;67:877-888.

CHAPTER 35

Chronic Pain

Kathleen M. Veloso and F. Michael Ferrante

Pain is defined by the International Association for the Study of Pain as "an unpleasant sensory and emotional experience associated with actual or potential tissue damage or described in terms of such damage." Pain is most often divided into two types, acute and chronic, based not only on duration but also on physiologic sequelae and behavioral adaptations.

Chronic pain persists beyond the normally expected duration of acute pain attendant to a given injury. Traditionally, pain of greater than 6 months' duration has been deemed to represent chronic pain. Moreover, chronic pain can occur spontaneously without a discernible organic cause. Second, many patients with chronic pain fail to display the autonomic responses typical of acute pain, such as increased sympathetic tone and altered neuroendocrine function. Third, chronic pain may be associated with behavioral adaptations that eventually become embodied in the patient's complex signs and symptoms and in the patient's persona. Patients suffering chronic pain may lose sleep and become depressed and socially maladjusted. Secondary gain may reinforce unwanted behavior. Lastly, speaking teleologically, acute pain serves an obvious protective function in warding off further injury; chronic pain serves no useful purpose.

Medical management of chronic pain requires distinguishing between the behavior and physiology of the pain experience, finding an etiology for the pain, and planning a rational treatment program to interrupt the cycle of chronic pain and disability. Often, care of the patient with chronic pain requires contributions from primary physicians, consultants from a wide range of disciplines, nurses, physical therapists,

and social workers. Anesthesiologists specializing in pain medicine may supervise the overall care of such patients or provide limited consultative services. Pain medicine is distinct as a subspecialty of anesthesiology and has its own nomenclature (Table 35-1).

Pathophysiology of Chronic Pain

Pathophysiologically, there are two types of pain: nociceptive pain (including somatic and visceral pain) and neuropathic pain. Somatic and visceral pain are similarly mediated by activation of nociceptors, nerves that generate or transmit electrochemical impulses in response to noxious stimuli. Neuropathic pain results from injury to neural tissue.

■ Nociceptive Pain

Somatic pain is well localized. Typical descriptions of somatic pain include "aching," "sharp," or "throbbing." Good examples of somatic pain are incisional pain after operation and bone metastases. In contrast, visceral pain is usually diffuse and poorly localized. Moreover, visceral pain may be referred to a location far distant from the site of tissue injury, as with the shoulder pain associated with diaphragmatic irritation. Typical adjectives used to describe visceral pain are "deep," "colicky," and "squeezing."

There are four physiologic processes associated with nociception:

1. *Transduction* refers to the process whereby noxious stimuli are translated into electrochemical impulses at sensory nerve endings.

Table 35-1

Terms Used in Pain Management	
Allodynia	Pain due to a stimulus that does not normally provoke pain
Anesthesia dolorosa	Pain in an area or region that is anesthetic
Causalgia	A syndrome of sustained burning pain, allodynia, and hyperpathia after a traumatic nerve lesion, often combined with vasomotor and sudomotor dysfunction and later tropic changes
Central pain	Pain associated with a lesion of the central nervous system
Dysesthesia	An unpleasant abnormal sensation whether spontaneous or evoked
Hyperalgesia	Increased sensitivity to noxious stimulation
Hyperpathia	Increase in the threshold of pain associated with increased pain to suprathreshold stimulation
Neuralgia	Pain in a distribution of a nerve or nerves
Neuropathy	A disturbance of function or pathologic change in a nerve
Nociceptor	A receptor preferentially sensitive to a noxious stimulus or to a stimulus that becomes noxious when prolonged
Paresthesia	An abnormal sensation, not unpleasant, whether spontaneous or evoked

Note: Addiction and tolerance (see Chap. 10) must be distinguished in pain management.

2. *Transmission* refers to the rostral propagation of the electrochemical impulses to higher centers within the central nervous system.
3. *Modulation* refers to the process whereby transmission is altered by the influence of discreet pathways containing endogenous analgesic neurotransmitters such as met- and leu-enkephalin, norepinephrine, and serotonin.
4. *Perception* is the final process whereby the subjective and emotional experience of pain is created.

While somatic and visceral nociception are not identical, they are sufficiently similar to allow discussion as a single entity. Nociception is mediated by C and A-delta fibers that end as unmyelinated free nerve endings in the periphery. Nociceptors respond to mechanical, chemical, and thermal stimuli. Potential injury can cause mechanical distortion or local disturbances in the chemical environment resulting in the synthesis and release of algesic substances. Through the incompletely understood process of transduction, these algesic substances activate and sensitize both C and A-delta nociceptors. Resulting nociceptor activity is then transmitted to second-order nociceptors in laminae I, II, and V of the dorsal horn of the spinal cord. From laminae I, II, and V, ascending relay neurons send axons that cross over to the contralateral side and form the spinothalamic tract. The spinothalamic tract ascends to form multiple synaptic connections with centers throughout the brainstem and thalamus. Subsequently, nociceptive transmission occurs to more rostral centers via thalamocortical projections.

Certain discreet areas, including the periventricular and periaqueductal grey matter, the pontine tegmentum, and the median raphe magnus, are rich in analgesic neurotransmitters such as endogenous opioids, norepinephrine, and serotonin. From diffuse areas of the rostral central nervous system, fibers containing these endogenous analgesic substances coalesce to form a descending tract called the dorsolateral funiculus. Fibers from the dorsolateral funiculus descend to synapse in the same laminae where afferent nociceptive transmission occurs.

The interactions between the physiologic processes of transduction, transmission, and modulation are embodied in the gate theory of pain. Factors that enhance transduction and afferent transmission "open the gate" and facilitate transmission through the dorsal horn of the spinal cord. Factors enhancing modulation act to "close the gate" by interdicting afferent nociceptive transmission.

■ Neuropathic Pain

Neuropathic pain is the result of injury to neural tissue that produces spontaneous ectopic discharges that result in the generation of pain. Neuropathic pain is associated with structural integrative changes in normal neurophysiologic processes, a process known as *neuroplasticity*. Neuropathic pain is divided into peripheral, central, and sympathetically mediated types.

In the periphery, nerve damage can result in formation of a neuroma. Neuromas are formed when several nerve endings fail to reunite during regeneration, forming a "tuft" of nerve fibers. Neuromas exhibit intrinsic spontaneous electrical activity and enhanced sensitivity to norepinephrine. At the level of the spinal cord, changes begin within minutes of nerve interruption as the receptive fields of the affected dorsal horn cells reorganize to amplify messages from the injured target tissue (neuroplasticity). Days later, there is further reorganization of receptive fields affecting dorsal horn cells that respond ordinarily only to inputs from adjacent undamaged peripheral nerves. These dorsal horn cells may respond spontaneously or when unaffected nerves are stimulated, so that injury to a nerve alters the behavior of other neurons to produce sensations that do not relate in an obvious way to the original injury.

When central nerve damage occurs, symptoms may represent chronic interruption of afferent transmission with spontaneous firing of higher-order neurons (deafferentation pain). Such "central" pain is accompanied by burning dysesthesia, hyperpathia, and hyperalgesia. Examples of central pain include postherpetic neuralgia, phantom limb pain, and pain after thalamic stroke (Déjerine-Roussy syndrome).

Neuropathic pain can be mediated by the sympathetic nervous system also. The classic example is reflex sympathetic dystrophy, which is discussed at length later in this chapter.

Psychologic Mechanisms in Chronic Pain

Patients' behavioral responses play an important role in determining the morbidity due to chronic pain. Over a period from 6 months to several years after the onset of pain, these may include mood changes, increased or decreased appetite, decreased physical activity, immobility, and gradual social withdrawal. More time is spent in doctors' offices, physical therapy, the home, and the pharmacy. Multiple drug prescriptions may compound symptoms.

Later, there appear vegetative changes such as disturbances of sleep, appetite, mood, bowel habits, and sexual function. Psychomotor retardation and a decreased pain tolerance may become evident. In addition to the central depletion of monoamines associated with chronic pain, maladaptive behavior is enhanced by secondary gain. Family members, physicians, and lawyers may reward pain-related behavior out of sympathy or to further their own goals. Pain becomes a "habit," and patients consent to procedures that reinforce the learned behavior.

Evaluation of Patients with Chronic Pain

Evaluation of the patient with chronic pain begins with a review of the entire medical history and all the physical findings. It is essential to discover treatable primary causes of pain, such as malignancy, before undertaking treatment for chronic pain.

■ History

Specific data required to evaluate a patient with chronic pain are listed in Table 35-2.

Table 35-2

The History from a Patient with Chronic Pain as a Chief Complaint

1. The history of the pain: when it began, associated injuries or illnesses, whether it is constant or intermittent.
2. The patient's choice of words to describe the pain: sharp, dull, burning, electric shock, cramp.
3. The severity of the pain as compared with other pain the patient has experienced and its effects on function, such as work, favorite activities, or sleep.
4. The location of the pain: location on a diagram of the body, depth, radiation.
5. The diagnoses the patient has been given before.
6. Previous treatment and its effect. What makes the pain better? What makes it worse?
7. The patient's previous history of chronic pain.
8. Litigation or Worker's Compensation actions.
9. History of numbness, paresthesia, weakness.
10. Range of motion of the affected parts.
11. Symptoms of sympathetic overactivity: sensations of heat or cold, sweating, skin and hair changes, skin temperature, color, galvanic responses.
12. Current medications, responses to previous medications.
13. The general medical and surgical history.

■ Measurement of Pain

Objective measurement of organ function is of great value in managing medical problems such as renal failure, lung disease, and liver disease. Unfortunately, pain by its nature is subjective, and reports of pain cannot be corroborated by external observation and measurement.

Simple standardized pain scales, such as the 11-point visual analogue scales and verbal descriptive scales, provide useful information. More elaborate tests such as the McGill Pain Questionnaire, the Minnesota Multiphasic Personality Inventory, and the Multidimensional Pain Inventory provide more in-depth data for analysis, but they are time-consuming. Their use is also limited by patients' misunderstandings of underlying concepts.

Although these tests are useful both practically and for scientific studies, the outcome of treatment of individual patients is best measured in terms of return to an active, functional life. Restoration of normal patterns of sleep, eating, and sexual behavior, the resumption of work duties, and an improved mental outlook are indications of successful chronic pain management.

■ Physical Examination

The physical examination for the evaluation of chronic pain begins with a neurologic examination, including reflexes, changes in sensitivity to pinprick, temperature, and light touch, and motor deficits. Swelling, changes in peripheral pulses, skin atrophy, loss of hair, and changes in skin temperature and color all contribute to the assessment of sympathetic neural activity. Tests of active and passive range of motion may demonstrate guarding. If the problem is limited to one side, comparisons are made with the normal side.

■ Nerve Blocks for Diagnosis: Differential Spinal and Epidural Anesthesia

Diagnostic nerve blocks for the evaluation of chronic pain can help determine the neural pathways involved by using a sequence of placebo, sympathetic, and complete somatosensory nerve blocks. Placebo responders gain relief from all blocks, even those performed with normal saline. If blockade with very dilute concentrations of local anesthetic that do not

produce numbness to pinprick is effective, then sympathetic mechanisms play a role in maintaining pain. If the patient gains relief from a profound sensory block only, then sympathetic mechanisms do not act alone. If such a block provides no relief, then central or psychological causes dominate.

Differential spinal anesthesia has been used to diagnose pain syndromes in the lower body. After a needle is placed in the cerebrospinal fluid (see Chap. 18), a dose of saline is followed by increasing concentrations of local anesthetic solutions (saline followed by 0.2%, 0.5%, and 1% procaine) injected in sequence to produce a progressively more profound block. Because the tracts of Lissauer are separated from the cerebrospinal fluid (CSF) by one cell layer, local anesthetic injection into the subarachnoid space results first in sympathetic preganglionic and corresponding C fiber neural blockade. Somatosensory axons are located more peripherally at each spinal cord segment than are motor fibers, so increasing concentrations of local anesthetic result next in sensory and then motor blockade.

The results of differential spinal anesthetics are often inconsistent and confusing because objective correlates of discrete sympathetic or somatosensory blockade were never developed or applied to clinical pain syndromes. A more common practice is to employ an epidural catheter through which placebo and local anesthetic solutions of graded concentrations can be infused. Patients who get no relief from an epidural anesthetic with motor block require therapy centering on their psychological adaptation to pain.

■ Nerve Blocks for Prognosis

A prognostic nerve block that precedes the permanent ablation of a nerve or a part of the spinal cord can give the patient a sense of the relief to be expected and the likely side effects. Some patients find the anesthetic effect of the block more disconcerting than the pain. Prognostic blocks also confirm the locations of nerves in case of anatomic variation.

Therapies for Patients with Chronic Pain

■ Overall Strategy

An understanding of pathophysiology allows the practitioner to devise a pharmacologic regimen in accordance with underlying mechanisms of pain. The use of multiple therapies to treat a single pain problem may be valuable if each treatment is directed at a particular mechanism for generation of pain. Some agents such as nonsteroidal anti-inflammatory drugs (NSAIDs) and opioids are relatively nonspecific analgesics and can be used for both nociceptive and neuropathic pain, with certain provisions (see below).

■ Opioids

Opioids are nonspecific analgesics, rendering excellent analgesia for somatic pain, except for mobility-induced pain. Opioids can be used for neuropathic pain, although they are not the agents of first choice; in general, neuropathic pain is more refractory to opioid analgesic than somatic pain.

Long-term opioid administration is most useful for chronic cancer pain and may be combined with nonsteroidal anti-inflammatory drugs, tricyclic antidepressants, and nerve blocks. Owing to progression of disease and sometimes acquired tolerance, large doses may be required. It is important not to set arbitrary limits on the amount prescribed but to limit doses only because of side effects such as somnolence and respiratory depression. Opioids may be employed in the treatment of chronic nonmalignant pain, but this use is controversial.

■ Sedatives and Antidepressants

Sedatives and hypnotics prevent normal sleep, exacerbating the sleep disturbance that accompanies chronic pain. Patients suffering from various pain states often benefit from treatment with small doses of a tricyclic antidepressant at bedtime.

Antidepressants are very effective in the treatment of neuropathic pain. The analgesic efficacy of antidepressants is derived from inhibition of presynaptic reuptake of serotonin and norepinephrine by the amine pump. The analgesic effect of antidepressants can be seen within 48 to 72 hours of drug administration. The antidepressant effect of these medications can only be seen after protracted use of these agents for 3 to 4 weeks. Side effects of antidepressant administration include muscarinic anticholinergic effects (dry mouth, constipation, difficulty with micturition), antihistaminic effects (sedation), and orthostatic hypotension.

■ Anti-Inflammatory Drugs

Inflammation is part of many chronic musculoskeletal and cancer pain syndromes. Nonsteroidal anti-inflammatory drugs (NSAIDs) achieve analgesia through inhibition of prostaglandin synthesis. NSAIDs specifically inhibit the action of the enzyme cyclooxygenase. As a group, NSAIDs are similar to opioids in that they are good general nonspecific analgesics with some action in neuropathic pain states.

Side effects of NSAIDs are prostaglandin- and nonprostaglandin-mediated. Gastropathy, nephropathy, and platelet dysfunction are prostaglandin-mediated and derived from removal of the protective effects of prostaglandins on the respective organ. Nonprostaglandin-mediated effects of NSAIDs include rare phenomena such as liver toxicity.

■ Membrane-Stabilizing Agents

Membrane-stabilizing agents include anticonvulsants and local anesthetics (intravenous and oral). These agents are used traditionally in neuropathic pain states. Older anticonvulsants such as phenytoin and carbamazepine achieve analgesia by the same mechanism as local anesthetics: blockade of sodium channels. Clonazepam is unique in that it is a benzodiazepine. Newer anticonvulsants with analgesic potential affect the gamma- aminobutyric acid pathways.

Intravenous local anesthetics (lidocaine and chloroprocaine) have been used for some time in the treatment of neuropathic pain, often with protracted analgesia after an infusion. Mexiletine is a congener of lidocaine that can be administered orally for treatment of neuropathic pain.

■ Exercise and Physical Therapy

Immobility and a progressively sedentary lifestyle commonly accompany chronic pain. The initial musculoskeletal reflexes associated with injury or visceral disease are exaggerated, and secondary muscular pain may eventually mask the initial problem. Daily exercises help restore a normal range of motion to dysfunctional muscle groups. Additional physiologic, psychological, and social benefits are realized when patients participate in daily exercise programs outside the home.

Nerve Blocks in the Treatment of Pain

In addition to establishing diagnosis and prognosis, nerve blocks are often successful in treating patients with chronic pain. Nerve blocks alleviate chronic pain by several mechanisms. First, simple interruption of sensory pathways may provide long-term relief. Second, a short course of anesthetic nerve blocks may abort the onset of self-perpetuating pain syndromes. This "preemptive analgesia" is most clearly effective in preventing the appearance of phantom limb pain and sympathetically maintained pain syndromes. Third, the analgesia produced by nerve blocks may be required to permit treatments such as physical therapy or manipulation. Fourth, corticosteroids added to the local anesthetic may contribute to pain relief by providing long-term anti-inflammatory effects. Fifth, sympathetic blocks may provide definitive therapy for sympathetically maintained pain, as described previously.

■ Neurolytic Blocks

Once it is established that a nerve block relieves the patient's pain, that the side effects are tolerable, and that a short series of repeated blocks produces only transient effects, it may be advisable to use a neurolytic chemical to produce longer-lasting relief, particularly in cancer patients. Agents such as alcohol and phenol denature neural proteins and extract lipid membrane components. They penetrate tissues poorly and must be deposited close to the peripheral nerve or into the subarachnoid or epidural space (Table 35-3). The effects of neurolytic agents are not permanent and last from days to months, so it may be required to repeat the blocks. Motor deficits or deafferentation pain may occur, and recurrent pain may be difficult to treat. In general, destructive nerve blocks are used for patients with cancer and are best avoided in patients with chronic nonmalignant pain. Fluoroscopy confirms needle placement and the extent of spread of the neurolytic agent.

■ Stellate Ganglion Block

A stellate ganglion block may be indicated in the treatment of acute herpes zoster or postherpetic neuralgia as well as sympathetically mediated pain of the head, neck, or upper extremity. The stellate ganglion is the fusion of the inferior cervical and first thoracic sympathetic ganglia and lies anterior to the prevertebral fascia, posteromedial to the vertebral artery and cupola of the lung, and anterior to the transverse process of C7. The postganglionic sympathetic supply to the face, upper chest, thoracic viscera, and arm traverses the stellate ganglion.

A direct approach to the stellate ganglion at C7 risks pneumothorax; depositing the local anesthetic within the fascial space containing the cervical sympathetic ganglia at C6 produces as effective a block. Furthermore, the risk of injection into the vertebral artery is greater at C7. Because phrenic or recurrent laryngeal nerve block may result as well, only one side is blocked at a time.

The patient lies with the neck extended over a pillow and looks up and behind at a spot on the wall. The mouth is open to allow relaxation of the sternocleidomastoid muscles. The operator's nondominant index and middle fingers retract the sternocleidomastoid muscle and vascular bundle laterally, with the carotid pulse beneath the index finger, at the level of the anterior tubercle of the transverse process of C6 (cricothyroid membrane). A short, thin needle (23 to 25 gauge, 1 to 1.5 in) attached to a 10-ml syringe is inserted perpendicular to the plane of the table on which the patient lies until the tubercle is reached a few millimeters below the skin surface. After aspiration to test for blood return, a test dose of no more than 1 ml 0.25% bupivacaine is injected. If there are no signs of intraarterial injection, the remaining 9 ml of solution is injected slowly. Sympathectomy renders the skin warm and dry and produces venodilation.

A successful block is confirmed by the presence of an ipsilateral Horner's syndrome, which includes ptosis, miosis, anhidrosis, enophthalmos, conjunctival injection, and unilateral nasal stuffiness. Complications from this block include seizure (injection into

---

Table 35-3

Neurolytic Agents that Directly Destroy Neural Tissue and Are Used in Nerve Blocks for Severe Chronic Pain

	Phenol	Ethyl Alcohol
Concentration	5–10%	50–100%
Pain on injection	No	Yes
Local anesthetic effect	Yes	No
Density relative to CSF	Hyperbaric	Hypobaric

the vertebral artery), subarachnoid injection at the dural cuff of the nerve root, pneumothorax, phrenic nerve block, recurrent laryngeal block, and hematoma.

■ Lumbar Sympathetic Block

A lumbar sympathetic block is indicated for treatment and evaluation of sympathetically mediated pain in order to differentiate between sympathetic or somatic components of pain and to increase blood flow to an extremity in the treatment of ischemia. Sympathetic outflow to the retroperitoneum, pelvis, perineum, and lower extremities can be blocked paravertebrally at L2 with a single injection. The patient is positioned laterally with the side to be blocked uppermost; a pillow beneath the iliac crest opens the space between the transverse processes of L2 through L4. A skin wheal is made halfway between the tip of the eleventh rib and the tip of the spinous process of L2. This corresponds to the lateral border of the paravertebral muscles and often lies just inferior to the tip of the twelfth rib.

For all but children and morbidly obese adults, a 5-in, 22-gauge spinal needle suffices. Starting from the point described, the needle is advanced toward the umbilicus. As the edge of the paravertebral muscle is encountered, there may be a slight contraction visible at the skin. As the quadratus lumborum is traversed, there is a slight loss of resistance upon leaving the muscle. Patients may then sometimes begin to experience paresthesias, first to the hip and later to the knee and below as the psoas is entered. At a depth of 4 to 5 in, the needle exits the psoas fascia. There are no further paresthesias (Fig. 35-1). A test dose (5 ml) of local anesthetic produces a sensation of pressure but no paresthesias.

If genitofemoral paresthesias are encountered, the needle is advanced 1 mm. If there is resistance to injection, the needle is advanced slowly until the prevertebral fascia is passed. If bone is encountered at 2.5 to 3 in of depth, the needle is repositioned cephalad or caudad to miss the transverse process. If the vertebral body is encountered at 3.5 to 4 in, the needle is angled more laterally while visualizing the relationship between the needle, the kidney, and the vena cava in order to avoid penetrating either of these structures. Fluoroscopy can confirm the position of the needle and the spread of the solution injected. Ten milliliters of dilute local anesthetic

(0.25% bupivacaine or equivalent) injected slowly produces a sympathetic blockade.

A successful block is demonstrated when the skin temperature increases without motor or sensory impairment after the block. Risks include epidural, subdural, intrathecal, intrarenal, and intravascular injection.

■ Celiac Plexus Block

An extended periaortic ganglion, the celiac plexus sends postganglionic sympathetic fibers to the abdominal organs and also receives nociceptive transmission from organs such as the pancreas. Blocks of the celiac plexus can be used to relieve visceral pain from structures extending from the distal esophagus to the descending colon.

To perform a celiac plexus block, the patient is placed in a prone position. After skin wheals are placed bilaterally 8 cm from the midline at the inferior edge of the twelfth rib, 22-gauge, 7-in needles are directed 45 degrees toward the vertebral body. After contact with the vertebral body, the needles are redirected at a steeper angle until the tips of the needles lie ventral

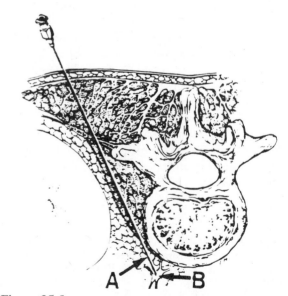

Figure 35-1

The relationship of the needle (*A*), the sympathetic chain (*B*), and the body of L2 during lumbar sympathetic block. *(Used with permission from Carron H, Korbon GA, Rowlingson JC:* Regional Anesthesia: Techniques and Clinical Applications. *New York: Grune & Stratton, 1984, p 138.)*

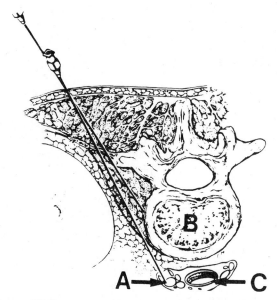

Figure 35-2

The placement of the needle adjacent to the celiac ganglia (A) the body of L1 (B) and the aorta (C) during celiac plexus block.

(Used with permission from Carron H, Korbon GA, Rowlingson JC: Regional Anesthesia: Techniques and Clinical Applications. *New York: Grune & Stratton, 1984, p 141.)*

to the vertebral body in the periaortic region (Fig. 35-2). Needle position can be confirmed with fluoroscopy and radiographic contrast or by computed tomographic (CT) scan. In increments of 5 ml, with aspiration to test for the return of blood or symptoms of local anesthetic toxicity, a total of 25 ml of local anesthetic solution is injected through each needle. Side effects or potential complications include hypotension and increased gastric motility (attendant to physiologic sympathetic blockade), retroperitoneal hematoma, vascular injection, kidney puncture, and blockade of somatic nerves.

Chronic Pain Syndromes

■ Sympathetically Maintained Pain (Reflex Sympathetic Dystrophy)

In 1864, S. Weir Mitchell used the term *causalgia* to describe the burning pain that followed peripheral nerve injury due to gunshot wounds. This and other clinical conditions such as reflex sympathetic dystro-

phy, Sudeck's atrophy, and shoulder-hand syndrome are examples of sympathetically maintained pain. All share the characteristics of burning pain, hyperesthesia, exaggerated sympathetic activity, allodynia, dystrophy, and eventual atrophy.

These syndromes begin with minor symptoms that may resolve or may progress through three stages. The first (acute) stage lasts approximately 3 months following the onset of symptoms that begin within weeks of injury. During the acute stage, the extremity becomes red, hot, dry, edematous, and hyperesthetic. Skin, hair, and nail growth may be accelerated. During this stage, diagnosis is confirmed when the patient experiences relief from sympathetic blockade, which may be produced by a nerve block or by phentolamine, an alpha-adrenergic antagonist administered intravenously in a placebo-controlled, blinded fashion.

In this first stage, successful treatment can be expected in most patients with physical therapy and sympathetic blockade, which can be accomplished with a series of nerve blocks. Orally administered alpha-adrenergic blocking drugs such as prazosin may be useful, as may tricyclic antidepressants. Physical therapy can be scheduled immediately to follow sympathetic blocks if patients cannot tolerate physical therapy otherwise.

The syndrome may progress to the second, or dystrophic, stage in the first 6 months following the onset of symptoms. Allodynia is prominent, indicating changes in central neuronal receptive fields. Hyperactivity of the sympathetic nerves renders the extremity cold, blue, sweaty, and stiff. Dystrophy progresses to include early subcutaneous atrophy, shiny hairless skin, slow-growing and brittle nails, and periarticular demineralization evident on radiographs. The patient protects the extremity assiduously.

In the second stage as in the first, treatment is aimed at restoring function through a combination of physical therapy and sympathetic blockade, but therapy is more prolonged and less likely to succeed. Repeated blocks of the sympathetic ganglia or continuous sympathetic and somatosensory blockade for up to a week at a time has been advocated in desperate cases. Vasodilators may be administered either orally or using a Bier block technique (intravenous regional anesthesia) to restore capillary blood flow.

A few patients enter the third, or atrophic, stage of reflex sympathetic dystrophy within 2 years after the onset of symptoms. The affected extremity becomes a useless, painful appendage. Psychologically based treatment emphasizes improved coping; nerve blocks are ineffective at this late stage.

■ Neuropathic Pain

Postherpetic neuralgia is a common neuropathic condition usually diagnosed in elderly or immuno-compromised patients. *Postherpetic neuralgia* is defined as pain that persists in a dermatomal pattern after the eruption from a herpes zoster infection has healed. The pain is severe and distressing. A wide variety of treatments have been employed, including anticonvulsants, systemic corticosteroids, regional blocks, sympathetic blocks, epidural injections, antiviral agents, local infiltration with corticosteroids and anesthetics, topical capsaicin, topical aspirin in chloroform, and surgical procedures. Sympathetic blocks during the acute phase of herpes zoster may be helpful, and some evidence (though controversial) exists that early sympathetic blockade may provide prophylaxis against the development of postherpetic neuralgia.

Of the cranial neuralgias, trigeminal neuralgia (tic douloureux) has been the most widely studied. Compression of the nerve peripheral to the nucleus causes deafferentation; some time after 4 weeks, central neuronal changes are established. Local anesthetic nerve blocks are useful in the diagnosis of the site of compression but do not predict favorable responses to destructive nerve blocks. Carbamazepine treatment is effective, although doses as great as 1600 mg/day may be required. Neurolytic blocks or surgical nerve decompression may be required for those who do not respond to medical therapy.

■ Phantom Pain

Amputation sometimes leads to phantom limb pain afterward; the mechanisms are similar to those involved in other peripheral nerve injuries. Blockade of the sympathetic and somatosensory nerves carried out before amputation may prevent phantom limb pain. For this reason, some recommend regional anesthesia for these operations, even if general anesthesia is also required for psychological reasons.

For trauma victims, treatment with regional anesthesia may begin promptly after amputation. As with other situations in which peripheral nerve injury results in central pain, peripheral neural blockade is helpful only during the 2 to 4 weeks following injury.

■ Cancer Pain

Pain in patients with malignancies is affected by the tumor type (solid tumors are more painful than lymphoma or leukemia), the site (invasion of bone or neural tissue increases pain), the stage of the disease, and the patient's mood. Pain is usually of a mixed type and may contain components of somatic, visceral, and neuropathic pain.

Seventy-five to ninety percent of patients with cancer receive effective analgesia with oral medications alone; opioids are the mainstay for cancer pain. Treatment progresses in sequence from nonopioids (e.g., NSAIDs) with or without adjuvants such as antidepressants or anticonvulsants, to mild opioids used for moderate pain (e.g., codeine, hydrocodone, oxycodone, etc.) with or without adjuvants, to opioids for severe pain (e.g., morphine, methadone, levorphanol, hydromorphone).

Oral therapy is abandoned when analgesia can no longer be achieved, dose-limiting toxicity intervenes, or the patient is unable to swallow or absorb oral medication. At this point, subcutaneous or intravenous administration of opioids, neuraxial drug administration, or neurolytic blocks may be used.

■ Myofascial Pain

Localized areas of hardened tender muscle, called *trigger points*, may arise spontaneously or after injury. Chronic pain associated with trigger points is called the *myofascial pain syndrome* and may include muscle spasm, tenderness, stiffness, limitation of motion, tingling, paresthesias, and weakness, along with symptoms referred to distant areas. Predisposing conditions include genetic factors, poor general physical condition, microtrauma, heat, cold, fatigue, and prolonged immobility. It is speculated that prolonged and inappropriate segmental muscle contractions result in ischemia and edema; trigger points may lie where a peripheral motor nerve fiber and the corresponding artery and vein pass between two fascial layers. Diagnosis is made from symptoms such as muscle stiffness associated with sharp shooting pain possibly radiating to a distant area and from physical findings such as restricted range of motion and tight bands or firm nodules that are tender on palpation.

Therapies include restoration of normal muscle range of motion, daily exercise, and correction of poor posture. Stretching of the involved muscles to restore range of motion after a coolant spray to inactivate trigger points is the mainstay of physical therapy. Improvement also results from placing a needle in the trigger point or injecting saline, local anesthetic, or a small amount of corticosteroid. Increased ability to exercise and to participate in physical therapy are the rationale for the injections, which are not continued if the patient does not participate in an exercise program.

■ Back Pain

Low back pain is the most common disabling problem of those of working age; about 14 percent of Americans have had an episode of low back pain lasting more than 2 weeks. Successful treatment of low back pain requires appropriate diagnosis of the source of the pain. In the acute phase, bed rest (limited to 2 days) and NSAIDs may be the only treatment necessary. Bed rest of more than 10 days duration owing to disk disease is associated with worsening of symptoms. When pain persists, or when there are neurologic deficits, further evaluation is necessary.

The causes of low back pain are varied and may arise from myofascial pain syndromes, irritated nerve roots, herniated intervertebral disks, lumbar facet disease, sacroiliac joint disease, spinal stenosis, compression fracture from osteoporosis, rheumatoid arthritis or osteoarthritis, or pain referred from an abdominal disease. Intervertebral disks may bulge, herniate, or leak onto spinal nerve roots. Once the need for operation to treat spinal stenosis or nerve compression has been considered and a simple program of bed rest has not given relief, patients require treatment for back pain.

Localized back pain and secondary paravertebral muscle spasm are treated with an exercise program. The epidural injection of depot steroids is sometimes used to reduce inflammation of nerve roots in patients with herniated disks and radicular symptoms. Ill effects include transient exacerbation of the pain and the risk of possible neurotoxicity from the depot steroid preparations inadvertently injected in the CSF.

Epidural steroids provide effective palliation for inflammatory pain, but results are limited and transient unless the patient takes advantage of the period of reduced discomfort to begin effective physical therapy.

Patients with herniated or leaking disks often have pain with forward flexion or straight leg raising, while those with facet disease have increased pain with back extension and lateral rotation. For the latter patients, facet nerve blocks with local anesthetic may allow exercise therapy.

BIBLIOGRAPHY

Bonica JJ, Loeser JD, Chapman CR, Fordyce WE, eds. *The Management of Pain*. Philadelphia: Lea and Febiger, 1990.

Carron H, Korbon GA, Rowlingson, JC. *Regional Anesthesia: Techniques and Clinical Applications*. New York: Grune & Stratton, 1984.

Cousins MJ, Bridenbaugh PO, eds. Clinical Anesthesia and Management of Pain. In *Neural Blockade,* 2nd ed. Philadelphia: JB Lippincott Co, 1988.

Stolker RJ, Vervest ACM, Groen GJ. The management of chronic spinal pain by blockades: A review. *Pain* 1994; 58:1.

CHAPTER 36

Hazards of Anesthesia

Frank L. Murphy

The Overall Risks of Anesthesia

Patients often ask whether anesthesia is safe. In one sense, this question is easy to answer: It is not completely safe. Complications of anesthesia range from frequently occurring annoyances that rarely do permanent harm, such as sore throat after tracheal intubation, to catastrophic events, such as airway obstruction, hypoxemia, and cardiac arrest, that can result in death or permanent brain damage. It is unlikely that anesthesia will ever be completely safe, for general anesthesia includes loss of consciousness, obtunded airway reflexes, depressed cardiovascular reflexes, respiratory insufficiency, and often muscle weakness or paralysis. General anesthesia will result in death in minutes if proper care is not provided. Spinal and epidural anesthesia cause hypotension and can result in cardiac arrest, seizures, and loss of consciousness. Even regional anesthesia and sedation can produce these complications.

If anesthesia is not completely safe, how risky is it, and what can be done to decrease these risks? These questions are difficult to answer. "Anesthesia" encompasses multiple drugs, techniques, and people, each of which influences the outcome. The risks depend on the patient as well: It is likely that valid estimates of risk can only be made for narrowly defined patient cohorts. Also, the relevant risk is that of anesthesia and operation combined. Patients never undergo anesthesia without an operation or diagnostic procedure; control groups of patients who undergo anesthesia without operation or who undergo operation without anesthesia are equally inconceivable. Instead, series of cases are analyzed in retrospect.

Serious risk is usually defined as the risk of dying, and the contribution of anesthesia to the outcome is determined through retrospective analysis by panels of experts. From these data, two general conclusions can be reached: First, investigators can estimate the likelihood of various complications. Second, analysis of the cases can point to mechanisms of injury and may suggest means to prevent complications.

The major limitation of such studies lies in the retrospective analyses, which are limited by the unrecognized prejudices and ignorance of the experts, the latter resulting from inadequate documentation of all aspects of care. Pathologic processes may go unrecognized (e.g., malignant hyperthermia in any studies conducted before 1960), and conclusions about causation are likely to be erroneous, at least when viewed in retrospect. This occurred in the early 1950s when Beecher and Todd found an increased death rate in patients receiving curare and concluded that the drug had an inherent toxic effect, missing the fact that inadequate postoperative ventilation was causative. As medical knowledge increases, deaths once attributed to patient diseases come to be seen as due to suboptimal management and, eventually, to inexcusable error. Our understanding of the hazards of anesthesia derives from studies such as these, from case reports, and from analyses of untoward events.

The overall death rate within the first 30 days after operation is approximately 1 percent. Of these deaths, the majority are attributed to the patients' diseases; a smaller fraction are said to be due to mismanagement; very few are attributed solely to anesthesia. In recent studies, the rates of death owing to anesthesia range from 0.01 percent (1 in 10,000) to 0.0005 percent (1 in 200,000), with a tendency for more recent studies to show improved death rates. Large series of anesthetics without deaths have been reported from outpatient surgery centers. Given the 20 to 25 million operations performed in the United States each year, there may be as many as 2000 or fewer than 100 preventable anesthesia-related deaths. These are many fewer deaths than are attributable to cardiovascular disease, cancer, or automobile accidents, but are more than the number caused by airplane accidents.

Studies that analyze the causes of death and near misses, such as the critical incident studies of Cooper and the ASA Closed Claims Project, have characterized the epidemiologic profile of death or major harm from anesthesia. The overall risk of dying varies a great deal; studies of death rates after repair of fractured hip report postoperative mortalities ranging from 6 to 25 percent. Equipment malfunction is not a common cause of death or critical incidents attributed to anesthesia, but human error is more common. Hypoxic gas mixtures, airway obstruction, errors in drug administration, and lapses in vigilance are often cited as the causes of death or near misses.

The overall death rate is greater for patients undergoing more invasive operations. The death rate from anesthesia appears not to be increased in the elderly but is greater in the ill, perhaps because they cannot recover as well from episodes of hypotension or hypoxemia. No convincing large-scale studies have shown a specific safety advantage for general or regional anesthesia, except when regional anesthesia alone can be used for peripheral operations in patients at great risk. However, global retrospective studies are unlikely to detect small differences in safety among various techniques, especially when patient populations are not carefully stratified by the types of operation or extent of coexisting disease. Although the death rate from anesthesia appears to be decreasing, the cause cannot be proven; improved training and equipment such as inspired oxygen analyzers and pulse oximeters undoubtedly have contributed.

When patients ask about the safety of a proposed anesthetic, the anesthesiologist can offer not only detailed information about the plans for anesthesia management but also general reassurance based on the information presented above and on comparisons with travel by automobile and airplane. The remainder of this chapter discusses some specific hazards not discussed elsewhere in this book.

Malignant Hyperthermia

■ Pathophysiology

Malignant hyperthermia is a rare inherited myopathy that is inapparent in daily life. After the affected patient receives anesthetics known to trigger the syndrome (potent inhaled anesthetics and nondepolarizing muscle relaxants), defective intracellular calcium control mechanisms in muscle may result in sustained muscle contractures. Apparently the massive muscle depolarization produced by succinylcholine overwhelms available mechanisms for uptake of intracellular calcium. Onset may be prompt or delayed after exposure to the responsible agent; the diagnosis is sometimes first made in the recovery room.

In the muscle, a hypermetabolic state develops, with or without marked increases in tone. This increased metabolism is manifested at first by increased CO_2 production, tachycardia, and increased cardiac output, mimicking light anesthesia. As the hypermetabolic state continues, body temperature increases, at times rapidly and to dangerous values (40 to 43° C). Anaerobic metabolism, metabolic acidosis, cellular hypoxia, muscle cell breakdown, hyperkalemia, myoglobinemia, cardiac failure, and renal failure follow. Early series reported mortalities as great as 70 percent; with better therapy and improved detection of the syndrome early in its course, mortality is now 5 percent or less.

■ Preoperative Evaluation and Diagnostic Testing

The incidence of susceptibility to malignant hyperthermia may vary depending on the makeup of the gene pool and perhaps the degree of inbreeding in the population studied. In one study, the incidence of fulminant malignant hyperthermia was 1 in 62,000 anesthetics that involved agents known to trigger the syndrome. A careful personal and family history often suggests an increased susceptibility to malignant hyperthermia. Sentinel events in the patient or a family member include a history of a previous episode, a history of unexplained fever in the operating room or recovery room, a history of an aborted anesthetic, Duchenne's muscular dystrophy, or other muscular dystrophies.

Malignant hyperthermia in swine is an autosomal

recessive disease physiologically identical to that in humans. It has been traced to a single point mutation affecting the ryanodine receptor, which forms part of the mechanism for release of calcium by sarcoplasmic reticulum. In some but not all affected humans, malignant hyperthermia appears to involve ryanodine, the gene for which lies on chromosome 19, near the site where malignant hyperthermia has been mapped. In humans, the disease behaves as an autosomal dominant trait, and it seems to represent a variety of genetic and physiologic defects having in common susceptibility to muscle hypermetabolism after triggering anesthetics. This heterogeneity, along with the fact that even susceptible patients may undergo several anesthetics uneventfully, makes the patient's history useful for suggesting susceptibility but not for ruling out the possibility of malignant hyperthermia.

The diagnosis of malignant hyperthermia depends on observing greater than usual contractile responses to halothane, caffeine, or a combination of the two in a freshly biopsied viable muscle specimen. Testing is performed at a limited number of centers,[1] and results are somewhat inconsistent. As a rule, testing is effective for ruling out malignant hyperthermia, but equivocal or false-positive results are not uncommon.

A telephone call to the North American Malignant Hyperthermia Registry[2] may provide information if the patient or a relative has been documented as having malignant hyperthermia previously.

Neuroleptic malignant syndrome occurs slowly, over days, following exposure (usually long-term) to phenothiazines or haloperidol and includes fever, muscle rigidity, acidosis, and rhabdomyolysis. Although there is no obvious inherited basis for this syndrome, muscle from these patients sometimes exhibits enhanced susceptibility in the halothane-caffeine contracture test used to diagnose malignant hyperthermia, suggesting that it is prudent to avoid the use of succinylcholine when these patients require

anesthesia for electroconvulsive therapy or other procedures.

■ Clinical Presentation and Early Detection

Malignant hyperthermia often presents in an insidious fashion; the hyperdynamic circulation that occurs in response to the increased metabolic rate resembles light anesthesia. The earliest reliable sign of malignant hyperthermia is excessive CO_2 production, manifested by increased end-tidal CO_2 during controlled ventilation, increased minute ventilation in a patient breathing spontaneously under anesthesia, or warmth and rapid exhaustion of the CO_2 absorbent. These are never normal findings and deserve immediate investigation. Fever is a late and inconsistent sign of hypermetabolism. Routine monitoring of temperature is of little use for very brief anesthetics but a necessary part of routine care for operations lasting more than a few minutes.

Masseter spasm may be the presenting finding with malignant hyperthermia, especially among children. After succinylcholine, the jaw is clenched and the mouth cannot be opened. If the anesthetic is continued, the jaw muscles may relax after the succinylcholine effect dissipates; the onset of clear signs of the hypermetabolic state may be delayed for 10 to 30 minutes. In several series, 50 to 60 percent of patients who developed masseter spasm exhibited positive caffeine-halothane contracture tests. However, not all patients with masseter spasm after succinylcholine have malignant hyperthermia. Other diseases, such as myotonia fluctuans, are associated with muscle spasm after succinylcholine. Some increase in the tone of jaw muscles (but not outright rigidity) after succinylcholine is a normal finding, and as many as 1 percent of all children receiving halothane and succinylcholine develop marked increases in masseter tone. These findings suggest that only those with marked masseter spasm should be treated as if they have malignant hyperthermia. There is a spectrum of severity in masseter spasm and a spectrum of recommendations as to how to proceed when this occurs. The more urgent the operation and the milder the masseter spasm, the more appropriate it is to proceed with the anesthetic, using nontriggering agents and monitoring carefully; the less urgent the operation and the more severe the spasm, the wiser it is to abandon the anesthetic and begin immediate treatment for malig-

[1]Malignant Hyperthermia Association of the United States (MHAUS), P.O. Box 3231, Darien, CN 06820, (phone: 209-634-4917, ask for "Index Zero" for a malignant hyperthermia consultant). MHAUS is an organization of patients and families involved with malignant hyperthermia. By calling the phone number, one can obtain immediate referral to physician experts.
[2]The North American Malignant Hyperthermia Registry, Department of Anesthesiology, Pennsylvania State University Medical Center, Hershey, PA (phone: 717-531-6936). The registry responds to inquiries about patients.

nant hyperthermia. After operation, these patients are referred for consultation and testing.

An anesthetized patient who shows signs of unexplained hyperdynamic circulation, increased CO_2 production, and increasing temperature (or one that is not decreasing as fast as usual for the temperature of the operating room and the size of the patient), with or without increased muscle tone and with or without masseter spasm, must be treated promptly for malignant hyperthermia to avert tissue damage and death resulting from the fully developed syndrome.

■ Treatment

Treatment of malignant hyperthermia consists of halting the anesthetic and the operation as soon as possible, eliminating the triggering agents immediately, administering dantrolene (which blocks calcium release), enhancing the monitoring (arterial and urinary bladder catheters, core temperature probe at the minimum), treating the biochemical abnormalities, and cooling the patient (Table 36-1). Sodium bicarbonate and hyperventilation are needed to treat

Table 36-1

Treatment of an Acute Episode of Malignant Hyperthermia

1. Discontinue all anesthetics; if the operation cannot be concluded immediately, narcotics and nondepolarizing muscle relaxants are safest.
2. Intubate the trachea and establish controlled hyperventilation to prevent hypercarbia and treat acidosis. Insert esophageal temperature probe at the same time.
3. Administer dantrolene 2 mg/kg intravenously every 5 minutes to a total dose of 10 mg/kg.
4. Administer sodium bicarbonate 2 to 4 mEg/kg; more may be required, depending on results of arterial blood gas analysis.
5. Apply ice to groin, axilla, and neck and iced irrigating solutions to stomach, bladder, and open body cavities as needed to maintain temperature below 40°C.
6. Insert arterial cannula, and draw blood for gas analysis, electrolyte determinations, glucose, BUN, creatinine, coagulation studies, acute CPK values, and urine and blood myoglobin and hemoglobin. Treat abnormalities as required.
7. Telephone the malignant hyperthermia hotline (209-634-4917, ask for Index Zero) for consultation as required.
8. Continue biochemical treatment as required, intravenous dantrolene, and monitoring in recovery room or intensive care unit at least overnight.

acidosis and hyperkalemia. Because of expected myoglobinuria, mannitol for diuresis is indicated. Cooling measures include administration of iced intravenous fluids, surface cooling with ice, gastric lavage with iced solutions, and heat exchange with a pump oxygenator. It has been recommended that the anesthesia machine be changed because of residual volatile anesthetic in the breathing circuit. This recommendation is not well founded, since the increased fresh gas flows (6 to 10 liters/min) quickly wash out residual anesthetic, and time spent obtaining an uncontaminated anesthesia machine is better spent on specific therapy. Appropriate supplies for treating malignant hyperthermia, including ice and iced solutions, dantrolene, and a flowsheet describing the appropriate therapy, must be maintained near all anesthetizing locations.

After the initial episode abates, intravenous dantrolene is continued at 12-hour intervals for at least 24 hours, and the patient is observed in a recovery room or intensive care unit because recurrence is possible. After the acute episode, an informative visit with patient and family and referral to the Malignant Hyperthermia Registry and a center where biopsies are offered are appropriate.

■ Anesthesia for Malignant Hyperthermia-Susceptible Patients

Patients known to be susceptible to malignant hyperthermia can be anesthetized safely. Prophylactic dantrolene, 2.5 mg/kg intravenously, shortly before beginning anesthesia (oral dantrolene is sometimes ineffective) blocks the onset of malignant hyperthermia. Anesthesia may be provided with nerve blocks, spinal or epidural anesthesia, or general anesthesia. The drugs recommended in Table 36-2 have established records of safety in humans and in malignant hyperthermia-susceptible swine. Flushing the anesthesia machine, ventilator, and breathing circuit with oxygen at moderate flows (10 liters/min) for an hour and removing or flushing until dry the vaporizers containing volatile anesthetics ensure that the inspired gas will not contain a triggering agent. Close monitoring of end-tidal CO_2 and temperature is required.

In some instances, a patient may have preoperative findings that suggest a possible susceptibility but do not warrant a biopsy. For example, a patient with bulky muscles and a family history of unknown

Table 36-2

Malignant Hyperthermia and Drugs Used in Anesthesia

Safe
  Barbiturates
  Etomidate
  Droperidol
  Opioids
  Nondepolarizing muscle relaxants (possible exception: curare)
  Anticholinesterases
  Local anesthetics, esters, and amides
  Nitrous oxide
  Antihistamines
  Propranolol
  Catecholamines and sympathomimetics
Known triggering agents, unsafe
  All inhalational anesthetics except nitrous oxide
  Depolarizing muscle relaxants: succinylcholine, decamethonium
Controversial or insufficient experience
  Curare
  Phenothiazines (increase intracellular calcium)
  Ketamine (likely a safe drug, but the hypertension and tachycardia of ketamine anesthesia would confuse the management of a patient susceptible to malignant hyperthermia)

difficulties with anesthesia in the distant past who requires a minor operation might not wish to obtain a biopsy. In these cases, anesthesia with an agent that does not trigger malignant hyperthermia is prudent, but prophylactic dantrolene is not warranted; monitoring of temperature and CO_2 production is required.

Toxicity of Anesthetics

Until relatively recently, it was thought that inhaled anesthetics were biologically inert; it is now clear that they all are metabolized to a variable extent and that they and their metabolites sometimes react with tissues to produce deleterious effects. Toxic effects are reproducible, dose-related, and predictable, whereas allergic reactions and those which depend on genetic predisposition (e.g., malignant hyperthermia) are not. The toxic effects of intravenous agents (e.g., etomidate and altered adrenal function) and the acute toxic effects of inhaled agents on the liver and kidney have been described previously. Other toxic effects have been proposed, usually

related to long-term exposure or to exposure during vulnerable periods of fetal development.

■ Carcinogenic Effects

Several surveys have raised the possibility that anesthesiologists, anesthetists, and dentists chronically exposed to small concentrations of anesthetics in the workplace may suffer an increased incidence of cancer. Many of these surveys are open to criticism for their design and show either no statistically significant increase in the incidence of cancer in exposed workers or small increases (50 percent increase in incidence, of borderline statistical significance). Nitrous oxide differs from the other inhaled anesthetics. First, it inhibits methionine synthetase, impairing synthesis of deoxyribonucleic acid (DNA) and producing bone marrow depression during prolonged exposure. Second, in a survey of dentists and chairside assistants, there was a marginally significant increase in the rate of cancer in those exposed to nitrous oxide.

The inhaled anesthetics are structurally similar to chemicals known to be carcinogens. In the initial animal testing of isoflurane, an increased incidence of liver tumors was observed in mice; this finding delayed the approval of isoflurane for human use by several years. However, it became apparent that the animals had been exposed to other known carcinogens, and the studies were repeated. These studies and others in which rats and mice have been exposed to the greatest concentrations of anesthetics they will tolerate over nearly their entire life spans have failed to show any carcinogenic effects from inhaled anesthetics.

At present, it is clear that patients are at no increased risk of cancer from therapeutic exposures to inhaled anesthetics. Although the risks of long-term exposure to trace concentrations of anesthetic for those in the operating room seem minimal, there is no reason to abandon the commonly used measures that reduce the contamination by anesthetics of the operating room atmosphere.

■ Teratogenesis and Anesthesia for Pregnant Patients

Some older anesthetics (divinyl ether and fluoroxene) alter DNA in vitro; of the current agents, only nitrous oxide and halothane have been found to have occasional weak effects in animal studies. No chromosomal aberrations have been found in patients or operating room workers exposed to anesthetics. These findings suggest that anesthetics are unlikely to alter genetic material.

Pregnant rats and mice exposed to anesthetics during the period that corresponds to the first trimester in humans produce an increased number of malformed fetuses. Similar effects for isoflurane, enflurane, and halothane occur only for prolonged exposures and very large doses. These findings of weak teratogenic potential suggest that human exposure to inhaled anesthetics during early pregnancy might result in fetal malformations.

Retrospective surveys among those who work in the operating room suggest small increases in the rate of spontaneous abortion (20 to 30 percent) but not in the rate of congenital defects. However, these studies depend on recall and do not differentiate between the effects of trace anesthetics and the effects of other elements in the operating room environment, including stress, activity, work hours, and radiation exposure.

Of the many surveys of the outcome of pregnancy in women exposed to operation and anesthesia, the most thorough involved a review of 2500 women in Manitoba, Canada, who underwent general anesthesia for operations during pregnancy. As compared with a matched cohort of pregnant women who did not undergo operation, the group of women studied suffered an increase in the rate of spontaneous abortion when operations and general anesthesia occurred during the first two trimesters, but there was no increase in the occurrence of congenital malformations among their babies. As with others, this study could not differentiate the effects of anesthesia from other effects of operation.

Thus there appears to be little risk of harmful effects on the fetus from exposure to typical amounts of inhaled anesthetics in patients or in those who care for them. Nevertheless, because of remaining uncertainty in the results of these studies, certain precautions are indicated in providing anesthesia for pregnant women. Because the risk of harm in animal models is greatest early in pregnancy, it is appropriate during preanesthetic evaluation to ask women of childbearing age whether they are likely to be pregnant. Elective operations can be postponed until after the pregnancy. More urgent operations can be performed safely. Especially later in pregnancy, management includes measures to ensure adequate uterine blood flow (see Chap. 26). Regional anesthesia may offer the advantage of minimal physiologic ef-

Table 36-3

Precautions to Reduce Environmental Exposure to Anesthetics in the Operating Room

1. Avoid leaks around face masks.
2. Use a waste gas scavenger to collect waste gas from breathing circuits and ventilators.
3. Conduct regular inspection and maintenance to detect and repair leaks in gas machines, piped gas supplies, connections, and fittings.
4. Assay to anesthetic gas concentrations in operating rooms detect problems.
5. Shut off vaporizer and nitrous oxide when the breathing circuit is not attached to patient.
6. Provide adequate operating room ventilation.

fects, but general anesthesia appears to be safe as well.

■ Preventing Occupational Exposure to Anesthetics

There are still no data that define safe concentrations of anesthetic vapors for those with prolonged exposures, such as operating room personnel. In surveys, some operating rooms have been found to have peak concentrations of nitrous oxide of 5000 parts per million (ppm) and of halothane of 50 ppm. By employing simple precautions (Table 36-3), these concentrations can be reduced to the levels that the government has recommended (but not required by regulation): 0.5 ppm for volatile agents and 25 ppm for nitrous oxide.

Infections

■ Infection of Patients

In the hospital, patients may acquire infections from other patients or from providers of care. This hazard is reduced in anesthesia practice by the routine use of aseptic precautions, gloves, and other elements of sterile technique, as well as disposable needles and other equipment for vascular access. An important precaution is to discard syringes and contaminated multidose vials at the end of each anesthetic. The prevention of the spread of infections via airway equipment is not so straightforward. Sterile, disposable endotracheal tubes and single-use oral and nasal airways are now standard. Whether breathing circuits used in anesthesia are sources of infection for patients

Table 36-4

Precautions to Prevent the Spread of Blood–Borne Viral Illness such as HIV or Hepatitis in Anesthesia Practice

1. Hepatitis B immunization.
2. Eliminate the use of needles as far as practical. Use stopcocks in intravenous sets instead of injection ports.
3. Safe handling and disposal of needles, scalpels, and other sharp objects.
4. Routine use of gloves for all procedures such as intubation, placing intravenous catheters, and handling patient's secretions. Avoid injury by patients' teeth.
5. Frequent hand washing.
6. Proper disposal of contaminated waste.
7. Effective methods of cleaning and sterilizing instruments and surfaces.
8. Goggles, eyeglasses, or other protection for eyes during awake intubation or during surgical procedures that scatter bone, blood, or tissue fragments.

is difficult to establish, but it is now standard practice to use disposable breathing tubes, to interpose a filter between the patient and the breathing circuit, or to wash the breathing circuit in germicidal solutions between uses. Laryngoscope blades require cleaning in germicidal solution between uses as well.

Varicella is a particular hazard to immunosuppressed patients, such as those with transplanted organs or human immunodeficiency virus (HIV) infection. It is important to protect patients from hospital personnel who might spread varicella virus.

■ Infection of Anesthesia Personnel

Although one can acquire almost any infection from a patient in the course of anesthesia practice, the two of greatest concern currently are hepatitis C and HIV. Although transmission of HIV from patient to anesthetist has not yet appeared as a major vector for this virus, the well-documented risk of hepatitis infection makes it appropriate to take precautions against both viral diseases (Table 36-4). Because not all infected patients can be detected, it is wise to manage all patient using these techniques (universal precautions).

Electrical Safety

Because of the large number of electrical devices attached during anesthesia and operation, patients are

vulnerable to electrical burns and shocks. A complete review of the physics of electric currents lies beyond the scope of this chapter, but the precautions required for safety are uncomplicated.

■ Microshock and Macroshock

The mechanisms of death from increasing electric current are arrhythmias, respiratory paralysis, and massive tissue injury from heating (rare except in industrial accidents or legal electrocution). The biologic effects of various currents are given in Table 36-5. Electrical effects on the heart depend on current density; whereas very small currents of a few microamperes delivered directly to the heart can produce electrical responses, much larger whole-body currents greater than 100 mA are needed before the current passing through the heart is great enough to do harm to that organ.

Macroshock in the operating room is prevented by attaching the chassis of the equipment to ground, by routine maintenance, and in some hospitals, by isolated power supplies. These devices consist of a

Table 36-5

Significant Electric Currents in Humans

Current	Biologic Effect in Humans
0.010 mA	Maximum leakage current allowed for devices in contact with the heart; designed to prevent microshock
0.050 mA	Probably lower limit of current that will produce fibrillation if applied directly to heart
0.3 mA @ 60 Hz	Threshold for sensation
1 mA @ 60 Hz	Threshold for pain
2 mA	Maximum current permitted by isolated power before line isolation monitor sounds alarm
10 mA @ 60 Hz	"Let go" current; subject is unable to relax grasp and let go of current source
100 mA	Usual whole-body resistance of 100 ohms; when connected to household current supply of 110 V, permits current of about 100 mA
>100 mA @ 60 Hz	Whole-body current required to produce ventricular fibrillation
100 mA/cm²	Current density (current per unit area) at which burns occur

mA = milliampere.

transformer interposed between the main power source and the distribution system for the operating room. In contrast to ordinary power distribution systems, neither of the arms of the circuit in an isolated supply is connected to ground. Thus, even if a patient or a worker touches a piece of equipment that has become "live" through a fault in the insulation, a circuit to ground is not completed. A line isolation monitor constantly monitors the system for failure of insulation between either arm of the circuit and ground; insulation faults that could allow currents of 2 mA or more trigger the alarm. When the alarm sounds, there is only the potential for an electrical hazard and the current is not shut off, but it is important to investigate immediately the cause of the fault and disconnect the responsible equipment. The alarm threshold of 2 mA is low enough to prevent macroshock but does not guarantee against possible microshock.

Microshock occurs when currents as small as a few microamperes pass through low-resistance pathways, such as pacemaker wires or saline-filled catheters, directly to the heart. Because these pathways offer so little resistance to current flow, very small potential differences may produce lethal currents. Devices that might cause microshock are now designed with internal isolated power supplies, high-impedance patient connections, and optically isolated signal paths to reduce the chance of this complication, which now seems to be rare. When external pacemaker wires are exposed or saline-filled catheters are used to obtain intracardiac electrocardiogram (ECG) signals, special care must be employed.

■ Electrosurgery

Radiofrequency electrosurgery units cut or coagulate tissue with electric current. Because the tip of the operating electrode is small, local current densities are great; the return electrode attached to the patient's skin with adhesive and a conductive gel is large, keeping current density below the threshold for damage to tissue. The current is supplied at 0.3 to 2 MHz to reduce the chance of ventricular fibrillation. Unwanted burns can occur at the site of an improperly applied return pad if the path for the return of current to the electrosurgical unit offers greater than usual impedance. In the same situation, high-frequency electrocautery currents may pass by capacitive coupling to ECG wires or other devices that offer a return path to ground, causing burns at these sites. Careful

attention when attaching the electrocautery ground pad and placing it as close to the operative site as possible help prevent burns.

■ Pacemakers

Patients with implanted pacemakers often require operations. Usually, no difficulties are encountered. However, current from the electrocautery may induce a signal in the pacemaker leads that a demand-type pacemaker may interpret as cardiac electrical activity, causing it to stop pacing; this induced current also may produce microshock, but this seems rare. Risks are minimized by using a bipolar electrocautery, in which current flows only between two small electrodes in the cautery wand. The anesthesiologist must be prepared to convert the pacemaker to fixed-rate operation if necessary.

Addiction

Addiction to opioids and other drugs does not seem to be a significant hazard for patients in the operating room, but there is risk of addiction among those who administer anesthesia. Listing addiction as a "hazard of anesthesia" implies that choosing anesthesia as a career increases one's liability to addiction. This proposition has not yet been proved; data about the true prevalence of drug abuse among the population at large, among physicians, and among anesthesiologists are so difficult to gather that it is impossible to state with certainty that anesthesiologists are more likely to be addicted than are other physicians or the general populace. There is also some indication that those who choose anesthesia as a career are more likely to have personalities that predispose them to becoming addicts. The addict may make anesthesia a career instead of the career making the addict. Indeed, survey of causes of death among anesthesiologists found a disproportionate incidence of suicide.

Nevertheless, the data that are available are worrisome. Anesthesiologists are disproportionately likely to be found in drug rehabilitation programs as compared with other physicians, and they seem to use a wider variety of drugs and to be more likely to take drugs intravenously. The anesthesiologist's work environment may increase the risk of substance abuse, both because of the tension and anxieties of providing or supervising anesthesia and because of the unique availability of drugs. Death owing to inadvertent or intentional overdose is frequently reported in surveys of drug abuse among anesthesiologists.

Departments of anesthesia and individual anesthesiologists can take steps to reduce the prevalence of the problem and the severity of its consequences. First, individuals can seek counseling when emotional problems seem overwhelming or when there is a temptation to experiment with drugs. Although this simple advice is notoriously futile (because of the strong effects of denial), it is worth giving and worth heeding. Second, departments can establish programs to detect and treat addicted individuals (an example of such a policy has been published by the ASA). The limits of these programs are established by the rights of the individual against unreasonable surveillance and, at the other extreme, by the anesthesia department's obligation to ensure that those who provide care for patients do so with their mental faculties unimpaired.

BIBLIOGRAPHY

Brown DL, ed. *Risk and Outcome in Anesthesia*, 2nd ed. Philadelphia: JB Lippincott, 1992.

Cooper JB, Newbower RS, Kitz RJ. An analysis of major errors and equipment failures in anesthesia management: Considerations for prevention and detection. *Anesthesiology* 1984;60:34-42.

Duncan PG, Pope WDB, Cohen MM, et al. Fetal risk of anesthesia and surgery during pregnancy. *Anesthesiology* 1986;64:790-794.

O'Flynn RP, Shutack JG, Rosenberg H, Fletcher JE. Masseter muscle rigidity and malignant hyperthermia susceptibility in pediatric patients. *Anesthesiology* 1994;80:1228-1233.

CHAPTER **37**

The Law and Anesthesia Practice

Alan J. Ominsky

Anesthesia Practice and The Law

Today, many who practice anesthesia can expect to be involved in legal action alleging malpractice, either as defendant or as expert witness. Even if one does not come to be part of a suit, the cost of malpractice insurance and the threat of legal action now influence the ways in which physicians practice, relations with patients, fee structures, and equipment purchases. This chapter reviews briefly some relevant legal principles (in the United States), the means of minimizing legal risk, and what to do in the event of an accident or untoward medical outcome.

■ Torts

Malpractice concepts are part of tort law. A *tort* is an action or inaction that society has declared to be unlawful through a series of decisions in court; these are wrongful acts even though no formal contract or statue is violated. For example, the courts have consistently required a professional to act "reasonably" and with the care required to similar members of the profession. Some courts also have held that failure to adopt a new procedure that would clearly increase safety at little or no risk is negligent, even if the new procedure is not yet widely used.

■ Variations Among States

Conditions of law under which malpractice suits may be pursued successfully vary among the states. Where the legislature has spoken by passing a statute, the courts are obligated to follow the clear language of that statute. For example, so-called statutes of limitations are virtually always laws passed by the state's legislature to define the permissible time after an alleged injury occurs during which a person retains their right to sue. This period varies considerably from state to state. Courts can effectively alter statutes by the process of interpreting that statute. Based purely on this process of judicial interpretation, in many states the period of time before the plaintiff first has reason to suspect that an injury has occurred does not count against the time during which a plaintiff still retains the right to file suit.

Because the plaintiff has the "burden of proof," plaintiffs often have considerable more choice about where a lawsuit is adjudicated than do defendants. This can be very important to outcome, since the forum selected can be important with regard to which state's law will govern the outcome, what types of pretrial discovery will be permitted, what rules of evidence will govern trial procedure, how soon the case is likely to come to trial, and whether the jury is likely to favor economic "haves" (usually the defendant physicians in a medical malpractice suit) or the economic "have-nots." If the suit is of sufficient financial magnitude and all plaintiffs come from a different state than do all the defendants, either the plaintiff or the defendant may be able to have the suit adjudicated in federal rather than state court.

■ Trials and Appeals

In theory, judges decide what the law is, and the jury decides what the true facts are. For example, the judge in some states will instruct the jury that as part of informed consent, a doctor will be required by the law to provide only that information which a "reasonable doctor" would provide. In other states, the judge will instruct the jury that a doctor must provide those facts which a "reasonable patient" would require to make an intelligent decision. This can turn out to be a quite different standard. If there is a dispute as to what facts a doctor did or did not provide, or about whether the facts provided were sufficient for a reasonable patient to make an informed decision, this dispute is resolved by the jury.

For the most part, only decisions about what the law is, rather than what the facts were, can be appealed. Except on the rarest occasions, courts of appeal do not second-guess the jury as to what the facts actually were, since the appellate judges are not able to listen to the witnesses and to weigh their credibility. While juries are generally given great deference about what was or was not "reasonable," this deference is not absolute, and both the trial and appellate judges occasionally overrule juries when their decisions are completely inconsistent with undisputed evidence. Nevertheless, it is by far the exception for either side to lose a civil case in court and then win it on appeal.

■ Nature of Malpractice

Malpractice, or to use the preferred term, *medical negligence,* consists of failure to employ methods, agents, or skills ordinarily considered appropriate, and having that failure result in harm. Unfortunately, any practitioner sooner or later does something negligent. Usually, these errors are discovered and corrected before they cause serious harm. Physicians who are sued when such a careless act does produce harm need not be completely unforgiving with themselves; none of us is without fault.

Just because a hoped-for result does not follow or complications occur after an anesthetic does not imply liability, unless the complication arises from improper care or the physician is foolish enough to have promised a specific result. Physicians must also recognize that they may be sued without merit. When that happens, they must not take to heart the inflammatory language of the usual legal complaint. These are only accusations, and are overstated for effect.

On the other hand, many malpractice actions are justified, particularly when results are both catastrophic and unanticipated. In a study of 104 cases drawn at random from an insurance company's files, 26 cases involved cardiac arrest during anesthesia or immediately after anesthesia; the anesthetic care afforded was unacceptable in all 26, and this group accounted for 99 percent of the total cost of the settlements and judgments rendered in the 104 cases.

Judgments concerning medical negligence hinge on the requirement of reasonable behavior by a physician, but what is reasonable depends on circumstances and the state of the art at the time. Thus, experts disagree on what is reasonable, and the result of a trial often depends largely on the jury's choice of which experts to believe.

Understandably, many physicians are uncomfortable when nonphysician jurors decide what constitutes reasonable professional behavior. However, physicians can take comfort from the fact that well over two-thirds of the medical cases brought to plaintiff lawyers for possible suit are rejected by the lawyers, after consultation with doctors, for obvious lack of merit. Further, well over two-thirds of the medical negligence cases that are tried result in a verdict in the favor of the defendant physician.

■ Settling Out of Court

Once begun, a medical negligence suit may be interrupted at any point. The plaintiff may learn through counsel's advice that there is no legitimate basis for a suit; the defendant may be forewarned that there is unquestionable liability and settlement is advisable; after hearing depositions, either party may make settlement; the plaintiff may not find experts to testify that there was malpractice; finally, a settlement can be arranged with the aid of the judge during the trial, prior to the jury's verdict. Plaintiffs may be motivated to settle by the guarantee of a financial return as opposed to the uncertainty of a trial. Defendants may be motivated to settle not only to avoid the uncertainty of a trial but also because the expense of defending successfully against a suit (defendant's expenses are not incorporated in the award through contingency arrangements, as are the plaintiff's expenses) can be as costly as an adverse verdict. Only a small proportion of malpractice suits proceed to trial and a court verdict.

■ Conflicts of Interest Between Physician and Insurer

Since January 1991, a federal statute has required every adverse judgment or settlement to be reported to a national registry. Every hospital is required to query that registry at the time of any new staff appointment or reappointment. Fear of an adverse entry in the registry might prompt a physician to defend against a suit despite the insurance company's recommendation that it might be less expensive to settle the case without trial. Some insurance policies specify that a suit may not be settled by the insurance company without the defendant physician's consent. A conflict between the physician and the insurance company also may arise when an insurer refuses to offer an amount equal to the limits of the policy to settle a meritorious case, thereby exposing the physician to personal liability in excess of insurance protection.

Even though it is the insurance company that is paying the defense attorney's bill, that attorney is required to represent the physician's best interests and to inform the physician of any possible conflict of interest between the insurance company and the defendant physician. In case of a significant conflict, the defense attorney is wise to suggest that the physician obtain independent representation. Failure to make such a suggestion when appropriate can expose both the defense attorney and the insurance company to legal liability. Physicians can also raise these issues themselves; if consultation with the defense attorney is not adequately reassuring, it is wise to seek independent counsel. Lawyers, just as do doctors, have the professional obligation to give their clients enough information to participate in informed decision making.

■ Proof of Malpractice: Expert Opinion, Res Ipsa Loquitur

Proof of malpractice can be established in several ways. Most commonly, the plaintiff and defendant produce expert testimony to establish the standard of care for the specialty involved. Once, physicians were

notably reluctant to testify against colleagues; today, more are willing to do so, especially when standards of patient care have not been met. Thus the accusation of a "conspiracy of silence" is of less merit now than it was previously. Sometimes, expert witnesses recruited by the plaintiff provide evidence in favor of the defendant and vice versa, but this is rare in court, except in fiction.

Because physicians were once reluctant to participate, the law developed the doctrine of res ipsa loquitur, which in certain cases, for practical purposes, eliminates the need for expert testimony. Literally, the res ipsa doctrine says, "the act speaks for itself." This usually has been applied in situations where harm could not possibly have occurred except through negligence. However, except when foreign objects are left in the body after a surgical or diagnostic procedure, expert testimony is still needed to establish the proposition that a given result would not have occurred except through negligence.

■ Patient Rapport and the Chances of Being Sued

The chance of a suit increases greatly when physicians fail to establish rapport with their patients. Anesthesiologists are at special risk, since opportunities for contact with patients outside the operating room are few and visits too often are completed hastily. If one anesthesiologist performs the preoperative evaluation and then another anesthetizes the patient without first having established rapport, the liability for misunderstanding is increased further. When a preoperative examination has been omitted and postoperative visits are not made, the patient may not remember the anesthesiologist at all until the bill arrives. Obviously, under these circumstances, a bond of understanding between patient and physician has not been established, and the stage is set for resentment if anything goes even a bit wrong.

Responsibilities of Medical Students, Residents, and Nurse Anesthetists

■ Students and Residents

Medical students and resident physicians are not immune to court action and must be protected by malpractice insurance. Rarely are they named as sole defendants; more likely, they are named as one of several, including the supervising anesthesiologist, perhaps the surgeon, and the hospital. Medical students pursuing courses for credit and registered with a university or college are usually protected against suit through the institution, sometimes by the hospital and occasionally by both, provided that they act under the supervision of a faculty member on the staff at the hospital.

However, students who are under preceptorships, who are taking elective courses not approved by the medical school, or who are training in hospitals or working with physicians unaffiliated with a medical school should inquire as to their protection rather than assume that they are protected and therefore bear no risk. House staff, likewise are protected through the hospital or medical center in which they are training, but they can inquire as to insurance protection and, if need be, secure it for themselves. Residents who engage in extramural part-time work must recognize that they are not protected outside the parent institution unless they have made prior arrangements with an insurance carrier.

■ Nurse Anesthetists

A nurse anesthetist can be held liable for negligence in the administration of anesthesia, and it appears that the incidence of malpractice cases against nurses is increasing. This person is assumed to be responsible for the technical administration of the anesthetic, for the observation and recording of vital signs, and for the welfare of the patient. Most certified registered nurse anesthetists (CRNAs) avail themselves of malpractice protection.

When a suit involves the actions of a nurse anesthetist, the likelihood is that legal responsibility for those actions will be shared at least in part by others. If a surgeon or anesthesiologist supervises a nurse in the administration of an anesthetic, under the "borrowed servant" doctrine, the nurse is an assistant of the physician, and the latter must assume responsibility. If an anesthesiologist or surgeon employs the nurse or advises the hospital as to the qualifications or conditions of employment, the anesthesiologist is responsible, even though not directly concerned in supervision at the time of an alleged act of negligence. Under the doctrine of "joint and several responsibility," where multiple defendants share any responsibility for negligence, a plaintiff is free to collect the entire judgment, if he or she wishes, from the defendant with the greatest resources ("deepest pockets," rarely the nurse or resident) even if that defendant bears relatively minor responsibility. The defendant who pays is then free to try to seek reimbursement from others for their proportional share, but that is of little practical importance if a more responsible defendant has few assets.

■ Hospital's Liability and Quality Assurance

The last two decades have seen an important expansion of two theories of law, *respondeat superior* and *corporate liability,* within the doctrine of hospital liability. The impetus for change came from the case of *Darling v Charleston Community Hospital* (1966), in which hospital liability was extended to include failure, through control of staff membership and clinical privileges, to monitor the care provided by attending physicians. To hold a hospital liable on corporate liability theory, a plaintiff must show that the hospital knew, or should have known, that the physician (and presumably the resident or nurse) whose negligence caused the plaintiff's injury was providing substandard care.

The implications of this doctrine include the need for hospitals, through their responsible physicians, to routinely survey the clinical privileges and clinical competence of professional staff. In a malpractice action against a southwestern for-profit hospital and a CRNA, the hospital made a large pretrial settlement on behalf of the brain-damaged plaintiff, acknowledging that its board of trustees neither established guidelines for quality control in hiring and overseeing CRNAs nor delineated the supervising responsibilities of surgeons and anesthesiologists for those CRNAs employed by the hospital.

Minimizing Legal Risk

■ Preparation for Anesthesia and Informed Consent

Pertinent points of the history must always be summarized on the patient's chart along with results of the physical examination and interview, including a statement of any unusual risk involved, the type of anesthesia planned, and the reasons for the choice if the choice has possible disadvantages. If such a procedure were always followed, many a lawsuit would be avoided.

The problem of *informed consent* must be considered at the time of the interview with the patient, and a notation made on the chart. Patients not only must sign a statement authorizing operation and anesthesia but also must thoroughly understand what is to be done. The patient is given the opportunity to ask questions or to make a choice if any is to be made. This does not mean that the anesthesiologist presents the patient with a "shopping list" of agents and techniques; few patients have the competence to make such a selection. Informed patient choices are more likely to involve regional versus general anesthesia, intravenous induction versus inhalation induction, premedication versus no premedication, and so on.

What constitutes adequate informed consent? The various states have different interpretations, some insisting that every possible complication be described to the patient, others recommending to speak only of likely complications and tempering what is said. In general, a physician may not withhold facts or even minimize risks to induce the patient's consent. At the same time, the physician must place the welfare of the patient first; this requirement may conflict with the need to inform the patient. One alternative is to explain to the patient every risk no matter how remote, risking alarming the patient and thereby doing harm. The other alternative is to recognize that each patient presents a separate problem, that the patient's mental and emotional condition may be crucial, and that in discussing the element of risk a certain amount of discretion must be employed. The physician may choose in unusual instances to share certain information only with the patient's family, but this must clearly be the exception rather than the rule.

The anesthesiologist must go into detail about possible complications if an unusual drug or technique is to be used or if the patient is susceptible to a particular complication, such as the dislodging of loose or diseased teeth during laryngoscopy. The note on the record includes a statement that the anesthesiologist has described the proposed anesthetic and that the patient understands. When new drugs or techniques are to be used, or when patients are in critical condition or are to undergo prolonged, complicated operations, it is best to have them sign for both understanding and consent.

■ Shared Responsibility with Surgeon

Once a patient has been delivered into the hands of the anesthesiologist, the anesthesiologist assumes responsibility for the patient, except when this is shared by the surgeon. Depending on the specific situation, positioning of the patient for operation may be the responsibility of the surgeon, the anesthesiologist, or both. In this and other matters of shared responsibility, differences of opinion are best resolved promptly, but without writing in the chart accusatory notes likely to harm all potential defendants, including the writer.

The surgeon is not usually responsible for the conduct of anesthesia because the anesthesiologist is in effect an independent contractor. However, both physicians have a duty to protect the patient, to the extent they can, against obvious negligence on the part of the other.

■ Legal Aspects of Monitoring

In the event that new techniques, equipment, or agents are employed, anesthesiologists should be able to substantiate their familiarity with these methods and an understanding of any complications that may arise from their use.

What monitoring devices are required during general anesthetic procedures? There is no unanimity on this question; this text's recommendations appear in Chapter 6, and the American Society of Anesthesiologists has approved standards for basic intraoperative monitoring. In the opinion of many experts, pulse oximetry and capnography are now so cost-effective at preventing catastrophe that routine failure to employ them might be considered presumptive negligence.

Anesthesiologists are not ordinarily responsible for maintenance of nonanesthetic equipment in operating rooms, although they must be certain that a routine preventive inspection program is in place. They are responsible for seeing that anesthesia equipment is regularly inspected and serviced.

Anesthesiologists are wise to point out to the hospital administration improper control of humidity and ventilation, inadequate disposal of waste gases, and obvious electrocution hazards associated with electrocautery, electrocardiography, and other devices. If anesthesiologists find that such equipment is defective and continue to use it, they are quite likely to be held liable for resulting accidents.

■ Records

The best protection an anesthesiologist can devise against suit is an accurate and complete anesthesia record with written observations at regular intervals as the operation and anesthesia progress. A record must never be altered after the fact. If items of information are recorded subsequently, these must be clearly indicated as additions. In at least some states it is a presumption of law that anything that would customarily be recorded but was not recorded, was not done.

■ Blood Component Infusion

The kinds and quantities of parenteral fluids given during operation are best determined by consensus between surgeon and anesthesiologist. The physician who starts a transfusion is responsible for identifying each unit of blood or component given and determining that it has been matched properly. The anesthesiologist must be aware of the hazards of blood transfusion and must be certain that the indications for transfusion are valid.

■ Postoperative Care

Responsibilities of the anesthesiologist do not cease when the patient is transported from the operating room; observation continues until care is assigned to another competent person. If dissatisfied with the patient's condition, the anesthesiologist is responsible for remaining in attendance. In most institutions, the recovery room is supervised by an anesthesiologist. A detailed record of the patient's progress in the recovery room is essential, and the release of a patient from the recovery room must be signed by a physician.

During postoperative visits, discussion of the anesthetic experience can be encouraged; if the patient is dissatisfied, this is usually apparent. It is the disgruntled patient not given the opportunity to express dissatisfaction who may ultimately sue. An appropriate note is written in the patient's record after each visit.

Testimony at Deposition or Trial

If called upon to testify at a deposition, a physician is well advised to set aside the time for one or more preparation sessions with the attorney, the first at least a week in advance of the deposition. Of the greatest importance is to tell the truth, but avoid speculation. What may seem like a helpful answer in context may be devastating if it is shown to be untrue or it is employed by the plaintiff's attorney in some unanticipated way. Cases with otherwise relatively minor damages have been converted into economic catastrophes for physicians when juries became convinced that those physicians had given false testimony or made a self-serving change in a record.

If called to testify at trial or at a video deposition, the physician's greatest enemy is likely to be any appearance of arrogance. A patient one makes unnecessarily angry is far more likely to sue; similarly, a jury can be antagonized by a defendant's manner. Doctors need good bedside manners to help stay out of court and to win when they cannot.

There are hard choices faced by an anesthesiologist called upon to provide expert testimony in a medical negligence case. Experts have an obligation to other members of their specialty to distinguish between a failure to follow their own particular preference and a failure to follow defensible practice. They also must distinguish between a breach in the standard of care that has no ill consequences and one that caused the harm of which a plaintiff complains. Frivolous malpractice cases are rarely initiated in the absence of frivolous or poorly thought out expert reports. However, when care is indeed improper, physicians with the time and expertise to do so have a moral obligation to testify on behalf of an injured plaintiff. Moreover, a physician who is willing to testify for plaintiffs when indicated is far more effective and believable when he or she appears as a defense witness in another case than is a physician who never testifies except for the defense.

In the Event of an Error or a Complication

Medicine cannot be practiced without accidents or complications. Most patients are understanding and are satisfied by a frank discussion of problems. However, if the physician belittles or ignores a complication or fails to impart sympathetic understanding, the stage is set for malpractice action.

In the event of an accident or complication definitely or possible related to anesthesia, the anesthesiologist must document the facts in the patient's chart in chronological order during or immediately following administration of anesthesia. The notes include the treatment employed and the consultative opinions obtained. Subsequent notes are made in the chart periodically during the remainder of the patient's course.

The anesthesiologist must immediately provide the hospital and the insurer with a complete account of an accident but must be aware that the contents of such reports may be discoverable by the plaintiff. Should a suit be threatened or legal inquiry made, the physician must also notify the insurer and, where appropriate, seek legal assistance. Many large hospitals now retain full-time attorneys, whose advice may be sought. Failure to carry out these obligations within a reasonable period has resulted in loss of protection from insurers.

The anesthesiologist's best protection against medicolegal action lies in the thorough and up-to-date practice of anesthesia, coupled with sympathetic interest in the patient and maintenance of detailed records on the course of anesthesia. One must keep in mind that sickness does not deprive the patient of legal rights and that physicians cannot impose what they think is advisable simply because they know what is in the patient's best interest. Patients and their families must be given the information on which to base their decisions.

BIBLIOGRAPHY

Peters JD, Fineberg KS, Kroll DA, et al. *Anesthesiology and the law.* Ann Arbor, Mich: Health Administration Press, 1983.

Weisbard AJ. Defensive law: A new perspective on informed consent. *Arch Intern Med* 1986; 146:860.

CHAPTER 38

The Further Study of Anesthesiology

Frank L. Murphy

Leaving school and embarking on a career in anesthesia demands that the student adapt to new ways of learning, significantly different from those used before beginning clinical training. To ensure progress in learning clinical anesthesia, the learner and the instructor must understand the nature of clinical education and make good use of the opportunities available for education. This last chapter offers direct suggestions for the study of anesthesia beyond the reading of an introductory text.

Learning Outside School

Anesthesia training differs from school because of several factors: the learners, the subject matter, the methods of learning, the teachers, and the environment.

Residents and nurses in clinical training are adults whose educational needs differ from those of the younger students found in schools. They are older, with less resilient and retentive minds; learning may come more slowly, and fatigue can be a problem. They carry financial and family responsibilities that compete for their attention. Motivation comes from within; adults are less likely to learn simply because they are told to do so. An anesthesia resident planning a career as a laboratory investigator has learning goals different from one with previous training in psychology who plans a clinical career in pain management. Further, adults often learn best if allowed to employ their own styles of learning as much as possible rather than being forced into a lock-step program.

Before clinical training, learning in school is perceived largely as cognitive: A body of information is to be learned. In addition to simply acquiring information, clinical trainees also must learn complex behaviors, the intellectual foundations of their knowledge, and an array of skills (for some this is the first opportunity to learn mechanical skills). To master this noncognitive material, classroom teaching is less useful, and on-the-job training and independent study are more important. Teaching is less structured, and responsibility rests jointly on both student and instructor to ensure that such informal instruction is productive.

As compared with those in schools, clinical instructors are not primarily teachers. They have no formal training as teachers and receive their salaries largely in return for clinical care or research, not for instruction. Although the instructor is likely to be an expert and to have a great deal of information to impart, the learner may have to contribute as much to the tutorial relationship as does the instructor.

The environment for learning clinical anesthesia differs markedly from school. A resident is an employee who receives a salary for providing the services of a physician; the job is so demanding, and the responsibility of taking care of patients is so important, that residents' roles as learners may be overlooked in day-to-day work. Similar perceptions affect nurse anesthetists in training. In addition, everyone around clinical trainees (operating room nurses, consultants, surgeons, supervisors, and peers) is likely to evaluate them for their clinical skills, not as learners. Fatigue, a constant factor in trainees' lives, not only robs them of the time and energy for formal study but also may prevent them from learning from clinical experience.

All these characteristics distinguish clinical learners from undergraduate students and clinical training from school. Clinical training in anesthesia more closely resembles continuing medical education for the practitioner than it does college, nursing school, or medical school. Successful trainees recognize the differences and adapt to the novel ways of learning.

Learning Anesthesia

Learning clinical anesthesia requires that the learner not only accept the instruction offered by the training program but also take advantage of situations that motivate learning and follow an overall plan that takes into account individual goals and learning styles. Some of these opportunities and plans are described below.

■ Reading

Reading is the most important and efficient means by which clinical trainees gain information. Readers may choose an appropriate level of instruction that takes into account their backgrounds and goals and can reread a passage until it is understood. Editorials, review articles, and scientific articles in journals and textbooks are written and edited with more care than all except the best lectures. Reading during and after training must become a regular habit; there is too much material to learn by any other means.

An appropriate reading program begins with an introductory text, completed in the first month of training, and progresses to one of the large comprehensive texts, read over the next 6 months. Even though not all this material is retained at first, familiarity with the specialty provides a framework for other reading. At present, no one comprehensive textbook is clearly superior to the others, because all are multiauthored texts; direct comparison of chapters dealing with the same subject shows that each book has its own strengths and weaknesses. The drawback to this suggestion is that motivation for daily reading

is weak. Other reading, begun at the same time, benefits from more immediate motivation.

First, at least one case each day should provoke additional reading to learn about a new anesthetic drug or procedure, an intercurrent disease, an incidental medication, or a new surgical procedure or to respond to an instructor's suggestion. At first, this study will involve one or more of the comprehensive textbooks; later, sources such as specialty texts, journals, and electronic databases become important. Material learned in this active way is retained better than that covered in routine or assigned reading. Second, similar motivation comes during subspecialty rotations (such as obstetrical anesthesia), when the student will find it easy to read and remember material from specialty texts. Third, learners can begin reading journals regularly at the start of the residency. In the United States, it is best to begin with two major journals, *Anesthesiology* and *Anesthesia and Analgesia*, both of which are provided as part of inexpensive resident memberships in the sponsoring organizations. Other journals and the periodicals that provide review articles can be valuable additions to a reading program, but they may require more time and money than trainees have to spend on them. To make the reading of journals more efficient, learners can read selectively, focusing on major scientific articles accompanied by editorial comment, medical intelligence articles, and the letters, which often expose the reader to a wide range of opinions expressed in a lively format. Before accepting the conclusions offered in an article, it is best to read it critically, making notes and filing them for later use (Table 38-1).

■ The Personal Library

At first, the expense of buying medical texts makes accumulating a useful library seem impossible. However, a personal collection of books and journals can be accumulated at relatively modest cost (Table 38-2). Books to be included in this library are those required for close study or for frequent reference. Less commonly used items may be found in departmental or hospital libraries. Access to electronic searching of the National Medical Library is essential and can be found at any medical library or obtained on-line through one's own computer. There are now numerous videotapes and computer-based offerings, ranging from programs that simulate anesthesia management or uptake and distribution of anesthetic gases, to videotaped lectures and learning programs, to text-

Table 38-1

Questions to Ask About a Scientific Article in a Medical Journal

1. What type of article is it?
   a. A report of a single case
   b. A report of a series of cases
   c. A retrospective study based on a series of cases
   d. A controlled clinical trial
   e. An in vivo laboratory study
   f. An in vitro laboratory study
2. What hypothesis did the study test? Do the findings validate or reject the hypothesis? Summarize the findings in a single sentence.
3. Why was the study undertaken? Does it provide new information that reinforces or contradicts what the reader already knows? How does this article compare with others on related subjects?
4. Under what clinical circumstances are the findings of this study important? How and when will the reader put this information to use? Here the reader must avoid the temptation to view animal studies as irrelevant while also resisting the urge to apply laboratory information uncritically, without first evaluating the validity of the animal model.

At first it will be difficult for the beginner to put studies in perspective; the discussion section of the paper, an accompanying editorial, and reference to textbooks will help. Answering these questions will help assimilate the information in an article. It may seem to the reader that the study did not provide a valid answer to an important question, this may be the fault of the study and not the reader.

books recorded on compact discs with useful searching programs included. At present, many of these interesting and useful items are worth consulting in the library, but all are beginning efforts, too incomplete, expensive, and underdeveloped to warrant a trainee including them in a personal library.

■ Learning from Cases

In clinical training, relatively little time is spent in formal instruction. Since most of the time is spent managing patients' anesthetics, this clinical experience must contribute to learning as much as possible. Each case begins with a thorough, problem-oriented note and a socratic discussion with the instructor. During this discussion, the instructor raises questions as in an oral examination and provides not only some of the answers but also guidance for reading. Learners can improve this experience not only by participating willingly but also by drawing out reticent instructors with suggestions for alternative plans for managing

anesthesia. Reading for the case also enhances learning, as does even a brief discussion with the supervisor after the anesthetic is concluded. Occasionally, something about the case suggests further study; from this beginning may arise a case report, review article, or a scientific study.

■ Lectures, Conferences

Compared with reading and individual study, lectures are inefficient means of conveying information to learners; there is not time enough to impart by lecture all the required information. Lectures are of greatest value when they convey a lecturer's unique insights, when their content is designed around local needs, or when they synthesize and make understandable material that is confusing or not presented clearly in available written material.

Interactive forms of group teaching, such as seminars and clinical case conferences, make learners into participants instead of spectators. These conferences, however, only reach their full potential when they are based on firm scientific information rather than simple recollections of prior experience. Clinical trainees can improve their learning by participating actively in these conferences. Journal clubs and opportunities to teach medical students provide the same benefits of active participation.

Table 38-2

A Minimum Personal Library in Anesthesia

1. An introductory text.
2. The most recent edition of at least one comprehensive text; two are better.
3. The current edition of a pharmacology text.
4. One of the texts describing the anesthesia management of patients with uncommon diseases.
5. Specialty texts (e.g., obstetrical anesthesia) according to the recommendations at the end of the various chapters in this book or faculty preference.
6. Journals
   Subscriptions:
   Anesthesiology
   Anesthesia and Analgesia
   New England Journal of Medicine
   Follow in library or subscribe as time and money permit:
   British Journal of Anaesthesia
   Canadian Journal of Anaesthesia
7. A comprehensive surgery text.
8. Access to a user-oriented automated database that allows searching the medical literature, such as OVID, or Grateful Med.

■ Learners Helping Teachers

Learners must contribute actively to the tutorial relationship. Usually, this simply requires that they participate in socratic teaching and be willing to use new anesthetic drugs and methods suggested by their instructors. Less often, a trainee may take the lead, drawing out a reticent instructor who may have much to offer when stimulated by a curious learner.

■ Scheduling Elective Time During Residency

The structure of anesthesia residencies is determined by the American Board of Anesthesiology (ABA), which certifies consultants in anesthesiology, and the Residency Review Committee (RRC) of the Accreditation Council on Graduate Medical Education (ACGME), which certifies residencies. Postgraduate training in anesthesia begins with the clinical base year (CBY; internship) and goes on to 3 years of clinical anesthesia training (CA-1, CA-2, and CA-3). Although programs have some latitude in scheduling, the CA-1 year is spent in learning the basics of anesthesia care, the CA-2 year in learning subspecialities such as cardiac anesthesia and obstetrical anesthesia, and the CA-3 year in advanced anesthesia training, including the more difficult or complex anesthetic procedures and care of the most seriously ill patients.

There are three general categories of study in the CA-3 year: The Subspecialty Clinical Track (SCT) requires spending the majority of the year in the study of one or two anesthesia clinical subspecialties; the Advanced Clinical Track (ACT) involves spending the year in more diversified but still advanced clinical assignments; the Clinical Scientist Track (CST) involves spending a minimum of 6 months in clinical work and up to 6 months in scientific studies. An alternate CST allows mixing equal portions of clinical and research work over 36 months of residency following completion of the CA-1 year. The program director consults with residents and then assigns each a schedule that fits one of the three tracks.

■ The ABA/ASA In-Training Examination

The annual In-Training Examination sponsored by the American Board of Anesthesiology and the American Society of Anesthesiologists is open to all residents-in-training in anesthesiology. The written component of the ABA certifying examination is based on a subset of the questions from the In-Training Examination; the candidate's performance on this subset constitutes the score for the written examination. Data returned to the resident or to the program director from the In-Training Examination include the subject matter of questions the resident answered incorrectly, individual scores, and data that allow comparison between an individual's performance or a department's performance and national results. This examination provides individual residents and their program directors with objective, comparative assessments of cognitive learning. The content outline of this examination represents the breadth of the specialty; it serves as an outline against which to compare personal and departmental education efforts.

■ Information Retrieval

Lecture handouts, notes, articles taken from journals, and other scraps of information soon accumulate to defeat casual storage and defy easy retrieval; storing and retrieving this sort of information are necessary for organized study and reference. Workable systems for individuals must be simple to administer and require as little clerical work as possible so that time can be spent in study and not in managing a filing system. Tempting though they are in prospect, complex systems involving elaborate cross-referencing or computerized database management do not meet this test and usually prove impractical. Computerized personal databases are especially unnecessary given the availability of easy-to-use databases that index the entire medical literature.

A workable scheme consists of a collection of file folders labeled according to subject. The subject outline can be taken from the index of a text or the ABA/ASA content outline, but a better scheme is the indexing system used in common by the journals *Anesthesiology* and *Anesthesia and Analgesia*. At the beginning of training, the number of folders is few, and subjects are broad (e.g., "ANESTHESIA, regional"). As the user's interests become better defined and entries accumulate, individual folders contain too many items to search easily (40 items seems to be an upper limit). When this happens, additional folders are added to accommodate subheadings (e.g., "ANESTHESIA, regional, brachial plexus"). This simple system requires little maintenance and answers the most common requirement for individuals, the need to review a given subject rather than to search according to authors' names, key words, or other criteria. Cross-references depend on the user's familiarity with the subject matter.

Searches of the literature can begin with a review of relevant articles in textbooks or recent reviews in journals. Also, automated searches of the National Library of Medicine are now made easy and inexpensive by user-friendly interface programs such as OVID, Colleague, or Grateful Med. The citations generated by this search usually are found in a local library; as more journals become available in electronic form, the articles themselves can be called to one's computer screen. These automated databases are already an important part of learning; they will soon be a routine part of practice.

■ Learning to Use New Drugs

Frequently, one is asked to use new drugs claimed by their makers to offer significant advantages over other similar drugs. Indeed, for new learners, every drug is a new drug the first time it is used. To put a new drug into use safely, first learn as much as possible about it, comparing it with more familiar drugs of the same class. Although manufacturers attempt to provide complete information, it is important to study the more scientific assessments found in the medical journals.

Second, begin with patients and operations for which awkwardness in using the drug will do no harm. Usually, these are healthy patients undergoing less demanding procedures. Third, if possible, begin with lesser doses of the drug, and study the effects carefully before progressing to greater doses. For example, a new muscle relaxant might be used first for a peripheral procedure expected to last several hours so that unexpected prolongation of effect will not delay the end of the anesthetic.

■ Learning Technical Skills

Learning technical skills is an important part of anesthesia training. Analogies with sports, mechanical trades, hobbies, or laboratory skills suggest how one goes about learning to do something instead of to know something. The hoary adage, "Watch one, do one, teach one," contains elements of truth but does not describe the best way to go about teaching or learning a skill.

Consider as an example learning to intubate the trachea using a curved laryngoscope. To learn this

efficiently, it is best first for the instructor or the text to break the task down into as many small, discrete steps as possible. For example, one step might be positioning the head, the next might be opening the mouth, and the next might be inserting the laryngoscope. Sometimes this sequence of steps can become a checklist (e.g., the checklist for preparing an anesthesia machine given in Chapter 5). This analysis of the task not only makes it easier to understand and demonstrate but also makes it easier for the learner and the instructor to assess performance at each stage. Also, even though few learners succeed at the entire task (intubating) at the first attempt, all will succeed at some portion of the task; this allows credible praise, providing the positive reinforcement that is more effective than negative reinforcement as a means of changing behavior. Another task of the instructor is to guarantee that the task will be completed safely and without undue delay; this allows the student to focus on learning. Even during residency, this sort of careful teaching may not be available; it is almost always unavailable to practitioners. Individuals can organize their own learning along these lines by preparing notes and checklists as needed.

Learning After Training

Those who adopt the active methods of learning described here will have little difficulty with continuing medical education. An individual reading program, learning from cases, and attending departmental meetings at which clinical care is discussed (a JCAHO requirement) will provide abundant continuing education. Just as in residency, at national meetings practitioners will find it most valuable to attend lectures, conferences, or seminars that provide more than simple recitations of facts. Indeed, at the ASA's annual meeting, panel discussions and interactive learning opportunities are consistently oversubscribed, probably because those who attend recognize the value of these conferences.

Most reading programs for practitioners involve the same journals read in residency: subspecialty journals or those designed for continuing education. An often overlooked source of reading material for continuing education is the comprehensive textbook. It may not cover areas of special interest as thoroughly as subspecialists might like, but periodic rereading of such a book is a good way to keep up a broad familiarity with anesthesiology in general.

During training, evaluation comes from the faculty and from examinations; it is a natural part of the resident's learning. Later, such evaluation is harder to obtain but is just as important. Recertifying examinations provide one source of assessement. Quality assurance programs are often perceived as threats or as bureaucratic nuisances, but they provide a possible avenue for such continued assessment. Even more important is one's own careful retrospective assessment of cases. Adverse outcomes and complications must never be accepted as inevitable; rather, they must provoke efforts to improve care.

BIBLIOGRAPHY

The American Board of Anesthesiology Booklet of Information, Available yearly. Office of the Board, 4101 Lake Boone Trail, The Summit, Suite 510, Raleigh, NC 27607-7506.

Anesthesia and Analgesia. Residents may join the International Anesthesia Research Society, Suite 140, 2 Summit Park Drive, Cleveland, OH 44131, at reduced rates and receive the journal.

Anesthesiology. Residents may join the American Society of Anesthesiologists, 515 Busse Highway, Park Ridge, IL 60068, at reduced rates and receive the journal.

Grateful Med. U.S. Department of Health and Human Services, National Institutes of Health, National Library of Medicine, Bethesda, MD.

Joint Council on In-Training Examinations. ABA/ASA In-Training Examination Content Outline. American Board of Anesthesiology, American Society of Anesthesiologists, 515 Busse Highway, Park Ridge, IL 60068.

Index

Page numbers in *italics* refer to illustrations; numbers followed by t refer to tables.

Prostaglandin E_1 analogues, preoperative, 31
Prostate, transurethral resection of, 420
Prosthetic devices, antibiotic prophylaxis with, 32–33
Protein binding, of drugs, 67
    aging and, 373
    in hepatic disease, 71, 310
    in neonate, 338
    in renal disease, 71
    local anesthetics, 204t, 205, *206*
  of thyroid hormones, 328
Protein-energy malnutrition, 323
Prothrombin complex concentrate, 183t, 184–185
Pseudocholinesterase, 113–114
Psychological trauma, to pediatric patient, 339, 340–341, 342, 346, 349
Pudendal nerve blocks, bilateral, *352, 354*
Pulmonary. See also *Lung* entries. *352, 354*
Pulmonary anatomy, 293, *294*
Pulmonary artery catheter, 53–56
    in critically ill patient, 445–446, 445t
    in pediatric patient, 344
    in shock, 390, 390t
      cardiogenic, 393
    intraoperative, with pulmonary or cardiac disease, 306–307
    right internal jugular cannulation for, 53, *54*, 55
Pulmonary artery occlusion pressure, 306
    monitoring of, 53, 55, *56*
    perioperative reinfarction and, 283
Pulmonary artery pressure, monitoring of, 53, 55, *56*
Pulmonary aspiration, in critically ill patient, 441
    in gravid patient, 352
    prevention of, in high-risk patient, 152–153, 153t
      routine, 30–31
Pulmonary complications, risk factors for, 18, 18t, 299–300, 299t, 300t
Pulmonary edema, 444
    from mechanical ventilation, 142, 449
    in renal disease, 316
Pulmonary embolism, 443–444
    alveolar dead space and, 306
    pulmonary vascular resistance and, 306
Pulmonary function, aging and, 366–368, *368*
    antineoplastic agents and, 425
    in critically ill patient, 440, 440t, 441–444
      monitoring of, in ICU, 444–446
    in hepatic disease, 310
    in neonate and infant, 332–334, *335*, 335t, *336*
    in pregnancy, 350
    in renal disease, 316
    inhaled anesthetics and, 82–83
    physiology of, gas exchange in, 294, 296, 297–299
      perfusion, 296, *297*
      ventilation, 293–296
    preoperative evaluation of, 14, 16, 18
Pulmonary function tests, 301, *301*
Pulmonary monitoring, in ICU, 444–446
    intraoperative, 305–307
Pulmonary oxygen toxicity, 127–128
Pulmonary perfusion, 296, *297*. See also *Pulmonary artery catheter.*
    monitoring of, 306–307
Pulmonary vascular resistance, 306
Pulmonary vasoconstriction, hypoxic, 296
    inhaled anesthetics and, 83
Pulmonary ventilation, 293–296, 298–299
Pulse oximetry, 58–59
    in critically ill patient, 445
    legal necessity of, 489

Pulse oximetry *(continued)*
    with mask ventilation, 141
Pulseless electrical activity, 269, *276*
Pyridostigmine. See *Anticholinesterases.*

Radial artery catheter, for blood pressure monitoring, 51–52
    in infant, 344
Radial nerve block, 240, *241*
Radial nerve injury, from anesthesia, 196
Radiology procedures, anesthesia for, 420–421
    for neurologic MRI, 409
Raman spectroscopy, for anesthetic gas monitoring, 57
Ranitidine, preoperative, 31
Rapid-sequence intubation, 152–153, 153t
Rebreathing bags. See *Reservoir bags.*
Receptors, for drugs, 71, 72
    for opioids, 99–100, 101t, *102*, 456–457
Record(s), anesthesia, 168–169
    intubation notes in, 156, 156t
    legal aspects of, 490, 491
Recovery. See *Emergence, from general anesthesia; Postanesthesia care.*
Rectal administration, of drugs, 66
Reference sources, 493–494, 494t
Reflex sympathetic dystrophy, 473–474
Regional anesthesia. See also *Epidural anesthesia; Nerve blocks; Spinal anesthesia.*
    in obstetric patient, *352*, 354–357
    in pediatric patient, 346–347
    in trauma patient, 398
    intravenous, 247–249
      for outpatient surgery, 382
    with cardiovascular disease, 282
    with respiratory disease, 303–304
Regurgitation. See also *Pulmonary aspiration.*
    rapid repositioning before, 142
    risk of, from airway obstruction, 141
Renal disease, mild, 315
    pharmacokinetics with, 70–71
Renal failure, anesthesia management with, 316t, 317–320, 319t
    hepatorenal syndrome, 310
    pathophysiology of, 315–317
    perioperative, 317
    protection from, by intraoperative fluids, 178
Renal function, aging and, 369, *369*
    anesthetic effects on, 317
    antineoplastic agents and, 425
    in infant, 336–337, 337t
    in shock, 386
    in trauma patient, 398
    inhaled anesthetics and, 84–85
    with hepatic disease, 310
Rendell-Baker Soucek pediatric mask, 143, *143*
Renin-angiotensin system, 326
Research, by anesthesiologists, 7
Reservoir bags, 40, *41, 42,* 43
Residency programs, structure of, 495
Residents, learning by, 492–493
    legal responsibilities of, 487–488
Residual volume, 294, *295*
Resistance, airways, 294–296
Respiratory acidosis, 21–22, 24, 25
Respiratory depression, by opioids, 102–103
    in neonate, 363
    postoperative, 437
Respiratory disease, intraoperative management of, 304–307
    postoperative management of, 307

ISBN 0-7216-6279-X